Health Status and Health Policy

Health Status and Health Policy
QUALITY OF LIFE IN HEALTH CARE EVALUATION AND RESOURCE ALLOCATION

Donald L. Patrick
University of Washington

Pennifer Erickson
National Center for Health Statistics

New York   Oxford
OXFORD UNIVERSITY PRESS
1993

Oxford University Press

Oxford New York Toronto
Delhi Bombay Calcutta Madras Karachi
Kuala Lumpur Singapore Hong Kong Tokyo
Nairobi Dar es Salaam Cape Town
Melbourne Auckland Madrid

and associated companies in
Berlin Ibadan

Library of Congress Cataloging-in-Publication Data
Patrick, Donald L.
Health status and health policy :
quality of life in health care evaluation and resource allocation /
Donald L. Patrick and Pennifer Erickson.
p. cm. Includes bibliographical references and index.
ISBN 0-19-505027-4
1. Medical policy—United States.
2. Medical care—United States—Evaluation.
3. Quality of life. 4. Medical care, Cost of—United States.
I. Erickson, Pennifer. II. Title.
[DNLM: 1. Cost-Benefit Analysis—methods.
2. Health Expenditures—United States.
3. Health Policy—economics—United States.
4. Health Resources—economics—United States.
5. Health Status—United States.
6. Quality of Life—United States. W 74 P314h]
RA395.A3P298 1993 362.1'0973—dc20
DNLM/DLC for Library of Congress 92-6173
Co-authored by Pennifer Erickson in her private capacity.
No official support or endorsement by the U.S. Department
of Health and Human services is intended or should be inferred.

987654

Printed in the United States of America
on acid-free paper

In memory of the vision and contributions of

J. W. Bush, M. D., M. P. H.

Preface

Over the past century, advances in public health and medicine, along with social, economic, and environmental progress, have improved the health of the public in the United States. Life expectancy has increased by some 29 years. Monumental gains have been made in identifying both the leading causes of death, disease, and disability and the means to prevent them. Yet many major health problems remain unresolved. Heart disease, stroke, emphysema, cancer, accidental injuries, addictive disorders, and violence continue to threaten the public's health. Providing access to health services for the 35 million uninsured Americans and reducing social inequalities in both access and health status for minority and special populations are major challenges.

Society's main response to these problems continues to be increased investment in health care, including preventive, caring, and curing interventions. Treatment, however, far exceeds prevention in its share of health care expenditures. Rapid advances in technology, increasing use of more intensive modes of therapy and diagnosis, and an aging population all contribute to this increase. Per capita health care expenditures in the United States are higher than those of any other nation, and spending on health care also increased more rapidly during the last decade than did spending in other developed nations. Yet the health-related quality of life of people in the United States is no higher than that for residents of Western Europe or Japan, where health expenditures are considerably lower. Mortality due to heart disease is 40 percent higher in the United States than in France or Switzerland, and treatment for heart disease costs Americans more than $70 billion a year.

As a nation, Americans look to health policy to help decide how to make health expenditures reap more benefits. Increasingly decision makers, providers, patients, and the public ask that every additional expenditure be justified according to expected outcomes. Health decision making has never been more important, whether to reduce inefficiency, eliminate ineffective medical procedures, increase competition, change reimbursement formulas, or ration services. To a large extent, *health policy in the United States is shaped, intentionally or unintentionally, by the way in which resources are distributed to competing programs.* With each change of resource expenditure comes the question of measuring benefits. Will cutting services to decrease expenditures result in lowered health status? With increasing investment in more expensive technology to treat disease or disability, will health and quality of life outcomes exceed those from an alternative resource investment like prevention? On what grounds can such decisions be made?

This book advocates the use of health and quality of life outcomes to measure the benefits of health expenditures. We focus on *health-related quality of life* as the most relevant and comprehensive outcome measure for comparing costs. Health-related quality of life is defined as *the value assigned to duration of life as modified by impairments, functional states, perceptions, and social opportunities that are influenced by disease, injury, treatment, or policy.* Because health-related quality of life incorporates social values, life expectancy, and a comprehensive description of health, it addresses the tradeoff between how long people live and how well they live.

Health-related quality of life as a concept and measurable construct addresses the major concerns of consumers, families, providers, and decision makers in evaluating the outcomes of disease and treatment. Even though we have retained the more familiar term of health status in our title, health-related quality of life is larger than health status, a term that tends to be focused more centrally on clinical outcomes and functioning. On the other hand, health-related quality of life is smaller in scope than the more general term "quality of life." Social, environmental, economic, and cultural characteristics, while determinants of health-related quality of life, are not always health concerns or the province of health professionals, even when people are ill.

This book has two major objectives. The first is to propose the Health Resource Allocation Strategy as a social and political process for comparing costs and outcomes of alternative policy options in the health and medical care arena to select interventions with greatest benefit in relation to cost (Chapters 1, 2, 10–15). The second objective is to provide a reference for state-of-the-art development and application of health status and quality of life measures for health care policy and research, including clinical applications (Chapters 3–9). Not all policy applications of health-related quality of life involve resource allocation. Thus we present guidelines to assessment for use in program evaluation, monitoring of health policy, clinical trials, and health services research.

Each chapter contributes to the building and application of the Health Resource Allocation Strategy using health and quality of life outcomes obtained either through primary data collection or secondary analyses. Our approach constitutes a "strategy" in that we present the conceptual, mathematical, and sociopolitical organization and processes for relating health care costs to outcomes. The Strategy is based on the theory of social choice and can be applied to a large number of resource allocation problems with different sociopolitical assumptions about scarce resources, rational decision making, and economic efficiency (Chapter 1). Equity and equality of opportunity for health care are the guiding principles for applying the Strategy within the prevailing political system and economic values.

In this book, health status and quality of life measures are presented in the context of health decisions and the multiple cultural, social, economic, and political forces that shape them (Chapter 2). From the societal perspective, the main stakeholder in health decisions is the community itself, including all the values held by residents for health care and its outcomes in relation to other goods and services such as education and housing. Individual stakeholders include decision makers such as legislators, administrators, and health care providers in addition to well and ill persons and their relatives and significant others. Not all stakeholders, however, have equal power in the decision process. Health decisions are made at different levels; at the most global level, eligibility and reimbursement policies are set by legislators and administrators, and at the most individual level, patients and clinicians make referral and treatment decisions.

The Health Resource Allocation Strategy involves eight distinct steps. These steps build a foundation for the sociopolitical consideration of cost and health-related quality of life data. The Strategy itself does not make health decisions; stakeholders in the decision make them through the political process. In fact, many health decisions are made through processes that bear little resemblance to a rational model based on research and data. The Strategy provides a systematic way of uncovering the assumptions made in allocating resources and in considering all available information on alternative uses of resources and the maximization of desired outcomes.

Additional foundations for the concepts and measures included in the Health Resource Allocation Strategy lie in major theories from psychology, economics, and sociology (Chapter 3). Using these theories as applied over the last two decades, we provide a classification, definition, and examples for core concepts, domains, and indicators of health-related quality of life (Chapter 4). This conceptual framework assists researchers and analysts in selecting the most relevant concepts to include in assessments, including those that implement the Health Resource Allocation Strategy or involve health services research that includes a quality of life component. We also propose a taxonomy of the different types of measures—single indicators, indexes, profiles, and batteries—that are currently available (Chapter 5). This taxonomy helps decision makers and analysts to identify the type of measure they need and select the appropriate measurement strategy for their purpose.

The Health Resource Allocation Strategy makes explicit the tradeoffs among different states of health and quality of life that determine whether a population is better or worse off with competing interventions. These tradeoffs are built on the basic notion that health state preferences reflect the perceived value assigned to *quality* and *quantity* of health. Alternative methods for assigning preferences to health states are identified to provide the means for making these tradeoffs between quality and quantity (Chapter 6).

The health-related quality of life of a population can be assessed using both primary data collection and secondary analyses. Major methodological and practical criteria already exist for selecting measures to use in collecting, analyzing, and interpreting health-related quality of life data (Chapter 7). These criteria are formulated as steps in the selection process and a guide to investigators. The Health Resource Allocation Strategy also can be applied using existing data in secondary analyses, particularly using national data (Chapter 8).

Quantity of health is the expected duration of survival, or life expectancy, of a population, as influenced by mortality and health status. This expected duration is *prognosis*. Assigning preferences to health states permits different domains of health-related quality of life to be combined with prognosis into a single index called *years of healthy life*. Years of healthy life are calculated by adjusting the expected duration of survival by the point-in-time estimate of health-related quality of life (Chapter 9).

In implementing the Health Resource Allocation Strategy, the analyst must estimate all costs attributed to each of the alternative courses of action, including out-of-pocket expenses and psychic costs incurred by recipients of health care services. We discuss issues involved in estimating both the direct and indirect health care costs of different policy or program alternatives (Chapter 10). Health costs and health-related quality of life outcomes are compared for each alternative by calculating the ratio of *cost per year of healthy life gained* for each alternative course of action. These ratios are ranked from low to high with the budget constraint included in the ranking. Ratios that are less than the budget constraint are considered cost effective. The strategy uses the methods of cost–benefit, cost–effectiveness, and cost–utility evaluation (Chapter 11).

The ranking of health care alternatives according to cost per year of healthy life gained is a technical procedure. Judgments of worth are not made by technical data; they necessarily use the prevailing cultural, political, and ethical values of the community and all stakeholders in the health decisions. Rankings must be reviewed by stakeholders and rankings adjusted to reflect the fullest possible range of community values before legislative and administrative decision makers, the final arbitrators, assign priorities and allocate resources. This sociopolitical process is essential and desirable in applying the strategy to health decisions that affect all members of the community (Chapter 11).

We illustrate how the Health Resource Allocation Strategy can be applied to resource allocation decisions in three health policy areas that are priorities for the 1990s: monitoring progress in achieving health promotion and disease prevention objectives for the year 2000 (Chapter 12), managing the implementation of health care technology (Chapter 13), and improving access to health care through rationing (Chapter 14). These are national policy problems as well as concerns at the state, county, or city level.

There are limits to rationality in implementing social choices such as the allocation of health resources. Budget constraints and the political process of allocation involve *rationing*, or the denial of benefits or access to desired services. Resource allocation can arouse the deepest fears of stakeholders because interests compete and people can lose valued benefits. The ethical implications of applying the Health Resource Allocation Strategy to the evaluation of prevention effectiveness, to deciding which technologies to implement, and to rationing of health care to improve access should be considered. In the final chapter we address the limits to rationality in examining the contributions of the Strategy, ethical and political challenges, and potential uses and abuses, and we consider the major unresolved issues (Chapter 15).

Even with all its problems, possible weaknesses, and potential for abuse, the Strategy promises to bring systematic information to decision makers. It uncovers heretofore hidden social values and assumptions involved in the allocation process. Stating these assumptions and values aids public debate of alternative uses of resources. Such debate is sorely needed to address the many problems in health care organization and delivery that face our nation. We intend this book to spur debate and controversy. The decisions before the nation about health care surely deserve as much informed debate as possible.

No single book puts together both health status measurement and health policy decisions. Ours is an ambitious task fraught with the challenge of presenting highly technical language and concepts in a simple and straightforward manner. Political, economic, and ethical minefields abound in traversing the field of health resource allocation. We have undoubtedly approached some of them. We hope that both our insights and our mistakes help in uncovering the formidable challenges to health decisions.

In bringing the two fields of health status and health policy together, we hope to (1) assist national, state, and local users of health status and quality of life information in the critical assessment of research results for health policy formulation, implementation, and evaluation; (2) to assist researchers of health-related quality of life to identify and use the major theoretical, methodological, and practical advances made over the past three decades in constructing or selecting measures for health policy research; and (3) to provide an introduction to the field of health status and quality of life assessment for use in graduate-level courses in health policy, health services research, and health administration.

The primary audience for this book includes health decision makers in the public and private sectors, health services and clinical researchers, and students in public health, social sciences, and clinical sciences. Health decision makers and researchers from other nations may find this book useful in their own health services context. Methods and measures from Europe are included.

The use of social choice theory, a formal strategy, and the technical language of socioeconomic evaluation can bewilder even the most interested and dedicated of readers. Sources of information about health-related quality of life measures and a glossary of terms are included to help readers learn the language and logic of the field. The major health status measures developed to date for applying the Health Resource Allocation Strategy are illustrated in Appendix I.

Important health decisions are going to be made as we move toward the next century. Rising expenditures, provision of basic health care to all, rationing of expensive technologies, inequalities in both access to services and health status, and the difficult tasks of promoting and protecting the nation's health require sound decisions based on deliberation of data and their implications. We hope this book will encourage the collection and use of health-related quality of life information to help shape these decisions.

Seattle, Wash.   D.P.
Hyattsville, Md.   P.E.
March 1992

Acknowledgments

Many years of research, discussions accompanied by table-napkin calculations, cross-country air trips, national and international conferences, workshops, heated debates, and restless days and nights culminated in this book. Many of the ideas put forth here in one place first arose in the late 1960s in early collaborative research between J. W. Bush, Donald Patrick, and Milton Chen and during the early 1970s in discussions between Pennifer Erickson and Dr. Bush in the development of the Clearinghouse on Health Indexes at the National Center for Health Statistics. Through the years that followed, active dialogue between Jim Bush and the authors continued until Dr. Bush's death in 1985. A large number of others, either personally or in their writings, contributed additional insight into the use of health status and quality of life information to inform health policy. Among those who have influenced our thinking the most are Marilyn Bergner, Anthony Culyer, Richard Deyo, Jack Elinson, David Feeny, Gordon Guyatt, Robert Kaplan, Rachel Rosser, Daniel Sullivan, George Torrance, Milton Weinstein, John Ware, and Alan Williams. Countless others have helped in working out the conceptual and technical problems in applying an economic model in the social and political context of health decision making. Barry Anderson, John Anderson, Thomas Hodgson, Donald Malec, Paige Sipes-Metzler, and Helene Starks have been particularly helpful. Kathleen Lohr deserves much praise for her matchless review and comment on the entire manuscript. We also thank David Grembowski and Thomas Wickizer for their thorough reviews of all the chapters.

Grants from the Henry J. Kaiser Family Foundation and the New England Medical Center have provided support to the University of Washington to complete this work. We owe special thanks to Alvin Tarlov, Barbara Kehrer, and Edward Schor for their encouragement. We also thank the Association for Health Services Research, which prompted our initial collaboration by inviting us to conduct a workshop on health status assessment at its first annual meeting in 1984.

The Department of Health Services at the University of Washington, chaired by Edward Perrin, contributed much needed space, help, and additional resources. Ronald Wilson at the National Center for Health Statistics was particularly encouraging. Lorene Neubauer prepared all the tables and figures, helped prepare the text, and provided the essential administrative and emotional glue for this venture. Christine Sexauer, Gloria Campbell, Molly Gerhard, and William Lin assisted in preparing the manuscript. Steve Jones, Louise Simpson, and Laura Larsson helped to retrieve large amounts of information. We must also acknowledge that without the help of communications technology—bitnet, fax, and express mail—this cross-country collaboration would not have worked. We are grateful to Robert Shimabukuro and Jeffrey Scott for keeping our computers and printers humming.

Without the faith and good-natured patience of Jeffrey House at Oxford University Press, we could not have seen this project to completion. For the tolerance of many hours away from home as well as for their understanding and most gracious endurance of moments of anxious emotion, we thank our family members, Shirley Beresford, Alistair and Mira Patrick, and Jeffrey Scott.

Contents

Tables

Figures

Health Status and Health Policy

1
Health Status and Health Decisions

THE CHALLENGE TO HEALTH DECISION MAKING

Most people care about their health and about what determines how healthy they are or they will be. Although sometimes taking actions that are harmful to health, most persons attempt to enhance health and avoid harmful effects to the greatest extent possible. Individuals, families, groups, communities, and entire nations attempt to improve or maintain their health through legislation, education, environmental modification, behavior change, and many other avenues.

Because of disease, injury, genetics, lifestyle, poverty, stress, and a number of other influences, people cannot always maintain health. When health breaks down and recognized illness results, people usually attempt to take care of themselves with the help of their families and friends. Many people eventually turn, however, to a special collection of personnel, facilities, services, and goods, that is, *health care*. People turn to health care with different objectives in mind: for a diagnosis to understand the meaning and prognosis of a symptom, for a cure that will restore them to good health, for relief of pain and other discomforts, for reassurance, for assistance and advice that will prevent further deterioration, for prevention of illness, or simply for comfort, particularly when there is little hope for finding an effective treatment to prolong life or restore health.

Health care is not confined to enhancing health and improving the opportunity for individuals to achieve life goals. The most important events in peoples' lives—birth, major illness or injury, and death—often involve health care. Although the occurrence of disease and illness may heighten one's awareness of its importance, health care has a special, sometimes symbolic and hidden, role to play in the lives of most people.

That health and health care play an important role in peoples' lives is evidenced by the willingness of societies to devote a large percentage of their economic resources to the production and distribution of health services. The United States and Canada as well as most Western European nations spend an increasing proportion of their economic wealth on health care. For the last three decades spending for health care in the United States has risen faster than either inflation or growth in the gross national product (GNP). In 1960, national health expenditures totaled $276 billion, or 5.2 percent of the GNP. The Health Care Financing Administration (HCFA) estimates that, by the year 2000, health care in the United States will be over a $1.6 trillion enterprise and will consume over 16 percent of the GNP (Sonnenfeld et al., 1991) (Figure 1.1).

Rapid increases in health care spending affect both government health programs and privately financed health care. The trust fund for the Federal hospital insurance pro-

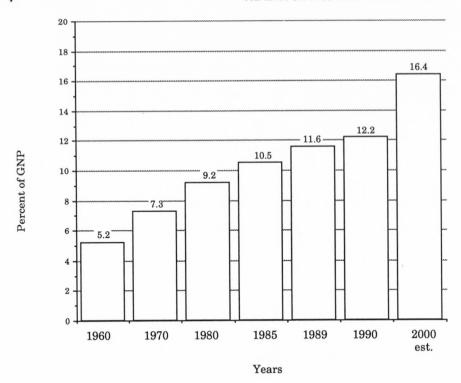

Figure 1.1 Health expenditures as a percentage of the U.S. gross national product, 1960–2000. *Source*: Levit et al., 1991; Sonnenfeld et al., 1991.

gram (Medicare Part A), which derives most of its income from payroll taxes, is currently projected to be exhausted in the year 2005 (Sonnenfeld et al., 1991). State-operated Medicaid programs, financed through a combination of state and federal taxes, are fiscally strained in face of increasing demand from unemployed and low-income residents. Employer payments for health care, including health-related payroll taxes, exceed after-tax profits (Levit et al., 1991a).

In the United States more is spent on health care than on either education or national defense. In 1988, six percent of the gross domestic product (GDP) was spent on national defense and 6.5 percent on education, while more than 11 percent was spent on health care (Barker et. al., 1991). In the last two decades, the proportion of the GDP spent for education and national defense has decreased, while the proportion for health care has increased 50 percent, even after adjusting for economy-wide inflation. This increase in health care outlays raises an important question facing the United States and many other Western countries: How much should the nation be spending on health care?

The answer to this important question leads to another fundamental question asked about most large investments: What are the realized and expected benefits? In comparing spiraling outlays to health outcomes over the last three decades, one might expect steep improvement in *health status*, paralleling the rise in expenditures. Unlike our use of the GNP to track health care expenditures, however, no GNP-like index of health

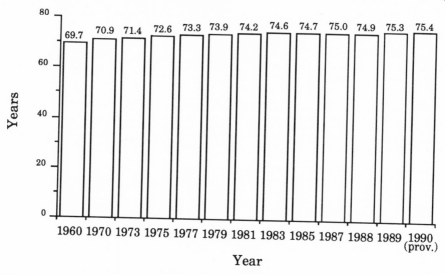

Figure 1.2a Life expectancy at birth, all races, United States, 1960–90. *Source:* National Center for Health Statistics, *Vital Statistics of the United States, 1985; Health: United States, 1991.*

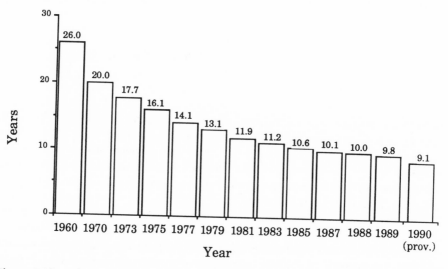

Figure 1.2b Infant mortality rates per 1,000 live births, all races, United States, 1960–90. *Source:* National Center for Health Statistics, *Vital Statistics of the United States, 1985; Health: United States, 1991.*

status is available for the U.S. population to compare expenditures and benefits directly.

Commonly used single indicators of national health status, that is, those derived from a single measure used by the U.S. National Center for Health Statistics, are illustrated in Figures 1.2a and b. *Life expectancy* for all persons in the United States increased from 69.7 years in 1960 to 75.4 years in 1990, a gain of 5.7 years. During

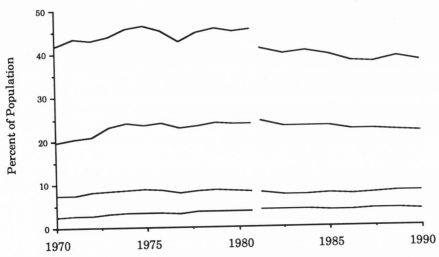

Figure 1.2c Trends in prevalence of any activity limitation by age group, United States, 1970–90. (Changes in survey definitions between 1981 and 1983 did not permit tabulation of results in 1982. See Pope and Tarlov [1991, p. 53] for a complete explanation of these changes.) *Source*: National Center for Health Statistics, Current Estimates from the National Health Interview Survey 1979–90.

the same interval, *infant mortality* dropped dramatically from 26 deaths per 1,000 live births in 1960 to 9.1 in 1990.

These two mortality-based measures indicate considerable improvement in preventing deaths in the total population. Average life expectancy and infant mortality rates, however, vary considerably for different population groups. White women have the longest life expectancy (79.2 years), and black men have the shortest (64.8 years). In 1989, infant mortality was twice as high for black infants (18.6 per 1,000 live births) as for white infants (8.1 per 1,000). Native Americans and Puerto Ricans also have markedly higher infant mortality rates than the national average. The benefits of increased survival are therefore not shared equally in the United States.

Mortality rates are also imperfect indicators of the health of the surviving population. Figure 1.2c shows the proportion of the population in different age groups reporting *activity limitations* between 1970 and 1990. Prevalence rates were relatively stable over the entire period, but increasing prevalence of activity limitations was observed in the early 1970s, particularly for those age 45–64. The actual number of people reporting any activity limitation, however, increased from 24 million in 1970 to an estimated 33.7 million in 1990. Lower-income persons (under $20,000) report activity limitations more frequently than higher-income persons ($20,000 or more). Overall, these data indicate that an increase in disability occurred during the same period as a decrease in mortality (Pope and Tarlov, 1991).

Figure 1.2d shows the percentage of people of all ages reporting good to excellent health in the National Health Interview Survey conducted by the U.S. National Center for Health Statistics. The period covers 1973 through 1990. *Self-reported health status*, the major available single indicator of "quality" of health, remained relatively constant over the 17-year period. The indicator increased slightly, from 87.8 percent in

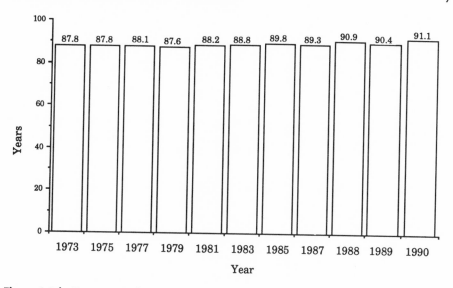

Figure 1.2d Percentage of persons of all ages reporting good to excellent health, United States, 1973–90 (adjusted for age). *Source*: National Center for Health Statistics, *National Health Interview Survey, 1973–90.*

1973 to 91.1 percent in 1990. Most Americans consider themselves healthy, although differences appear when examining different population groups. Similar to the mortality data, black persons and persons with lower incomes report poorer health much more frequently than do white persons and persons with higher incomes.

Comparison of these U.S. expenditure and health status data shows that as health care outlays increased, fewer deaths occurred, but many Americans reported increasing disability and did not report large improvements in health, particularly persons in minority groups and persons with low income. Because expenditures and outcomes are not on a common scale or unit of measurement, some analysts might consider these comparisons invalid. Activity limitations and self-rating of health status also may not be the most comprehensive and sensitive outcome measures to use in relation to changes in health expenditures, although people's perceptions of their own health correlate well with their actual health status and with their use of health services. The comparison does suggest, however, that increases in important domains of health status other than survival have not necessarily paralleled increases in health expenditures. As Verbrugge (1984, 1989) posed the question: Do Americans have longer life but worsening health?

In this chapter we explore the reasons for rising health care expenditures and different approaches to controlling spending. The resource allocation strategies of medical effectiveness evaluations and rationing are put forth as policy alternatives that emphasize health care outcomes in relation to inputs to the system. At the outset, these two policy alternatives involve sociopolitical processes and ethical implications that we examine. We then introduce three major health policy questions for the 1990s that illustrate the application of costs and outcomes to resource allocation and rationing. We also define what we mean by the concepts of health status, quality of life, and health-related quality of life, the term adopted for use in this book. The final section of the chapter surveys the different objectives and applications of health-related quality of life assessment to identify which applications are most relevant for health policy.

Why the Rising Expenditures in Health Care?

Hospital expenditures account for 40 percent of total health care costs.* Increasing hospital expenditures, in turn, have been attributed to rising incomes, growth of insurance coverage, technological advances, and an aging population (Aaron and Schwartz, 1984; Aaron, 1991). Americans want, and many feel entitled to, the best technology and medical care possible, regardless of cost. Physicians and other health professionals as well as hospitals and other health care organizations want to deliver high-quality health care. High-quality care often involves technology, and almost all technological innovations will increase health expenditures in the future, because these innovations represent the development of new procedures rather than labor-saving processes. Finally, the shift from infectious diseases to chronic diseases as major causes of death and the combination of an aging population coupled with the high cost of care during the last year of life suggest that the upward trend for health expenditures will continue.

Although technological advances, chronic illness, and an aging society account for a sizable portion of the increase, other system-wide processes—third-party reimbursement systems, a growing supply of physicians, continuing patient and professional demands for high-quality, technologically sophisticated care with little regard to cost, and diverse organizational arrangements lacking coordination—also force expenditures upward. The billions of dollars available through private and public health insurance programs fuel expenditure growth by increasing eligibility of participants and by reducing incentives to achieve production and consumption efficiency. Patients have incentives to consume costly care and providers have incentives to deliver such care.

As Aaron and Schwartz (1990) point out, patients paid, on average, only about 10 cents of each dollar devoted to hospital care and 26 cents of each dollar paid to physicians in 1987. When insurance plans pay more of the cost than do consumers, some consumers may elect more treatment than others believe they need. Insurance can distort the behavior of both providers and consumers by encouraging the use of services that cost more than the value of expected benefits. The health care system in the United States gives neither providers nor patients incentive to control expenditures, since insurers pay the majority of the bills (Aaron and Schwartz, 1990).

Public expectations for health and health care undoubtedly play a major role in increasing health care costs. When an individual's life is endangered and effective rescue measures are available, community values mandate treatment in most instances. This proclivity to treat has been called the "Rule of Rescue" by Jonsen who observes that those technologies that stave off death pose a particularly daunting problem for resource allocation (Jonsen, 1986). Even the "most evangelical utilitarian" will eventually face this duty-based imperative that cannot be "expunged from our collective moral conscience."

Consumer reluctance to forgo expensive treatments—some life-sustaining—also

---

*Although economists distinguish between costs meaning opportunity costs and expenditures meaning accounting costs or charges, the terms are sometimes used interchangeably in this book.

indicates that anticipations are high for technology in health care (Danis et al., 1988). Some Americans may also have a "rescue fantasy" in which technology will come to the rescue when prevention fails or treatment is not followed. In addition, an increasing number of survivors at all ages with permanent impairments and disabilities place demands on health care providers for treatment that will prevent further deterioration in function and increase opportunity for full participation in society. These demands suggest increasing hopes for longer and better quality lives—not a surprising state of affairs. Such rising expectations put constant pressure on resources to match these demands for health care and high quality of life.

Inefficiencies in the production and delivery of health care services also increase expenditures. The price of labor has risen in the health sector faster than in the rest of the economy; growth in productivity has been slower (Aaron and Schwartz, 1990). So-called defensive medicine and malpractice litigation may also contribute to costs by requiring more time, more visits, and more technological evidence of morbidity or the lack of it. Duplication of services and excess capacity also increase the level of expenditures.

Health technologies and practices undoubtedly benefit large numbers of people by improving the quality and outcomes of health and medical care. The increasing investment in health, in fact, is based on the premise that health expenditures produce benefits. The belief that the benefits are worth their cost, however, faces increasing skepticism from legislators, insurers, consumers, and the public at large. Medical professionals also express growing concern about the appropriateness and effectiveness of some medical interventions. Legislators and administrators question the effectiveness of entitlement and health programs. Finally, employers ask whether the increasing cost of health benefit packages improves employee health care and health status. These concerns have led to diverse approaches to control expenditures and the notion that the United States is experiencing a "crisis" in health care. Clearly many are no longer willing to invest an increasingly high percentage of economic wealth in health care; hence a crisis, that of conflicting priorities, persists and dominates much health policy debate.

"Fixes" to Control Health Care Spending

Increases in health care spending have convinced public and private payers to demand that health care expenditures be contained. Despite a broad consensus that limits and cost containment are needed, major disagreement exists over the content and focus of containment policies. Many observers warn that American society must be willing to make difficult choices concerning what kind of health care will be provided and to whom (Fuchs, 1974; Feldstein, 1988; Aaron and Schwartz, 1990; Callahan, 1990).

Fixes to control health care spending are numerous and complex; it is impossible to explore each one in detail here. A brief listing of proposed solutions can be outlined:

1. Improving management and increasing efficiency through using managed care providers, reducing the number of physicians, using intermediate-level practitioners, and related approaches.
2. Increasing competition among providers by disseminating statistics on costs, quality, and outcomes or by soliciting competitive bids among providers.

3. Regulating hospital costs by reducing admissions and average lengths of stay and by controlling provider payment through price control programs, diagnostic-related groups (DRGs), and other means of shifting costs outside the hospital.
4. Reducing health care capacity by curtailing growth in investments and requiring certificates of need.
5. Evaluating medical practices and limiting reimbursement to those procedures and practices that show evidence of effectiveness.
6. Rationing services by denying health care to persons who cannot afford to pay or by limiting access to services or procedures regardless of eligibility or ability to pay.

Many of these fixes concern the supply side of health care spending. Improving management, increasing competition, regulating hospital costs and provider payment, and reducing health care capacity are strategies for changing *inputs* to the health care system. Although potentially effective in the short term, these supply-side solutions are unlikely to have long-term effects on expenditure growth.

Innovations in management, for example, may reduce spending when first introduced but have little effect on growth rates in the long term. Savings achieved through reductions in hospital admissions and lengths of stay were significant in the 1980s. If further drops in inpatient days are accompanied by increases in ambulatory care including home health care, savings are likely to decline and total costs can be expected to rise (Schwartz and Mendelson, 1991). Other measures need to be applied if hospital cost containment is to be sustained.

Regulation of provider payment has shown considerable promise in curtailing health care spending. Vigorous monitoring of provider payment is necessary, however, to prevent changes in diagnostic practices, charging, and other unintended consequences of regulation. The savings accrued from regulating provider payment, that is, limiting increases or reducing reimbursement, may be considerably reduced because of the costs in administering the regulatory program.

The final two strategies for controlling health care spending—medical effectiveness evaluations and rationing—are based on *outputs* of the health care system rather than inputs. Medical effectiveness evaluations and rationing, both examples of resource allocation, are the major policy alternatives addressed in this book. *Medical effectiveness evaluations* concern the elimination of unnecessary practices and the distribution of resources to interventions that are shown to produce the most benefit. Interventions may be evaluated only on the basis of effectiveness, defined as health status outcomes, without formal comparisons with expenditures. Evaluations of health programs, clinical interventions, and regulatory practices are examples. The major goals of effectiveness evaluations are (1) to establish the magnitude of effect, if any; (2) to disseminate the results of the evaluation; and (3) to eliminate ineffective interventions through changes in practice or administrative behavior, such as changes in benefits or reimbursement formula. Eventually, in theory, a reallocation of resources will occur through inclusion of only effective interventions in benefit packages.

Outcomes may also be related formally to costs. Analysts conduct cost–benefit, cost–effectiveness, and cost–utility analyses of health interventions to compare health outcomes and health care costs. The cost and outcome of different interventions for a single condition may be compared, for example, back surgery may be compared to medical treatment. Alternatively, multiple interventions may be included within one costs and outcomes analytic framework, for example, coronary artery bypass graft surgery and heart transplantation within an entire array of heart disease treatments. The results of these analyses can be used for distributing resources to interventions with a lower ratio of costs to outcomes. These methods play a central role in the allocation strategy presented in this book.

Rationing refers to the distribution of resources to services or individuals according to rules based on one or more of the following: (1) *personal characteristics*, such as age, gender, and ethnic identity, sexual preference, and lifestyle behaviors including smoking, alcohol, and drug abuse; (2) *socioeconomic status*, such as income, poverty level, or employment; (3) *disease status*, such as diagnosis and prognosis; (4) *cost of intervention*, such as organ transplantation or dialysis; and (5) *outcomes*, such as physical, mental and social functioning. The rules that govern rationing in the United States may be explicit, such as the eligibility criteria that exclude persons from benefits and services, a major example being the federal poverty level used to determine Medicaid eligibility. On the contrary, rules may be implicit, such as inequality in the rates of coronary artery bypass grafting (CABG) between white and black Medicare patients. Nationally the sex- and age-adjusted CABG rate in 1986 was 27.1 per 10,000 for whites (40.4 for white men and 16.2 for white women), but only 7.6 for blacks (9.3 for black men and 6.4 for black women) (Goldberg et al., 1992).

Rationing is not a new concept; in the United States, people are denied benefits or services on the basis of ability to pay (as in fee-for-service), age (as in Medicare), residence (as in urban and rural), ethnic identity (as in Indian Health Service, a part of the U.S. Public Health Service), gender (as in inequalities in use), and other characteristics. Rationing occurs whenever health care resources are insufficient to make them available to all who might benefit. Explicit rationing on the basis of cost and outcome comparisons, however, is receiving increasing attention as a means for containing health care expenditures. The debate prompted by Callahan (1987) on how to devise a fair, humane, and sensitive plan to limit health care for aging persons and the program designed by the State of Oregon to provide universal access to care for all state residents under age 65 (Kitzhaber, 1989) are recent examples of proposals for rationing services and procedures.

Medical effectiveness evaluations may also be considered a form of rationing in that resource-centered criteria are employed to determine which health care resources will be made available to beneficiaries. Resource-centered criteria therefore ignore differences between persons and instead emphasize rationing decisions on features of health services themselves (Jecker and Pearlman, 1992). For example, preventive health care may be emphasized over acute care services. Resource-centered rationing thus avoids controversy by focusing on comparisons of services rather than on comparisons between persons.

Person-centered rationing is based on the characteristics of persons. For example, liver transplants may be denied to persons who have a history of alcohol abuse. Decisions based on resource-centered rationing will eventually involve persons, in that providers and patients negotiating treatment must consider the range of treatments considered effective, particularly when affected by reimbursement systems. Services may be denied to persons that are likely to receive the least health benefit or on some other criteria such as income eligibility or health need.

Medical effectiveness evaluations and rationing share an emphasis on and rediscovery of health care *outcomes*. Among the expected benefits from health care spending are improved health status and quality of life. Spending may be constrained depending on the benefits expected from the investment of resources. Allocation decisions usually set the constraints within which rationing occurs, that is, the total amount of resources available to meet the demands of those eligible to consume them. Rationing then distributes available resources by determining eligibility to consume them according to a defined set of rules.

HEALTH POLICY AS COSTS AND OUTCOMES

The two resource allocation strategies of medical effectiveness evaluation and rationing suggest a definition of health policy based on costs and outcomes. To a large extent, *health policy in the United States is shaped, intentionally or unintentionally, by the way in which resources are distributed to competing programs*. Heretofore most health policy decisions have not been made using an explicit set of economic and sociopolitical criteria. Given unwillingness to accept increased spending on health care, health decisions should be made with some estimate of the costs and benefits of each alternative. Information for making such cost–benefit comparisons is not always available. Thus, discussion and debate center on assumptions, estimates, or other information about the relationship between costs and outcomes.

Allocation of health resources also raises larger questions of how society makes social choices and social arrangements. One can characterize human society as a cooperative endeavor aimed at achieving a better life for all through various social arrangements and joint labors. This cooperative venture can be further characterized as a set of individual interests, the union of which sometimes produces conflict when working toward the greatest good. Maximizing social or community good may well conflict with individual wishes or demands.

Decisions on allocating health resources are informed by social choice theory, pioneered by Kenneth Arrow, an economist, in his monograph *Social Choice and Individual Values* first published in 1951. Social choice theory deals with the aggregation of individual interests or preferences into some aggregate notion of social welfare or social choice. The fundamental problem is how to make choices for the welfare of society, given the expressed views and preferences of its members. Social choice theory examines how a state of affairs can be improved from the social point of view. In allocating resources to health care, social choices are made, beginning with the assumption that these choices will improve the social well-being of the community.

A necessary prerequisite to all medical effectiveness evaluations and rationing initiatives is the cultural acceptance that everyone can't have everything he or she wants. Thus, some means must be found to determine which benefits and services are going to be made available and which persons are going to receive these benefits. Some sociopolitical process is necessary to define universal entitlement and rules of distribution, both of which have important assumptions and ethical implications behind them, as described next.

The Assumption of Scarce or Finite Resources

Within a society, the health sector is not the only one demanding available resources. Education, defense, transportation, housing, and other sectors command considerable public expenditures to maintain the welfare of the society. Resource allocation and rationing strategies assume that there are insufficient funds to provide every health intervention to meet every demand.

An argument is often made that resources from other sectors, most notably defense in the United States, could be made available to the health sector. The "guns versus health" argument asks: If we can afford to spend hundreds of billions for national defense, why should we cut back or hold down health care expenditures? Transfers of revenue from one sector to another would indeed be a short-term solution, particularly with the changes in defense prompted by global political changes. Political pressures in the United States, however, make such shifts of resources between sectors in the economy unlikely. In the long run, transfers of resources from other economic sectors are also unlikely to solve the problem of scarce resources available to health.

Allocation of health resources is based on the assumption that some finite amount of economic resources should be devoted to health care. This amount may be larger or smaller than the current estimated 13–15 percent of the GNP to be spent on health care in the next few years. The assumption is that some limit to health care spending is necessary. Thus, health decision makers must make tradeoffs to allocate resources among competing interventions on one basis or another.

The Assumptions of Rationality and Economic Efficiency

Another major assumption of resource allocation and rationing strategies is that individuals in society can and do make choices in a rational manner. As discussed in Chapter 2, many health decisions in the United States do not follow a clearly defined rational process. Our pluralistic health care system is a mixture of public and private benefits, services, and payers. The public system is a mix of federal and state programs with different levels of responsibility and authority. The private system operates in many different organizational forms and under regulatory constraints that vary state by state. No comprehensive plan for controlling health care costs exists. No single government body or social institution has the authority to make and enforce resource allocation and rationing decisions for the entire population.

The lack of centralized decision making with a single source of funds implies that separate allocation and rationing decisions will be made for different population groups. In the public sector, federal decisions may be made for persons age 65 and over participating in the Medicare program, for federal government employees, and for veterans. States, with federal approval, allocate resources to low-income persons eligible for Medicaid and for a myriad of different state-sponsored programs. In the private sector, third-party payers make decisions concerning benefits and reimbursement for individuals with health insurance through their employers or through self-insurance.

Thus, resource allocation and rationing strategies at present can operate only within the patchwork organization of health delivery in the United States.

Rational behavior in resource allocation and rationing implies the selection of one alternative over another based on relative benefits, the notion of *economic efficiency*. An economically efficient allocation of resources means that no one in the community can be made better off without making someone else worse off. Although an allocation may be efficient according to this "optimality" criterion, put forth by Vilfredo Pareto in 1917, it may not be equitable. An allocation that grants all of society's resources to a small group and no resources to a large number may be economically efficient given that distribution of income while failing in an equitable distribution of resources according to normative criteria for equity.

Conceptions of Justice and the Problem of Equity

Economic efficiency does not include any principle of equity in health resource allocation. Inequities can come about in a number of ways. As one example, if information in the decision process is biased, perhaps being collected only from people who obtain medical treatment or have private insurance, resources will be allocated among the diseases and health conditions experienced by the subgroup of service users. Resources would be made available to the remainder of society only to the extent that their perceived needs and demands overlapped with those with access or insurance or who sought and obtained medical care. In this example, the poor and people without health insurance might receive a disproportionately small allocation of resources.

Similarly, people with rare diseases and health conditions may receive fewer resources than those with common diseases. For example, more resources are allocated to prevention and treatment strategies for heart disease than for psoriasis. A third situation that could bias allocation of resources might occur if the preferences of different groups in society differ in important ways from those of the decision makers.

The cost and outcome ratio for health interventions targeted at younger people may be lower than for health interventions targeted at older people because of the incorporation of life expectancy in the ratio. People born in 1988 had, on average, 74.9 years of life remaining. By contrast, people 65 years and older had 16.9 years of life remaining (National Center for Health Statistics, 1991b). As a result, cost–effectiveness ratios for health promotion programs would be lower for younger than for older persons. For example, a low-cost polio immunization program would result in a relatively small cost and outcome ratio because the years of healthy life gained are large. On the other hand, an equally low-cost pneumonia immunization program for older adults will have a larger cost and outcome ratio because the years of healthy life gained are small. This difference in ratios of cost per years of healthy life gained is largely due to the inclusion of quantity as well as quality of life.

The bias toward youth is not universal across all interventions. Duration of life becomes significant in costs and outcomes comparisons when considering the additional years of healthy life to be gained because of the intervention under consideration. Some interventions aimed at older adults may result in greater health benefits than interventions aimed at younger people. Assuming that costs for these interventions were the same regardless of the age of the target population, the intervention for older people would be more cost effective than that for the younger age group. For example, a physical activity program for older adults compared to a home care program for severely disabled children might result in more years of healthy life gained for the older population. As a result, the cost and outcome ratio would be lower for the physical activity program than for the home care program. Assuming that only one of these two programs can be funded, the desirability of funding the home care rather than the physical activity program would depend on community values.

The allocation of health resources therefore involves a conception of justice. Conceptions of justice are held by individuals and implemented by institutions, and different conceptions exist, including global or local theories and end-state or procedural theories. Global theories concern the overall design of society, and they may be end-state or procedural. Utilitarianism (Williams and Sen, 1982; Sen, 1982), egalitarianism (Dworkin, 1981), and John Rawls's theory of justice (1971) are global end-state theories, and the best known procedural global theory is that of Robert Nozick (1974).

These global theories concern one "good" to be allocated through a redistributive system using a single principle of redistribution. Global theories are intended for the design of basic institutions in society and not for the solution of specific allocation problems. Health care can be viewed as a primary good for distribution according to a single principle of justice. Conceptions of local justice involve a variety of different goods that are allocated by a number of different principles, for example, admission to college, allocation of military service, and allocation of scarce medical resources (Elster, 1991). Different principles may be used in the allocation process, such as absolute equality or allocation on the basis of status, productivity, social worth, or some other criterion or mechanism.

Allocation of health and medical services, organ transplants, and mammography exams, for example, are different health care goods that may be distributed according to different principles or a single principle. Distributing health resources for only one group in society may lead to inequities. High-cost interventions, such as organ transplants, might be denied to the poor while those able to pay for the intervention would have access.

Alternatively, resources could be allocated according to other ethical principles, such as the principles of justice put forth by John Rawls (1971) in *A Theory of Social Justice*. In this theory, Rawls recognizes that rules and procedures must be designed that will reconcile conflicts between individual and social interests. Basic rules of justice, according to Rawls, arise from an "original position" in which individuals are under a "veil of ignorance," such that no one knows what those interests are, only that their interests may collide with others.

In such a position, Rawls postulates two major principles: (1) each person is to have an equal right to the most extensive total system of equal basic liberties compatible with a similar system of liberties for all; and (2) social and economic inequalities are to be arranged so that they are to the greatest benefit of the least advantaged and they are attached to positions and offices open to all under conditions of fair equality of opportunity. In Rawls' view, these principles are universal, in that any rational, self-interested person would accept them as the just basis of social decisions in the original position.

Using these principles of justice, society should maximize the expected welfare level of the worst-off person in society. Thus, when conflicting interests occur, effective health care would be distributed to those who are worst off or get the least.

Robert Nozick (1974, p. 149) dismisses "distributive justice" by noting that "we are not in the position of children who have been given portions of pie by someone who now makes last minute adjustments to rectify careless cutting. There is no central distribution, no person or group entitled to control all the resources, jointly deciding how they are to be doled out." Nozick offers an entitlement theory wherein the history of the distribution of goods and services must be considered. To Nozick there are only different individual people with their own individual lives. Thus there is no social entity that has the *right* to decide how everything is to be divided up.

The problem of justice and equity thus invokes questions concerning the rights of communities or social entities to make decisions for others and their commitments to caring for others. As Larry Churchill (1987) phrases the question of social justice in health: Are we willing to care for the needs of strangers? How health care is distributed and to whom in the United States are answers to this question.

A major ethical challenge to health resource allocation is how to involve the community in making difficult health care decisions. Some members of the community may have to do without desired services to provide services that benefit other members more. These limitations in choice must be made for the sake of the social good, that is, maintaining or increasing the overall level of health given the resources the community is willing to devote to health.

Equality of Opportunity

One of the major effects of resource allocation and rationing is the impact of resource shifts on equality of opportunity for health care in a given community. Equal opportunity means, theoretically, equity in access to health care and equity in health outcomes. Equity in access to health care, however, is a substantially different goal than equity in health-related quality of life. Equal access does not guarantee equal health outcomes because medical care cannot be assumed always to be effective (Levine et al., 1983). By affecting access to the benefits of health care, however, resource allocation also affects equity in health outcomes.

These sociopolitical and ethical issues indicate that resource allocation and rationing operate within a given culture, including the prevailing political systems and economic values. Use or abuse of such strategies depends on the ethical principles, moral values, and political goals of the analysts and decision makers who use it.

HEALTH POLICY QUESTIONS FOR THE 1990s

Costs and outcomes are involved in a large number of health policy decisions in the United States. The focus of much public health policy is on allocation of resources to prevention. Another policy debate concerns the distribution of resources to technology. Finally, contemporary health policy decisions in the United States often concern access to health care services and measures to improve that access. These questions are the basis of our examination of how health outcomes and costs can be used in allocating resources to competing health care alternatives.

Which Health Promotion and Disease Prevention Objectives Should be Given Priority?

In the mid-1970s, policymakers began to reemphasize the long tradition of health promotion and disease prevention activities as a way of increasing the health status of the entire population. In the United States, the framework for action targeted three areas: lifestyle, environment, and services. *Healthy People* (Department of Health, Education and Welfare, 1979) developed and set forth national goals and objectives.

Whenever possible, these goals were expressed in terms of positive health. One example is a goal for older adults calling for a 20 percent reduction in restricted-activity days. Similar goals were set for other age groups. Experience has shown, however, that reported increases in activity limitations are not the most sensitive indicators of lifestyle changes. This is especially true when people cut back on smoking, alcohol consumption, or physical activity because of chronic conditions.

Most recently the goals and objectives for improving the nation's health reflect an increased emphasis on preventing ill health and disability, reducing health disparities between population groups, and improving the quality—not just the quantity—of life (Department of Health and Human Services, 1990). The purpose of *Healthy People 2000*, the national statement of health objectives, is to increase the proportion of Americans who live long and healthy lives. By the year 2000, health promotion and disease prevention policies should

1. **Increase the span of healthy life for Americans** to at least 65 years from estimated baseline in 1980 of 62 years.
2. **Reduce health disparities among Americans** by increasing years of healthy life among African Americans to at least 60, among Hispanics to at least 65, and among people aged 65 and older to at least 14 years of healthy life remaining.
3. **Achieve access to preventive services for all Americans** to increase years of healthy life to at least 65.

These measurable goals consider more than mortality and require data on the health status and quality of life of the U.S. population.

Strategies for achieving these national goals include improving surveillance systems, increasing services and protection, and improving professional and public awareness to reduce health risks. Each strategy implies resource expenditure to produce an anticipated health status benefit. Although health outcomes are an important part of *Healthy People 2000*, cost estimates are not included. Different prevention strategies, however, clearly have varying degrees of cost and potential for producing measurable outcomes. We discuss *Healthy People 2000* as a major approach that decision makers in the United States have adopted to address the issue of cost containment (Russell, 1986).

How Can the Effectiveness of Health Technologies Be Evaluated?

With increased development and application of health care technology, health care costs have risen. Innovations that extend the capabilities of existing technologies are generally more expensive to operate than those they replace. For example, computed tomography (CT) scans are replacing X-rays and magnetic resonance imaging (MRI) is replacing CT scans, both at increased costs. Similarly, new but more expensive pharmacologic agents are replacing previously accepted medicines. General consensus exists that technological innovation is cost-increasing, although theoretically it can be cost-decreasing or cost-saving, if a less expensive technology is substituted for a more expensive one (Scitovsky, 1985; Hodgson, 1988). The net result is that survival is no longer the only important outcome; rather, quality of life and associated costs have become important to both consumers and providers.

In evaluating health care technologies, the decision maker must balance the costs and benefits for both the consumer and provider. We discuss the allocation of resources to constant and continuous care of the critically ill newborn as a major example of the tradeoff between costs and quality of life in a highly expensive health technology. We also consider treatment for angina, including coronary artery bypass graft surgery, as an example of cost and outcomes comparisons for a moderate-cost technology that is available to a large number of persons in the United States and elsewhere.

What Can Be Done to Improve Access to Health Care?

Lack of universal access to an agreed-upon standard of health care in the United States is a major social problem. A growing number of states are proposing or establishing health programs to increase access to health care for low-income or uninsured residents. Based on the premises that health care access is a "right" and that decreased access to health care leads to decreased health status, health care access for everyone has been a major policy debate for over three decades.

The 1990s is not the first time the adequacy of access to health care has been questioned in the United States. For over two decades, access to health care has been monitored in periodic surveys. In 1987 the Robert Wood Johnson Foundation's *Special Report on Access to Medical Care* reported that all communities in the United States had made significant progress in improving access to health services. Despite this progress, significant barriers remain. Many different analyses of the problem and potential solutions have been offered to achieve the goal of providing a satisfactory standard of health care to all. There are two major policy questions. First, to what extent can improvements in access to health care be achieved by different strategies, such as expansion of state Medicaid programs and federal health benefit programs or employer-mandated or universal health insurance. Second, how will improved access to health services affect health disparities or inequalities in health status?

These questions are particularly important given the current ineffectiveness of efforts outside the health sector to decrease socioeconomic inequalities. The health status of low-income groups—working poor people, black persons, Hispanic persons, migrant farm workers, and rural residents—has improved over the last three decades. In the United States, however, minority and disadvantaged groups still experience more than their share of ill health and death (Department of Health and Human Services, 1985).

One of the major strategies to reduce health disparities among Americans in *Healthy People 2000* is to provide equal access to preventive and other health care services for all. Many incremental strategies have been attempted, primarily by states, to increase health care access to persons with low income, families and persons without health insurance, people with high-risk medical conditions, and other vulnerable populations. Proposals for major reform are being debated at both the federal and state levels.

As one major example, the State of Oregon has proposed a program to provide universal access to care for all state residents under age 65 Kitzhaber, 1989). This program includes changes in the state's risk pool, Medicaid coverage, and employment-based coverage. The essential question addressed by Oregon is: What state-funded services and procedures should be provided to raise the level of health-related quality of life of all Oregon residents? The Oregon plan involved explicit costs and outcomes comparisons as described in this book.

These three policy questions—priorities for health improvement objectives, methods to evaluate effectiveness of health technologies, and strategies to improve access—pose a formidable challenge to health decision making in the 1990s. Debate over optimal strategies will undoubtedly concern the comparative costs and outcomes of different policy options. In the next section, we define the concepts of health and quality of life that constitute these outcomes.

HEALTH STATUS, QUALITY OF LIFE, AND HEALTH-RELATED QUALITY OF LIFE

Health Status

Concepts of health often lack clarity. The terms used to define health include positive states—"wellness" and "normal"—and negative states—"disability" and "illness." These terms do not specify what health is; neither do they indicate where it begins or ends. The ambiguous nature of these concepts, however, is only part of the definition problem. The notion of disability or of illness as distinct from health is a value judgment. Illness definitions usually contain assumptions about what states of physical being are desirable or undesirable, normal or pathological, damaging or benign. What separates the "healthy" from the "unhealthy" and the "sick" from the "well" is a subjective interpretation of what is "good" or "bad," "desirable" or "undesirable."

One of the major difficulties in health status measurement and discussions about health and illness is the lack of attention to this underlying value problem. Whatever the basic perspective of health and disease—biological, psychological, social, or cultural—values exist that identify deviation from some standard of fitness or acceptable state of being. There are almost as many definitions of health and illness as there are states of being. All citizens, including health experts, humanists, scientists, and philosophers, have some notion of what is good health or high quality of life. Attempts to define conditions of health are influenced by people's deepest aspirations and fears. The variety of health concepts indicates that there is no unified entity but rather a combination of complex phenomena.

Perhaps the best example of a general definition is the oft-quoted World Health Organization's (WHO) definition of health as "a state of complete physical, mental, and social well-being, and not merely the absence of disease or infirmity" (World

Health Organization, 1948). This proposition fosters the ideal of positive health but does not encompass physiological phenomena or define which states of well-being are healthier than others. Another major problem with the WHO definition is defining well-being, particularly social well-being. What is or isn't part of health? Does social well-being refer to the social and economic environment of the society in which the individual resides or does it refer to social interaction and social integration, concepts more closely related to functional status? Although there is a lack of clarity to the concepts, WHO's popular definition encompasses most of the usual meanings given to health status, including functional status, morbidity, and well-being. With the addition of physiological outcomes (Brook et al., 1979), the definition describes well the content of health status.

Quality of Life

The term "quality of life" also has many meanings. These meanings reflect the particular knowledge, experience, and values of each individual. Aristotle (circa 335–323 B.C./1976) recognized this question in his definition of happiness in the Nichomachean Ethics:

> When it comes to saying in what happiness consists, opinions differ, and the account given by the generality of mankind is not at all like that of the wise. The former take it to be something obvious and familiar, like pleasure or money or eminence, and there are various other views, and often the same person actually changes his opinion. When he falls ill, he says that it is his health, and when he is hard up he says that it is money.

To some, quality of life may mean aesthetics or beauty; to others, the satisfaction of a close family life or a spiritual understanding of existence. Others, suffering from disease or disability, see quality of life as centering on the malady and its effects.

Quality of life is a concept that invokes the notion of value. Rene Dubos (1976) agrees that "quality of life involves highly subjective value judgments" and equates it with "profound satisfactions from the activities of daily life." Research and measurement of quality of life have encompassed both objective and subjective indicators. Social indicators researchers have commonly used objective indicators such as percentage of unemployed, percentage under the poverty level, home ownership, and overcrowding. Others classify populations in terms of income, food intake, access to transportation, occupational status, and living conditions.

Other researchers use a subjective approach to quality of life to investigate how people feel or think about their life. Social indicator researchers at the University of Michigan (Andrews and Withey, 1976; Campbell et al., 1976) have focused on subjective indicators such as global happiness and overall satisfaction with life, as well as satisfaction with specific life domains. These researchers assessed the importance of each domain and the importance of specific components to overall satisfaction with the domain. Level of well-being or happiness was then correlated with specific social, geographical, and demographic characteristics.

Clearly, quality of life involves a wide array of experiences, states, and perceptions. Cultural, psychological, interpersonal, spiritual, financial, political, temporal, and philosophical dimensions may be incorporated into various definitions (Calman, 1987). Because quality of life is such a global concept, it is generally advisable to ask for a listing of domains when the term is used.

Certain widely valued aspects of human existence may be considered apart from health status and well-being. These include a safe environment, adequate housing, a guaranteed income, respect, love, and freedom (Maslow, 1943; Andrews and Withey, 1976). The health care system and its providers usually do not assume responsibility for these more global human concerns, even though they may adversely affect or be affected by disease or treatment.

For example, people with respiratory disease, arthritis, or cardiac disease may experience changes in occupational mobility and income, require barrier-free housing, or be forced to live in a dry, warm climate. Some patients may also associate illness with extreme dishonor, disappointment, shame, or guilt. These social, economic, and cultural aspects of life are important considerations for patients, families, medical practitioners, and society. The main concern of health decision making, however, is in health-related quality of life. Although health status and health services influence and are influenced by the broader environment, not every aspect of human life is necessarily a health or medical concern.

Health status and quality of life are often used to describe an individual's or a group's functional status at a single point in time. Duration of life and estimates of future capacity to function are often separated from the definition of functional status. For example, mortality indicators, readily defined and developed from available data, are often used to measure "health." By health and quality of life, people often implicitly mean both present and future state; that is, most people do not consider dying people "healthy." Health, therefore, can be viewed as some combination of life and death. Indeed, mortality indicators can be conceptualized as binary (0/1) assumptions of value; that is, is it better to be alive than dead (Patrick, 1976)? This assumption may have widespread agreement, but the indicator begs the question of preference for life under all conditions. How much better is life at a higher level of health than at a lower one? Can one ever have enough good health? Some mutual understanding of what constitutes health status and quality of life is important to considering specific methods for assessing quality of life for health decisions.

Quantity and Quality of Life

Quantity and quality of life can be viewed as distinct but related concepts used to evaluate the present and future state of an individual or a group of people (Patrick and Elinson, 1984). Taken together, these concepts should represent a complete picture of the individual or group. Quantity of life concerns length of survival, for example, the number of days that a patient survives after undergoing heart transplantation or receiving pharmacologic agents such as azidothymidine (AZT) or zidovudine. These may prolong the life of people with human immunodeficiency virus while at the same time producing toxic effects.

Although it is relatively easy to measure quantity of life objectively, prognosis for survival can only be estimated, often without great accuracy. In addition, the value attached to a day of life, under the best of circumstances, will differ from one person to another (Patrick et al., 1973b). For some, death is preferable to coma, profound pain, or chronic depression (Torrance, 1987).

Health-Related Quality of Life

Because "quality of life" represents the broadest range of human experience, use of this general term in the health field has led to considerable confusion, particularly because of the overlap with the older, more specific concept of health status. To make the meaning more specific and still retain the important aspects of life quality, the term "health-related quality of life" is both useful and important. *Health-related quality of life is the value assigned to duration of life as modified by the impairments, functional states, perceptions, and social opportunities that are influenced by disease, injury, treatment, or policy.*

This definition covers five broad concepts that fall along a continuum of health-related quality of life shown in Figure 1.3. This continuum is anchored at the top by an optimal level assigned arbitrarily the value of 1.0 and at the bottom by a minimal level assigned arbitrarily the value of 0.0. Often the two ends of the continuum are labeled with the optimal level defined as "perfect health" and the minimal level defined as "death." Perfect health is an abstract notion meaning "health as good as it can be

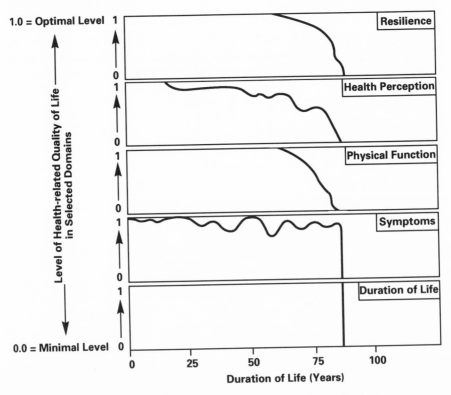

Figure 1.3   Health-related quality of life profile for a prototype individual.

imagined" or "free of all disease, symptoms, dysfunction, or unwellness." Although death may be considered the minimal level of health for many people, states of health such as coma, constant pain, or severe cognitive dysfunction may be considered worse than death, or some negative value below 0.0. Thus a minimal level might be assigned a negative value such as -1.0.

The specific domains of survival, impairment, functional state, perceptions, and opportunities fall along this broad continuum from optimal to minimal. Figure 1.3 illustrates the health-related quality of life for a prototypical individual over his or her lifetime. The duration of life for this person was 82 years; symptoms began at age 25; physical function began a steep decline at age 60. This individual's self-perceptions of health were variable. The individual's ability to withstand major stress or undergo organ system decline was excellent until age 60, when a heart attack occurred leading to declining function. Death for this individual occurred at 82.

Domains of the five health-related quality of life concepts may be negatively or positively valued when compared to each other, for example, physical compared to mental functioning or symptoms compared to satisfaction with health. The value assigned to a particular combination of the five attributes—an individual's health state—defines *quality* of life. Thus, health-related quality of life combines duration and quality into a single value. When an entire lifetime is considered, one can calculate the *years of healthy life* for an individual, as seen in Figure 1.4. The area under the curve represents the duration of this individual's life, as modified by the decrements in health and well-being.

Quantity and quality of life can also be combined to form an estimate of the health-related quality of life for a population or group of individuals. Figure 1.5 illustrates years of healthy life for a prototype group of individuals. Health-related quality of life is the average duration of survival modified by the average level of quality of life

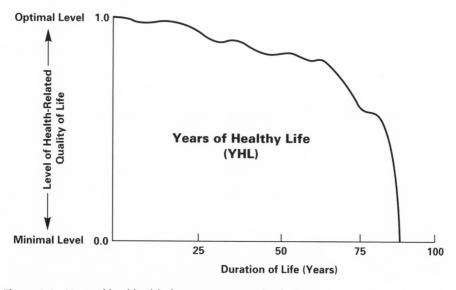

Figure 1.4 Years of healthy life for a prototype individual.

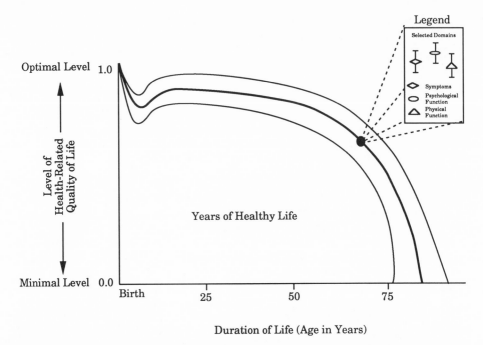

Figure 1.5 Years of healthy life for a prototype cohort. The area under the curve represents years of healthy life for a cohort defined by average health-related quality of life scores at each age. The heavy curve in the middle depicts the average health-related quality of life scores. The lighter curves on either side represent confidence intervals for these scores. The average health-related quality of life scores are calculated from scores on different domains, as shown in the legend.

(symptoms, function, perceptions, and opportunity) represented in Figure 1.5 as the mean value of symptoms and of functional status. The inset indicates that each point on the average line consists of several domains of health-related quality of life, in this example, symptoms, psychological function, and physical function. Each of these domains is subject to various sources of error, such as measurement and sampling errors, in addition to individual differences.

The variability observed in a group of individuals on each of these domains is represented by the vertical lines in the inset. This variability is present for each point along the horizontal axis. The lighter lines above and below the heavy line, which represents the mean function level, depict this variability through time, that is, upper and lower confidence intervals. A vertical line drawn at any point along the horizontal axis allows us to estimate the average health-related quality of life for the group. For example, persons 25 years of age have an average level of health-related quality of life of about 0.85. According to the confidence intervals, the score varies between 0.80 and 0.90. The average number of years of healthy life for the cohort is the area under the curve represented by the heavy line. Areas under the two lighter lines represent the upper and lower bounds of the years of healthy life for this cohort.

A complete representation of health-related quality of life involves (1) specification of relevant states and/or domains; (2) values or preferences assigned to these states; and (3) duration or probability of survival in different states. This definition of health-related quality of life is similar to the health state utilities approach developed over the last two decades by an increasing number of research groups (Fanshel and Bush, 1970; Rosser and Watts, 1972; Patrick et al., 1973b; Torrance et al., 1973, Kaplan et al., 1976, Torrance, 1976a; Weinstein and Stason, 1977a; EuroQol Group, 1990).

OBJECTIVES AND APPLICATIONS OF HEALTH-RELATED QUALITY OF LIFE ASSESSMENT

As indicated, measures of health status and quality of life have been used to assess outcomes of the medical care process and to track the level of health of communities and nations. In general, health status and quality of life outcomes are used in

1. **Clinical practice** to select treatments and monitor patient outcomes.
2. **Clinical and epidemiologic investigations** to identify determinants of health, investigate the course of disease and illness, and test the efficacy of treatments.
3. **Program evaluation and policy analysis** to establish priorities, examine the effectiveness of health policies and programs, and allocate resources.
4. **Population monitoring** to track trends in levels of health, risk factors, and use of services.

Categorizing measures of health-related quality of life according to the type of application for which they have been developed is one form of organizing structure. We have chosen this format and the foregoing terms because they are sufficiently broad to encompass most measures and their applications and are generally familiar. A number of other terms that relate to applications of health-related quality of life may be encountered in the literature. For example, clinical decision making and nursing assessment are terms that you might see in the clinical literature. Depending on the context, patient care or clinical research would fit in one of the first two applications listed here. Terms such as program planning, economic research, medical and preventive effectiveness, outcomes management, disability prevention, and technology assessment are most likely to appear in health policy discussions; thus these would be included in the program evaluation and policy analysis category.

Different applications require health status measures of differing levels of sophistication. For example, for monitoring the health of a population, a single indicator such as the prevalence of limitation of major activity may be sufficient. To select treatments and monitor patient response, however, more detailed health status information may be needed. In addition to overall, or generic, data on individual functioning, the clinician will need to know about symptoms and other side effects that may represent adverse consequences of the selected treatments.

For both population monitoring and clinical practice applications, it may not be necessary to combine different domains to arrive at an overall summary measure. Clinicians and patients usually make decisions that affect the patient directly and the family and clinician indirectly. In such decision-making settings, multiple domains of health-related quality of life will be integrated by the individuals involved, either implicitly or explicitly.

When using health status and quality of life measures for setting policy, however, a measure that summarizes multiple domains and can be used to compare across different health policy alternatives is needed. Such a measure includes tradeoffs between the different domains in the decision process and thus substitutes for the integrated decision making that occurs at the individual level. It should be possible, however, to disaggregate an overall measure such that analysts and decision makers can assess the relative contribution of individual domains to the overall value.

Incorporating health-related quality of life into clinical practice, epidemiologic investigation, policy analyses, and population monitoring involves definition and measurement. Whereas the assessment and interpretation process flows from the problem, users, objectives, and application, many definitions and measurement issues are held in common. All users of health status and quality of life measures may find common ground in application of these measures to resource allocation.

To address the health care crisis in the United States a comprehensive strategy is needed that incorporates *both* costs (inputs of care) and outcomes (effectiveness of care). This strategy needs to consider an equitable distribution of care even at the sacrifice of some economic efficiency. Without this inclusion of distributive justice, any "fix" is bound to fail. People need to be convinced that decision makers are concerned about their well-being and health-related quality of life. Without public confidence in the allocation process, people will not be willing to accept tradeoffs and possibly lose some benefits in the allocation of health care resources to improve everyone's opportunity for health. Chapter 2 describes a strategy for allocating health resources in the context of the health decision process in the United States.

2

A Strategy for Allocating Resources to Health Care

In Chapter 1 we defined health policy as decisions concerning resource expenditure on competing health programs in relation to anticipated benefits. This idealized definition of health policy implies that decisions are made by comparing costs and outcomes of different policy options and choosing those options that maximize health benefits for the populations of interest. The actual health decision process, however, is considerably more complex and less systematic than simply comparing costs and outcomes to make a one-time decision. Cultural, social, economic, and political forces, as well as individual interests and power, influence the decision process. In this chapter we explore the health decision process and propose an eight-step Health Resource Allocation Strategy to help health policy analysts and health decision makers evaluate the tradeoffs that society faces in health care. This chapter describes the crucial first step of the strategy: specifying the health decision in its social, political, and economic context. Subsequent chapters then lead the analyst or decision maker through the remaining steps of the strategy.

NATURE OF THE HEALTH DECISION PROCESS

Both the academic and popular image of decision making is that an "event" occurs (Weiss, 1986). A group of authorized decision makers assemble at a particular place and time. They review a problem, consider alternative courses of action, value the advantages and disadvantages of each, weigh the alternatives against their goals or preferences, and then select an alternative that seems most likely to achieve their goals. The result is a decision (Bachrach and Baratz, 1963). This image of decision making, often called "rational," is characterized as bound in time and location, purposive, calculated, significant, and sequential.

Indeed, some but not many policy decisions do resemble such rational processes. National decision analysts sometimes think about policy in terms of a rational policy model; that is, they attempt to understand events as purposive choices given a particular strategic problem. Allison (1971) offers a classic account of the "essence of decision" by President Kennedy and his advisers in considering American response to the Cuban missile crisis. Rational policy model analysts attempted to show that the Soviet installation of missiles in Cuba was a reasonable act from the point of view of the Soviet Union, given Soviet strategic objectives. Given the "rationality" of the decision from the Soviet perspective, the U.S. government was prepared to engage in counterplanning using a similar decision process.

Some health decisions may also follow a process that roughly fits the image of rational decision making. A hospital board's decision to construct a new wing might involve considering potential capital investment costs in relation to anticipated income from the new wing. Alternative policies regulating reimbursement to physicians under Medicare might also be compared by the Health Care Financing Administration using estimates of the savings associated with each alternative.

Many health decisions, however, are made through processes that bear little resemblance to a traditional, rational model. Health decision making most often takes place incrementally through diffuse, sometimes unrecognizable processes. Decision makers may not even be conscious that they are making decisions, and the "event" can appear to be a fait accompli similar to sending out a memo announcing a new administrative regulation.

In the U.S. Congress, policy options are often expressed as alternative bills supported by opposing interest groups. Alternative versions of Medicare and Medicaid legislation and the numerous alternative plans for national health insurance are examples of complex health policy options. Legislators can be familiar with only portions of a lengthy bill or with only one among many. A great deal of behind-the-scene activity, sometimes involving political tradeoffs, takes place without public knowledge. Authority is thus fragmented, and a jumbled political process replaces any formal comparison of costs and potential outcomes. It can even be difficult to identify formal stages or identify key actors in the complexity of government policy-making.

Yet policy decisions do get made. Policy analysis illuminates a number of key characteristics of decision making (Weiss, 1986). Six of these characteristics are particularly relevant to health decisions:

1. **Innovation within customary and implicit rules.** In the process of doing what agencies traditionally do, new policies are made by subsuming the decision within the already familiar. Reimbursement formulas for health providers are a prime example of such innovation. Rules of reimbursement may be rewritten that represent new policy directions, such as eliminating coverage for specific services, adding a new benefit to a health insurance plan, or changing levels of deductions or copayments.

2. **Mutual adjustment.** When decisions are made by one office or arm of government, other offices often reach decisions by reacting explicitly to those already made. In the United States, for example, down-the-line adjustment takes place when the Executive Office of Management and Budget makes decisions about health legislation and appropriations, such as granting waivers for special health service demonstrations. The Congress and the White House influence the Office of Management and Budget, which, in turn, makes decisions that influence the Department of Health and Human Services and the Health Care Financing Administration, which influences whether a new health services demonstration gets implemented.

3. **Bargaining.** Overt conflicts occasionally arise over boundaries of authority, such as departments of health and departments of social services, or between overlapping federal agencies such as the Health Care Financing Administration

and the Agency for Health Care Policy and Research. Direct negotiation may then take place between the interested parties, often using tradeoffs of past decisions ("you owe me one"), perceived advantages, and obligations. The consequences of these arrangements can tip the balance in favor of one policy option or another. For example, when health programs are shifted from one department to another, decisions may be made that change eligibility for services. Staffing patterns may also change. Maternal and child health programs may reach different clientele using different staff when placed in a social services department rather than in a health department.

4. **Move and counter move.** Bargaining isn't always acceptable to all parties in a dispute. When bargaining fails, one agency takes unilateral action. A department of health, for example, may decide to establish a needle-exchange program or close the "gay baths" in a city to influence high-risk behavior and prevent AIDS. The mayor or city council, however, could thwart these decisions through legal maneuvers and insistence on traditional public health education rather than "regulating" behavior. An entire series of moves and countermoves occur until bargaining is possible or the decision is shifted to higher levels, in this example, most likely the courts.

5. **The solution precedes final recognition of the problem.** Policy options often sit around for years or even decades before a window appears in which the problem finally is confronted and a decision gets made. Consider proposals for universal health insurance or a national health system. Not infrequently, a decision results from the commitment of one or more interested parties in putting their pet idea into action. These partisans wait until the right "window of opportunity" appears in which to get a solution accepted. Proposed solutions to the health care "crisis" appear and reappear as health care costs and problems of access continue to escalate. A state may consider implementation of universal health insurance under one administration, then throw this proposal out when a new administration enters office.

6. **Unanticipated consequences.** Merton (1968) identified another route by which policy is made as the "unanticipated consequences of purposive social action." Because one decision is made to achieve a desired result, other unintended outcomes occur. The passage of Medicare legislation, for example, improved access to health services for persons age 65 and over and some disabled persons, but it also spawned an era of health care cost inflation (Pauly and Kissick, 1988). Subsequent cost-containment policies, such as diagnosis-related groups and mandatory second-opinion programs, can be viewed, in part, as the unintended consequence of the successful decision to improve access to health services for older adults. Shifts in pricing, personnel distribution, and technology may also lead to unintended decisions.

In addition to these characterizations of decision making, there are other routes to policy decisions, some as yet unrecognized. These processes indicate that decisions can be and are made without formal assessment that uses a rational process to review research data or projected costs and outcomes. Informal decisions will sometimes be formalized by legislation or executive order giving the appearance that the decision process is more considered than it is. Legislation or administrative regulation may simply ratify a decision that has already been made. As Weiss notes, "At some periods and in some areas it is only a slight exaggeration to say that ratification of the status quo, and allocation of funds to support it, is a main function of legislation" (1986, p. 225).

We propose that using the Health Resource Allocation Strategy in health decision making will *improve* the political process. Described in the next section, the strategy provides a step-by-step structure for specifying decision alternatives, for collecting and/or analyzing data on costs and outcomes, and for incorporating this information into the political process.

THE HEALTH RESOURCE ALLOCATION STRATEGY

The Health Resource Allocation Strategy is both a conceptual and mathematical representation that provides a systematic framework within a sociopolitical process for comparing health outcomes with health care costs across all programs in the health sector of the economy. Unlike previous "fixes" to control health care spending, the strategy explicitly addresses tradeoffs that must necessarily be made between improving health status and controlling costs for the society as a whole.

The Strategy emerges from a large number of theoretical and methodological traditions including economics, medicine, political science, psychology, public health, and sociology. At least four teams of investigators have identified one or more of the steps in building the strategy and have contributed substantially to its application over the last two decades: Bush and his colleagues with the Quality of Well-Being Scale and General Health Policy Model (Patrick et al., 1973a; Bush, 1984a; Kaplan and Anderson, 1988; Kaplan, 1989); Torrance and his colleagues with the Health Utilities Index and Cost–Utility Analysis (Torrance, 1986); Rosser and her colleagues with the Disability/Distress Classification and Index as used in British economic appraisal (Williams, 1985; Rosser, 1988); and the EuroQol Group currently developing an instrument for conducting cost–utility analyses in several Western European nations (EuroQol Group, 1990; Brooks et al., 1991; Nord, 1991).

As shown in Table 2.1, the Health Resource Allocation Strategy involves eight major steps outlined here and discussed in detail in subsequent chapters.

Step 1. Specify the Health Decision

The single most important step in applying the Strategy is the initial statement of the policy problem. In common with most decision processes, the question asked affects the information collected and the decision to accept or reject a particular policy alternative. Health decisions may involve choosing between different entitlement criteria for health insurance programs or allocating resources to several competing health interventions. The decision context might involve the allocation of a global budget for a national, statewide, or local constituency, including all federal, state, or local services. Other decisions may be more specific and include assessing different technologies or evaluating a single health promotion program. Regardless of the situation, specifying the health decision involves five tasks.

Table 2.1   Eight steps in the Health Resource Allocation Strategy

1. **Specify the health decision** by

   Describing the sociocultural and health services context of the decision;

   Identifying alternative courses of action under consideration;

   Identifying stakeholders;

   Defining stakeholder values for outcomes of alternatives;

   Recognizing the assumptions used in the socioeconomic evaluation; and

   Specifying the budgetary constraints to be considered. (Chapter 1)

2. **Classify health outcomes as health states** by

   Identifying relevant concepts, domains, and indicators of health-related quality of life;

   Listing the hypothesized relationships among concepts, domains, and indicators; and

   Selecting combination of domains to be included in the health state classification. (Chapters 3,4,5)

3. **Assign values to health states** by

   Identifying population of judges to assign preferences;

   Sampling health states to be assigned preference weights;

   Selecting a method of preference measurement; and

   Collecting preference judgments and assigning preference weights to health states. (Chapter 6)

4. **Measure health-related quality of life of target population** using primary data collection or secondary analysis to

   Classify individuals in target population into health states;

   Assign a preference weight to the health state of each individual; and

   Average scores of all individuals to obtain a point-in-time estimate of the target population's health-related quality of life. (Chapters 7,8)

5. **Estimate prognosis and years of healthy life** by

   Calculating expected duration of survival (life expectancy) of target population; and

   Calculating years of healthy life by adjusting duration of survival by the point-in-time estimate or observed differences in health-related quality of life. (Chapter 9)

6. **Estimate direct and indirect health care costs** by

   Identifying all organizing and operational costs attributed to each of the alternative courses of action; and

   Specifying out-of-pocket expenses and productivity losses incurred by the recipients of each alternative. (Chapter 10)

7. **Rank costs and outcomes of health care alternatives** by

   Calculating the ratio of costs per year of healthy life gained for each alternative course of action;

   Ranking the ratios from low to high with the budget constraint included in this ranking; and

   Identifying ratios that are less than the budget constraint as cost effective. (Chapter 11)

8. **Revise rankings of costs and outcomes** by

   Reviewing rank order of each alternative course of action with stakeholders in the decision;

   Adjusting the rank order based on stakeholder challenges and community consensus on the values and goals of health care; and

   Recommending the revised rank order to political decision makers. (Chapter 11)

Describe the sociocultural and health services context in which the decision will occur. Our approach to describing the social and cultural context in which decisions occur is to provide an analytic framework for identifying the potential determinants of health-related quality of life that may influence outcomes, such as the economy, lifestyle behaviors, genetic endowment, and health services. Theoretically, all factors, processes, and organizational structures that might influence outcomes should be identified, and the evidence for these influences should be considered. These determinants can be viewed from the policy perspective as causal hypotheses about the role of health care in producing better health. Identifying the possible determinants of health assists in estimating the potential effectiveness of health care interventions under consideration in producing improved health-related quality of life. Analyzing determinants also emphasizes the importance of the potential effects of factors or processes other than health care in limiting disease and promoting health.

Identify all the alternative courses of action under consideration and the stakeholders involved in the decision process. Alternative courses of action involve decisions "to intervene or not to intervene." At the microlevel of clinical decision making, this may mean deciding between surgery and watchful waiting for a patient with a particular medical condition (back pain, cataracts, knee replacements, etc.). At the macrolevel of population-wide resource allocation, alternatives are all the services and procedures possibly included under an entitlement program. For example, the Health Care Financing Administration may recommend to Congress which preventive services should be included as a benefit of the Medicare program. In between, decisions are made for special population groups and procedures such as neonatal intensive care for newborns. In this case, the alternatives are different levels of intervention, for example, aggressive versus nonaggressive treatment for very low birth weight infants where success is questionable.

Identify the stakeholders. This description includes all the groups interested in the decision, when they are interested, and why. Stakeholders most often include persons or patients in the target population, their relatives or significant others, and providers, although other groups may have an interest in the decision as well. In deciding the level of treatment for low birth weight infants, stakeholders obviously include the infants, their parents, and other family members. Neonatologists and other professionals are also invested in the decision. Administrators and legislators are stakeholders as well as decision makers. From the societal perspective, the entire community has a stake.

Define stakeholder values for outcomes of alternative actions. These values are the beliefs, cultural notions, norms, and other organizing principles that form the basis for social decisions. For example, parents and families of low birth weight babies may hold values about the sanctity of life and love for their offspring. Providers may blend concern about the effectiveness of treatment with compassion for the infant. Administrators may have special interest in the cost of treatment. Society might be concerned with equal opportunity for all newborns and the cost of treatment. Identifying these values for each stakeholder group provides a foundation for deciding what groups should be involved in the allocation model and what information is needed.

Identify the specific method of socioeconomic evaluation. The Health Resource Allocation Strategy incorporates the cost-utility method of socioeconomic evaluation, specifically estimating the cost per year of healthy life gained for each policy option. Other methods of cost-effectiveness might be used such as those based on life years that rely on mortality or duration of life and do not estimate quality based on assigning utilities to health states.

Specify the budget constraint. The amount of money available for resource allocation must also be identified as a constraint on the decision. Legislators and the executive branch of government specify the budget that ultimately constrains what services are provided and to whom.

Step 2. Classifying Health Outcomes or States

Health states are combinations of one or more concepts, domains, or indicators of health-related quality of life: survival, impairment, functional status, perceptions, opportunities, and so on. The potential number of states is almost limitless because each individual may be described by a different combination of the attributes used to define health and quality of life. In practice health states are limited to the concepts and domains with broad agreement on importance to health and widespread use in health status measures, namely, symptoms and the domains of physical, mental, and social function.

Identify all relevant concepts, domains, and indicators. Each possible major health outcome can be described in terms of health states. For some investigations, there may be only a few health states. For example, in a study of kidney dialysis and transplantation, Torrance and his colleagues (1973) used only four states because there were only four distinct health outcomes: kidney transplant, hospital dialysis, home dialysis, and death. When Torrance and others evaluated neonatal intensive care (Torrance et al., 1982; Boyle et al., 1983), however, 960 states were required because of the large number of potential outcomes.

Hypothesize relationships among concepts, domains, and indicators. In general, we view the concepts and domains of health-related quality of life moving from disease processes outside the individual through individual characteristics "beneath the skin" to behaviors, processes, and opportunities involving membership in a particular culture, society, or community. The relationship among domains may be straightforward; for example, a given level of impairment such as symptoms of chest pain may be associated with a particular level of functional status, such as confined to bed and to a particular level of perceived health status, such as poor rating of health. In other instances, impairment may not translate so easily into functional status, perceptions, and opportunities. Hypothesizing in advance of measurement what the expected relationships are will help in the interpretation of measures used in any application or model of health-related quality of life outcomes.

Select combination of domains for health state classification. Figure 2.1 shows an example of the possible range of content in describing health states. At the most

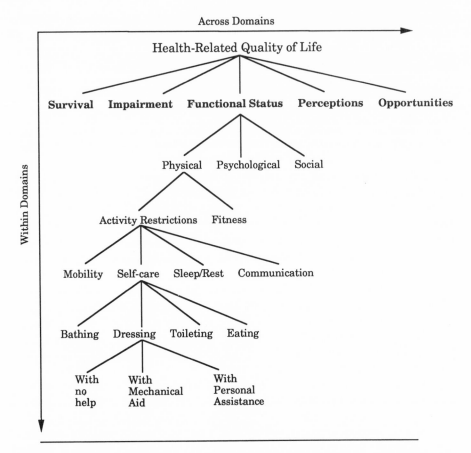

Figure 2.1 Examples of concepts and domains for a health state classification system. In a health state classification system, concepts of health-related quality of life are broken down into domains, e.g., functional status is divided into physical, psychological, and social function. Each function can be further broken down into more specific constituent domains. Health states are created from the classification system by combining different domains and levels within domains. *Source*: Adapted from Torrance, 1986.

comprehensive level are the five broad concepts of health-related quality of life including functional status. Within functional status are the domains of physical, psychological, and social function. Physical function has two subdomains, activity restrictions and fitness. Activity restrictions include activities used to describe physical function: mobility, self-care, sleep/rest, and communication, for example. Self-care activities are bathing, dressing, toileting, and eating. At the lowest level of the hierarchy are the actual activities and the amount of assistance needed to perform them: dresses with no help; requires mechanical aid to dress; or requires personal assistance to dress.

Within each concept and domain, the classification system should be mutually exclusive and exhaustive. This permits every individual to be classified at any point in time on each attribute into one and only one level of health-related quality of life. Every combination of levels, however, represents a unique multiattribute health state, which illustrates the large number of potential states. For that reason, most multiattribute health state classifications are limited to a small number of concepts and domains considered most critical to health status assessment. These include symptoms and physical, emotional, and social function.

Step 3. Assign Values to Health States to Create Levels of Health-Related Quality of Life

Once health states have been defined, the problem becomes how to compare one health state with another. As Moriyama (1968) pointed out, total counts of cases lead one to question how "one equates a case of coryza with a case of primary lung cancer, or a case of congenital anomaly with a case of senile psychosis." All these conditions may be described with different health states: which health state is "better" or "worse." The frequency of the occurrence of health conditions or health states gives no indication of the relative importance of the condition or health state.

The problem of tradeoffs also occurs in assessing health status over time. Take, for example, an individual with arthritis assessed at baseline; supposed she is having difficulty dressing herself, but she can lift a jar down from her kitchen cupboard. At follow-up, however, she reports that she can no longer lift the jar down from her kitchen cupboard but has no difficulty dressing. Is she better off at follow-up than she was at baseline (Paterson, 1984)? The qualitative as well as the quantitative aspects of health states must be taken into account to assess tradeoffs in health-related quality of life. Both the frequency and preference or relative desirability of the health state is important in assessing overall health status. Preferences are therefore assigned to health states to permit measurement of the level of health-related quality of life.

Identify who is going to assign preferences. Patients, family members, respondents living in the community, and health professionals can assign preferences to health states. In clinical practice and in studies of individual patient treatment decisions, patients are asked to assign preferences to their own state of health and potential outcomes of treatment. In the Health Resource Allocation Strategy, members of the community assign preferences to health states as a representation of the whole society or community involved in the allocation process.

Sample health states for assigning preferences. Comprehensive health state classification systems contain a large number of potential states, thereby requiring a sampling strategy for selecting states for preference assignment. One approach is to sample a sufficiently large number of comprehensively defined states covering the range of all domains to permit estimation of preferences for all potential states in the system. Another approach is to use multi attribute utility scaling of individual attributes to build a preference weighting system that estimates preferences for all potential health states. The first approach requires a sampling of health states, whereas the second approach does not. Multi attribute methods are most often used with classification systems built on seven or more domains.

Select a method of assigning preference weights. Different methods exist for assigning preference weights or utilities to health states so that one health state can be considered "better" or "worse" than another, for example, category scaling, standard gamble, time tradeoff. Preferences can be measured on an ordinal, interval, or ratio scale (see *measurement* in the glossary). Ordinal weights, as in the case of disease-specific functional classifications, often are insufficiently descriptive of small changes in health status, although they are commonly understood and can describe major shifts (The Criteria Committee of the New York Heart Association, 1964). Interval and ratio preferences reflect the strength of preference for one or another health state. Economists refer to cardinal measures as those that have either interval or ratio properties.

Preference measurement techniques are used to obtain the value of each health state for individuals or groups. In cost–utility studies, individual values are usually grouped into a collective utility. In the Health Resource Allocation Strategy, aggregation is achieved by measuring all individual utilities on the 0/1 scale representing minimal and optimal value of the health states. The arithmetic mean of individual utilities is used to calculate an aggregate utility weight for health states.

Collect preference judgments and assign preference weights. Assigning preferences to health states involves extensive instrumentation such as the use of visual aids, interviewer training, response recording, data entry, and statistical analysis. Standardized methods are available for collecting and assigning preference weights to health states, including direct and indirect scaling methods, utility methods, and social valuation.

Step 4. Measure Health-Related Quality of Life of Target Population

Measuring health-related quality of life in the strategy involves classifying individuals into health states and assigning preference weights to these states. Scores are averaged for all individuals in the population.

Classify each individual into one health state. To measure the health-related quality of life of a target population, one needs to design a questionnaire or some other standard way of collecting information about individual health status. That is, information in the classification system needs to be translated into a format for data collection. In primary data collection, the investigator can either choose an existing questionnaire, such as that for the Quality of Well-Being Scale, or can design his or her own. In secondary data analysis, the analyst selects a data set and a classification system that are comparable; items from the existing data are structured as if they had been collected using the questionnaire associated with the classification system.

Assign a preference weight to each individual's health state. Whether conducting primary or secondary data analysis, each respondent in the survey is classified into one and only one health state in the classification system. For example, when the Health Utilities Index is used, a respondent may have the following health state: able to get around the community without help, have some limitation in walking, able to perform his or her self-care but limited in performing work activities, anxious yet has an active social life, and has no health problems or complaints. In the Health Utilities Index Classification System, this person would be assigned a health state with the weights 0.91, 0.94, 0.86, and 1.00 for each domain; when combined according to the formula, these weights yield a score of 0.62.

Average scores of all individuals. The average health-related quality of life for any target population can be found by summing over the scores of the individuals in the group and dividing by the number of individuals. As illustrated in Appendix I, the Health Utilities scores for eight individuals might be 1.00, 0.87, 0.66, 0.61, 0.47, 0.14, −0.14, and −0.21 These scores are typical of those that might be obtained by applying the foregoing procedures in either primary or secondary data analysis. Using these eight scores, the average health-related quality of life is 3.4 divided by 8, or 0.425. This process generalizes for any target population and gives an estimate of the current, or point-in-time, level of health.

Step 5. Estimate Prognoses and Years of Healthy Life.

Prognosis is the foretelling of survival, recovery, or deterioration in a person's condition once it has been diagnosed and analyzed. In populations, prognoses are measured as the probabilities of moving from one level of health-related quality of life at one point in time to another level at one or more subsequent points. In the Health Resource Allocation Strategy, the analyst is interested in incorporating prognosis into the estimate of health-related quality of life of the population through calculation of years of healthy life.

Calculate expected duration of time in a health state. The Health Resource Allocation Strategy involves both the current level of health of an individual or a population and the probability of transition to other levels. Movement from one level of health-related quality of life to another involves both one's current level and characteristics that may influence the current level. Together the current level and the influencing characteristics determine whether the level of health-related quality of life will increase, stay the same, decrease, or vary through time.

The most common way of incorporating prognosis into the estimation of the level of health-related quality of life is through the use of transition probabilities. These probabilities can be obtained from studies in which people in various health states are monitored over time, that is, as they move from one state to another. From these observations it is possible to form estimates of health state transition probabilities.

Calculate years of healthy life. Dynamic health status is the expected value of the point-in-time health-related quality of life scores associated with levels of health-related quality of life multiplied by the transition probabilities. For example, with two time periods and three health states, if we know a person's current level of health-related quality of life and the transition probabilities associated with moving from the current state to the three possible health states in the next period, then we can estimate this person's health-related quality of life over this time interval.

Calculation of dynamic health status can be illustrated using three health states from the Health Utilities Index Classification: optimal health (1.0), a health state with dysfunction only in the social-emotional domain (0.86), and the example health state used previously (0.62). Assume the example individual is in the state with the intermediate score, 0.86. Also assume the probability of being in the health state with a higher score at the second time period is 0.15, and the probability of being in the health state with a lower score is 0.35. Then the expected level of health-related quality of life for this person at the second time interval is 0.797, that is, $(1.0 \times 0.15) + (0.86 \times 0.50) + (0.62 \times 0.35)$.

If a second individual in the study was at the optimal level of functioning at the first time period and moved to the intermediate level at the second time period, one could calculate this individual's dynamic health status in a similar way. Assume for this example that the transition probabilities for staying the same or moving to a lower health state were 0.85 and 0.15. Then the expected health status for this individual is 0.979. For this sample of two individuals, the average (or expected value) is 0.888.

Most often we lack data to calculate dynamic health status for individuals. Instead, we use estimated probabilities and statistical modeling to calculate the expected health status of groups of individuals. The most frequently used technique is the standard life table. In this approach, life table estimates are adjusted by the mean level of health-related quality of life for each age to calculate years of healthy life. The result is a statistic that gives a composite estimate of a group's health status, combining both quantity and quality of life.

Step 6: Estimate Direct and Indirect Health Care Costs

In developing estimates of health care costs for resource allocation, it is the notion of economic, or opportunity, cost rather than accounting cost that is important. In economics, the cost of a resource is defined in terms of its value in an alternative use. For example, the cost of a renal dialysis center is determined as the value of all of the resources—personnel, facilities, patient transportation costs to the center, materials, and so on—that could be applied to other programs. Health care costs are usually referred to as either direct or indirect costs, both of which should be included in any cost and outcome analysis. Even though it may be impossible to measure all of the costs of a health intervention, the most important and relevant ones need to be identified and measured to obtain meaningful cost estimates to use for efficient and equitable allocation.

Identify all organizing and operational costs. These costs include physician services as well as the services of other health care providers and equipment needed for making diagnoses, for patient care, and for rehabilitation services. Some of the costs included in this category may be considered as fixed costs, for example, capital and operating expenses. Other costs may be considered as variable costs, for example, time and supplies. These costs are referred to as direct medical care costs.

Specify out-of-pocket expenses and productivity losses. Direct personal costs include out-of-pocket medical expenses for items such as both prescription and nonprescription medication as well as medical devices and appliances. People may also incur direct nonmedical costs as a part of undergoing treatment. Such costs include the modification of one's home to accommodate health care needs of the patient and care provided by relatives and friends.

In addition to direct costs of health care, patients and their families can also incur costs that are usually described as productivity losses due to ill health. These indirect costs include time lost from work and psychic costs and may include leisure time lost and reduced levels of output while at work.

Few economic evaluations take into account a third type of costs, namely, those that are external to the health care sector, individuals, and their families. A new insurance or employee benefit program can raise the price of the product or service offered by an employer. This increased price is a cost of the intervention that is borne by those who do not use services covered under the benefit package.

Step 7. Rank Costs and Outcomes of Health Care Alternatives

In comparing costs and outcomes it is the present value of both additional cost and the additional years of healthy life gained that are of interest. That is, the policymaker is interested in learning the additional cost C with a given intervention compared to the cost without the intervention, or $C_w - C_{wo}$, and the additional health benefits attributable to the intervention, $YHL_w - YHL_{wo}$, where YHL is years of healthy life. Since many health programs result in expenditures and health benefits not only in the current period but also in future periods, the general practice is to convert both into present-value terms.

As shown in Figure 2.2, four costs and outcomes combinations result. Ideally, health interventions will produce better health-related quality of life at reduced cost (lower left quadrant). Medical treatment for back pain (versus surgery) and new drugs to limit benign prostatic hyperplasia might produce such results. Rationing, capping reimbursement, and other cost-containment methods may result in worse health-related quality of life at lower costs (lower right quadrant). Higher cost and worse health-related quality of life (upper right quadrant) are to be avoided, though some life-extending treatments such as ventilation and nutritional support might well fall into this category. Most health interventions, including technological innovations, probably result in better quality of life at higher cost (upper left quadrant).

Calculate ratio of cost per year of healthy life gained. Although such fourfold comparisons allow for the identification of interventions that are more or less costly for either improvement or worsening of health-related quality of life, they fail to inform the decision maker as to how much better one intervention is than another in terms of costs and outcomes. Thus, analysts have begun to calculate the ratio of additional costs

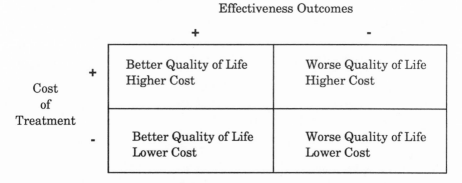

Figure 2.2 Cost and outcome results in evaluating treatment effectiveness.

of a given intervention to the additional years of healthy life gained from the intervention. This type of analysis is frequently referred to as cost–utility analysis.

The ratio of cost per year of healthy life gained is generally formed by dividing the net cost, $C_w - C_{wo}$ by the net health effect $YHL_w - YHL_{wo}$. This ratio indicates the additional cost per year of healthy life that can be attributed to the health intervention of interest. By using a standard way of calculating years of healthy life, these ratios can be compared for different health interventions. This across-intervention, or societal, perspective can be used by decision makers with overall responsibility for health, such as administrators and legislators, to choose among competing demands for resources.

Tables 2.2, 2.3, and 2.4 show the estimated cost per year of healthy life gained from selected health interventions or programs using the Disability/Distress Index, the Health Utilities Index, and the Quality of Well-Being Scale, respectively. Three separate tables are presented to illustrate that comparisons between interventions using the Health Resource Allocation Strategy are valid only if the same classification system and method of estimating preferences are used to calculate years of healthy life. Otherwise, relative rankings of similar programs might vary because different methods have been used for obtaining estimates of years of healthy life. In addition, possible cultural differences (United Kingdom, Canada, and the United States) among these three classification systems and preferences suggest that single-system comparisons are most appropriate. With additional empirical research, we may eventually be able to compare the ratios of cost per year of healthy life for health interventions that have been evaluated using different classification systems and/or preferences.

Table 2.2   Estimated cost per year of healthy life gained using the Disability/Distress Index

Program (reference)	Reported cost/YHL gained in British pounds (year)	Adjusted cost/YHL gained in British pounds (1989)
Advice to stop smoking (Williams, 1988b)	200 (1987)	225
Pacemaker implantations for atrioventricular heart block (Williams, 1985)	700 (1985)	860
Total hip replacement (Williams, 1985)	800 (1985)	990
Valve replacement for aortic stenosis (Williams, 1985)	900 (1985)	1,110
Coronary artery bypass grafting for severe angina and left main vessel disease (Williams, 1985)	1,000 (1985)	1,230
Action to control severe hypertension (Williams, 1988b)	1,700 (1987)	1,930
Action to control total serum cholesterol levels (Williams, 1988b)	1,700 (1987)	1,930
Scoliosis surgery ideopathic adolescent (Gudex, 1986)	2,600 (1986)	3,100

Table 2.3 Estimated cost per year of healthy life gained using the Health Utilities Index

Program (reference)	Reported cost/YHL gained in U.S. dollars (year)	Adjusted cost/YHL gained in U.S. dollars (1989)
Postpartum anti-D gamma globulin (Torrance and Zipursky, 1977)	<0 (1977)	<0
Antepartum treatment of primiparae and multiparae (average) (Torrance and Zipursky, 1984)	1,223 (1983)	1,517
Neonatal intensive care of low birth weight infants, 1,000–1,499 grams (Boyle et al., 1983)	2,800 (1978)	5,325
Neonatal intensive care of very low birth weight infants, 500–999 grams (Boyle et al., 1983)	19,600 (1978)	27,767
Continuous ambulatory peritoneal dialysis (Churchill et al., 1984)	35,100 (1980)	52,820
Hospital hemodialysis (Churchill et al., 1984)	40,200 (1980)	60,495

Rank ratios from low to high. Programs, or health interventions, in Tables 2.2 to 2.4 are ranked according to the cost per year of healthy life gained. Lower ratios indicate more cost-effective programs than do higher ratios. Table 2.2, reporting studies using the Disability/Distress Index, indicates that advice to stop smoking which is given in doctor's offices in Britain cost £200 per year of healthy life compared to £2,600 for scoliosis surgery.

The screening programs for postpartum anti-D and (Rh) gammaglobulin phenylketonuria shown in Tables 2.3 and 2.4, both have negative cost–effectiveness ratios. Further analyses of these programs indicate that costs associated with each program are less than those without the program and that each program results in increased years of healthy life compared to the situation without the program. Thus these interventions would be considered to have saved money. In general, the data in Tables 2.2 to 2.4 indicate that screening and prevention programs have lower cost per year of healthy life gained ratios than do chronic disease interventions. In contrast, high-technology interventions tend to have high ratios. For example, in Table 2.3 hospital hemodialysis is the least cost effective; that is, this program has the highest cost per year of healthy life gained ratio.

Identify ratios that are less than budget constraint as cost-effective. Until the present the Health Resource Allocation Strategy and other types of cost–outcome comparisons have been used primarily in research settings. These studies, some of which are summarized in Tables 2.2 to 2.4, were designed to demonstrate the role of such comparisons in policy-making. These studies, however, do not show estimated ratios in the context of prospective resource allocation, that is, the case where the policymaker faces a budget constraint and must decide from among a set programs which to fund and which not to fund given the constraints. *Cost per year of healthy life gained*

Table 2.4 Estimated cost per year of healthy life gained using the Quality of
Well-Being Scale

Program (reference)	Reported cost/YHL gained in U.S. dollars (year)	Adjusted cost/YHL gained in U.S. dollars (1989)
Phenylketonuria screening program (Bush et al., 1973)	<0 (1970)	0
Parasite screening and treatment (Anderson and Moser, 1985)	5,415 (1985)	7,123
Screening for serum thyroxine (T4) (Epstein et al., 1981)	3,600 (1977)	9,430
Oral gold in rheumatoid arthritis (Thompson et al., 1987)	12,059 (1991)	10,130
Diet in non-insulin dependent diabetes mellitus (Kaplan et al., 1988)	10,870 (1987)	12,474
Exercise program for chronic obstructive pulmonary disease (Toevs et al., 1984)	10,834 (1984)	15,145
Tuberculin testing program (Bush et al., 1972)	5,760 (1968)	28,083
Alkaline Phosphatase Test (Amberg et al., 1982)	85,400 (1980)	170,230
Total hip replacement (Liang, 1987)	293,029 (1991)	246,144
Neonatal circumcision (Ganiats et al., 1991)	[a]	[a]

[a] A ratio has not been calculated because the program produced less than 1 day of additional benefit.

ratios may be used to allocate resources across a wide range of potential health
interventions.

Kaplan and Bush in 1982 suggested that programs with a ratio of less than $20,000
per year of healthy life are "cost effective by current standards." Those with a ratio of
$20,000 to $100,000 per year of healthy life gained may be "controversial but are
justified by many examples." Programs over $100,000 were considered questionable
in comparison with other potential health expenditures. Where to draw the line, that is,
how to decide which programs have acceptable cost per year of healthy life gained
ratios, is a sociopolitical and ethical judgment.

Step 8. Revise Rankings of Costs and Outcomes
for Allocating Resources to Health Care

The ranking of health care alternatives according to Steps 2 through 7 is a technical
procedure which does not directly consider the sociocultural or political context of the
policy decisions considered in Step 1. The ranking of health care alternatives according
to their relative cost per year of healthy life gained does not answer the question before
the decision maker: Is the gain in years of healthy life for a particular health care

alternative worth the extra expenditure? The answer to this question is not precise, mathematical, or objective. Rather it is a value judgment to be made at the end of the allocation process by decision makers, both administrators and legislators. Once health alternatives have been ranked according to their cost per year of healthy life gained, the proposed rankings need to be subjected to a formal sociopolitical process for comparison with the prevailing values of the community.

A published summary of the preliminary rankings should be made available to as many persons as possible who have a stake in the decisions to be made. Political negotiation of the value to be placed on different alternatives must take place, including input from the community. This final step is conducted to assure that the final ranking recommended to legislators reflects, to the greatest extent possible, society's preferences for the totality of interventions to be included in any benefit package and supported as part of the policy decision.

Review rank order of each alternative course of action with stakeholders in the decision. The ranking of health interventions in terms of cost per year of healthy life gained should be reviewed by persons and groups who stand to be affected by the interventions that are funded or those that are considered to have a cost per year of life gained that may exceed available resources that is, the budget constraint. This review is needed for two reasons. First, there are inherent deficiencies in the methodology of calculating cost per year of healthy life gained for different interventions. Real-life health care programs do not produce easily indexed outcomes (Warner and Luce, 1982). Programs have multiple outcomes that are not easily measured, weighted, and summed into the single years of healthy life index. Data on program outcomes are often unavailable, and thus analysts use estimates of program effects. Cost data are also difficult to obtain and must be estimated. These estimates may lead to calculated cost–outcome ratios with high variance. Thus, the final ranking may be unstable, that is, the estimates may not be robust.

Second, the rankings resulting from Steps 3 to 7 of the Health Resource Allocation Strategy are based solely on ratios of cost per year of healthy life gained. These ratios will not incorporate all of the community values for health care that drive the resource allocation process. For example, bone marrow transplants for children with cancer might well fall below the budget constraint, but community compassion for children would place this intervention "above the line." Nor will the ranking based on ratios accurately reflect the preferences of all stakeholders in the community. Patients with terminal diagnoses or people with disabilities would clearly be concerned about treatments for the diagnoses that are not included in the funding package. Thus, they will advocate for changes in the ranking based on their own interests.

Adjust rank order to reflect community values. To account for the disparities that arise from either methodological deficiencies or stakeholder disagreement, the ranked list of cost outcome ratios needs to be adjusted to arrive at the rank ordering informed as much as possible by community values and sociopolitical debate. To organize the debate within an identifiable value context, the proposed rank ordering should be reviewed in two ways: (1) challenges to the validity of the published estimates of the costs, health outcomes, preferences, and prognoses, the four major data elements contained in the cost per year of healthy life gained ratio; or (2) challenges that the preliminary rank order does not represent community consensus on the value of the alternatives.

In the first instance, stakeholders would challenge the list by stating their disagreement with the estimates, for example, costs are underestimated or expected health outcomes are greater than estimated. Stakeholders should provide, if possible, alternative estimates supported by data or expert opinion and consensus, which should be inserted into the recalculations to determine what impact, if any, the adjustment has on the rankings. Political debate will likely ensue, since stakeholders, whether individuals or groups, will desire a reordering of the list of interventions according to their own particular values. Any adjustments to the rank order would depend on the consensus that results from an evaluation of the technical procedures used in the strategy.

In the second instance, stakeholders could challenge that the preliminary rank order does not reflect the consensus of the community on the value of particular interventions or treatments for specific conditions, such as organ transplants, treatments for end-stage disease, or cosmetic surgery. If data are available on stakeholder or community values, these should be shared. If not, challenges should be described and folded into the final decision process by administrators and legislators.

Recommend revised rank order to the decision process. Political and bureaucratic decision makers are the final arbitrators of the rankings. The initial and revised rank order should be submitted to the decision makers empowered by the political process to review and produce the final priority ranking based on the revised cost and outcomes ratios and their perceptions of community values. The political authority, most likely the legislative body, will ratify the final priority ranking and set the budget constraint that determines which services will be included in the funding package, that is, those services that society is willing to fund. The final list of priority interventions should be published to permit examination of the changes that occurred between the initial and revised ranking based on costs and outcomes ratios and the final priority list that reflects all the values of the community as expressed by stakeholders and interpreted by administrators and legislators.

This final step of the Strategy links the allocation process back to the initial identification of the health decision, including stakeholders, the values of stakeholders, and community values and goals for health interventions. The technical procedures for estimating cost per year of healthy life gained to assign priorities to health services is therefore embedded in a sociopolitical process that concerns the entire community. The next section describes Step 1 of the Strategy in greater detail.

SPECIFYING HEALTH DECISIONS

To describe health policy decisions in specific terms as Step 1 of the Health Resource Allocation Strategy, analysts and decision makers should (1) list the causal hypotheses concerning all the potentially relevant determinants of health-related quality of life that may influence the decision; (2) identify all the policy options and stakeholders in the decision process and their values for alternative courses of action; and (3) specify the logic and assumptions involved in any socioeconomic evaluation, including budgetary constraints.

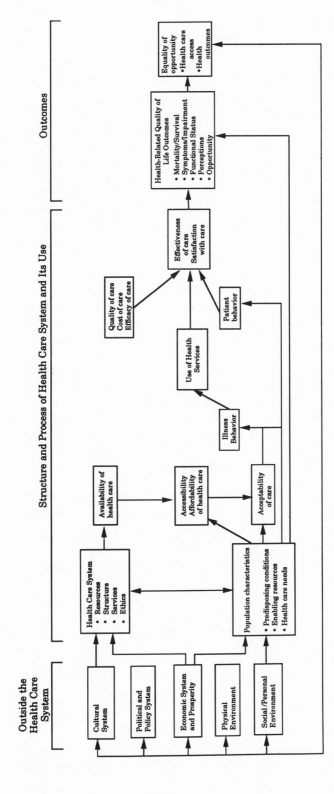

Figure 2.3 Determinants of health-related quality of life in the Health Resource Allocation Strategy. *Source:* Adapted from Patrick, Stein, et al., 1988.

Causal Hypotheses Concerning Determinants of Health-Related Quality of Life

Evans and Stoddart (1990) suggest there is a growing gap between our understanding of the determinants of health and the primary focus of health policy on the provision of health care. The analysis and use of health-related quality of life data are often limited by the lack of an organizing framework for examining known and hypothesized relationships among social and cultural circumstances, health services, and health outcomes. Identifying and describing health-related quality of life and health services concepts and processes within a comprehensive system provide the means for putting health decisions and outcomes in a social and political context. A comprehensive view of the inputs into the health services delivery system and health outcomes can also assist research efforts to evaluate the effectiveness of different health and social programs.

The determinants of health-related quality of life outcomes are shown in Figure 2.3. The arrows and their position in the figure indicate our current understanding of potential causal and often multidirectional relationships among different determinants. Analysts and decision makers should use this analytic framework (1) to state assumptions about the determinants and the production of health involved in a particular decision process, (2) to develop causal hypotheses about the interaction among different factors, processes, or structures inside and outside the health care system that influence health-related quality of life, and (3) to identify the data needed to test these hypotheses.

For example, a particular medical procedure such as transplantation of artificial organs might extend the life of individuals with organ failure. However, religious beliefs, societal values, or personal preferences might make artificial organ transplants unacceptable, thus influencing health outcomes. Both health-related and non-health-related determinants should be considered in developing causal hypothesis for application of the Health Resource Allocation Strategy.

Determinants Outside the Health Care System

Many determinants of health-related quality of life exist outside the personal health care system. These determinants are related to the cultural, political, and economic system as well as to the physical, social and personal environments of the individual or group. Examples of such outside influences are as follows:

Culture: values, beliefs, rituals, and their meanings in a particular society or community

Political system: public health policy, private sector health policy, and community organization

Economic system and prosperity: income distribution, housing, employment, and environmental conditions

Physical environment: carcinogens, air pollution, toxic waste

Social/Personal environment: gender, social class, social support, life-style, diet, exercise, substance use

Structure and Process of the Health Care System

Cultural, political, economic, physical and social-personal influences are major determinants of health. They influence health outcomes directly without working through the health care system. Sociocultural, political, economic, and geographical systems also affect the structure and process of the health care system. From a broad perspective, the political economy of a particular nation, whether a welfare state or free market economy, may determine the structure of the health care system, the amount of resources invested in health, and the principles by which services are provided. Health care may be considered a "right" provided to all citizens or a "privilege" extended to those who are able to pay. From a narrower perspective, culture and the social environment help to define what is considered a health care need within a particular society and how these needs are met. A particular health care system can be described briefly using the following elements:

Resources: facilities, personnel, and equipment/technology
Structure: finances and organization
Services: preventive, curative, and support
Education and promotion: mass media, community interventions, and personal services
Geographic distribution: national, regional, urban, or rural
Current practice standards: professional standards reviews, audits, and utilization reviews

The role of health care in relation to health and quality of life outcomes is controversial. It has been persuasively argued that the major advances in general health over the last century have occurred through improvements in living standards, diet, and sanitation rather than through medical care (McKeown, 1976). Public health and economic development are viewed as the most important determinants of population health. Medical care has also been charged with creating sickness (Illich, 1976) and with producing no beneficial effects (Carlson, 1975). Regardless of these claims, medical care and, more broadly, health care and preventive services have been and continue to be regarded as strategies for improving health-related quality of life. The structure of the health care system influences and is influenced by the characteristics of the population it serves.

As proposed by Aday and Andersen (1975), population characteristics can be viewed to include

Predisposing conditions: risk factors for declining health and mortality—demographics, living conditions, nutrition status, and health beliefs
Enabling resources: insurance and poverty status
Health care needs: comparative need

Health care "need" in this context refers to comparative need. Comparative need is based on the principle of equality that corresponds to territorial justice (Daniels, 1985). If x and y have similar health characteristics and y receives a good or service not received by x, then x is perceived to be in need. Comparative needs are determined by socially defined principles of equity, that is, equality of opportunity for health care and, in the long term, for health and quality of life. Such principles provide the basis for equity and rationing decisions affecting different population groups.

The relation between need and health-related quality of life is not consistent across social groups. People with similar health status do not have similar perceptions, nor do they make similar demands of health care. Differences in health beliefs, illness behavior, social networks, willingness or ability to pay for a service, and other sociopsychological, economic, and cultural processes affect how needs are perceived and translated into demand for health care. Needs assessment is not simply a matter of defining population health status and distributing available resources. It must also consider the social, economic, and political environment of individuals and populations.

The distinction between need and health status is often blurred. Health status as a measure of service need can be primarily, but not exclusively, limited to subjective health. Self-perceived ill health that is reported to others, and thus becomes a social phenomenon, can be viewed as a need for prevention, cure, or comfort. Self-reported health status and satisfaction with health, at the level of both the individual and populations, can be indications of need.

Health perceptions may also be viewed as indicators of outcomes. In Figure 2.3, health-related quality of life outcomes include individual conditions, behaviors, subjective states, and socioculturally defined states (see Chapter 4). Many of these outcomes—social role limitations and activity restrictions—are reported by the people involved. The ability to perform usual social roles—to work, to attend school, to play, and to enjoy recreation—are central objectives of the health care system. Thus, health status can be both a *predictor* and an *outcome* of access to services.

The concept of access to health services has been notoriously difficult to define. At least the following four "levels of health care coverage" are implied by the term:

Availability of health care: provision of staff and facilities—the ratio of providers to population or presence of health care in a community

Accessibility: provision of insurance, eligibility, entitlement, and ease of using a service

Affordability: ability to purchase insurance or care

Acceptability: perceived value of obtaining care and of the care obtained

The actual process of health care is exceedingly complex: a progression of health, illness, and sick role behaviors from health habits such as smoking through recognized ill health such as chronic obstructive pulmonary symptoms to patient status and release of social role obligations such as sickness absence or disability compensation. These behaviors have been identified in many studies and analyses of the use of health services (Rosenstock and Kirscht, 1979). The quality, cost, and efficacy of health care are clearly important determinants of both effectiveness of health care and patient satisfaction with care. Efficacious medical treatments, high quality of medical care delivery, and affordable cost may increase effectiveness and produce high patient satisfaction. Treatments that do not work, care that is considered low quality, and rationing according to increased charges tend to be associated with low effectiveness and satisfaction.

Health outcomes in Figure 2.3 cover the five major concepts of health-related quality of life defined in Chapter 1 and indicators of which are further described in Chapter 4. The final box in Figure 2.3 proposes *equality of opportunity* as the ultimate goal of the health care system. This opportunity includes equitable access to health care services for all as well as equality in health-related quality of life to the greatest extent possible. That is, no group in society should experience disadvantage because of health or lack of health care in relation to any other group. Reducing inequalities in access to health services and disparities in health status between population groups is therefore a major objective of health care.

Figure 2.3 also illustrates that inequalities in opportunity for health and health care affect determinants outside the health system—the cultural, political, economic, social, and personal environment. Disparities in access to health services and health status are one aspect by which societies are characterized in political and economic terms. These disparities also influence economic development and the political process, through labor force participation, need for government subsidy, and voting behavior. In this normative model, the extent to which the inequalities in access to health care and to health status are recognized and reduced defines whether the entire society can be considered "better off."

The complexity of Figure 2.3 and the ambitious scope of its content and meaning make clear that identifying the determinants of health-related quality of life is not a simple task. Such a complex diagram, however, serves a major purpose in identifying determinants and the point at which these determinants are relevant to a particular policy decision. For example, population health status measures involve all the influences shown in Figure 2.3, whereas evaluation of specific medical treatments usually involves a more limited causal chain. Figure 2.3 also helps in the analysis of health outcome data by locating which determinants and outcomes are included in a data set. The diagram thus helps guide the organizing of relationships among determinants and suggests causal hypotheses.

Causal hypotheses should be listed as a first step in specifying a health decision. The Institute of Medicine study of the Medicare End-Stage Renal Disease Program is used to illustrate this step (Rettig and Levinsky, 1991). In the early 1970s, the U.S. Congress had to decide whether the Medicare program administered by the Health Care Financing Administration (HCFA) should cover end-stage renal disease. The major causal hypotheses were that increased access to treatment for people with the disease would (1) increase survival and (2) return them to their usual activities. The Social Security Amendments of 1972 created an entitlement to Medicare for persons of all ages with a diagnosis of permanent kidney failure, regardless of income.

The End-Stage Renal Disease (ESRD) program is the only one in which the U.S. government tries to provide treatment for every person (and spouses and dependent children) eligible for benefits under Social Security who has a disease, regardless of income. In addition, both ESRD patients and providers depend on Medicare reimbursement policy to a greater extent than in any other domain of medicine. The number of patients under treatment for ESRD has grown over time. There were approximately 10,000 eligible persons with kidney disease in 1973, when entitlement became effective and dialysis treatments were so costly that hospitals limited access to scarce dialysis machines. Today HCFA pays for treatments for 150,000 persons at an annual cost of nearly $4 billion. In the year 2000, it is projected that the ESRD program will serve a quarter of a million patients.

Although access to treatment was considered the major determinant of health outcome in the deliberations of Congress in passing entitlement legislation, the primary diagnoses of diabetes and hypertension along with incidence in the population are also important determinants of outcomes. More diabetic and hypertensive patients, and a disproportionate representation of black and Hispanic patients, have characterized the ESRD program in recent years. Other determinants of health-related quality of life outcome included lifestyle and the availability of social support; cultural acceptance of life-sustaining treatment over long periods of time; and geographic availability of treatment centers and personnel.

One major determinant of outcome, unexpected in the deliberations of the 1970s, was the aging of the population in combination with the availability of treatment centers and health care workers and the number of hours of treatment. The number of persons 65 years and older increased from 5 percent of the total Medicare ESRD population in 1973 to 27 percent in 1988. National expenditures for this program have been controlled by progressively lowering real costs per dialysis treatment, by successful transplantation programs, and by some shifting of payment responsibility to private payers. Regardless of these impressive cost controls, the steadily growing number of patients has led to program costs more than ten times what was expected.

Because of drops in financing, services and staff have been reduced, and patients are receiving fewer hours of treatment than before. The Institute of Medicine study (Rettig and Levinsky, 1991) suggests that this drop in hours of treatment may have caused an increase in morbidity and mortality among those treated. Thus the current status and future of the ESRD program raises national concerns about presently known and future determinants of health-related quality of life outcomes in relation to expenditures.

Components of Health Decisions: Alternatives, Stakeholders, and Community Values

Components of health decisions can best be specified by identifying (1) alternative courses of action under consideration; (2) all the stakeholders—groups interested in the decision—and when and why they are interested; (3) the values of stakeholders for each alternative course of action; and (4) the values of the total community for health care. Alternative actions or interventions can be identified through a review of treatments. Policy analysts should describe these interventions as completely as possible, including budgets, organizational structure, target population, and relevant health outcomes. When Medicare coverage for end-stage renal disease was being considered, treatment included hospital dialysis only. Hospital hemodialysis still predominates (60 percent), although peritoneal dialysis (10 percent) and transplantation (25 percent) are other treatment modalities.

The alternative courses of action were to (1) leave all insurance coverage to private carriers and private payers; (2) require fee-for-service payments for renal dialysis treatments; (3) broaden coverage for renal treatment to all persons under a new universal health insurance program; and/or (4) finance insurance by expanding Medicare coverage for everyone with end-stage renal disease regardless of age. Congress attempted to estimate the potential costs for each of these alternatives. The organizational structure was hospital-based care financed by Medicare. The target population included everyone eligible for Social Security, regardless of age, with end-stage renal disease. Thus, the ESRD did not establish a universal benefit. Medicare-certified dialysis facilities reported 6–7 percent of their patients as not eligible for benefits, and this proportion increased to 7.5 percent in 1989 (Rettig and Levinsky, 1991). Relevant health outcomes identified by Congress were survival and return to work or other major social role activity.

Groups of stakeholders interested in the decision included patients with end-stage renal disease and the families of these patients; clinicians who treat and make the decision of whom to treat; congressional representatives with constituents who have end-state renal disease; the Health Care Financing Administration, which administers

Medicare; and all contributors to Medicare. Some of these stakeholders—patients, families, and clinicians—clearly have more interest in the decision than others. Contributors to Medicare through Social Security payments or special taxes might be interested when they stand to benefit directly or when a program they want is not funded because of resource allocation to end-stage renal disease.

Stakeholders' values include those broad social and cultural attitudes incorporated in the overall resource allocation process and those associated with alternative courses of action. These values may be elicited in focus groups and meetings with advocacy groups for decisions concerning specific groups or in community meetings and public hearings for decisions concerning an entire community. A large number of values might be involved in the allocation process, including equality of opportunity, duration of survival, other health-related quality of life outcomes, probability that treatment will be effective, cost of treatment, community compassion, perceived responsibility for the problem, and age, gender, and ethnicity. In implementing the Oregon Plan, for example, 13 community values elicited from community meetings and public hearings were organized into three categories: (1) overall value to society of providing health services: prevention, cost effectiveness, impact on society; (2) value to individuals at risk of needing the services: ability to function, length of life, quality of life; and (3) value to a basic level of health care: prevention, cost effectiveness, quality of life (Oregon Health Services Commission, 1991).

The process of eliciting stakeholder or community values incorporates the perspectives of community organization and community activation. In these perspectives, the people affected by a problem are involved in defining the problem and planning, instituting, and maintaining steps to resolve the problem. By involving stakeholders and the community, the health allocation process promotes the principles of participation and ownership (Mills, 1959; Olson, 1965; Kahn, 1982). Large-scale social change requires the persons affected have a sense of responsibility for and control over the change, so that they will continue to support change after the initial organizing effort. Participation and ownership follow the premise that social decisions are more likely to be successful and permanent when the people affected are involved in initiating and promoting the change. This perspective currently enjoys resurgence in community health decision making and in community health promotion programs (Bracht, 1990; Green and Kreuter, 1991).

Each stakeholder group consulted may place different values on the health care alternatives under consideration. For example, Congress expected that dialysis would help persons with end-stage renal disease return to a productive life, including employment. Thus, high value was placed on reducing work disability and on functional status. For patients and their families, however, a high premium was placed on survival itself, given the poor prognosis for the disease without dialysis. Happiness, life satisfaction, and overall well-being were also important.

Specifying all courses of action, identifying groups interested in these actions, and determining the values associated with the alternatives is a complex sociopolitical process requiring the investment of time and other resources. Eliciting stakeholder values in focus groups or community meetings and public hearings, however, is an important political process that shapes allocation decisions. Insufficient attention to this process will lessen the fit between the decision and prevailing community values and may result in vigorous challenges to decisions, which can be avoided. Outlining a policy decision in this detail also uncovers the relevant health-related quality of life outcomes involved in decisions.

Identifying health status and quality of life outcomes makes it easier to incorporate these data into the decision process. Specifying the values of different interest groups brings a political and ethical dimension to the decision. Systematic analysis is further enhanced by incorporating the assumptions and logic of socioeconomic evaluation described in the next section.

Methods and Assumptions of Socioeconomic Evaluation

Socioeconomic evaluation is the comparison of costs and outcomes under the assumption of finite resources. The strategy requires cost–utility analysis as the method of socioeconomic evaluation in order to use years of healthy life to assess the benefit of health interventions and to maximize health outcome for a given level of expenditure.

Cost–utility analysis is closely related to two other methods of socioeconomic evaluation, cost–benefit and cost–effectiveness analysis (Drummond et al, 1987). In fact, both cost–effectiveness and cost–utility analytic methods derive from the original methods of cost–benefit analysis that were introduced in the early 1900s for the purpose of allocating resources to projects in which the benefits were not valued in the marketplace. Table 2.5 summarizes these three types of socioeconomic evaluation. As shown in the table, costs are estimated in the same way for the three types of evaluation. The measurement of outcomes, however, varies for each method. In each example the subscripts refer to alternative health interventions, one of which may be the no-intervention alternative. Although this table illustrates the simplest case, the number of

Table 2.5   Comparison of three types of economic evaluations

Type of study	Measurement of costs (C)	Identification of outcomes (O)	Measurement of outcomes	Comparison of costs and alternative intervention outcomes[a]
Cost–benefit analysis	Dollars	Single or multiple outcomes that may be achieved to different degrees by alternative health interventions	Benefits in monetary terms (B)	$(C_1 - C_2) - (B_1 - B_2)$
Cost–effectiveness analysis	Dollars	Single effect of interest which is common to both alternatives but achieved to different degrees	Effects expressed in natural units, e.g., life years, disability days saved (E)	$\dfrac{C_1 - C_2}{E_1 - E_2}$
Cost–utility analysis	Dollars	Single or multiple outcomes which may be achieved by different degrees by the alternatives	Years of healthy life (YHL)	$\dfrac{C_1 - C_2}{YHL_1 - YHL_2}$

[a] Subscripts 1 and 2 designate two alternative health interventions, one of which might be the status quo.

alternatives can be extended for any condition or disease. Also, the situation becomes more complex when alternatives for more than one health condition are evaluated simultaneously. This simple case shown in Table 2.5, however, generalizes to multiple outcomes and conditions.

In *cost–benefit analysis (CBA)*, treatment costs and benefits are compared in terms of monetary units to determine net benefits. These benefits are obtained by first subtracting the costs of one program (or the status quo) from the costs of the alternative $(C_1 - C_2)$. Then the outcomes of one program are subtracted from the outcomes of the alternative $(B_1 - B_2)$. Net benefits result from the subtraction of the difference in benefits $(B_1 - B_2)$ from the difference in costs $(C_1 - C_2)$.

In applying cost–benefit analysis to social and health programs, analysts encountered the difficulties of translating such health benefits as changes in health-related quality of life into monetary units. Such a translation requires that a money value be assigned to an individual's life. Various methods, including the human capital approach, willingness to pay, and revealed preferences, have been used for this purpose. Although each method has it proponents and has proved useful, conceptual and practical concerns have prevented any single method from becoming widely accepted.

The difficulty of using monetary units to compare costs and outcomes led to the development of cost–effectiveness analysis. In *cost–effectiveness analysis (CEA)*, benefits are expressed in any one of a number of units, including life years saved, number of disability days saved, number of cases of disease averted, and number of cases treated. For example, Steinberg et al. (1988) used life years gained to assess the cost effectiveness of thrombolytic therapy for treatment of acute myocardial infarction (AMI). This study examined the additional cost of streptokinase and recombinant tissue–type plasminogen activator (TPA) when compared to conventional therapy. The cost per additional life year gained when streptokinase was used for treating AMI was approximately $53,000; for TPA, the corresponding cost was approximately $57,000.

Other studies, for example, those by Nissinen et al. (1986), Oster et al. (1986), and Rees (1985), have also used life years gained as a measure of health benefit to analyze the cost effectiveness of hypertension, smoking cessation, and cancer prevention. In addition to using life years to represent health benefits, Cantor and colleagues (1985) used behavioral variables, such as ability to comply with a medication schedule, ability to keep health care appointments, and ability to control blood pressure, to assess the effect of a hypertension control program.

These examples illustrate that units of outcome in cost–effectiveness analyses are dependent on the particular health condition under investigation. When different units of measure are used to assess health outcomes, it is impossible to compare the costs and outcomes of different health interventions. This limits the use of cost–effectiveness methods in policy applications.

Cost–utility analytic methods emerged in the 1980s as a form of socioeconomic evaluation that allows for the comparison of costs and benefits derived from diverse interventions, for example, coronary artery bypass graft surgery, phenylketonuria screening, and hospital hemodialysis, in a standard outcome measure, namely, years of healthy life. In *cost–utility analysis (CUA)*, net benefits of health care interventions are expressed in terms of the common denominator of years of healthy life. *Utility* refers to the value of a particular health state or improvement in health status. Utilities are measured by assigning the preferences of individuals or society to health states (Step

3). Analyses that use utilities as the measure of net program effect are therefore called cost–utility analyses.

The costs and outcomes comparisons shown in Tables 2.2 to 2.4 illustrate the wide range of socioeconomic evaluations that have applied cost–utility analyses to health. Cost–utility analyses emerge as the analysis of choice because using years of healthy life allows the comparison across health interventions. Although cost–benefit analysis also allows this comparison, the difficulty of placing a money value on life has precluded its widespread use.

Incorporating cost–utility analyses demands yet another assumption to the Health Resource Allocation Strategy in addition to the assumption of finite resources and economic efficiency discussed in Chapter 1. This additional assumption, called the *interpersonal comparability of utility*, concerns the nature of preference and aggregation of utilities across individuals. Kenneth Arrow (1951), in his seminal book *Social Choice and Individual Values*, proposed the viewpoint that interpersonal comparisons of utilities have no meaning; that is, combining individuals' preferences or choices is impossible. In simpler terms, the impossibility can be stated: one person's happiness will never be another person's happiness. Arrow thus restricted social choices to the ordinal preferences of individuals. Subsequent treatments of this problem have relaxed the restriction to ordinal utilities, although the problem of obtaining a "correct" representation of social values remains (Seabright, 1989).

Cost–utility analyses involve aggregation of interval or ratio level individual utilities to define net benefit of a health intervention. In aggregating preferences across individuals, we contradict Arrow's well-established impossibility theorem. Thus, the Health Resource Allocation Strategy makes the assumption that the utility of one individual can be combined with the utility of another in assigning preferences to health states and calculating years of healthy life. In relaxing Arrow's impossibility theorem, we also recognize that there is a distinction between aggregating the preferences of individuals about what would be good for themselves and aggregating individual judgments about what would be good for society.

Specifying the Budgetary Constraint

The Strategy may be used in rationing when the size and intensity of the program is the main consideration. In this case, the decision is one of how extensively a program should be made available, that is, the number of services to provide or the number and characteristics of the people to receive the service. Eligibility criteria for a program may determine the size and intensity of the program. For example, all patients with end-stage renal disease might be considered eligible for Medicare versus only those ESRD patients who have contributed to Social Security. Persons at different stages of diseases such as cancer and AIDS might be eligible for different types of services, such as active treatment versus hospice care. This type of decision differs from deciding whether to fund a program or sets of programs.

If the aim of the analysis is to determine whether to fund one program or another, that is, an "all or nothing" decision, then the cost–utility ratio is based on differences in *overall* costs and outcomes measured in terms of years of healthy life. On the other hand, if the goal is to determine the size and intensity of the program to fund, then the ratio of *marginal* costs and effects is the relevant measure (Kamlet, 1990).

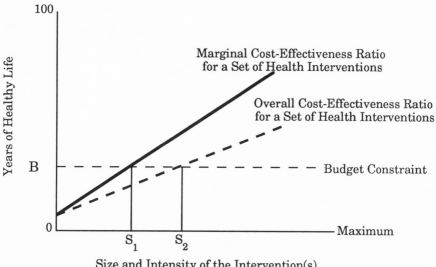

Figure 2.4 The budget constraint and the Health Resource Allocation Strategy. S_1 = cost-per-year-of-healthy-life ratio when the alternative is how much of the program (size and intensity) to fund. S_2 = cost per year of healthy life ratio when the alternative is to fund or not to fund intervention. *Source*: Adapted from Kamlet, 1992.

Figure 2.4 compares the overall and marginal cost–effectiveness ratios for a set of health interventions that have been ranked in order of increasing cost–utility ratios. The horizontal line, labeled B, represents the *budget constraint* set by policymakers; this is the total amount of money available for allocation to the set of interventions. This line differentiates between interventions with acceptable and unacceptable ratios. Those that fall below B are cost effective relative to other programs included in the comparison. Ratios falling above B represent health interventions that are not cost effective.

If more health care resources are made available, then the level of B in Figure 2.4 would rise and a greater selection of health interventions would be judged cost effective. If the amount of resources were reduced, then the level of B would be lower and fewer programs would be judged cost effective. As shown in Figure 2.4, a health intervention of the size and intensity that corresponds to the intersection of the budget constraint line B and the marginal cost–effectiveness curve S_1 is cost effective. That is, S_1 represents the cost-effective size and intensity of the intervention.

If the policy issue is whether to fund an intervention or to stay with the status quo, the S_2 identifies the cost-effective level. Interventions where cost/YHL ratios fall between S_1 and S_2 are considered to be cost effective only if the alternative is to do nothing. Such programs provide sufficient additional benefits to justify the expenditures.

Regardless of the policy issue, specification of the budget constraint boils down to identifying how much money is going to be made available for allocation to health care interventions. Government budgets generally provide the dollar amounts available in the coming year. In nations, states, or local governments where deficit spending is allowed, the proposed budget may not reflect the actual amount of available resources. Where spending on health care cannot exceed income and the allocation of monies to the health care sector, the budget constraint is easily identified.

RESOURCE ALLOCATION IN THE HEALTH DECISION PROCESS

The Health Resource Allocation Strategy goes beyond cost–utility analysis in several ways that have significant implications for policy-making. First, it brings the policy context directly into the health decision process. Step 1 of the Strategy requires the analysis of socioeconomic and political environments in which resources are to be allocated. By requiring that policy analysts identify the concerns of different stakeholders in the decision process, the Strategy provides a systematic way of incorporating the important cultural and political factors that influence the allocation of resources across health interventions.

Step 8, the final step, also goes beyond simple cost–utility analyses by offering stakeholders in the decision, as well as policymakers, the opportunity to adjust the ranking that obtains from using cost–utility methods. This is an important step since ranking health interventions on the basis of cost per year of healthy life gained ratios contains important assumptions and can produce decisions biased in favor of one population group over another. For example, one source of bias may result in comparing interventions designed to benefit children with those designed to benefit adults. Since children generally live longer than adults, any intervention that improves the years of healthy life of children may result in more benefit than a comparable intervention designed for adults. Similarly, interventions that involve prevention generally are less costly than those involving complex medical technologies. Thus, preventive interventions that do not require advanced technology are more likely to result in low cost per year of healthy life gained ratios. The review and adjustment process involved in Step 8 of the Strategy helps to identify and address these and other biases that result from costs and outcomes comparisons.

Another way the Health Resource Allocation Strategy goes beyond the traditional formulation of cost–utility analysis is in its more precise specification of the inputs to the comparisons of costs and outcomes. Cost–utility analysis has been used primarily for research to demonstrate the potential role of socioeconomic evaluation in policymaking. The Strategy encourages health decision makers to use systematic analyses of costs and years of healthy life for allocating resources across a wide range of health interventions. Therefore, the Strategy requires that all cost per year of healthy life ratios be based on the same set of preferences, or tradeoffs, for levels of health-related quality of life. Without uniform values or preferences assigned to the health states used in evaluating the outcomes of different health interventions, differences in relative ranking of cost per year of healthy life ratios may be attributed to the methods used in assigning preferences rather than in the outcomes of alternative health interventions.

The Health Resource Allocation Strategy is a simplification of the reality surrounding the health decision process. The Strategy embeds logic and assumptions not shared by all analysts and decision makers. Although less than optimal, the logic and assumptions are integral to applying rational choice theory to social decisions. To accept the impossibility of aggregating individual preferences for health states, for example, implies that collective decision making based on social choices is untenable. In our view, social choices must be made explicit in the decision-making process, and a systematic step-by-step strategy should be used to guide the health decision process.

Theories of social choice are not the only theoretical underpinnings for the Health Resource Allocation Strategy. Social choice theory defines the nature of the health decision and the incorporation of socioeconomic evaluation methods into the Strategy. The definition and measurement of health-related quality of life is also theory bound. Chapter 3 describes these theoretical foundations to the development and application of health-related quality of life measurement in the Strategy.

3

Theoretical Foundations for Health-Related Quality of Life

All measurement processes include assumptions about the nature and value of the constructs used in the measurement, yet the role of theory in developing health-related quality of life measures and in interpreting data is often neglected (Patrick and Gutt-macher, 1983). Theory, in fact, guides implicitly or explicitly both the selection of content and the measurement process. Even though users and analysts may not identify a particular theory or set of theories in selecting the concepts and domains to be included in the measurement of health-related life quality, the choice itself reflects the investigator's ideological and cultural notions and those of the society in which he or she lives.

The measurement operations used to assign numbers to concepts and domains of health-related quality of life also reflect theoretical assumptions. Measurement theories differ on how the nature of the phenomena under investigation is perceived and on how numbers are assigned to constructs using specific rules. Because of these theoretical differences in conceptualization and measurement, different measurement strategies and instruments may yield different data and conclusions, thereby sending patients and providers as well as analysts and decision makers down different paths.

In measuring health-related quality of life, analysts use *constructs*, or theoretical ideas based on observations of what we cannot observe directly. Different kinds of health-related quality of life constructs are *domains* that distinguish different ideas or concepts into groups. Finally, the measurement operations result in a set of *indicators* of these constructs that indicate the presence, absence, or degree of health-related quality of life.

The Health Resource Allocation Strategy is a decision process based on the global theories of social choice. In this chapter we present the major social and behavioral science theories that underlie the conceptualization and concepts of health-related quality of life used in the Strategy and in other applications. We also identify major measurement theories that govern the rules for assigning numbers to the constructs used in creating indicators; these include health states based on the different concepts and domains of health-related quality of life. In the final section, we discuss how these concepts and domains may be organized into different conceptual frameworks for expressing their interrelationships. We offer this additional theoretical background to help analysts, decision makers, and others uncover the implicit assumptions involved in using health status data in health policy.

THE CONTRIBUTIONS OF THEORY

Two major problems arise with the supposedly "atheoretical" use of measures in collecting and analyzing health-related quality of life data. First, unless the investigator considers the possible determinants of health-related quality of life discussed in Chapter 2, it is difficult to interpret results. This is particularly true in nonrandom research designs. Many cultural, political, and social processes influence the meaning and measurement of health-related quality of life. The analyst must consider these influences to understand how respondents react to health-related quality of life questions and to analyze data in a manner consistent with measurement assumptions.

A second problem is the difficulty that arises in interpreting relationships among different health-related quality of life concepts. Clinical indicators, such as blood pressure measurement, may be associated with physical, psychological, or social functioning. Functional status, in turn, may be associated with satisfaction with health. When the concepts are contained in a theory of biological, psychological, and social process that specifies the system of relationships connecting the concepts, the investigator can analyze the change in one measure as related to change in another measure. For example, when blood pressure changes significantly, what are the expected changes in physical and psychological function? At a more social level, when access to health care improves, what changes in health-related quality of life can be expected?

Theory also permits combining different health-related quality of life domains into analytic indexes (Land and Spilerman, 1975). These indexes vary with changes in social conditions: if the index changes in the "right" direction while other things remain the same, the population is considered "better off." For example, self-ratings of health (excellent, very good, good, fair, or poor) obtained from national survey samples have improved over the last decade while reports of restricted activity and bed disability have increased (Wilson and Drury, 1984). Combining these different concepts in a measurement system requires specifying the theoretical relationship between general health perceptions and reported disability. One might postulate, for example, that expectations for health have increased because of the saliency of health to the population, the diffusion of technology into American life, or changes in even deeper cultural traditions, such as the Protestant work ethic, that underpin American society.

Such specification among indicators is also of strategic importance in determining the content and construct validity of health-related quality of life indexes. The items of a questionnaire should adequately represent the theoretical domain generally considered to be relevant; the content should be valid. Since no one measure can be considered a criterion, construct validation of health indicators is necessary (see Chapter 7). The major method used to provide evidence of construct validity is to compare one measure to another using a hypothesized relationship between different concepts (Kaplan et al., 1976; Bergner et al., 1981; Parkerson et al., 1981; Charlton et al., 1983; Nelson et al., 1991). In the process of providing evidence for construct validity, for example, an analyst might hypothesize that the number of chronic conditions and the number of symptoms should be highly correlated or perhaps that reports of physical dysfunction should increase with age.

Theoretical relationships between disease and functional status are not difficult to specify; however, relationships between quality of life measures of attitudes or behaviors (feelings of positive well-being and activities of daily living) are often difficult to predict. For example, emotional well-being might well improve with advancing age. A variety of social theories have been invoked to help specify the interrelationships among different indicators of health-related quality of life.

Four major theories or sets of theories—functionalism, positive well-being, utility, and psychophysics—underlie much conceptualization and measurement of health-related quality of life, particularly those measures used in the Health Resource Allocation Strategy. These theories are derived from anthropology, economics, philosophy, psychology, sociology, and related fields. No single theory appears sufficient to encompass the myriad concepts or operations involved in defining and measuring health-related quality of life.

The principal theoretical bases for defining health and life quality states are the functionalist theory from sociology and anthropology and theories of positive well-being and quality of life from psychology. The conceptual framework for weighting health states is provided by utility theory from economics and the decision sciences and by psychophysical theory from psychology. Although these are not the only "theories" of health and quality of life that have been invoked, they are the principal ones used in developing, applying, and analyzing the predominant measures of health-related quality of life.

TALCOTT PARSONS AND FUNCTIONALISM

Functionalism involves the analysis of social and cultural phenomena in terms of the functions they perform in a sociocultural system. In functionalism, society is viewed as a system of interrelated parts in which no part can be understood if isolated from the whole. The development of functionalism, as its focus suggests, came from the model of the organic system found in the biological sciences.

Durkheim (1897/1951), often credited with founding functionalism, was concerned with social integration and the concepts of normality and deviance. He perceived "normal" to be those social conditions most generally distributed. Other conditions he called "morbid" or "pathological." Normal equated to average type, and every deviation from this standard was considered to be a morbid phenomenon. Using Durkheim's conception, the common denominator of all ill health is this deviation from an ideal of well-being imposed by any disease process on any person, no matter what his or her social role.

In contemporary theoretical sociology, functionalism has been in disrepute because of its inherent conservatism and closed-ended systems approach. Social theorists concerned with the reality of social systems in terms of social interdependence or differentiation, however, have contributed a major theoretical perspective to defining states of health and quality of life. Structural functionalism focuses on a whole, relatively autonomous social unit, called a culture by anthropologists or a society by sociologists (Moore, 1978).

This conception of normality/deviance or function/dysfunction contributed to the classical analysis of health and illness by the Harvard circle revolving around Talcott Parsons. Parsons, in *The Social System*, defined illness as "a state of disturbance in the normal functioning of the total human individual including both the state of the organism as a biological system, and of his personal and social adjustments" (1951, p. 431).

Health, in this viewpoint, is "the state of optimum capacity for the effective performance of valued tasks" (Parsons, 1958, p. 168). Illness is a deviation from the social expectation that a person perform the functions associated with his or her social role. Although not all ill health is associated with role function—for example, consider physiological status, symptoms, and pain—it is at the level of role performance that illness becomes a significant problem for the social system.

This sociological perspective has been the basis for health and quality of life indicators of function, often defined as the capacity to perform the usual daily activities for a person's age and major social role (Patrick et al., 1973b). The norm from which deviation is noted is the productive role of wage labor, school, housework, or ability to care for one's personal needs. Limitations in major activity, restricted-activity, or cutdown, days, bed-disability, and work-loss days are examples of indicators based on these roles. A person is "well" if he or she is able to meet the norms or standards for functional behavior that would usually apply to him or her. Thus, quality of life indicators, such as life satisfaction, are often based on people's ability to perform the social roles and activities that they want to perform as well as the degree of satisfaction derived from performing them (Levine and Croog, 1984).

Functionalist theory has significantly influenced the description of states for health indicators and indexes. As a result, descriptions of role functions have been developed in terms of performance and/or capacity. Performance descriptors are the actual behaviors of individuals—"does not walk freely" or "walks only with the help of an aid." Capacity descriptors are the potential abilities of the individual—"cannot walk freely" or "can walk only with the help of an aid." The distinction between performing and the ability to perform is the problem of social control or society's regulation of an individual's commitment to standards of behavior. Not all persons in a society meet or indeed "want" to meet the standards of behavior expected by others.

The legitimation of illness or society's evaluation of the adequacy of role performance is not in the usual objective of the developers or users of health-related quality of life indicators, although it is a significant sociological problem. Legitimation, usually in the form of release from usual social role obligations, may occur, however, using the same concepts and indicators developed to assess health-related quality of life. Deviation from the performance of usual activities, rather than capacity, is most commonly incorporated in health indicators because of concerns about the reliability of the respondent reporting and the potential for "underreporting" when capacity wording is used (Anderson et al., 1977; Patrick et al., 1981; Bush, 1984b).

Functionalist definitions of health focus on the "major" social roles that people perform in Western societies. These roles encompass work, school, housework, and the independent performance of activities of daily living to care for one's personal needs. Such definitions implicitly operationalize the ideology and culture of our society (Patrick and Guttmacher, 1983). Definitions of health based on productive functioning may devalue those population groups that do not or cannot "produce" in the roles of wage labor, school, housework, or independent functioning. Persons with severe physical, mental, or emotional impairments may not be able to hold a job, attend a regular school, maintain a household, or care for themselves independently. They may, however, engage in meaningful activity, learn, and attend to daily activities within a supported environment.

Determining who receives the support of society and who is released from usual expectations for role performance presents a dilemma. Society faces the problem of deciding when inability to produce is legitimate. This problem of legitimizing sickness and dependency is inherent in most disease or illness benefits, such as disability income maintenance or worker's compensation (Stone, 1984). Even though it is not explicitly addressed in health indicator construction, the analysis of disability trends by age, gender, color, and income raises important policy questions of inequalities of health (Wilson and White, 1977), expectations for health (Colvez and Blanchet, 1981; Verbrugge, 1984), and the role of the state in providing for its dependent citizens (Stones and Kozma, 1980).

THEORIES OF POSITIVE WELL-BEING AND QUALITY OF LIFE

Functionalist theory has been the basis for definitions of disability and dysfunction; other theorists and investigators have attempted to define positive health and quality of life, often viewed as concepts and domains located on the upper end of the health–illness continuum. Many of these attempts have been in the mental health field, since mental or psychological well-being constructs are central to our notions of positive health. Models of psychological well-being guide the assessment of quality of life by exploring subjective reactions to life experiences (Diener, 1984). These models are numerous, ranging from personality-type theories, social learning theory, and theories of personal control to theories of specific subjective phenomena such as happiness, elation, or optimism.

Zautra and Goodhart (1979) review four psychological models that have contributed concepts to health-related quality of life: the epidemiologic model of stressful life events (Cassel, 1975), the crisis-management model of coping (Rappaport, 1977), the competency model emphasizing self-mastery (Jahoda, 1958), and the adaptation-level model. Together these four models suggest two sets of human needs: (1) to avoid and/or adjust to painful life experiences and (2) to develop and sustain life satisfaction by increasing competence, skills, and mastery over the environment. Quality of life is viewed as enhanced to the degree that both adjustment and competence needs are fulfilled. Thus a person with a chronic disease or impairment might have a high quality of life, avoiding depression and mastering independence or use of personal assistance, and a person without disease or impairment might have a low quality of life, being depressed and dissatisfied with his or her situation.

The linkage of personality types and emotional reactions to health and illness derives from Greek notions of the four humors within the body. These humors correspond to physical states. Freud (1920) and Fromm (1979) made major contributions to this theory with the concepts of neurosis and egoreceptive states. Alexander (1950), another psychoanalytic therapist, was influential in trying to link physical symptoms with constellations of personality traits (e.g., asthma with repression and peptic ulcers with oral dependency needs). He failed to support this link, because symptom patterns and a specific disease could not be matched with a specific personality type, since there were many individuals with a particular disease who had a personality type that did not match. Strickland (1984) notes that the assumed relationships between emotional states and physical health or disease have not been clearly demonstrated. Furthermore, other concepts and ideas, including physical, psychological, and social paradigms, are necessary to explain individual reactions and their concomitants.

Another conceptual focus for positive health research centers on concepts of the self: the unique attitudes and cognitive characteristics of individuals. Numerous attempts have been made to define and measure self-esteem (Rosenberg, 1979). However, there is little consensus on a definition of self-esteem, and the measurement techniques often do not yield comparable findings.

Another more promising direction of investigation concerns self-efficacy, the perception of oneself as effective and competent (Bandura, 1982). Although self-efficacy usually refers to behaviors and not health states, Kobasa (1979) put this concept into an existential framework by describing characteristics of commitment, control, and response to challenge. In her study of middle-management executives under high stress, Kobasa found that the executives who did not fall ill had a strong sense of values, goals, and capabilities—a hardiness that functioned as a resistance-to-illness resource in the event of stress.

Theories of personality, self-concept, and subjective well-being are prominent among the growing number of investigators studying behavioral health or behavioral medicine (Matarazzo et al., 1984). These theories are often used to explain health or illness behaviors. Such behaviors, in turn, can be viewed as an intermediate outcome or variable in a causal analysis of health-related quality of life outcomes. Equating behavior itself with health or quality of life ignores the larger social and cultural factors that both define and influence behavior and health. In the future, these social psychological theories will be most important in developing a conceptual framework for understanding self-conception and for providing the basis for construct validation of positive health measures.

Theories of happiness or subjective well-being have existed since the ancient Greeks. Diener (1984) reviews telic, activity, top-down and bottom-up, associationistic, and judgment theories of happiness, all of which link happiness to different levels of human experience. Maslow's telic or end-point theory related states of well-being to environmental or ecological systems. In this theory, subjective well-being results when individuals fulfill the needs at their particular levels such as physiological needs, safety needs, love needs, esteem needs, and self-actualization needs (Maslow, 1943). Even though need theory is often cited in relation to quality of life research, little empirical evidence exists linking the constructs derived from this theory to health and quality of life.

Andrews and Withey (1974) invoke a top-down or personality-based approach to happiness; they amass data to suggest that the accumulation of positive experiences (from the bottom up) does not necessarily predict global life satisfaction. Other psychological theories of subjective well-being have seldom been used in developing health-related quality of life indicators, although judgment-based theory bears a striking relationship to utility theory (reviewed later).

Psychological theories of subjective well-being differ substantially in their treatment of happiness or quality of life as a *personality trait* versus a *psychological state* and in the different constructs employed. Constructs of happiness have been neither rigorously defined nor subjected to a hypothetico-deductive process where theory and data interplay in repeated studies.

Adaptation theory stresses the satisfaction derived from experiences and people (Brickman and Campbell, 1971). Satisfaction is a pivotal concept in quality of life. Although wide agreement exists about the major categories of fundamental life needs, satisfaction is experienced only by the person with that need. Nevertheless, concepts of satisfaction are often involved in normative measures of health-related quality of life. Along the lines of Maslow's theories, important needs include material, physical, psychological, social, and spiritual well-being as well as a sense of satisfaction with one's opportunity for access to the total environment, education and training, and employment. Little is known about the relationship of need satisfaction to other health-related quality of life outcomes. In some populations, functional status correlates only moderately with satisfaction with health or perceived quality of life (Patrick, Danis et al., 1988). This lack of correlation suggests that satisfaction must be considered separately from behaviors often contained in functional status measures.

Concepts of subjective well-being, however, are clearly consistent with the notion that quality of life can be defined as the performance of social roles and activities that people want to perform as well as the degree of satisfaction derived from performing them. The desire to become all that one is capable of becoming appears universal.

Appreciation of the importance of this positive underpinning to health characterizes the efforts to define "high-level wellness" as part of the national health indicator agenda. In 1947, Halbert Dunn, then chief of the National Office of Vital Statistics, chaired an Ad Hoc Committee of the National Committee on Vital and Health Statistics to consider problems of defining and measuring positive health. The committee defined freedom from illness as the "largely uncharted and undifferentiated area of good health . . . which is indicated as peak wellness" (Ad Hoc Committee of the National Committee on Vital and Health Statistics, 1958). Although high-level wellness did not remain a program of research in positive health, this pioneering effort set the stage for developing health indicators separate from illness indicators—a challenge that remains today.

Functionalism and theories of positive well-being are not the only theoretical examinations of what people mean by health and quality of life. Anthropologists, sociologists, and qualitative researchers from many different fields repeatedly discover that health and illness have particular meanings in different cultures, ethnic groups, and population groups within and outside a single country. The notions of functioning in social roles and satisfaction with function appear to exist in most, if not all, cultures, although the meaning of dysfunction and dissatisfaction may vary. Social and psychological domains will continue to appear in health-related quality of life definitions and measures precisely because doing what is expected or acting like others and feeling good about it are important to most people.

VALUES AND UTILITY THEORY

Theories of functionalism and positive well-being have been used to define various multidimensional states of health-related quality of life ranging from death to maximum health or wellness. Utility theory and psychophysics deal with the selection of one state over another whereby the perceived benefits from one health state exceed those from another (Pearce, 1983). Utility theory and psychophysical theories can be used to order health states along the value continuum of health-related quality of life. These theories provide the conceptual basis by which different levels of functioning within the states can be combined to give an overall assessment of life quality associated with health status.

Measures of health-related quality of life that incorporate explicit values in the ordering of health states are referred to as utility-weighted or preference-weighted measures. These measures contrast with those that use statistical weighting to define the magnitude of dysfunction or health of individuals and groups. Values are fundamental to the Health Resource Allocation Strategy because it incorporates social preferences for health states.

Value terminology and preference measurement have become prevalent in a broad range of social and behavioral sciences. Western sociology has shown particular interest in values since the publication of *The Polish Peasant in Europe and America* in 1918 (Thomas and Znaniecki, 1958). In economics, efforts to develop measures of utility go back to the eighteenth century, as in "indifference curve" analysis, and to define various types of value, such as value-in-use and value-in-exchange. Anthropologists developed the concept of values within the context of dominant cultural patterns. Finally, psychologists have explored value concepts in relation to attitudes, beliefs, opinions, and decision making. Fechner's 1860 publication of the *Elemente die Psychophysik* marked the beginning of modern interest in the quantification of judgment (Jones, 1974).

There is considerable confusion and controversy surrounding the precise placement of values in the sociopsychological domain of attitudes, needs, beliefs, cognitive orientations, lifestyles, norms, motives, sentiments, and preferences. The measurement of health state preferences follows in the tradition of treating *values* as standards of the desirable which influence selective behavior. In this view, "a value is a conception, explicit or implicit, distinctive of an individual or characteristic of a group, of the desirable which influences the selection from available modes, means and ends of action" (Kluckhohn, 1951). This definition focuses on the relationship between values (conceptions of the desirable) and selective behavior (the choice between alternatives).

Values are presumed to exist in advance of and independent from the context in which they are studied and measured. At this more abstract level, values are identified as attitudes, orientations, or belief systems which are organizing conceptions of a person's world. In studying behavior, however, values can be narrowly conceived as preferential judgments, responses, or choices that arise from human experience and may be influenced by anything that affects experiences. Thus values are synonymous with judgments of the desirability of a particular set of outcomes or situations that describe what is labeled "good" or "bad." The term *preference* is used to connote the exact meaning of value, desirability, or utility.

Assignment of weights explicitly requires that representative individuals, sometimes referred to as judges, be confronted with options incorporating concepts based on functionalist, positive health, and quality of life theories. The developers of health-related quality of life measures have assumed that health states can be ranked; that is, if presented with health state *A* and *B*, people can meaningfully say whether they prefer *A* to *B* or *B* to *A*, or whether they are indifferent. To satisfy this criterion, the analyst must clearly define the states and their operational components so that between any two function levels the individual can clearly express a preference for one level over the other or can clearly recognize his or her indifference between any two function levels. Researchers have borrowed theoretical constructs and the resulting techniques developed by economists, psychologists, and other decision scientists to explain how individuals select between different options.

One widely used approach for obtaining weights for health-related quality of life measures is utility theory. The classical theory of utility was derived from the eighteenth-century work of Jeremy Bentham. He formulated the utility principle that all individuals and society, as an aggregate of individuals, are directed toward a single end—to increase pleasure and decrease pain (Bentham, 1789/1948). Bentham asserted that people choose actions that increase pleasure. According to this utilitarian philosophy, preferences can be cardinally measured, that is, measured on an interval or ratio scale. As discussed in Chapter 2, it is possible to construct a cardinal utility scale, but it is difficult to aggregate interpersonal utilities. To overcome the difficulties in measuring utility up to a cardinal scale, economists in the early twentieth century developed the notion of ordinal utility. With this type of utility, people report how much of one commodity is equal to standard amounts of a second commodity. This method of ranking preferences differs from classical utility in the point of origin and the arbitrary units of scale. It obtains many of the same results, however, as the classical theory while overcoming the difficulty of measurement (Blaug, 1983). Thurstone, a psychologist, measured ordinal utility indirectly by plotting indifference curves (1959).

Utility theory, whether classical or ordinal, assumes that choices can be made with certainty. In 1944, von Neumann and Morgenstern developed the notion of *expected* utility as a way of incorporating uncertainty into preference judgments. As von Neumann and Morgenstern showed, if A and B states (health) are presented as gambles, and if certain axioms are satisfied for expressions of preference, then such preferences can represent the underlying mental structure as a cardinal utility function. Gambles lead to utility functions in contrast to value functions, and utility functions are seen as necessary in prescribing behavior with respect to risky options. Expected utility theory, appropriate for decisions with uncertain prospects, is a normative or prescriptive model for rational decision making, a theory of *ought*, not a theory of *is*. The von Neumann and Morgenstern theory does not describe how persons actually make decisions or behave under uncertainty. Rather, the theory describes how persons ought to make decisions under rationality.

Game theory, as von Neumann and Morgenstern described their theory, centers on the assumption that the utility of two objects or outcomes is reflected by the relative expectations for the occurrence or acquisition of the two outcomes. Thus, the issue of assigning utilities to outcomes expands to the problem of assigning values to *gambles*, which are choices about outcomes that are not a sure thing. By constructing various game situations, the investigator can determine the value or expected utility of gambles and outcomes. The concepts of game theory have suggested many new directions for experimentation in utility measurement. However, these methods of measurement, although appealing because of their logic and mathematical rigor, are difficult to apply to preference measurement studies concerned with outcomes not usually associated with gambles or risks.

Three axioms of rational behavior govern game or expected utility theory. Letting $\geq$, $>$, and $\simeq$ stand for the notions of weak preference, strict preference, and indifference:

1. Preferences for outcomes exist and are transitive (ordering axiom), that is,

    If $A > B$ and $B > C$, then $A > C$.

    If an individual prefers walking A to moving independently in a wheelchair B, and moving independently in a wheelchair B to being confined to bed C, then the individual prefers walking A to being confined to bed C.

2. Preferences for a risky prospect are independent of whether it has one stage or two (independence axiom), that is,

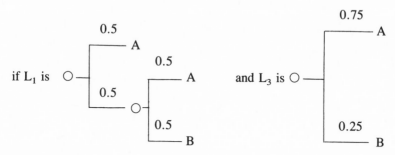

then $L_1 \simeq L_3$

There is a continuity of preferences (standard gamble), that is

$$\text{if } A > B > C \quad \text{then } B \simeq \bigcirc \begin{array}{l} \xrightarrow{\ p\ } A \\ \xrightarrow{\ 1-p\ } C \end{array}$$

The fundamental theorem of expected utility theory is that an individual's preferences should satisfy the three axioms. A corollary theorem predicts preferences for outcomes. If an individual wishes to make a decision consistent with the axioms of expected utility theory, then he or she should determine the utilities for the outcomes using axiom 3 and should select the risky prospect with the highest expected utility.

As with ordinal utility, expected utility theory results in ranks stated on a scale that has up to interval properties. Although the results are referred to as utilities, the concept differs from classical or ordinal utility, because expected utilities are numbers. These numbers play a special and well-defined role either in decision theory under uncertainty or in game theory (Torrance, 1987).

Conventional decision-analytic theories and procedures distinguish between riskless and risky events. Not all decision theorists accept the distinction between utility functions based on gambles and value functions based on riskless or certain outcomes (von Winterfeldt and Edwards, 1986). Both utility and value functions are constructed with error. Different procedures for eliciting utility functions using expected utility theory and for eliciting value functions using certainty methods produce different errors, and sizable differences may result in comparing the results of the two sets of procedures and resulting functions. The utilities or values are therefore theory- and method-bound, without the means to determine whether one is "better than" or "worse than" another.

We present both methods and their assumptions to help readers form their own opinions.

Expected utility theory is the basis for standard gamble and time tradeoff preference measurement methods discussed in Chapter 6. The elegance of expected utility theory has attracted many health status researchers to develop measures of utility for health states (Torrance, 1986). The theory also has considerable influence on the study and practice of medical decision making in predicting how individuals make choices between alternative medical treatments.

A different contribution to decision making has come from welfare economics. At about the same time British economists were incorporating Bentham's utilitarian views into nineteenth-century economic theory, a French engineer, Jules Dupuit, was proposing the notion of consumer surplus. He was searching for a measure of social benefit obtained from the development of collective goods, such as roads and bridges. Dupuit observed that the price people were willing to pay for such goods was, in most cases, greater than the price actually paid. Alfred Marshall refined Dupuit's original work, linking it with the economists' notion of utility or satisfaction (Blaug, 1983). This fundamental subset of modern welfare economics is used along with the concept of Pareto optimality—no one can be made better off without making someone else worse off—in societal evaluations of the relative merits between the status quo and some alternative (Fischer, 1979). A link therefore exists between utility theory used in weighting health states and the theory of social choice that underpins the Health Resource Allocation Strategy.

Another approach used by economists to obtain market-based estimates of willingness to pay is to analyze the wage rates and risks for various occupations. This approach assumes that the higher wages paid to individuals working in a hazardous environment reflect the risk of increased morbidity and mortality. Differences in wage premiums according to hazardous risk are assumed to indicate the value individuals place on incremental increases in the probability of dying in a given time interval (Thaler and Rosen, 1975). For two decades economists have combined the concepts of consumer surplus and willingness to pay with survey methodology to develop direct measures of consumer preference (Acton, 1973; Lipscomb, 1982; Thompson et al., 1984).

PSYCHOPHYSICS AND THE MEASUREMENT OF VALUE

Gustav Theodor Fechner (1801–1887) was the founding father of *psychophysics*, the study of the relationship between physical stimuli and psychological sensation or perception. Most commonly, psychophysics is concerned with the correlation between physical measurements of different stimuli and reactions to these stimuli, for example, decibels of sound intensity and perceptions of loudness. Rules of measurement play a large role in psychophysical theory.

Science is a complex interchange between theory and observation with measurement as the language or means of communication. On one side are conceptions of the world expressed in constructs like that of functional status, and on the other are controlled observations or records of events that provide ordered knowledge about these conceptions. Measurement operations relate the two sides and provide the order.

Measurement is "the assignment of numbers to aspects of objects or events according to a rule of some kind" (Stevens, 1968). Assigning numbers to health and quality of life is a less than ideal process. Like most constructs in the social and behavioral sciences, no physical device exists for measuring the values assigned to different descriptors of health-related quality of life. The measurer uses an arbitrary measure or derives one from an already established measure. Nevertheless, stable relationships among social and behavioral constructs can be as important as fundamental measures such as length, mass, or electrical resistance.

That the measurement of health-related quality of life must rely on human yardsticks or those not as familiar as a thermometer does not detract from the scientific nature of such measurement. Measurement theory provides the basis for assigning numbers to health states and for manipulating these numbers with mathematical operations. The rules by which a given magnitude of measurement is defined or theorized are types of scales: nominal, ordinal, interval, and ratio. Most health-related quality of life measurement occurs at the ordinal level and above, although classifications such as the International Classification of Diseases (Commission on Professional and Hospital Activities, 1978) assign numbers at a nominal level.

Measurement theories for social and behavioral constructs have been developed in different social sciences. The psychological research tradition provides a set of theories, psychophysics being one of the most important for measurement of health-related quality of life. Psychophysics has a long and varied history beginning with the publication of Fechner's *Elemente der Psychophysik* in 1860, continuing with the successive development of measures of physical sensations, and coming to the use of psychophysical methods in the measurement of social consensus. In the development of the preference measurement strategy, this tradition or base of empirical knowledge made it possible to adapt old methods to a new problem and to make a formal evaluation of the results.

Fechner's problem, and the task of traditional psychophysics, is to find numerical laws that relate psychological dimensions to physical dimensions. These laws take the form

$$\Psi = f(\Phi)$$

where Ψ is the psychological dimension, Φ is the physical dimension, and f is a numerical function that expresses a lawful or invariant relation between the mental and physical dimension. The psychophysical approach to solving this problem is to establish special psychological procedures for measuring sensations.

Fechner's procedures for measuring psychological sensations were based upon work by Ernst Weber on difference thresholds, or "confusability" between stimuli. According to Weber, confusability is proportional to the stimulus magnitude at which it is measured. Using this principal, Fechner conjectured that if two stimuli were just noticeably different, then regardless of changes in physical energies, the psychological difference must be equal. For instance, if one can distinguish between physical stimuli X_1 and X_2 50 percent of the time and between physical stimuli X_3 and X_4 50 percent of the time, then the psychological difference between the stimuli must be equal:

$$\Psi(X_1) - \Psi(X_2) = \Psi(X_3) - \Psi(X_4).$$

Employing the *just noticeable difference* (JND) as his unit of psychological magnitude, Fechner established his psychophysical law:

$$\Psi = k \log \Phi$$

where Ψ is expressed in JND units, Φ is expressed in physical units according to the dimension being measured, and k is a constant that also varies according to the nature of the phenomena being measured.

Fechner's law has generated more than a century of controversy over the appropriate psychological law relating subjective magnitude to stimulus magnitude. Fechner himself commented upon the power of his presentation: "The tower of Babel was never finished because the workers could not reach an understanding on how they should build it; my psychophysical edifice will stand because the workers will never agree on how to tear it down" (Stevens, 1957). Some workers, however, did not wish to destroy Fechner's "psychophysical edifice."

His work and logic found an able and willing disciple in L. L. Thurstone (1927), who developed the use of confusions among stimuli as psychological units of measurement. Thurstone ventured to extend Fechnerian methods to the general mental measurement problem where there is no physical variable. Techniques were developed to measure attitudes, values, interests, and other psychological constructs based on Thurstone's interpretation of Fechner (Thurstone, 1959). Not all psychologists, however, were convinced of the validity of Fechner's and Thurstone's methods.

S. S. Stevens (1961) spent over 50 years putting forth an alternative theory in hopes of repealing Fechner's law. Using numerical estimation methods such as ratio estimation, fractionation, and magnitude estimation, Stevens conducted experiments that yielded results different from those obtained by Fechner. Stevens asserts that these methods confirm what is known as the power law, the psychophysical law for the "new" psychophysics:

$$\Psi = \Phi^n$$

where Ψ is psychological magnitude expressed in terms of the estimation scale, Φ is the physical magnitude, and n is a unique exponent that varies in size with the property being measured. The simple statement of this law is that psychological magnitude increases in geometric progression. With physical continua, application of the power law generally consists of measuring the power exponent that characterizes a particular modality or set of continua. With nonphysical stimuli, application lies in the methodology used to describe the power law and the controversy between Fechnerian psychophysics and Stevens.

The significance of this controversy is not in its statement of the "correct" form of the psychophysical law, that is, whether it is a logarithmic or a power function, or the relative merit of Fechner and Stevens. In fact, a case can be made against power functions on the grounds that they do not describe subjective sensory magnitudes appropriately and that sensory dimensions do not have exponents of unique size and may not be comparable (Poulton, 1989). The importance of the controversy lies in the disparate results obtained by two different measurement methods. Using the numerical estimation method of category rating to approximate Fechner's scale and magnitude estimation as the comparison method, Stevens and others studied a number of physical and nonphysical continua by plotting one scale against the other.

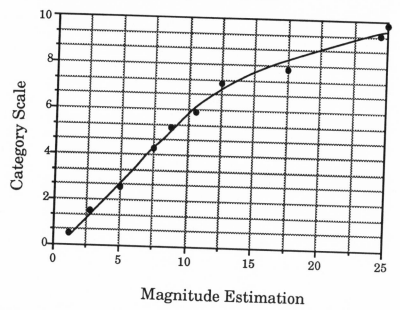

Magnitude Estimation

Figure 3.1 Comparison of category rating and magnitude estimation judgments. *Source:* Adapted from Stevens, 1968.

Generally these investigators have established that the expected form of the relation between category and magnitude scales is usually curvilinear or logarithmic. The result is that the mean category values plotted as a function of the means of magnitude or ratio estimates in arithmetic coordinates yield a function that can be described as concave downward. That is, the curve representing the relation between the category scale and the magnitude scale, as illustrated in Figure 3.1, is negatively accelerated. This nonlinearity disappears when the category scale is plotted against the magnitude estimation scale in log-log coordinates.

A great deal of uncertainty surrounds the theoretical interpretation of the relation between category and magnitude scales. Many experimentalists account for the results in terms of a systematic bias in one or both procedures. Otherwise, they would have to assert that there is more than one psychophysical law. The usual approach is to account for the difference in terms of a systematic distortion in the category scale.

It has been postulated that category methods give nonlinear results in relation to ratio methods whenever the respondent's sensitivity to stimulus differences is not uniform across the scale. In other words, at one end of the scale, discrimination is good and judges tend to make the categories narrow. Near the other end of the scale, stimulus differences appear less easy to detect. Fine distinctions, therefore, are not made among stimuli, and the categories broaden. As a consequence, the function slope is steep at one end and flattened at the other. With stimuli that have a corresponding physical continuum, discrimination tends to be better at the lower end of the scale; as the magnitude of the stimulus increases, sensitivity decreases and subjective variability increases.

Stevens and Galanter (1957) used the relation between category and magnitude scales and the principle that variability increases with stimulus magnitude to distinguish between two classes of psychological continua, *prothetic* and *metathetic*. For prothetic continua, a category scale is concave downward when plotted in linear coordinates against a magnitude scale, as in Figure 3.1. For metathetic continua, the relation is linear or closely approaching linearity. For prothetic continua, subjective variability increases with subjective magnitude, whereas for metathetic continua, it is uniform or constant. The distinction is often made in terms of "quantity" (prothetic) versus "kind" (metathetic), although it seems likely that any given attribute such as health state values will have a degree of quantifiability or "protheticity" rather than being strictly one or the other.

The importance of the prothetic–metathetic distinction and the category–magnitude scale comparison is that continua which do not have an established metric, such as preference for function, can be studied and classified on the basis of how they "behave" when the two methods are compared. Empirical determination of the nature of the continuum gives added confidence or validity to the outcome of a scaling experiment. Previous use of these methods in studies involving attitudes about the church, preferences for wristwatches, the aesthetic value of handwriting, responses to drawings and music, occupational preferences, degree of liberalism or conservatism, and the seriousness of offenses indicates the potential for these methods in the investigation of sociopsychological reactions to sociological phenomena and the extent of social consensus.

How numbers are assigned to states of health-related quality of life is critical to its measurement and interpretation. Chapter 6 takes these basic principles of measurement from utility theory and psychophysics and applies them to the assignment of numbers to different health states.

BUILDING A CONCEPTUAL FRAMEWORK

Theoretical concepts of health-related quality of life have been organized using different frameworks or models to express the interrelationships among concepts. While seldom drawn explicitly as a formal conceptual model, one commonly used framework is the continuum of health-related quality of life ranging from negative or minimal to positive or maximal, clearly implying that definitions of health and quality of life must be broad enough to include the positive aspects of health but narrow enough to distinguish the "healthy" from the "sick." Existing health-related quality of life measures have been criticized repeatedly for including concepts at the negative or illness end of the continuum while neglecting concepts at the more positive end.

Figure 3.2 is another model proposed for illustrating relationships among health-related quality of life concepts. This series of concentric boxes shows disease in the center and personal functioning, psychological distress/well-being, general health perceptions, and social/role functioning in surrounding boxes (Ware, 1984a).

This model indicates that health-related quality of life moves from characteristics at the center, or intrinsic to an individual, to characteristics outside the individual in a behavioral and a social and cultural perspective that links the experience of disease and treatment of the possibilities of intervention at the level of the individual, the immediate social environment, or the larger society. Relationships among different concepts and their measures are less well-specified, for example, how pain and symptoms are

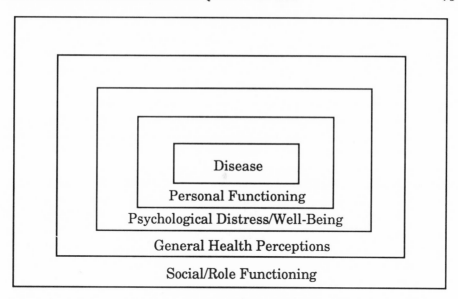

Figure 3.2 Framework for discussing disease and its impact. *Source:* Ware, 1984a.

related to restrictions in activity, health perceptions, and satisfaction for different impairments. Even within disease categories, such as arthritis, little is known about how disease maps into pain and the consequences of pain for different individuals.

A major challenge faces developers and users of health-related quality of life measures—the need to establish a testable theory of the expected relationships among the different concepts and domains. The problem is not confined to the relationship between physiological measures and behaviors or perceptions, for example, blood pressure and functional status. Measures of various dimensions such as symptoms, psychological function, and satisfaction have been shown to be only loosely associated or entirely dissociated within the same sample.

Figure 3.3 depicts hypothesized relationships among different health-related quality of life concepts in a simple linear progression from disease and impairment to opportunity (Patrick and Bergner, 1990). The concepts are bounded by environmental determinants that influence disease and its consequences and prognoses for improvement, maintenance, or decline in health-related quality of life. The World Health Organization (1980) trial classification of the consequences of disease in terms of impairments, disabilities, and handicaps is a similar conception.

The simple causal model suggested in Figure 3.3 does not represent the complexity or strength of the expected relationships among health-related quality of life domains. For example, a person can have an asymptomatic disease that affects prognosis without affecting functional status, perceptions, or opportunity. A person with hypertension or hypercholesterolemia may not have restrictions in activity but still may experience disadvantage in fear of a stroke or death. Similarly, not all persons with impaired physiological capacity have psychological dysfunction. Persons with rheumatoid arthritis or congestive heart failure may have high satisfaction with their health and positive well-being despite their physical limitations.

Figure 3.3 also indicates that the causal relationships among concepts can be re-

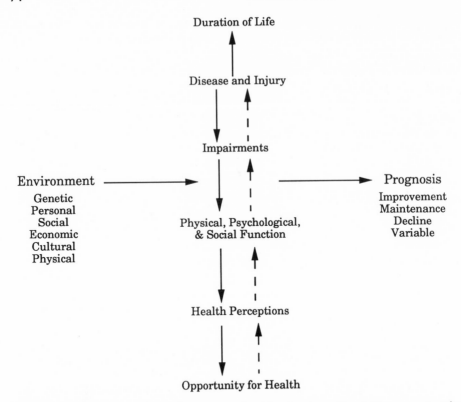

Figure 3.3   Theoretical relationships among health-related quality of life concepts. The solid arrows indicate a causal direction from disease through impairments to functional status, perceptions, and opportunity for health. This causal pathway is not a linear sequence; one may be impaired but not dysfunctional, as with a cosmetic disfigurement. Disfigurement may, however, cause a lower perceived health status and reduced opportunity because of stigma. Thus, the sequence may be interrupted or incomplete. The dashed arrows indicate that this causal sequence may be reversed, e.g., reduced health perceptions may affect function. Disease and all its consequences are shown to influence duration of life. *Source*: Patrick and Bergner, 1990.

versed; for example, functional limitations and perceived health can be viewed as influencing impairment or physiological measures of chronic disease (Patrick, 1987). Reversing the causal chain permits testing the variable course of chronic disease, which may cause impairments to become permanent and lead to changes in behavior and perceptions that, in turn, influence symptoms or level of impairment. The notion of an interplay between the psyche and body states is as old as medicine itself. Psycho-physiological processes such as disruption in the regulation of blood volume and control of blood pressure by the kidneys can be invoked to explain sociobehavioral influences on disease processes. This evidence may not be sufficient to convince the most skeptical biomedical researcher, but the hypothesis that perceptions and behavior can influence physiological processes has moved well beyond mere speculation (Kandel, 1979).

At present, researchers tend to approach the relationship among endpoints inductively by collecting data and examining the correlation among measures. Little hypothesis-based or deductive reasoning is involved in either the selection of measures or the analysis of results. A priori hypotheses and head-to-head comparisons of different domains are important for determining the association between specific disease states or disorders and their behavioral, perceptual, and social consequences. Testing hypotheses about expected changes in health-related quality of life measures is particularly important. Increasing our understanding of these relationships will help to realize the potential of health-related quality of life measures for identifying the intervention strategies that address the most important concerns of clinicians, patients, their families, policymakers, and society in general.

The theoretical foundations for the conceptualization and measurement of health-related quality of life set the stage for examining specific concepts, domains, and indicators that are contained in existing measures. It is important that these theoretical origins of our notions of health status and quality of life be studied and recognized, because they provide many of the implicit assumptions behind the data obtained from different measures and interpretation of those data. Too often the theories behind health-related quality of life measures are hidden from the user. Once development of a measure is associated with the conceptual theories and measurement traditions on which it is based, users of measures can better appreciate the strengths and weaknesses of a particular measure and the probable assumptions or biases that may arise from its use.

4

Concepts of Health-Related Quality of Life

In Chapter 1, we defined *health-related quality of life* as the value assigned by individuals, groups, or society to the duration of survival as modified by impairments, functional states, perceptions, and social opportunities influenced by disease, injury, treatment, or policy. This definition covers five broad concepts that combine the quantity and quality of life on a value scale or continuum. The five concepts are defined further by *domains*, which are states, attitudes, behaviors, perceptions, other spheres of action and thought in health-related quality of life.

In this chapter, we define all the concepts and domains used in our global definition of health-related quality of life. We identify indicators for each domain and illustrate how these indicators are used in developing measures and in assessing health status and quality of life. Whenever possible, we use national data to illustrate the five basic concepts and their domains and indicators. We discuss other domains and concepts of health and quality of life that are relevant to special situations or populations, including the concept of states of health considered worse than death. Finally, we describe how different concepts and domains may interact in classifying health states.

CONCEPTS, DOMAINS, AND INDICATORS

Table 4.1 lists the five broad health-related quality of life concepts—opportunity, health perceptions, functional states, impairments, and death or duration of life—domains of these concepts, and proposed indicators or measures of the concepts and domains. Table 4.1 is arranged with the concept and indicators of death and survival at the bottom and concepts, domains, and indicators of opportunity at the top as though placed on the value continuum from least desirable to most desirable. Individual domains and indicators, however, cannot be easily located hierarchically on the value continuum of health-related quality of life ranging from minimal to maximal. Different levels of symptom severity may cover the entire range of the continuum. Combinations of domains and indicators, such as physical function and health perceptions, interact and can be considered as different levels of health-related quality of life. For example, minor symptoms may not affect psychological or social function, although major impairments and symptoms may cause profound psychological and social dysfunction. Perceived satisfaction with health may be low even though physical, psychological, and social function are high.

Analysts and investigators will find Table 4.1 useful in considering which concepts and domains to use in developing a health state classification system or in assessing

Table 4.1 Core concepts and domains of health-related quality of life

Concepts and domains	Definitions/indicators
Opportunity	
Social or cultural disadvantage	Disadvantage because of health; stigma; societal reaction
Resilience	Capacity for health; ability to withstand stress; physiologic reserves
Health perceptions	
General health perceptions	Self-rating of health; health concern/worry
Satisfaction with health	Satisfaction with physical, psychological, social function
Functional status	
Social function	
Limitations in usual roles	Acute or chronic limitations in usual social roles (major activities) of child, student, worker
Integration	Participation in the community
Contact	Interaction with others
Intimacy and sexual function	Perceived feelings of closeness; sexual activity and/or problems
Psychological function	
Affective	Psychological attitudes and behaviors, including distress and well-being
Cognitive	Alertness; disorientation; problems in reasoning
Physical function	
Activity restrictions	Acute or chronic reduction in physical activity, mobility, self-care, sleep, communication
Fitness	Performance of activity with vigor and without excessive fatigue
Impairment	
Symptoms/subjective complaints	Reports of physical and psychological symptoms, sensations, pain, health problems or feelings not directly observable
Signs	Physical examination: observable evidence of defect of abnormality
Self-reported disease	Patient listing of medical conditions or impairments
Physiologic measures	Laboratory data, records, and their clinical interpretation
Tissue alterations	Pathological evidence
Diagnoses	Clinical judgments after "all the evidence"
Death and duration of life	Mortality; survival; years of life lost

health-related quality of life. Investigators can identify outcomes by (1) reviewing the five concepts, eighteen domains, and multiple indicators and (2) selecting concepts, domains, and indicators relevant to their health decision and/or assessment objective. For example, psychological function domains include affective attitudes and behaviors and cognitive function. A health intervention such as a health promotion program for older adults might affect both aspects of psychological function. Affective attitudes and behaviors are further subdivided into indicators of distress and happiness, because these positive and negative aspects of affect have been shown to be distinct from each other. Cognitive function is divided into general alertness, disorientation, and problems in reasoning. Reasoning problems would be those tasks included in a mental status examination. In a health promotion program evaluation, assessment of psychological function might involve affective attitudes and behaviors and cognitive functions as well as all indicators of these domains. Investigators planning on primary data collection must choose those concepts, domains, and indicators that fit their assessment objective, health decision or problem, and resources.

We derived the concepts and domains contained in Table 4.1 from the theoretical perspectives discussed in Chapter 3. Cultural, social, psychological, and biomedical perspectives have implicitly or explicitly prompted many researchers to develop measures of these concepts. Other investigators have proposed different classes of outcome variables (World Health Organization, 1948, 1980; Sanazaro, 1965; Donabedian, 1966; Starfield, 1974; Patrick and Elinson, 1979, 1984; Brook et al., 1979; Ware, 1984a; Bergner, 1985). The concepts, domains, and indicators shown in Table 4.1 build on these previous efforts to provide a comprehensive definition ranging across the continuum of health-related quality of life.

DEATH AND DURATION OF LIFE

Concepts of death and duration of life are obviously necessary for assessing disease and treatment outcomes. Length of life and time of death are of intense interest to individuals as well as of considerable importance to their family, friends, and caregivers. Length of survival has long been a primary endpoint in assessing disease burden and treatment effectiveness in medical effectiveness evaluations. In population studies, mortality rates for specific populations, diseases, and conditions are important in identifying need, allocating resources, and monitoring progress.

Life expectancy is not the only criterion patients, families, and clinicians use, however, when deciding about life-threatening treatments such as heart transplantation or chemotherapy. *Quality* of life (how well one lives) is considered along with *quantity* of life (how long one lives). In this instance, quality of life might be used in its broadest sense, including both health- and non-health-related aspects. When survival is at stake because of disease or injury, many aspects of the patient's life may become health-related that once were not defined as "health" or "well-being." For diseases or conditions with more favorable prognoses and where pharmacologic or nonpharmacologic treatments are available, mortality is not generally a sensitive indicator of therapy effectiveness. Other health status and quality of life issues must be considered to fully address health-related quality of life.

Death rates are most readily and accurately determined for populations where such rates are least valuable in assessing the population's health. In parts of the world where death rates are still high, incomplete records and uncertain population bases thwart measurement accuracy. When death rates are relatively low, they tend not to be very serviceable indicators in assessment of health services (Moriyama, 1968). For example, in countries with low death rates, 99 percent of the population lives in markedly varied degrees of health. In such countries, death rates are relatively insensitive indicators except for special population subgroups with higher than average mortality. These subgroups often include minority groups, neonates, people with significant disabilities, and persons living in poverty. For assessing equity in health status, death rates continue to be the most important indicator of health status differences and of gaps in socioeconomic status.

Mortality-based measures, including the total death rate, condition-specific death rates, infant mortality, maternal mortality, life expectancy at birth, potential years of life lost, and remaining years of life at various ages are the most frequently used indicators of health. Survival and life-table mortality experience models produce actuarial measures of life expectancy for different age groups, sexes, or races. These measures have been widely used and analyzed (Kleinman, 1977; Manton and Soldo, 1985). The Health Resource Allocation Strategy incorporates life expectancy or duration of survival in estimating health-related quality of life.

Deaths per 100,000 population in the United States have declined considerably over the last century and over the last few decades. Age-adjusted death rates for all causes fell from 841.5 in 1950 to 523.0 in 1989 (National Center for Health Statistics, 1992). Fundamental improvements in socioeconomic status with accompanying improvements in nutrition, transportation, agriculture, and sanitary conditions have helped prevent deaths.

Since the turn of the century, Americans have added more than 27 years in life expectancy, an increase from 47.3 years in 1900 to 75.2 years in 1989 (National Center for Health Statistics, 1991). The racial gap in life expectancy is narrowing. According to 1989 provisional data, life expectancy for blacks was 69.7 years compared with 75.9 for whites. The main cause of life expectancy improvement is the decline in the cardiovascular disease death rate during the last decade.

Two trends in mortality and duration of survival have important implications for health policy and the allocation of resources. The first trend concerns the change in mortality rates and life expectancy in the population of adults age 65 and over. In 1980, older adults were 11.1 percent of the total population. By the year 2000, they will constitute 13.2 percent of the population. By 2020, children born in the post–World War II baby boom will be 60 to 69. Older adults will constitute 17.2 percent of the population.

Figure 4.1 shows the life expectancy of persons at 65 years of age by color and gender for selected years between 1900 and 1989. Life expectancy for both genders at this age rose from 11.9 years at the turn of the century to 17.2 years at the close of the 1980s. White females 65 years of age can expect to live an additional 18.9 years, while black males at age 65 in 1989 can expect only 13.8 additional years of life.

The major reason for improved life expectancy is illustrated by the downward trend in age-adjusted death rates for the five leading causes of death (Figure 4.2). Death rates at all ages for heart disease fell from 286.2 per 100,000 resident population in 1960 to 155.9 in 1989. Heart disease remains the leading cause of death for persons 65 years of age and over, followed by malignant neoplasms and cerebrovascular diseases (National Center for Health Statistics, 1992). Figure 4.2 shows that deaths at all ages from heart disease and stroke have declined, while cancer deaths have increased slightly from 125.8 in 1960 to 133.0 in 1989.

Improved survival leads to concern over just how healthy older people will be in the future (Verbrugge, 1989). Will there be longer life but worsening health or will there be an increase in active life expectancy when longevity is coupled with better health? As the survival curve for older adults becomes more rectangular and a higher percentage of

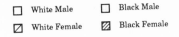

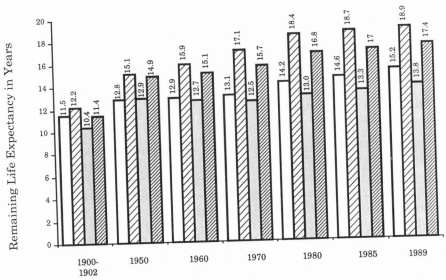

Figure 4.1 Life expectancy at 65 years of age by color and gender, United States, selected years, 1900–1989. *Source*: National Center for Health Statistics, 1991a, Table 15, p. 67.

older adults survive to 85 and above, this question assumes even greater importance. At present, most older U.S. residents live in the community, are cognitively intact, and are fully independent in their daily activities. Many report major activity limitations, however, due to chronic conditions.

The second mortality trend that has a major impact on health policy is that for premature deaths among youth. In the United States, the dominant causes of premature death, measured by years of potential life lost, are related to trauma. Many leading causes of childhood deaths—unintentional injuries, homicide, suicide, child abuse and neglect, lead poisoning, and developmental problems—are largely preventable. Preventive measures include swimming pool and spa covers and childproof enclosures; child-resistant packaging for prescription drugs and other hazardous materials; safer playground equipment; and smoke detectors (Department of Health and Human Services, 1991). Increased public awareness, improved safety measures, and early intervention programs have reduced fatalities among children age 1 through 14.

The age group from 15 to 24 is the only one in the United States to show an increase in mortality in recent years. Accidents, homicide, and suicide accounted for three-fourths of all deaths in this age group. The leading cause of death among white youths is motor vehicle accidents, and the leading cause among black youths is homicide. Approximately half of all motor vehicle crashes and homicides involve alcohol. These causes of death, potentially preventable, have deep roots in the social and cultural life of our nation.

The most important risk factors for chronic disease in later years frequently have their origins in behaviors developed in adolescence and early adulthood. Prevention of injury and violence and the promotion of healthy lifestyles, including special attention to tobacco, alcohol, drugs, and sexual behavior, are the major prevention targets in this age group. Preventive efforts range from policy or legislative initiatives to regulating the sale of firearms to programs emphasizing individual behavioral change through education and counseling. Clearly, an organized, targeted national health policy for children and adolescents will be needed to affect these deeply disturbing trends.

The establishment of the National Death Index (NDI) has advanced the use of mortality data in research, particularly in relation to population morbidity. The National Death Index is used to determine whether persons in prospective studies have died. If so, investigators obtain names of the states where the deaths occurred and the corresponding death certificate numbers. Demographic items recommended for linkage with the National Death Index include last name, first name, middle initial, social security number, month and year of birth, day of birth, father's surname, gender, race, marital status, state of residence, and state of birth. An index user can then obtain copies of death certificates from state vital statistics offices to establish cause of death (Department of Health and Human Services, 1981). In its population-based surveys,

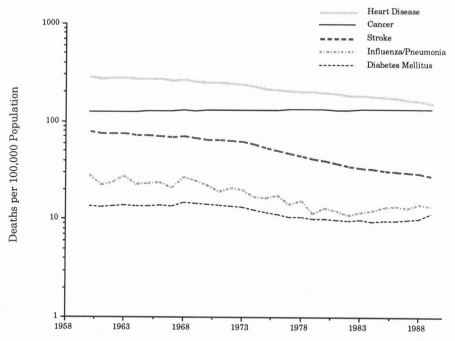

Figure 4.2 Age-adjusted death rates for total United States population, according to the five leading causes of death, 1960–89. *Source*: National Center for Health Statistics, *Vital Statistics of the United States. Volume II— Mortality, Part A*, 1962–90.

the National Center for Health Statistics now includes all the information required to use the National Death Index.

IMPAIRMENTS

The concept of impairment includes most of the familiar category of *morbidity*, for example, the number of sick persons or cases of disease in relationship to a specific population. Thus impairment is at the center of the professional appraisal of the presence or absence of abnormalities within the individual. These abnormalities may be present at birth or acquired later through pathologic processes or injuries. In the medical model of disease, morbidity includes both pathologic changes that have not yet been recognized and those that have become evident. Morbidity domains thus encompass both disease and impairment or any loss or abnormality of psychologic, physiologic, or anatomic structure or function (World Health Organization, 1980).

Technical distinctions have been made between the various domains of impairment and the methods for measuring them (Patrick and Elinson, 1979, 1984; World Health Organization, 1980). Although professionals have different etiologic, anatomic, and physiologic criteria for the evaluation of disease, at least six impairment domains can be distinguished: symptom or subjective complaints, signs, self-reports of disease, physiologic measures, tissue alterations, and diagnoses. The relative emphasis placed on each type depends on the health decision under investigation, on the assessment objectives, and on how the evidence is obtained.

Symptoms and Subjective Complaints

Complaints reported by respondents are often not directly observable by an interviewer or evaluator. Reports of physical and psychological symptoms, sensations, pain, health problems, or other feelings of abnormality are best known to the person who has them, although useful inferences can often be made by objective observers. Headache, backache, nasal congestion, cough, and tiredness affect millions of Americans annually. In a national poll asking Americans about the types of pain they experienced over the preceding 12 months, headaches (73 percent), backaches (56 percent), muscle pains (56 percent), and joint pains (51 percent) were most commonly mentioned (Taylor and Curran, 1985).

In one national survey (the National Health and Nutrition Examination Survey–1, hereafter NHANES-1), 78 percent of respondents reported at least 1 of 12 selected symptoms of psychological distress. These included headache, dizziness, and palpitating heart (Sayetta, 1980). Another survey estimated that Americans restrict their activities because of symptomatic experiences an average of 9.7 days per year and visit physicians an average of 2.7 times per year (National Center for Health Statistics, 1979). Clearly, physical symptoms and sensations profoundly affect people's feeling of health.

Four types of complaints are commonly assessed: physical symptoms, health problems, impairments, and pain. Condition and symptom checklists are in almost every questionnaire used in national health surveys. These checklists are most useful for identifying condition-specific subgroups for analysis; however, no comprehensive severity index has yet emerged for weighting medical conditions and symptoms obtained from checklists. Thus, many analysts use the overall number of conditions or symptoms reported to approximate an overall measure of impairment. In the Health Utilities Index and Quality of Well-Being Scale, the different symptom–problem complexes have been weighted along with the other domains to provide an overall health-related quality of life score.

Pain is commonly included in health state classifications, because it is both frequently reported by and important to people. For example, in the National Health and Nutrition Examination Survey–I Epidemiologic Follow-Up Study, back pain was reported by 9.1 percent of all male respondents and 10.9 percent of all female respondents. Pain is a highly subjective experience, "an unpleasant sensory and emotional experience associated with actual or potential tissue 'damage' " (IASP Subcommittee on Taxonomy, 1979). The behavioral effect of pain is even more intense if it is chronic, a term usually applied to describe a pain that is benign in origin and is present on a constant, daily basis for longer than six months (Sternbach et al., 1974). Pain is the result of a complex interplay of neurophysiological, behavioral, and psychological factors. The psychology of pain and study of its origins have produced a voluminous literature (Sternbach, 1978; Skelton and Pennebaker, 1982; Bonica, 1990).

There are also numerous approaches to assessing other physical and psychological symptoms. Examples of physical symptom measures are the Symptom-Distress Scale (McCorkle and Young, 1978) and the Symptom Rating Test (Kellner and Sheffield, 1973). Psychological symptoms are usually measured by a self-response checklist; one comprehensive scale developed for identifying psychological symptoms is the Hopkins Symptom Checklist (Derogatis et al., 1973, 1974).

Signs

Objective, observable evidence or signs obtained through physical examination add to self-reports of symptoms. Bleeding or overweight can be signs as well, because examination can confirm self-report. Data obtained by clinical examination under standardized conditions are generally considered to be less susceptible to potential nonresponse bias than data provided by the individuals themselves (Pearce, 1985). The earlier National Health Examination Surveys (NHES) and, more recently, the National Health and Nutritional Examination Surveys have collected and used data obtained by direct physical examination, clinical and laboratory tests, and related measurement procedures. In these surveys, examination record forms are combined with physiologic measures and self-reported interview and questionnaire data.

One major example of the combined use of physical examination and self-report is the nation's monitoring of high blood pressure and high blood pressure control. Figure 4.3 shows the prevalence of hypertension among people 20–74 years of age by race and gender for three time periods (1960–62, 1971–74, and 1976–80). These data are based on physical examinations of a sample of the civilian noninstitutionalized population. People with high blood pressure have blood pressure equal to or greater than 140 mmHg systolic and/or 90 mmHg diastolic and/or report taking antihypertensive medication. Percentages are based on a single measurement of blood pressure to provide comparable data across the three time periods. The prevalence of hypertension was higher among black males and females than among white males and females. Just over

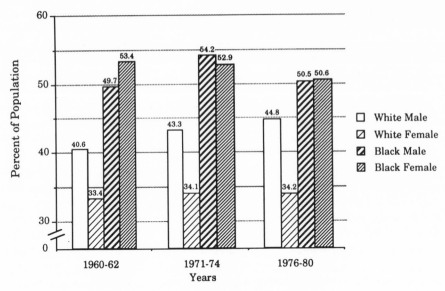

Figure 4.3 Age-adjusted prevalence of hypertension among persons 20–74 years of age according to color and gender, United States, 1960–62, 1971–74, and 1976–80. (Note that females exclude pregnant women.) A person with hypertension is defined by either having elevated blood pressure (systolic pressure of at least 140 mmHg or diastolic pressure of at least 90 mmHg) or taking antihypertensive medication. Percentages are based on a single measurement of blood pressure to provide comparable data across the three time periods. In 1976–80, 31.3 percent of persons 20–74 years of age had hypertension, based on the average of three blood pressure measurements, in contrast to 39.7 percent when a single measurement is used. *Source*: National Center for Health Statistics, National Health and Nutrition Examination Survey, Health United States 1990, NCHS 199a, Table 61, p. 131.

50 percent of black persons between 20 and 74 were detected as having hypertension in the 1976–80 survey.

Blood pressure control is defined as maintaining a blood pressure less than 140 mmHg systolic and 90 mmHg diastolic. The control may be through either pharmacologic or nonpharmacologic treatment such as weight loss, low-sodium diet, or alcohol restriction. Long-term blood pressure control can help to reduce the incidence of and death caused by cardiovascular diseases such as coronary heart disease, hypertensive heart disease, and stroke. Although the last nationally representative survey (1976–80) showed that only 11 percent of hypertensive adults were under control, the Seven States Study (represents the medians of data from California, Colorado, Georgia, Maine, Maryland, Michigan, and South Carolina) showed a larger percentage under control (24 percent) in 1982–84. These data suggest a progressive increase of hypertensive persons under control in the United States. Antihypertensive agents and nonpharmacologic interventions aimed at changes in dietary behavior and exercise are increasingly employed to bring high blood pressure under control.

Self-Reported Disease

As noted, survey respondents commonly report that they have or have had heart disease, cancer, respiratory disease, or some other disease. These reports may be made by patients who have been told by a physician that they have a disease and even by those who have not been told. It is a good idea to determine whether the patient has been told because this provides useful information about patient perceptions of disease and illness. Respondents reporting "diagnoses" unconfirmed by health professionals have evaluated the evidence for themselves, and the evidence on which these reports are based is unknown.

The National Health Interview Survey contains an extensive list of medical conditions. The list covers a group of chronic conditions classified according to the organ or body systems approach commonly used by clinicians. These systems include the skin and musculoskeletal, sensory-motor, digestive, glandular-blood-nervous-genitourinary system, heart and circulatory, and respiratory systems. This body systems approach was adopted to provide more thorough reporting and an increased number of conditions for which estimates of prevalence could be made. Since 1978, representative subsamples of respondents have been asked one of six condition lists to provide national estimates for the six body systems for each interview year. For example, in 1983–85 the prevalence of chronic back conditions was 77.5 per 1,000 people. This breaks into 17 per 1,000 for intervertebral disk disorders, 19.7 per 1,000 for curvature of the back or spine, and 40.8 per 1,000 for other impairments of the back. In 1983–85, chronic back conditions rivaled arthritis and heart disease as a major cause of activity limitation.

Self-reports of medical conditions can be biased estimates of prevalence because the reporters are influenced by use of medical care. Persons who see health professionals are more likely to report "diagnoses" than persons who do not (Wilson and Drury, 1984). These reports may also be sensitive to cultural variation. Researchers have found that cultural and ethnic groups differ in the subjective experience and interpretation of symptoms and pain (Zborowski, 1969).

Physiologic Measures

Clinicians use a vast number of physiologic measures to detect abnormalities such as blood count, glucose tolerance, and forced expiratory flow. Records from these tests are observed and interpreted. These records may be single readings or an extensive series of measures, such as prolonged electrocardiographic monitoring to determine the efficacy or toxicity of a drug prescribed to treat cardiac rhythm disturbance.

To detect abnormalities physiologic measures are included in the National Health and Nutrition Examination surveys. Examples are blood count, the nitrite test for bacteriuria, and electrocardiographic tracings. Physiologic measures are used in policy analyses to help define prevention targets and to monitor progress in achieving these targets. Body measurements, dietary interviews, physician exams, and other laboratory tests provide population baseline and follow-up measurements.

For example, the body mass index (BMI) for people aged 20 and older helps to define overweight. The BMI is calculated by dividing weight in kilograms by the square of height in meters. Overweight is defined as a BMI greater than 27.8 for men and 27.3 for women. Overweight affects a large proportion of the United States population, and its prevalence has not declined among adults for two decades. The *Healthy People 2000* risk-reduction objective is to reduce overweight to no more than 20 percent among people aged 20 and older and to no more than 15 percent among adolescents aged 12 through 19 (Department of Health and Human Services, 1991b).

Tissue Alterations

Alterations in body tissue may be detected by means of pathologic evidence obtained either at autopsy or in examination of tissues collected during a surgical procedure. For example, microscopic examination of the heart of a patient with atherosclerotic coronary heart disease can detect pathologic processes such as necroses of cardiac muscle. Although this kind of evidence may be important in clinical investigations of disease process and their complications and in some clinical trials, such data are infrequently collected to monitor the health status of populations.

Diagnoses

History, observation, physical examination, symptoms, and physiologic measures are used to arrive at both the diagnosis and the prognosis of disease or medical conditions for individual patients. Many clinical trials incorporate these diagnostic elements in a systematic protocol that defines diagnostic criteria. Such criteria can be important in identifying comparable experimental groups exposed to different treatments.

Few population surveys systematically incorporate all this evidence. Data collected in the National Health and Nutrition Examination Surveys have diagnostic potential for individuals who participate in the survey, but it is the policy of the National Center for Health Statistics to refrain from making clinical diagnoses on participants. Instead, in the case of abnormal readings and examination, the person's physician is notified so that the results can be verified and treatment prescribed as needed. Data from these examination surveys are used, however, to arrive at diagnoses for groups of participants to do disease-specific epidemiologic analyses.

FUNCTIONAL STATUS: PHYSICAL, PSYCHOLOGICAL, SOCIAL

The World Health Organization (WHO) defined health in its constitution as a "state of complete physical, mental, and social well-being and not merely the absence of disease or infirmity" (WHO, 1948). From this precedent have come a large number of measurement efforts focused on functioning in the physical, mental, and social areas of life. Although the WHO definition was not accompanied by operational methods for measuring "well-being" in these three areas, the comprehensiveness of the definition has set a standard by which many measurement efforts have been judged. Indeed, Ware (1987) recommends including physical, mental, social, and perceptual health measures in assessment efforts as a minimum standard for health measures claiming to be comprehensive.

Physical Function

Physical function is particularly important for assessing the impact of chronic disease and for evaluating rapidly emerging technologies and their effects on the course and outcome of chronic diseases such as kidney ailments, chronic respiratory conditions, and cardiovascular disease. Measures of health-related quality of life are particularly important for population groups dependent on others for essential activities of daily living—people 85 and those with severely limiting impairments and chronic conditions. Measures of physical function can be classified into two domains: activity restrictions and fitness.

Activity Restrictions

Concepts of physical function are commonly used by clinicians in obtaining a patient's history or listening to accounts of the patient's problems. Commonly reported disabilities are restrictions in body movement (e.g., difficulty in walking or bending over), limitations in mobility (e.g., having to stay in bed or not being able to drive a car or use public transportation), or interference with self-care activities (e.g., bathing, dressing, or eating without assistance). Reduced ability to carry out these activities of daily living is also among the most frequently measured concepts of health and well-being in population studies (Katz and Akpom, 1976). This is understandable because the capacity to perform daily routines and tasks determines personal independence, a widely shared value in our society.

The National Health Interview Survey uses the terms *activity limitations* and *activity restrictions*. Activity limitations are long-term reductions in a person's capacity to perform the average activities associated with his or her age group. Activity restrictions refer to selected behaviors associated with reduced activity because of long- or short-term conditions. Limitations thus refer to what a person is generally capable of doing; they are discussed in the section on social function as limitations in usual social roles. Restrictions ordinarily refer to a relatively short-term reduction in a person's activities below his or her usual capacity.

Four types of restricted activity are commonly assessed in national surveys. *Work-loss days* are days reported by currently employed people 18 and older who have missed more than half a day from a job or business. *School-loss days* are days reported by students from 5 to 17 who have missed more than half a day from the school in which they are currently enrolled. *Cut-down days* are days reported by a person who has cut down for more than half a day on the things he or she usually does. *Bed days* are those in which a person reports staying in bed more than half a day because of illness or injury. All inpatient hospital days are counted as bed days even if the patient was not in bed more than half a day.

Work-loss, school-loss, and cut-down days refer to the short-term effects of illness or injury. Bed days, on the other hand, may measure long- or short-term disability, depending on whether the bed day was associated with chronic or acute illness. *Restricted-activity days* refer to the number of days a person experienced any one of the four types of activity restriction. Each day is counted only once even if more than one type of restriction was involved.

As mentioned earlier, a major health objective for older adults is to make the

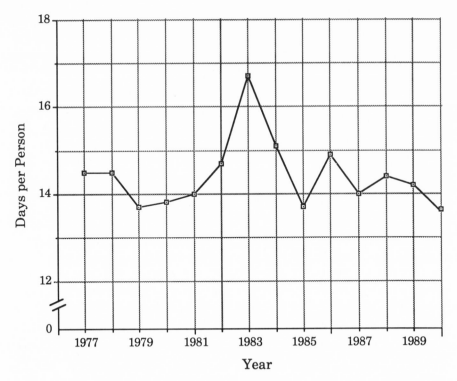

Figure 4.4   Bed-disability days for persons 65 years of age and over, United States, 1977–90. The increase in bed days for 1983 is attributed to the increased prevalence of influenza that occurred during that year. *Source:* National Center for Health Statistics, Current Estimates from the *National Health Interview Survey, United States, Vital and Health Statistics,* 1978–91, Table 69.

remaining years of life as healthy, active, and enjoyable as possible. Restricted-activity days and bed days are two frequently used measures to assess the health and activity of older adults. As shown in Figure 4.4, adults 65 and over reported an average of 14.5 bed days due to acute and chronic conditions in 1977; in 1983 this measure reached an 11-year high of 16.7 bed days.

A partial explanation for this dramatic peak is the greater prevalence of influenza and respiratory conditions reported in 1983. Another plausible explanation is change in the description of the period of time constituting a bed day after 1982. Specifically, in 1982 "days of disability" were described for respondents as days in which they stayed in bed for "more than half of the day." This differed from the phrase used in the bed day question before 1982: "all or most of the day." Such changes in wording, coupled with other changes occurring in 1982, such as the order of the disability day questions, could have contributed to an increased estimate (National Center for Health Statistics, 1985). Since 1983, however, the reported number of bed days shows a downward trend. In 1990, the average number of bed days reported by older adults fell to 13.6. This example illustrates the difficulty facing the analyst attempting to analyze trends in single indicators of health status.

Difficulty in performing personal care activities is another commonly used indicator of functional independence in older adults. Information on basic and instrumental activities of daily living are available from the 1984 Supplement on Aging to the National Health Interview Survey. In this supplement, respondents were asked about difficulty in performing daily living activities attributable to a health or physical condition. When difficulties were reported, respondents were asked about the level of difficulty in performing these activities without help or use of special equipment. Activities of daily living included walking, bathing, getting outside, getting in an out of bed or chair, dressing, using a toilet, and eating. The most frequently reported limitation in these activities of daily living was difficulty walking followed by bathing and getting outside (LaCroix, 1987).

Fitness

Fitness measures assess energy, endurance, speed, and the more "positive" nature of physical activity. Physical fitness is thus closely related to the concept of resilience classified under the broad category of opportunity that follows. Fitness is increasingly used as a measure of health-related quality of life. It is prominent in health promotion efforts to improve the performance of activity with vigor and without excessive fatigue.

Individual measures of fitness include such items as the ability to run the length of a football field or the speed with which one can walk ten yards. The Canadian Fitness Survey measures leisure-time energy expenditure calculated from questions on the frequency and average duration of sports and conditioning activities in the preceding two weeks (Stephens et al., 1986). Overall physical activity measures such as those based on the work of Paffenbarger et al. (1986) are currently being developed to study the health effects of physical activity. Measures of physical fitness are difficult to apply across entire populations because different norms apply to different age, sex, and disease groups. What defines physical fitness for a group of people disabled by respiratory disease, for example, differs from that for nondisabled persons. Nevertheless, there are increasing attempts to assess the "optimal" level of fitness by which to evaluate medical and nutritional interventions.

Table 4.2 shows the relationship between self-rated and observed physical fitness in persons 10–69 years of age from the 1981 Canada Fitness Survey (Stephens and Craig, 1989). In the total sample, 32 percent met the recommended standards applied to aerobic test results. Of those who rated themselves as "more fit," 43 percent met recommended aerobic standards, compared to 18 percent of those who gave a rating of "less fit." Just under a third of respondents in this survey refused aerobic fitness testing in each of the self-rated categories, and 10–18 percent were excluded from fitness testing based on one or more screening procedures.

Psychological Function

The domain of psychological function is sometimes restricted to affective indicators of happiness, distress, morale, or positive affect. *Psychological status*, however, pertains to or derives from the mind or emotions and includes cognitive aspects such as alertness, confusion, or impaired thought and concentration as well as affect. Both the affective and cognitive domains of health-related quality of life are important because

Table 4.2 Self-rated versus measured physical fitness in persons 10–69 years of age,
Canadian Fitness Survey

Self-rated fitness[a]	Total	Aerobic test results:[b] Percent of sample				
		Meeting recommended level	Meeting minimum level	At undesirable level	Screened out[c]	Refused testing
More fit	100	43	15		11	31
As fit	100	34	22	2	12	30
Less fit	100	18	29	5	18	30
Total	100	32	23	2	13	30

Source: Adapted from Stephens and Craig, 1989

[a] In response to the question "Comparing yourself to others of your own age and sex, would you say you are. . . ."

[b] Recommended = 65–70% of average maximum aerobic power for same sex 10 years younger; minimum = 65–70% of average maximum for same sex, same age; undesirable = 65–70% of average maximum for same sex, 10 years older.

[c] Excluded from fitness testing because of health history or current health problems.

they are influenced significantly by disease processes and treatment and, in a reversal of causal direction, they may affect disease and treatment.

Affective Functioning

Psychological distress and well-being have been usefully distinguished in theory (Bradburn, 1969; Veit and Ware, 1982). The relationship between positive and negative indicators, however, is not completely understood. Numerous scales have been developed to measure psychological dysfunction and distress, particularly depression and anxiety (Zung and Durham, 1965; Beck, 1967). A number of these scales are used to evaluate psychiatric symptomatology (Dohrenwend et al., 1980) or to produce psychiatric diagnoses according to the American Psychiatric Association Diagnostic and Statistical Manual (Spitzer et al., 1970). Another large collection of literature concerns the theory and measurement of well-being, and many advances have been made in this field over the last few decades (Gurin et al., 1960; Andrews and Withey, 1976; Diener, 1984).

Recent findings from the Medical Outcomes Study (Wells, Stewart, et al., 1989) indicate that patients with either current depressive disorder or depressive symptoms tend to have worse physical, social, and role functioning. They also have worse perceived health and greater pain than do patients with no chronic conditions. These findings underscore the importance of assessing depression, even when depressive disorder is not present. Depressive symptoms and chronic medical conditions interact, resulting in poor functional status.

Because of limited interview time and problems of respondent burden, it is often impossible to include separate, multi-item scales to measure aspects of psychological distress and well-being. Single-item scales tend to be less reproducible over time. In addition, the internal consistency and variance due to wording of specific items cannot be investigated. Thus, brief measures of emotional well-being composed of several important components are needed.

The General Well-Being (GWB) Schedule developed by Dupuy at the National Center for Health Statistics (Dupuy, 1973, 1974, 1984; Fazio, 1977) is an example of an emotional well-being measure that has been used in large surveys. This 18-item measure provides an index of self-representations of intrapersonal affective or emotional states. These reflect a sense of subjective well-being or distress in six states: freedom from worry about health, energy level, interest in life, cheerful mood, relaxation, and emotional and behavioral control. The scale has been validated against both self-reports on other instruments and clinician ratings (Fazio, 1977). Six subscales contain three to five items each, and these subscales, as well as scoring, administration, validating, reliability, and generalizability, are reviewed by Dupuy (1984). Data on the General Well-Being Schedule are available for 25- to 74-year-old noninstitutionalized adults resident in the United States. These data were obtained through inclusion of the GWB in the National Health and Nutrition Examination Survey–1. The GWB was also used in a large community sample of persons aged 14 and above who were interviewed in the Health Insurance Experiment (Ware et al., 1979).

Table 4.3 shows the mean levels of General Well-Being Scores from 10 of the 18 items administered at follow-up for persons age 55–84 in the National Health and Nutrition Examination Survey–I Epidemiologic Follow-Up Study (Costa et al., 1990). The 10 General Well-Being items were grouped into scores for negative affect, positive affect, and health concerns. Women reported significantly lower well-being on all subscales, indicating that they were more depressed. Older persons scored significantly lower on positive affect and significantly higher on health concerns. No significant age trend was noted for negative affect.

The Center for Epidemiologic Studies Depression scale, known as the CES-D, is another widely used measure of psychological function incorporated in population

Table 4.3 Mean levels of general well-being scores at follow-up for respondents to National Health and Nutrition Examination Survey–I Epidemiologic Follow-Up Study (NHEFS)

Gender, age (numbers of participants)		Negative affect	Positive affect	Health concern	Total well-being[a]
Men					
55–59	(407)	9.3	13.3	3.5	50.6
60–64	(388)	8.1	13.4	3.5	51.8
65–69	(326)	7.6	13.4	3.8	51.9
70–74	(261)	7.4	13.1	3.6	52.2
75–79	(449)	7.9	12.5	3.8	50.8
80–84	(252)	8.2	11.8	3.6	50.1
Total	(2,083)	8.1	12.9	3.6	51.2
SD		6.2	3.9	3.9	11.8
Women					
55–59	(536)	10.3	12.5	3.6	48.5
60–64	(497)	9.8	12.6	3.5	49.3
65–69	(384)	9.9	12.4	4.2	48.3
70–74	(352)	9.7	12.0	4.1	48.2
75–79	(628)	10.1	11.6	4.4	47.1
80–84	(392)	10.0	11.1	4.6	46.5
Total	(2,789)	10.0	12.0	4.1	48.0
SD		6.9	3.9	4.1	12.7

Source: Costa et al., 1990.

[a]Total well-being = positive affect − negative affect − health concern + 50.

Table 4.4 Depression status at initial survey (NHANES-I) and at follow-up (NHEFS) for persons age 55–84 years[a]

	Number (%)[b] with stated follow-up status			
	Women		Men	
Initial status	Depressed	Nondepressed	Depressed	Nondepressed
CES-D cut point of 20				
Depressed	19 (3.6%)	39 (7.4%)	10 (2.3%)	17 (4.0%)
Nondepressed	35 (6.6%)	437 (82.5%)	24 (5.6%)	379 (88.1%)
CES-D cut point of 16				
Depressed	41 (7.7%)	41 (7.7%)	13 (3.0%)	29 (6.7%)
Nondepressed	57 (10.8%)	391 (73.8%)	38 (8.8%)	350 (81.4%)

Source: Costa et al., 1990.

[a]Respondents were age 55–84 at the time of NHEFS.

[b]Percentages are given within gender. All corrected χ^2 are significant at $p < 0.001$.

NHANES-1 = National Health and Nutrition Examination Survey–1; NHEFS = National Health and Nutrition Examination Survey-I Epidemiologic Follow-Up Study; CES-D = Center for Epidemiologic Studies Depression Scale (Radloff, 1977).

surveys. Twenty items are scored on a four-point scale from "never" to "most or all of the time (5 to 7 days in the past week)." The CES-D produces scores ranging from 0 to 60 (Radloff, 1977). Alternative cutoff points of 16 or more or of 20 or more have been used to screen persons who "would likely have a disorder severe enough to require professional intervention" (Himmelfarb and Murrel, 1983).

Table 4.4 summarizes the depression status at initial survey and at follow-up for 960 people age 55 and older (Cost et al., 1990). Using the cutoff point of 20 to define cases of probable depression at follow up, 7.9 percent of men (2.3 percent depressed and 5.6 nondepressed at initial survey) and 10.2 percent of women (3.6 percent depressed and 6.6 percent nondepressed at initial survey) were classified as "probably depressed." Using the lower cutoff point of 16, 11.8 percent of men (3.0 percent depressed and 8.8 percent nondepressed at initial survey) and 18.5 percent of women (7.7 percent depressed and 10.8 percent nondepressed at initial survey) can be considered as "probably depressed."

Numerous attempts have been made to measure happiness or the more positive aspects of affective function (Bradburn, 1969). Sample surveys in many different countries have included questions concerning overall happiness, for example: "Taking everything together, how happy would you say you are? Would you say you are very happy, pretty happy, or not too happy?" Striking differences exist in comparing the response distributions from different countries. Ratings of happiness tend to be lower in developing countries than in industrialized nations: happiness is highest in the Netherlands (2.48 on the 3-step scale) and lowest in India (1.43) (Ouweneel and Veenhoven, 1989). Explanations for these differences include cultural bias, that is, the questions have different meanings in different countries, and variation in societal quality, that is, the questions reflect real differences in the life quality in different nations.

Cognitive Functioning

Cognitive functioning is also a major component of psychological well-being. For example, advanced congestive heart failure may decrease cerebral blood flow and metabolism, thereby producing confusion and difficulty in judgment or reasoning. Clinicians may observe impaired thought and concentration in many patients, particularly elderly ones, because of a wide variety of cerebral processes or therapies. Memory and the ability to carry out intellectual behaviors are of great importance to many people. The loss of cognitive function because of a treatment or disease can produce great psychological distress.

Mental functioning, often measured in children and older adults, can be assessed using unstructured "mental-status examinations" administered by clinicians, semi-structured interviews that permit scores to be derived from responses of the subjects and observations of the interviewer, self-completed questionnaires, observer ratings, and formal psychological tests (Kane and Kane, 1981). Extensive psychological tests are available to assess intellectual functioning, although these are most often prohibitively costly, beyond the skill of clinicians, and inappropriate for many study objectives. Change in intellectual functioning is often important to assess, given the importance of mental status to the independent performance of activities of daily living.

The Mental Status Questionnaire (MSQ) has been used extensively in geriatric research and practice, as well as in health surveys to identify the need for surrogate respondents to interviewer-administered or self-administered questionnaires (Kahn et al., 1960). The MSQ consists of ten questions scored as follows:

1. What is this place?
2. Where is this place located?
3. What day in the month is it today?
4. What day of the week is it?
5. What year is it?
6. How old are you?
7. When is your birthday?
8. In what year were you born?
9. What is the name of the president?
10. Who was president before this one?

Score shows severity of brain syndrome:

0–2 errors = none/minimal
3–8 errors = moderate
9–10 errors = severe

These ten items are straightforward orientation items, although the final two questions on the name of the president and immediate past president assess awareness of current events and memory for more distant events. The test–retest reliability of the MSQ is reported to be better than 0.8 with an internal consistency reliability coefficient of 0.84.

The MSQ was administered to respondents age 60 and above in the Epidemiologic Follow-Up Survey to the first National Health and Nutrition Examination Survey cohort, 25–74 years of age. The MSQ was used to identify dementia and also to determine if the respondent was capable of answering the questionnaire. Questions 1, 2, 6, 7, and 8 were administered to all respondents 60 years of age and over. If the respondent received a score of less than 3, the interviewer immediately administered questions 3, 4, 5, 9, and 10. If the respondent scored less than 8 on both parts of the MSQ, interviewers enlisted the aid of a proxy respondent, usually a relative or close friend, to help complete the rest of the questionnaire.

Of 4,085 respondents (age 60–84 years) to the MSQ in the National Health and Nutrition Examination Survey–1 Epidemiologic Follow-Up Survey, 96 percent were classified as having no or mild mental impairment (97 percent of males and 95 percent of females) (National Center for Health Statistics, unpublished data). Respondents with moderate impairment included 4 percent of the total sample (4 percent of males and 5 percent of females). Severe impairment was noted for 0.1 percent of sample respondents (0.1 percent of males and 0.2 percent of females). These results suggest that mental status and cognitive function should be included in any health-related quality of life assessment of respondents age 60 years and above.

Mental status items have also been included in general health status measures. Items describing thought and concentration have been included in the Sickness Impact Profile and the McMaster Health Index Questionnaire (Bergner, Bobbitt, Kressel et al., 1976; Chambers, 1982). Impaired alertness, disorientation, and reasoning difficulties are significant problems in their own right, but they also group with other psychosocial components in aggregated measures (Bergner et al., 1981; Charlton et al., 1983).

The relationship between affective and cognitive measures of psychological well-being is not well understood. In older adults, cognitive and affective function may be particularly hard to distinguish, because the two constructs overlap. The relationship between cognitive and social function may also be difficult to separate operationally, because both mental status and social function are products of the environment. Thus, measures of affective and cognitive function are commonly used in conjunction with measures of social functioning or well-being.

Social Function

Exactly what was meant by "social well-being" in the WHO definition of health status as complete physical, mental, and social well-being is not clear. Social well-being in its broadest sense can be both a component and a determinant of a person's quality of life. Therefore, it is difficult to provide an exact operational definition for the social domain without evaluating the individual's external environment. From a reductionist viewpoint (i.e., social behavior seen as reducible to psychological or physiological explanations), social support and health status are confounded by biologic effects (Broadhead et al., 1983).

In a broader view, social well-being can be derived from individual perceptions, motivations, attitudes, and behaviors and from circumstances external to the individual. These may include aspects of quality of life that may or may not be related to health, such as community life, physical environment, transportation, and financial resources.

Social well-being can also be defined in reference to social relationships. Social support has been operationalized in diverse ways, with considerable confusion between social networks and the support or benefits derived from one's network. Thoits (1982) notes the following: *quantity* of connections (number of people in the network), *quality* (having people one feels close to or can trust), *utilization* (actually spending time with people), *meaning* (the importance of social relationships), *availability* (having people or animals there when needed), and *satisfaction*.

Little consistency exists in the way these concepts have been measured and interpreted by different researchers and analysts (Bruhn and Philips, 1984). Social networks and social supports may be highly interrelated with health status. Thus, the description, measurement, and analysis of these constructs should be kept distinct from other domains of health-related quality of life.

Despite this conceptual confusion, social function remains an important concept in assessing health-related quality of life. Four types of social functioning—limitations in usual social roles, social integration, social contact, and intimacy—are important domains described more fully later.

Limitations in Usual Roles or Major Activity

Many health definitions focus on the capacity for or performance of usual social roles. Holding a job, going to school, parenting, managing a house, engaging in leisure pursuits, and maintaining relationships with friends are important to most people.

The National Health Interview Survey routinely includes questions concerning limitations in activities caused by chronic conditions. Two types of activity are covered: major and other. The term *major activity* refers to a person's participation in daily activities in the workplace, in the household, or at school. Social role identification and major activity are classified according to age groups that correspond to the natural status transitions from infancy to old age:

Below 5	Preschooler	Engage in ordinary play
5–17	Student	Attend school
18–69	Employee or householder	Work/keep house
70 and over	Householder	Capacity for independent living (able to bathe, shop, dress, eat, etc., without needing additional help)

People 18–69 who are classified as keeping house are also classified by their ability to work at a job or business. The term *other activities* also relates to age and refers to all activities not classified as major that a person in a particular age group might do on any given day. These might be participating in clubs, athletics, extracurricular activities, and so forth.

Persons included in the National Health Interview Survey are classified into one of four groups according to their responses to questions concerning major and other activities caused by chronic conditions: (1) unable to perform the major activity; (2) able to perform the major activity but limited in the kind or amount of major activity; (3) not limited in the major activity but limited in the kind or amount of other activities; and (4) not limited in any way. Total limitations in activity refer to limitations in any one of the three categories 1–3. People are not classified as limited in activity unless one or more chronic conditions are reported as causing the activity limitation. If more than one condition is reported, the respondent is asked to identify the major cause of the limitation.

Figure 4.5 shows the percentage of the population and the percentage of two major age groups (under 18 and 65 and over) reporting limitations in major activity (usual social role) between 1970 and 1990. For all persons, limitations in major activity varied from 8.9 to 9.3 percent during this time period. Reports of limitations in major activity increased from 1.3 to 3.6 percent for people under 18. Those 65 years and over showed considerable decreases from earlier years in reported limitations in major activity. In 1985 and after, about 23 percent of the population over 65 years reported limitation, compared to about 40 percent in 1980 and earlier.

This decrease in limitations in major activity for older adults in 1985 and later can be attributed to changes in the way major activity limitations are collected in the National

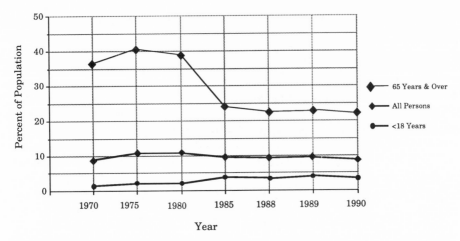

Figure 4.5 Limitations in usual social role (major activity) due to chronic conditions, United States, 1970–90. The drop in limitations in usual social role for persons 65 years and over, between 1980 and 1985, is due to the change in the criteria for determining activity limitation that occurred in 1982. Previously, persons 65 years and older who did not report their major activity as keeping house were classified according to their ability to work. The revised version after 1982 bases major activity limitation for all persons 71 years of age and older on (1) the ability to manage personal care needs and (2) the ability to handle other routine needs. This revised concept, which replaces work with activity more commonly associated with older persons, was introduced to provide more realistic classification criteria for this age group. *Source*: National Center for Health Statistics, Current Estimates from the *National Health Interview Survey, United States, Vital and Health Statistics*, 1971–91, Table 67.

Health Interview Survey. Before 1982, perceived ability to work was the basis for classifying limitations in major activity for older adults. Older males were asked if they were able to work, even if they were retired, and females were asked about their ability to keep house. Beginning in 1982, all persons 70 years of age or over have been asked about their ability to take care of their personal care needs and their ability to handle other routine needs, including everyday household chores, doing necessary business, shopping, and getting around for other purposes. This revised concept, which replaces "work," was introduced to provide more realistic classification criteria for this age group (National Center for Health Statistics, 1985).

The conditions that cause activity limitations are complex and difficult to summarize and interpret, particularly because the patterns shift according to the age group concerned. As shown in Figure 4.6, mobility limitations (e.g., those caused by spinal cord injuries, orthopedic impairments, and paralysis) are responsible for most of the activity limitations among young adults age 18–44 years. For middle-aged and older adults, chronic diseases, especially heart and circulatory problems, are the predominant causes of activity limitation. Intellectual limitations are important for persons under 18 and 85 years and above. In all age groups, a wide variety of conditions contribute to the prevalence of activity limitations.

Activity restrictions and limitations in social role performance may be unrelated to the presence of disease or each other. Furthermore, not all such disability is an indica-

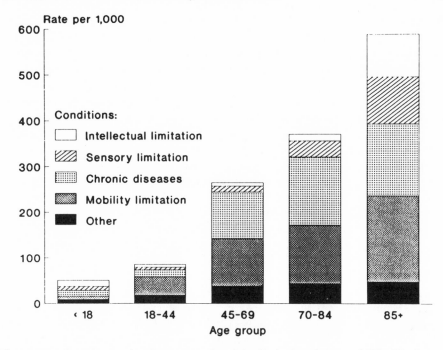

Figure 4.6 Prevalence of main causes of activity limitation, by age, 1983–85. *Source*: Pope and Tarlov, 1991, as calculated from LaPlante, 1988.

tor of physical well-being. For example, work-loss days may be measures of job satisfaction or conformity, as when workers take sick days because of tiredness or fatigue, because it is their "right," or because of alienating work conditions. Alternatively, persons who show evidence of severe disease processes and have limitations in mobility may still perform their desired social roles satisfactorily.

These activity limitation data indicate that disability, defined as interference in life activities, is a major social issue that affects a substantial proportion of the American population. About 35 million Americans (one in every seven) have some activity limitation, and more than 9 million people have physical or mental conditions that keep them from being able to work, attend school, or maintain a household. Of the current 75-year life expectancy, a newborn can be expected to experience an average of 13 years with an activity limitation (Pope and Tarlov, 1991). As technology and public health advances improve life expectancy at birth for severely impaired infants and lengthen life for older adults with impairments, the need increases to prevent disability and disadvantage and improve the quality of life for persons with disabilities. The challenge is to design and evaluate interventions that emphasize rehabilitation, the prevention of secondary conditions, and the enhancement of satisfaction and opportunity for disabled persons with the goal of community participation and integration. This challenge places increased emphasis on quality of life as an outcome measure.

Social Integration

Emile Durkheim's classic study of suicide (1897/1951) has stimulated a great deal of thinking and research. His work emphasizes the importance of close social ties and the

effects of the breakdown of social integration because of the emergence of an industrialized, highly technical society. *Anomie*, or the loss of social integration, was considered by Durkheim to be harmful to psychological well-being. Some people believe
active participation in the community through membership in social, civic, political, or
religious organizations is highly important to quality of life. Social participation may
also confer a high degree of emotional well-being, particularly for people who do not
have close family or friendship ties.

Social ties provide psychosocial and instrumental support to people with disabilities
(Morgan, 1989). Psychosocial support derived from social contact provides sympathy,
encouragement, and a sense of self-esteem, whereas instrumental support may take the
form of practical assistance, financial aid, advice, and guidance. The latter are particularly important for those who require assistance with daily living activities. Social ties
may be particularly important influences on survival, on recovery, on the course of
disease, and on other health outcomes (Kasl, 1983). In this sense, social support is a
predictor of social well-being, along with other aspects of health-related quality of life.

Social Contact

Social contact—the frequency of visits with friends or relatives, the number of meetings and community activities attended, or types of social interaction—is another well-
recognized component of social well-being (Donald and Ware, 1982). The importance
of social contact for different components of health status has not been systematically
determined. Mental health outcomes have, however, been implicated most frequently
(Brownell and Shumaker, 1984). The absence of a close, confiding relationship is an
important influence on depression, particularly in women (Brown and Harris, 1978;
Brown et al., 1987).

Social isolation and feelings of loneliness are particularly important for seriously ill
persons. The histogram in Figure 4.7 illustrates the aggregate social isolation score on
the Nottingham Health Profile for patients before and after human heart transplantation. The social isolation items consist of five statements concerning contact, social
relationships, intimacy, loneliness, and feelings of burden. The actual statements in
this domain and the weights applied to them are also presented in the figure. Patients
answered "yes" or "no" to each statement, and a domain score was calculated for each
patient and for the overall group; lower scores indicate lower dysfunction.

This figure shows that the social isolation of these patients increased before transplant. Sharp improvement occurred three months after the transplant operation, and
this improvement appears to be maintained thereafter. These data suggest that life-
threatening illness and life-sustaining treatment have significant effects on social well-
being. Family support programs such as transplant groups and individual counselling
are interventions designed to address the social isolation of seriously impaired persons.

Intimacy

Some people in an individual's network may provide a feeling of closeness and trust.
Such intimacy can be an important determinant of emotional well-being in patients
facing serious illness or death. Social contact and intimacy, of course, are not mutually
exclusive; both can be provided by the same person or persons in a social network.

Sexual function and dysfunction are important concepts of social functioning that
seldom appear in national health surveys or in national data sets obtained through

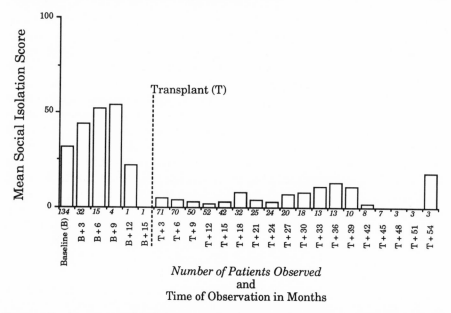

Figure 4.7 Average social isolation scores by three-month periods on Nottingham Health Profile for patients before and after heart transplant. The social isolation score is derived from respondents' answers to five yes/no statements. Each statement has been assigned a weight using the paired-comparisons scaling techniques developed by Thurstone. The maximum dysfunction score adds to 100. The five social isolation statements and their associated weights are as follows:

I'm finding it hard to get on with people	15.97
I'm finding it hard to make contact with people	19.36
I feel there is nobody I am close to	20.13
I feel lonely	22.01
I feel I am a burden to people	22.53
Total	100.00

Source: Adapted from O'Brien et al., 1988.

government funds. Those who object to including sexual questions on a survey often cite embarrassment on the part of respondents, biased answers, and interviewer sensitivity to asking the questions. Although questions concerning sex elicit refusals or result in missing data more than other survey questions, sensitive interviewing and well-constructed questionnaires can minimize missing data.

Sexual function or dysfunction can be assessed using a variety of measures, although the assessment of human sexual function is hindered by a surprising paucity of brief, self-report measures with reported reliability and validity (Conte, 1986). One comprehensive and thoroughly evaluated measure of sexual function is the Derogatis Sexual Function Inventory (DSFI) (Derogatis, 1980). As the term "inventory" implies, the DSFI provides operational measures of 10 constructs obtained from 245 different items: sexual knowledge, sexual behavior, drive, attitudes, psychologic symptoms, affect, gender identity, sexual fantasy, body image, and satisfaction. Test–retest reliabilities range from 0.42 to 0.96, and internal consistency reliability coefficients range from 0.56 to 0.97. Similar psychometric properties have been reported for the Brief Sexual Function Questionnaire (BSFQ), a 21-question self-report inventory of male sexual functioning based on the four domains of sexual activity/performance, interest, satisfaction, and physiological competence (Reynolds et al., 1988).

Often social networks or the availability of social support are considered as concepts and indicators of social function. Particularly in assessing social function, it is important to maintain the distinction between determinants of health-related quality of life and the terminal value assigned to the outcomes of these determinants. Thus distinctions should be made (1) among subjective perceptions, social behaviors, and external circumstances; (2) between social networks, social support, and their outcomes; and (3) between the quantity and quality of social ties. The concept and domains of social function remain ambiguous primarily because measurement has preceded development of an adequate conceptual framework.

As described in Chapter 5, many generic and composite measures of health-related quality of life include domains of social function. Among them are the Health Utilities Index, the Sickness Impact Profile, the Short-Form Health Survey, and the Nottingham Health Profile. These measures assess social function by measuring number and perceived quality of social contacts with family and friends, participation in community activities, and/or sexual activity.

HEALTH PERCEPTIONS

Szalai (1980) points out that when someone asks "How are you?" he or she is, in effect, asking for a personal judgment on your quality of life. That subjective judgments of life quality are made every day emphasizes the saliency and importance of the concept of health perceptions, although how these overall evaluative judgments are made is not well understood. For one person the evaluation may vary in different life situations; likewise, two people may evaluate a similar life situation in vastly different ways. Subjective judgments, however, capture both the personal evaluative nature of health and the more positive aspects of the quality of life.

General Health Perceptions

The measure of subjective health status most often used is *self-rating* of health: "excellent," "very good," "good," "fair," and "poor." Such judgments are considered ratings because they reflect individual differences in evaluating health. Self-assessed health status, like more comprehensive and lengthy measures of general health perceptions, include the individual's evaluation of physiologic, physical, psychological, and social well-being and the effect of health on other aspects of life such as opportunity and respect (Davies and Ware, 1981).

Perceived health is an indicator of the value of medical care in reassuring patients and reducing uncertainty. Self-ratings are important predictors of mortality, even after controlling for physical health status at baseline (Mossey and Shapiro, 1982; Idler and Kasl, 1991). The predictive power of self-evaluations of health status go above and beyond the contribution to prediction made by indexes based on the presence of health problems, physical disability, and biological or lifestyle risk factors. Thus, self-evaluations appear to have an independent ability to predict an individual's survival.

There are no straightforward explanations of why self-evaluations of health status predict future mortality. Sufficient studies and methodological evaluations have been conducted to suggest that the association is *not* a spurious one or a methodological artifact. Perhaps self-perceptions affect survival because they affect later health status; perhaps global health ratings are, in some way, expressions of expectations for personal survival (Idler and Kasl, 1991). Regardless of the precise explanation, what people perceive and report about their health clearly has importance for the respondents themselves and for those to whom these evaluations are given.

General population surveys conducted for the National Center for Health Statistics have included self-ratings of health since 1970. The original four-point scale of "excellent," "good," "fair," or "poor" was recently expanded to include a fifth point, "very good," in order to provide a finer classification of well people at the positive end of the health continuum. Adding this fifth category does not affect responses to the "fair" or "poor" categories.

The distribution of rating responses to this single question varies according to the placement of the question in the National Health Interview Survey schedule (Danchik and Drury, 1985). Single-item self-assessed health status is highly associated with many other aspects of an individual's health status and use of health care services. The item should be placed either at the beginning of the questionnaire or at the very end. Other health status questions such as symptom checklists should not be placed directly before self-ratings of health. In 1990, almost 70 percent of the noninstitutionalized American population rated their health as excellent or very good (Adams and Benson, 1991). As shown in Figure 4.8, self-assessment of health status differs by color. Black persons are more likely to rate their health as "fair" or "poor" than are their white American counterparts.

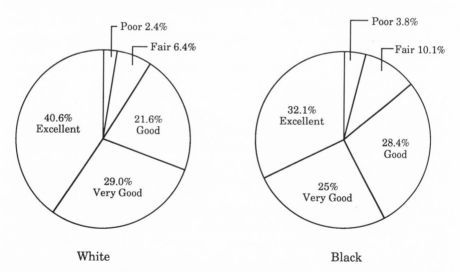

Figure 4.8 Self-assessment of health by color, United States, 1990. *Source*: Adams and Benson, 1991, Table 70.

Because this single-item rating of general health has been shown to be an important indicator of subjective health status, developers considered it desirable to explore this domain of health in further detail. The General Health Perceptions Scale, developed by Davies and Ware (1981), is one approach for obtaining more information about an individual's self-perception of health. These general health rating items score six dimensions: (1) past health, (2) current health, (3) future health, (4) health-related worries and concerns, (5) resistance or susceptibility to illness, and (6) the tendency to view illness as part of life. The instrument is easy to administer and has been tested for validity, reliability, and generalizability (Ware, 1984b).

Satisfaction with Health

The satisfaction derived from activities, relationships, moods, or other states of being is a pivotal concept in health-related quality of life. The level of satisfaction explains how people behave, make choices, communicate with professionals, follow treatment regimens, or accept the inevitable (Najman and Levine, 1981). The concept of satisfaction implies that quality of life is a mixture of the individual's objective resources, behaviors, and affects, and of his or her subjective satisfaction with those resources, behaviors, and affects. Satisfaction is a measure of the extent to which an individual's needs or aspirations are fulfilled. Only the person with a need can experience the actual satisfaction of that need (Hornquist, 1982).

Researchers agree that major categories of life needs include material, physical, psychological, social, and spiritual well-being. The individual must have a sense of satisfaction with personal access to the total environment, education and training, and employment. Little is known about the relationship of need satisfaction to other health-related quality of life outcomes. Some evidence suggests that lower levels of functional status are not necessarily correlated to lower levels of satisfaction and vice-versa (Patrick, Danis et al., 1988).

Satisfaction is an elusive concept that raises many methodological and theoretical problems. This is particularly true in comparison to related concepts such as happiness and morale. Campbell, (1981) stated that "there is no doubt that happiness and satisfaction have something in common [but] there is also a difference." Satisfaction, in his view, involves an act of judgment and is not the "spontaneous lift-of-the-spirits" that characterizes happiness. All three concepts have been distinguished by Stones and Kozma (1980): life satisfaction is "gratification of an appropriate proportion of the major goals of life," happiness is "an activity or state in the sphere of feelings," and morale is a "moral condition as regards discipline and confidence." Whereas these conceptual differences can be debated at length (George and Bearon, 1980), satisfaction can be viewed as a discrete and important domain of health-related quality of life.

Life satisfaction measures have been used most widely in gerontologic studies (Neugarten et al., 1961; George, 1981; George and Landerman, 1984). Satisfaction with *health*, however, has been a general health status concept proposed in several previous classifications of health outcome variables (Sanazaro, 1965; Shapiro, 1967; Starfield, 1974).

Figure 4.9 shows how respondents participating in the General Social Survey evaluated satisfaction with their "health and physical condition" between 1972 and 1991. The General Social Survey questionnaire is administered by the National Opinion

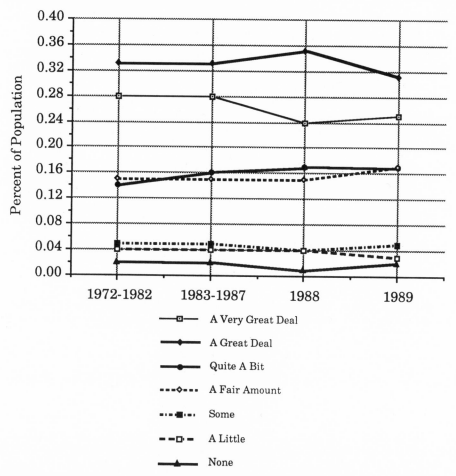

Figure 4.9 Satisfaction with health and physical condition, General Social Survey, United States, 1972–91. *Source*: National Opinion Research Center, 1991.

Research Center to national samples using a standardized questionnaire. The major goal of the Survey is to function as a social indicator program using items that have appeared in previous national surveys. As shown in Figure 4.9, over half the respondents to these surveys indicate "a very great deal" or "a great deal" of satisfaction with their health and physical condition. Less than 5 percent of the sample indicated "none" or "a little" satisfaction over the 17-year period.

OPPORTUNITY

Opportunity is defined as the potential for an optimal state of health or "being all that one can be." Opportunity is integral to many definitions of life quality. Calman (1984) suggests that quality of life is the difference between the hopes and expectations of the individual and the individual's present experience. In other words, quality of life is an assessment of potential for growth or improvement. Capacity or potential, an elusive concept to measure, can be viewed both in the negative term of disadvantage and the positive term of resilience.

Social or Cultural Disadvantage

A major social principle for people with disease, impairments, or disabilities is that all aspects of life should be accessible to them. These aspects include physical and social access to the environment, to education and training, and to employment. People with a disease or disability who are denied opportunities to acquire or use the fundamental elements of living that are generally available in a community experience a disadvantage. For example, patients with chronic renal failure who require dialysis may find it difficult to obtain or keep employment. People with congenital heart disease, a history of rheumatic fever, or following a regimen of steroid drugs may find it difficult or impossible to get life insurance or to meet premium requirements. Patients with moderate impairment may also experience difficulty in meeting eligibility requirements for disability income maintenance through social insurance programs.

Disadvantage is a social and cultural phenomenon. Health disadvantage is assessed in relation to people who do not have a particular condition or significant illness. Disadvantage can be affected by a disease, its treatment, or environmental factors. For example, vocational disadvantage because of health may depend not only on the individual's impairment and dysfunction but also on employers' attitudes, the demands of the job, availability of employment, and the range of vocational options. These factors, in turn, depend on age, intelligence, emotional stability, education, and past work experience.

Disadvantage is most often assessed indirectly. The analyst must estimate three values:

1. What is the social norm or average status of the group to which an individual belongs? For example, what is the employment rate of persons age 45–64 in a particular society?
2. Which individuals have health problems or disabilities that prevent them from achieving this norm? That is, who is prevented from working or limited in the kind or amount of work done?
3. What opportunities are available for achieving the normative status? What employment is available to people with and without disabilities? What is the ratio of labor force participation for the two groups?

Analysts can use questions from the monthly Current Population Survey conducted by the United States Census Bureau to assess the work disability status of persons in particular age, color, and gender groups. As shown in Figure 4.10, work disability rates for males increase with age. The rate of work disability for men 50–54 years of age has increased since 1970, suggesting that more males are leaving the work force for reasons of health. A possible explanation for the significant decrease in the rate for males age 65–69 between 1980 and 1990 is the change in definition of major activity that occurred in the National Health Interview Survey in 1982–83 (see footnote in Figure 4.5).

Adults with a work disability who are looking for work but unable to find it are

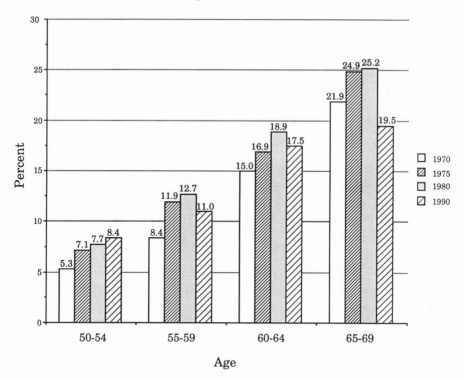

Figure 4.10 Percentage of males, for selected age groups, reporting inability to work because of health, United States, 1970, 1975, 1980, and 1990. *Source*: National Center for Health Statistics, Current Estimates from the *National Health Interview Survey, United States, Vital and Health Statistics*. Unpublished data.

difficult to identify using such data. The health researcher can more directly locate those unable to obtain employment, education, housing, or insurance because of health by conducting community surveys or examining eligibility or waiting lists. More direct approaches are needed to assess the opportunity of individuals and groups with health-related problems. Although many previous health status surveys have included restrictions in work activity or limitations in performing work roles, they have not routinely asked about the inability to obtain a job because of health. The following questions would be useful additions to health surveys: Are you able to work but unable to obtain a job due to your health? Are you unable to read or to obtain an education due to your health?

The domain of social and cultural disadvantage also includes the concepts of *social reaction* and *stigma*. The personal identity of persons with health conditions may be "discredited" by the negative responses of others. People with disabilities have described repeatedly the guarded references, changes in social relationships, and negative reactions of others to the "differentness" of disability. Being in a wheelchair, speaking with a slur, having a facial disfigurement, having cancer, and behaving "inappropriately" are among the many different health states that arouse curiosity, fear, pity, and a host of emotional and social reactions.

Goffman (1963) suggested the term "spoiled identity" to describe the potentially negative influence that societal stigmatization can have on one's self-image. The effects of stigma on the persons affected are rarely assessed directly. Instead, we rely on measures of attitudes toward people with disabilities and evaluations of physical access and environment to infer the disadvantage experienced by people of different abilities or behaviors. Nevertheless, stigma and the disadvantage that arises therefrom are important concepts and domains of health-related quality of life.

Individual Resilience

Opportunity can also be viewed as resilience or the capacity for health. Here resilience is defined as a desirable deviation from expected or usual functions, activities, or perceptions that constitute daily life. The definition of opportunity as resilience is consistent with the concept of physiologic reserve (Patrick and Bergner, 1990). Physiologic reserve is the unused capacity of the organism that can be called upon in times of stress, crisis, or increased activity. It decreases with age regardless of an individual's overall health. Individuals differ in their levels of physiologic reserve. Some of these differences may be genetic in origin; some may result from health-promoting states, interventions, or behaviors.

Unfortunately, physiologic reserve, in its positive sense, is difficult to observe or assess. We assume this reserve exists in people who resist or recover rapidly from stress or illness. However, we have no reliable way to estimate the reserve before the stress or illness passes. It is somewhat safer to estimate physiologic reserve by examining health decline. For example, we know that individuals with immunosuppressive diseases have poor physiologic reserve, as do those who are sedentary or obese.

Researchers face similar prediction problems when they assess health-related quality of life in terms of resilience. Capacity for health or resilience is most often measured by the ability to cope with or withstand stress or to maintain emotional equilibrium. This approach recognizes that people adjust differently to life situations altered by disease or treatment. Qualitative methods are often used to describe the dimensions of coping or adaptation.

The Ways of Coping Scale (Folkman et al., 1986) is one example of a quantitative measure. It consists of 66 items concerning a wide range of thoughts and acts used to deal with internal and external stress. Eight scales can be derived from responses to these items: confronting coping, distancing, self-controlling, seeking social support, accepting responsibility, escape-avoidance, planful problem solving, and positive reappraisal. Although resilience is a difficult domain to assess because capacity is neither directly observable nor easily reported, coping behavior and adaptive tasks are nevertheless important to health maintenance with or without disease and illness (Moos, 1977).

OTHER RELEVANT CONCEPTS AND DOMAINS

Duration of life, symptoms/impairments, functional status, perceptions, and opportunity are the core concepts of health-related quality of life found in current measures, including those used in the Health Resource Allocation Strategy. No single measure can begin to cover all the domains and indicators for these five organizing concepts. Even with this broad conceptual canvas, other concepts and domains can be relevant to the health-related quality of life of all persons and to specific populations and applications.

Selected concepts and domains outside the core have potential significance for new research directions and conceptualization of health-related quality of life. These concepts—dependency on persons or machines, meaning and purpose of life, and spiritual well-being—concern states of health and quality of life of particular relevance to persons undergoing serious illness, receiving life-sustaining treatments, or experiencing death. These concepts are also relevant to well persons but are often not assessed formally or routinely in general populations.

Confrontation with death—whether through disease, treatment, or contemplation—often gives new meaning to everyday activities and experiences. Persons confronting death and those loved ones and others around them may define the broader area of quality of life and the narrower area of health-related quality of life differently from those not yet facing imminent death. Thus, quantity and quality of life are viewed through different lenses.

People have long recognized that death sometimes may be preferable to a life of constant pain or suffering. They often make tradeoffs between quality and quantity of life using domains of the five core concepts to decide when the anticipated benefits of life prolongation are small and the marginal costs are high. As discussed more fully in Chapter 6, several researchers have observed that there are states of health-related quality of life that some people consider worse than death, such as unbearable pain, persistent coma, and severe cognitive deficit (Rosser and Kind, 1978; Pauker et al., 1981; Torrance, 1986). These states are described by the most severe level of the domains of symptoms and cognitive functioning. Other domains, however, may be identified in making decisions concerning the relative value placed on extending life versus immediate death.

Dependency on Persons and Machines

Modern medicine has enjoyed considerable success in averting the death of many people who encounter life-threatening diseases and injuries. For example, transplantation of the kidney, liver, and heart have extended the lives of many persons experiencing end-stage disease. Kidney dialysis has improved the prospects of many with renal failure; the artificial heart is in rapid development and should be available by the turn of the century. Infants born with serious birth defects or under 1,000 grams in weight did not survive in earlier decades, whereas today these severely impaired and low birth weight babies are being saved in neonatal intensive care nurseries across the country.

Survival often depends on high-technology medicine and/or the availability of relatives and others willing to provide the support necessary to undergo treatment and to prolong survival. Willingness to depend on others to provide care is one consideration mentioned in patients' decisions to undergo life-sustaining treatments and to prolong survival (Danis et al., 1988). Whether on "caregivers" or on "machines," the affected person is dependent.

Caregiver burden and the quality of life of those who support seriously impaired and disabled persons are areas of enquiry on their own (Thompson and Doll, 1982; George and Gwyther, 1986). Caregivers have been shown to have low morale and to be angry, sad, depressed, and tired much of the time.

In a study of the development and potential use of the artificial heart (Hogness and Van Antwerp, 1991), dependency on medical device technology was considered as particularly significant to the patient's quality of life. The artificial heart *replaces* rather than *assists* a natural organ, and the organ replaced is highly symbolic in American culture. The experience of a machine heart may raise some of the more philosophical aspects of health status such as "the whole person" or the separation of mind, body, and soul, as well as the feeling of emotions symbolized as being centered in the natural heart.

Dependency on persons can perhaps be encompassed in definitions of social well-being. Dependence on technology, on the other hand, may be a new area of enquiry with important relevance to the allocation of resources. The value placed on the extension of life with machine dependency deserves further consideration and enquiry.

Meaning and Purpose of Life

When faced with serious illness, people may find the value they place on different aspects of life shifting. Holding a job or being useful to others may no longer be necessary to define quality of life. An overriding emphasis may be given to personal dignity and the sense that life has meaning under any and all conditions (Frankl, 1990). Some individuals may have this sense of personal dignity throughout their lives; others tend to develop it or become more aware of it when experiencing physical or emotional trauma. Meaning and purpose of life have been recognized as being important considerations to life quality, but more work is needed on conceptualization and measurement.

A Meaning in Life Scale (ML) has been developed to allow patients to report their assessment of the worth of life remaining (Warner and Williams, 1987). Items in this measure cover domains included in existing instruments such as "being around people" (social contact), "coming to terms with illness" (coping), and "doing things for myself" (physical function). Other concepts concern more abstract and philosophical notions such as "will to live," "philosophy of life as a guide," and "looking forward to each new day." Some items concern spiritual well-being, another domain of potential relevance to all persons and particularly the seriously ill.

Spiritual Well-Being

The concepts of religion, religiosity, and spirituality have been distinguished by researchers (Ellison, 1983; Blazer, 1991). Health-related quality of life may be affected by religious beliefs, and spiritual well-being itself may be a significant domain for different people and treatment groups.

Spiritual well-being, from an ecumenical perspective, is the "affirmation of life in relationship with a God, self, community, and environment that nurtures and celebrates wholeness" (defined by the national Interfaith Coalition of Aging and quoted in Blazer, 1991, p. 62). Blazer proposes other domains of spiritual well-being to include self-transcendence (the crossing of a boundary beyond the self to a sense of the spirit of the universe), self-determined wisdom (possessing knowledge that integrates and stabilizes the person in the context of his or her physical and sociocultural environment), and acceptance of the totality of life (taking comfort in all experiences of one's unique life and having no despair). These domains are particularly relevant to older adults, although they may also hold significance for persons facing imminent death and for persons whose values center on a religious or spiritual life.

The concepts of meaning and purpose of life and spiritual well-being share common ground with the core concept of opportunity or the difference between what one values and the potential for obtaining or realizing it. As Abraham Maslow (1943) defined it, the process of "self-actualization," or becoming all that one is capable of becoming, is an important human need that may describe an individual's health-related quality of life.

Further conceptualization of health-related quality of life is likely to focus on individualistic and introspective domains as discussed here and social and cultural domains related to disadvantage and social well-being. Where "health" begins and ends in quality of life considerations will be argued, and the distinction between quality of life and its determinants will be blurred. Health and quality of life are ancient concepts that find new meaning and definitions for each generation of thinkers, researchers, and the public at large. Our continued efforts to define, classify, and measure will undoubtedly add both confusion and clarity to our understanding.

CLASSIFYING HEALTH STATES

The Health Resource Allocation Strategy is based upon a classification system encompassing all mutually exclusive states of interest. Appendix I contains the classification systems used in the Disability/Distress Index, Health Utilities Index, Quality of Well-Being Scale, and EuroQol Index. The content of these four systems varies according to the number of organizing concepts included and the domains covered within the concepts.

Disability/Distress Index

Rosser and colleagues in England (Rosser and Watts, 1972; Rosser and Kind, 1978; Rosser, 1983b; Rosser, 1990) developed an operational definition of health status, originally in an attempt to measure the performance of hospitals. The researchers asked a group of doctors to describe various illnesses. Next the doctors were asked to describe the criteria they used to decide on the severity of a patient's illness, considering only the present state of the patient. Two principal components of severity emerged from these discussions: observed *disability* (loss of function and mobility) and subjective *distress*. All other conditions were included within this framework. This descriptive system was then used to classify 40 patients. Further refinement was made after discussion with the doctors.

A second group exercise was conducted with economists and health administrators.

Participants were asked to recall two individuals they considered to be ill and two individuals they considered healthy. The most frequently cited characteristics were disability (impaired mobility and function) and distress (pain). Rosser concluded that both medical and nonmedical groups supported similar classification systems.

The resulting classification, reproduced in Appendix I, consists of 8 classes of disability and 4 classes of distress totaling 32 possible classes. One class is the absence of disability and distress. This class is not necessarily equated with perfect health. It distinguishes between the observable state of the patient's disability and his or her subjective feelings of distress. The original disability/distress states were redefined later as 175 combinations of disability, discomfort, and distress. Rosser and colleagues are currently preparing a more elaborate instrument called the Index of Health-Related Quality of Life (IHQL) that subsumes all possible combinations of 107 descriptors (Rosser, personal communication).

Health Utilities Index

Torrance and his colleagues at McMaster University (Torrance et al., 1972; Torrance, 1984; Drummond et al., 1987) developed a health state classification system to be used for program planning and resource allocation. This multiattribute system evolved over time; different classifications have been used for specific applications. Appendix I contains a classification system for people two years old and over. It includes the four domains of mobility and physical activity, social-emotional function well-being, role function (self-care and *role activity*), and health problems. This classification was originally developed for the economic evaluation of neonatal intensive care (Boyle et al., 1983) and later modified slightly for use in the general population (Drummond et al., 1987).

The Health Utilities Index classification system has six levels of mobility and physical function and five levels of self-care and role activity. Each level defines functional abilities and the need for help to perform daily activities. Four levels of *emotional well-being* and *social activity* are used. Emotional well-being is defined in terms of happiness, anxiety, and depression; social activity is defined by number of friends and contacts with others. Eight health problems are included ranging from minor physical deformity to loss of the sense of sight, hearing, or speech.

Recently, the Health Utilities Index classification system has been expanded to encompass nine health domains. These include vision, hearing, speech, ability to get around, use of hands and fingers, feelings, memory, thinking, and pain and discomfort. These nine domains are used in an interviewer-administered survey conducted in 60,000 households in Ontario, Canada, in 1990 (Ontario Ministry of Health, 1990). This health status survey will permit comparisons of general status between different sections of the population—geographical areas, age, gender, socioeconomic status, and the like.

Quality of Well-Being Scale/General Health Policy Model

Bush and colleagues developed a health state classification system for the New York State Health Planning Commission under PL 93-641, the Comprehensive Health Planning Act. The system was to be used for health planning and resource allocation. It consists of a comprehensive construct of health status and includes two components: (1) level of well-being and (2) prognosis (Fanshel and Bush, 1970; Patrick et al., 1973a). "Well-being" represents health-related quality of life and is comprised of 23 broad symptom–problem complexes combined with three attributes or domains of *function status*. This classification system for the Quality of Well-Being Scale is presented in Appendix I.

The symptom–problem complexes in the Quality of Well-Being Scale were based on the method of symptom description developed by White and Murnaghan and on a symptom checklist used by the Brown University Population Laboratory (White and Murnaghan, 1969; Organic and Goldstein, 1970; Patrick, 1972). These complexes do not explicitly indicate diagnosis, severity, or prognosis; rather, each complex relates to multiple health conditions. The complexes cover a variety of illness experiences, body systems, and risk factors ("overweight for age and height" and "breathing smog or unpleasant air"). The number of psychological and mental symptoms is lower than the number of physical symptoms. Psychological function was not included as a domain because of lack of consensus on a "normative" standard of mental health (Patrick, 1972).

The three attributes were based on variables used to describe function status in standard information-gathering mechanisms in the late 1960s. The two primary data sources were the National Health Interview Survey conducted by the National Center for Health Statistics and the Survey of the Disabled administered by the Social Security Administration (Haber, 1970; National Center for Health Statistics, 1970). In addition, the following community health and social surveys were examined: the Alameda County Population Laboratory, the Washington Heights Community Master Sample Survey, and the Brown University Population Laboratory (Hochstim, 1964; Gell and Elinson, 1969; Organic and Goldstein, 1970). The variables selected to describe function status were body movement, travel and confinement, and major activity. Body movement refers to walking, standing, stooping, sitting, or other physical movements of the trunk and extremities. Travel and confinement refer to the range and freedom of travel from one place to another. Major activity represents the activities usual for a person's age and social role.

EuroQol Instrument

Recently the EuroQol Group, a consortium of investigators in Western Europe, conducted postal surveys in England, the Netherlands, and Sweden using 14 different health states classified using a system with 6 domains: mobility, self-care, main activity, social relationships, pain, and mood (EuroQol Group, 1990; Brooks et al., 1991; Nord, 1991). The resultant descriptive system defines a theoretical universe of 216 states. The classification system was developed through review of existing classification systems. The EuroQol group intend to refine this instrument based on the experience of using it in different European countries. It is likely that other classification systems will be developed by various groups in the future to meet the needs of clinical and policy decision making.

Which definition of health-related quality of life to adopt and which concepts and domains to include in a particular inquiry usually depend on the following: the objectives of measurement, the political motives of funding sponsors, and the particular concerns of the users, including patients, clinicians, researcher, and policy analysts. The content of commonly used measures are examined in Chapter 5. These measures are introduced and described as part of a taxonomy of health-related quality of life assessment.

5

Types of Health-Related Quality
of Life Assessments

During the last three decades, researchers developed many measures to assess the concepts, domains, and indicators of health-related quality of life defined in Chapter 4 (Rosser, 1983a). Four of these measures—Disability/Distress Classification, Health Utilities Index, Quality of Well-Being Scale, and EuroQol Instrument—have been applied in the Health Resource Allocation Strategy (see Appendix I). Many additional measures are used in health decision making. Epidemiologic and clinical investigations, population monitoring, program evaluations, and resource allocation have been conducted with a wide array of health status and quality of life measures. In this chapter we present a taxonomy of these measures to help investigators select the one or more measures most appropriate to meet their objectives in health-related decision making and research.

A TAXONOMY OF HEALTH-RELATED QUALITY OF LIFE MEASURES

The taxonomy of health-related quality of life measures shown in Table 5.1 can be used to select measures according to the application and objectives of assessing health status and quality of life. The measures are classified according to (1) the type of scores produced, reflecting the level of aggregation across concepts and domains; (2) the range of populations and concepts/domains covered, including the different diseases, health conditions, and populations to be assessed and the breadth of concepts and domains included in the measure; and (3) the weighting system used in scoring items and in aggregating different domains (Guyatt, Veldhuyzen Van Zanten et al., 1989). The strengths and weaknesses of each type are summarized to help the user make selections among those measures available in each category.

Decision makers and analysts should first identify the health decision or problem, stakeholders in the decision, and the objectives of measurement. With this information, they can then identify the desired characteristics of existing measures to be included in the health-related quality of life assessment. The health decision or research problem dictates which measurement characteristics and types of measures are needed. Most health related quality of life assessments follow directly from the statement of the problem and purpose of assessment.

Table 5.1 provides a means for identifying these characteristics. For example, monitoring the health-related quality of life of populations and communities demands

Table 5.1 A taxonomy of health-related quality of life measures

Measure	Strengths	Weaknesses
Types of Scores Produced		
Single **indicator** number	Represents global evaluation	May be difficult to interpret trends
	Useful for population monitoring	May not be responsive to change
Single **index** number	Represents net impact	May not be possible to disaggregate contribution of domains to the overall score
	Useful for cost effectiveness	
		May not be responsive to change
Profile of interrelated scores	Single instrument	May not be responsive to change
	Contribution of domains to overall score possible	Length may be a problem
		May not have overall score
Battery of independent scores	Wide range of relevant outcomes possible	Cannot relate different outcomes to common measurement scale
		May need to adjust for multiple comparisons
		May need to identify major outcome
Range of Populations and Concepts		
Generic: applied across diseasees, conditions, populations, and concepts	Broadly applicable	May not be responsive to change
	Summarizes range of concepts	May not have focus of patient interest
	Detection of unanticipated effects possible	Length may be a problem
		Effects may be difficult to interpret
Specific: applied to individual disease, condition, population, or concept/domain	More acceptable to respondents	Cannot compare across conditions or populations
	May be more responsive to change	Cannot detect unanticipated effects
Weighting system		
Utility: preference weights from patients, providers, or community	Interval scale	May have difficulty obtaining weights
	Patient or consumer view incorporated	May not differ from statistical weights that are easier to obtain
Statistical: items weighted equally or from frequency of responses	Self-weighting samples	May be influenced by prevalence
	More familiar techniques	Cannot incorporate tradeoffs
	Appears easier to use	

global evaluations across a number of conditions and different age, gender, and ethnic groups. The evaluator may want a single indicator or index number to describe the health status of the population being assessed. This indicator could be obtained by using a generic measure weighted by assigning social preferences or by using statistical weighting. Cost–utility analyses of different interventions require a single index number obtained from a generic measure that is preference weighted. Epidemiologic investigations commonly include a battery of independent scores, often using specific measures that are weighted statistically.

Table 5.1 can be used in the selection process for primary or secondary analyses. Sources of information about different health-related quality of life measures are listed in Appendix II. Because developers tend to change instruments and measures over time, questionnaires and scoring instructions should be obtained directly from the developers. Their addresses are listed in the compendiums and monographs in Appendix II or in current journal articles on progress in measurement development.

INDICATORS, INDEXES, PROFILES, AND BATTERIES

The first way to classify health-related quality of life measures is by the number and range of scores they produce for analysis and interpretation of effects. The type of score reflects both the metric used in scoring each component domain of the measure and the level to which concepts and domains are aggregated. Measures may produce (1) a single number obtained from a single item (indicator); (2) a single number summarizing multiple concepts or a classification of health-related quality of life (indexes); (3) multiple numbers on the same metric (profiles); or (4) multiple numbers on different metrics (batteries).

Single indicators cover one concept or domain, such as a visual analogue pain scale, limitation in usual social role activity, or self-rating of health. *Health status indexes* are expressed as single aggregated numbers summarizing multiple domains similar to the consumer price index (CPI). The term *health profile* refers to those measures in which each domain is assigned a summary score on a metric that can be compared with other domains. Health profiles may also provide an overall or index score that summarizes all component domains. *Health batteries* are collections of different health status and quality of life measures that are scored independently using different metrics and reported as individual scores.

Single Indicators

Single indicators may be used to assess any one of the five broad concepts or domains of health-related quality of life. The mortality rate is the one most frequently used. Commonly used single indicators of impairment and function are counts of diseases or medical conditions and restricted-activity, bed days, and work-loss or school-loss days. Traditionally used measures of the incidence or prevalence of specific diseases can also be considered single indicators. In population surveys single indicators are obtained most frequently from single-item questions, from a series of questions on a single topic, or from checklists of acute or chronic conditions and impairments.

Reports of symptoms are important single indicators of health-related quality of life. Standardized symptom classification schemes have recently been developed as alternative coding schemes, and these are becoming more widely used (National Center for Health Statistics, 1979). A single question concerning "reason for visit" is included on the patient record forms in the National Medical Care Ambulatory Survey. It asks the Patient's Principal Problem(s), Complaint(s), or Symptom(s) this visit (in patient's own words). Participating physicians list the most important reason and other reasons for a sample of patients seen during a randomly assigned week of practice.

The reason-for-visit classification in the National Ambulatory Medical Care Survey uses a modular structure that categorizes patients' reasons into seven modules: symptoms, diseases, diagnostic/screening/preventive, treatment, injuries/adverse effects, test results, and administrative. The symptom model contains complaints, symptoms, or problems grouped by body systems with a general symptoms section for those symptoms that cannot be assigned to a body part or system. Distinguishing which of these reports are symptoms or diseases is a tenuous and difficult problem. The reason-for-visit classification generally includes reasons as symptoms rather than diseases.

Table 5.2 shows the ten most important symptoms included in the reason-for-visit classification by age groups and gender. Not surprisingly, commonly reported reasons for medical care visits for all age groups, but particularly for children under 5 years, are symptoms of upper respiratory infections and gastrointestinal problems. Skin conditions are important for adolescents and young adults, while headache and back symptoms are common reasons for visit among persons 25–64 years of age. In older adults, symptoms related to aging such as vision, chest pain, and leg symptoms are commonly reported. Because the perception of symptoms is important in determining illness behavior, many health-related quality of life assessments should contain checklists of commonly reported symptoms or symptoms related to the specific condition or treatment under evaluation.

The incidence of acute conditions has been published annually for the United States since 1957, and no long-range patterns or trends have occurred; over this time interval, the reported level of all acute conditions has been approximately 180 for 100 persons each year. In contrast, the prevalence of most fatal diseases and some prominent nonfatal diseases has increased for a variety of reasons (Wilson and Drury, 1984; Verbrugge, 1989). Morbidity has increased for fatal diseases such as diseases of the heart, diabetes, and cerebrovascular disease as well as for nonfatal diseases such as arthritis and musculoskeletal conditions.

The rapid decline in mortality accounts for some of this trend; a larger percentage of persons are surviving with chronic conditions over their lifetime. Some of this increase can be attributed to the increase of chronic conditions contained in the lists used in the National Health Interview Survey. Asking respondents about more conditions has resulted in a marked increase in reporting conditions that in the past were not always volunteered by respondents. Greater use of health services in which conditions may be diagnosed and more willingness to report chronic conditions may also contribute to the increase. Also, aging of the population may account for a "true" increase in the prevalence of morbidity.

Single-item disability measures are used to assess the impact of both acute and chronic illnesses. Measures of mobility and activity limitation are often used to assess the long-term impact of chronic illness. Disability days alone, however, are questionable indicators of health status change attributable to shifts in the prevalence of either acute or chronic conditions. During the past three decades, the proportion of persons with long-term limitation of activity due to chronic illness has increased markedly (Wilson and Drury, 1984). A number of competing hypotheses may explain this increase.

One explanation is that changing attitudes toward disability and sickness, as well as increasing attention to health and illness in our society, make people more willing to label themselves as "disabled." Another is that increased disability benefits encourage people to leave the work force because of their "disability." Yet another explanation

Table 5.2 Leading symptoms reported as reasons for visit to physicians in the National Ambulatory Medical Care Survey by age and gender, 1985

Males			Females		
Rank	Symptom		Rank	Symptom	
		Under 5 years			
1.	Cough	15.0	1.	Cough	15.0
2.	Fever	14.1	2.	Fever	13.9
3.	Nasal congestion	9.0	3.	Nasal congestion	8.4
4.	Earache, ear infection	7.7	4.	Earache, ear infection	7.8
5.	Head cold, upper respiratory infection	6.8	5.	Head, upper respiratory infection	7.4
6.	Other ear-related symptoms	5.1	6.	Skin rash	5.0
7.	Skin rash	4.3	7.	Vomiting	4.0
8.	Diarrhea	3.3	8.	Other ear-related symptoms	3.0
9.	Vomiting	3.2	9.	Throat-related symptoms	3.5
10.	Throat-related symptoms	3.2	10.	Diarrhea	3.5
11.	All other symptoms	28.3	11.	All other symptoms	27.7
		5–24 years			
1.	Throat-related symptoms	10.4	1.	Throat-related symptoms	11.1
2.	Cough	6.3	2.	Cough	6.3
3.	Earache, ear infection	5.0	3.	Earache, ear infection	5.0
4.	Fever	4.9	4.	Fever	4.3
5.	Acne or pimples	4.0	5.	Headache, pain in head	3.3
6.	Skin rash	3.8	6.	Skin rash	3.0
7.	Headache, pain in head	3.6	7.	Acne or pimples	2.7
8.	Nasal congestion	3.2	8.	Nasal congestion	2.6
9.	Allergy (not otherwise specified)	2.9	9.	Abdominal pain, cramps, spasms	2.6
10.	Knee symptoms	2.5	10.	Head cold, upper respiratory infection	2.5
11.	All other symptoms	53.4	11.	All other symptoms	56.6
		25–44 years			
1.	Back symptoms	5.2	1.	Headache, pain in head	4.3
2.	Throat-related symptoms	3.8	2.	Throat-related symptoms	4.1
3.	Cough	3.4	3.	Back symptoms	3.4
4.	Skin rash	3.3	4.	Abdominal pain, cramps, spasms	3.2
5.	Headache, pain in head	3.0	5.	Cough	3.0
6.	Low back symptoms	2.9	6.	Depression	2.9
7.	Knee symptoms	2.8	7.	Anxiety, nervousness	2.7
8.	Depression	2.7	8.	Neck symptoms	2.1
9.	Chest pain or related symptoms	2.5	9.	Nasal congestion	1.9
10.	Neck symptoms	2.2	10.	Vaginal symptoms	1.9
11.	All other symptoms	68.2	11.	Skin rash	1.9
			12.	All other symptoms	68.6
		45–64 years			
1.	Chest pain and related symptoms	4.4	1.	Cough	3.8
2.	Back symptoms	4.3	2.	Back symptoms	3.4
3.	Cough	3.6	3.	Headache, pain in head	3.0
4.	Vision dysfunction	3.1	4.	Abdominal pain, cramps, spasms	2.9
5.	Leg symptoms	3.1	5.	Anxiety and nervousness	2.8
6.	Shoulder symptoms	3.0	6.	Vision dysfunction	2.8

(continued)

Table 5.2   *(Continued)*

Males			Females		
Rank	Symptom		Rank	Symptom	
7.	Knee symptoms	2.6	7.	Leg symptoms	2.4
8.	Headache, pain in head	2.6	8.	Chest pain and related symptoms	2.3
9.	Neck symptoms	2.5	9.	Depression	2.3
10.	Abdominal pain, cramps, spasms	2.2	10.	Knee symptoms	2.2
11.	All other symptoms	68.6	11.	All other symptoms	72.1
		65+ years			
1.	Leg symptoms	4.2	1.	Vision dysfunction	5.0
2.	Cough	4.0	2.	Vertigo, dizziness	4.0
3.	Vision dysfunction	3.9	3.	Leg symptoms	4.0
4.	Chest pain and related symptoms	3.2	4.	Chest pain	3.2
5.	Shortness of breath	3.2	5.	Cough	3.1
6.	Back symptoms	2.9	6.	Back symptoms	3.0
7.	Vertigo, dizziness	2.6	7.	Shortness of breath	2.4
8.	Abdominal pain, cramps, spasms	2.5	8.	Abdominal pain, cramps, spasms	2.2
9.	General weakness	2.3	9.	Abnormal sensations of the eye	2.1
10.	Skin lesions	2.1	10.	General weakness	2.1
11.	All other symptoms	69.1	11.	All other symptoms	68.9

Source: National Ambulatory Medical Care Survey, 1985 (unpublished data).

attributes the increase to variations in health services use and susceptibility to age-related and environmental influences outside the health sector. Modifications to questions about activity limitations may also contribute to increased reporting of activity limitations. While the evidence to support one or more of these hypotheses is lacking, the fact remains that reports of both chronic conditions and disability are increasing at the end of the twentieth century.

Single indicators are useful for comparing different populations within a single country or across countries. International comparisons in health status are made most frequently using single indicators of mortality such as life expectancy and infant mortality. Less use has been made of self-assessments of health and disability indicators such as limitations in major activity due to chronic conditions. These single indicators are most useful in more developed countries where chronic disease contributes most to the pool of morbidity and causes of mortality.

Another reason for the continued use of single indicators is that they are sensitive to inequities among different population groups. Excess mortality among minority groups, that is, more deaths than would be expected if these groups had the same age and gender-specific death rates as the nonminority population, is used in planning interventions to close the gap. Deaths from cancer, cardiovascular disease and stroke, chemical dependency (cirrhosis), diabetes, and homicide and injuries are leading causes of excess mortality observed among black persons and other groups (Department of Health and Human Services, 1985). Single indicators, however, are not the most sensitive measures of population "health" and "well-being" because each assesses only one domain of health. As a result, *composite* measures (indexes, profiles, or batteries) that cover more detailed health states and aspects of well-being have been developed to detect health changes and to classify individuals.

It is difficult to incorporate all the domains of survival, impairment, functional status, perceptions, and opportunity into a single composite measure. As discussed in Chapter 1, the concept of "quality of life" can embody many facets of objective and subjective life, sometimes arousing our deepest fears as well as our strongest aspirations. Many persons continue to resist the idea that "health" or "quality of life" can be captured in a single number or that such notions can be measured at all.

Indexes

Over the past three decades, researchers have worked to combine mortality with other measures of health-related quality of life to form health status indexes. Sullivan (1966) was among the first to identify the conceptual and methodological problems in developing health status indexes. Sanders (1964) proposed combining measures of "functional adequacy" (the number of days each year individuals could fulfill their social roles) with mortality rates to create a modified life table. In reviewing data from Kit Carson County, Colorado, Sanders noted that although the community had higher than national estimates for many chronic diseases, traditional health status indicators suggested that health care needs were being met. For example, death rates for all diseases were lower than the national averages when adjusted for differences in age and gender. These lower rates raised the question of whether additional health care would reduce the prevalence of chronic conditions.

Thus, Sanders saw the use of life table methodology as one way of allowing health professionals to assess mortality and morbidity simultaneously. Sanders proposed a measure of "effective" life years that reflects the current health of the population in terms of mortality and the effects of morbidity. Although Sanders did not work out this method in detail, his idea of combining these data through survival analysis or life table procedures led to further efforts to develop single indexes of health. Linder (1966), as director of the National Center for Health Statistics, called for an overall index of health similar to the gross national product. The proposed "gross national health deficit" was to blend disability days with days of life lost through death and/or lack of intervention.

For the Indian Health Service, Miller (1970) developed the Q index for ranking diseases affecting the American Indian and Alaska Native population according to potential response to intervention and days lost due to premature death, hospitalization, and clinic visits. The index is expressed as

$$Q = MDP + 274 \frac{A}{N} + 91.3 \frac{B}{N}$$

where

Q = a numerical index for the program priority of a given disease
M = age- and sex-adjusted disease-specific mortality rates for the target population (American Indians and Alaskan Natives) as a ratio to the same rates for the U.S. population
D = crude disease-specific mortality rates for the target population

P = years of life lost because of premature death

274   = 100,000/365, a conversion factor to convert A to years per 100,000 population

A = number of inpatient days due to the disease

N = target population

91.3 = 274/3, a conversion factor weighting an outpatient visit as a loss of one-third of an inpatient day (3 outpatient visits are equated in time to 1 hospital day), to convert B to years per 100,000 population

B = number of outpatient visits due to the disease

When the Q index was computed for each of 17 classes of disease affecting American Indians and Alaska Natives (Miller, 1970), the five most important classes, in order of their importance, were as follows: (1) accidents, poisonings, and violence; (2) infective and parasitic diseases; (3) diseases of the respiratory system; (4) diseases of the digestive system; and (5) symptoms and ill-defined conditions. The computed Q values correlated closely with professional judgments of Indian Health Service administrators on the impact of disease upon the target population. Miller concluded that the Q index was a valuable tool for the political process of determining program priorities.

The Q index was one of the first single indexes to use existing data, a significant advantage in index construction. Although the index excluded a wide number of concepts and the method for combining the different concepts into a single score was atheoretic, this index was among the first to demonstrate the possibilities that indexes have for assisting in the selection of health programs and for program budgeting. Chen (1973, 1976) constructed a number of similar indexes to quantify unnecessary disability and death.

Research sponsored by the National Center for Health Statistics contributed to the creation of a national health index. Chiang (1965) proposed a technique for combining mortality and morbidity rates into a single index based on mathematical models of illness frequency, illness duration, and mortality. This single-index technique made an important contribution to the development of composite measures: it weighted the rapidity with which individuals in various health states returned to a state of perfect health. These weights could be obtained from incidence rates calculated from national population surveys.

Sullivan (1971) was the first to apply Sanders's suggestion and demonstrate the usefulness of a concept of combined mortality and morbidity that fulfilled the desirable properties of a composite measure as recommended by Moriyama (1968). Sullivan described two related indexes based on a life table model: the expectation of life free of disability and the expectation of disability.

These indexes are computed by subtracting the duration of bed disability and inability to perform major activities from life expectancy using data collected from the National Health Interview Survey. Based on a 1965 current life table, the average life expectancy at birth was 70.2 years. Adjusting this for time lost due to disability, where all types of disability were assigned a weight of 1.0, Sullivan estimated that a person born in 1965 would have 64.9 years of life free of disability and 5.3 years with disability.

Figure 5.1 compares ordinary and disability-free life expectancies by color and

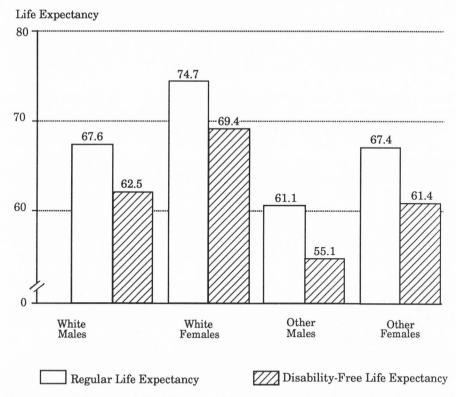

Figure 5.1 Ordinary and disability-free life expectancies by color and gender, United States, mid-1960s. *Source*: Sullivan, 1971.

gender for the United States population in the mid-1960s. Sullivan used this mortality/morbidity index to demonstrate that whites and females have greater expectation of life free of disability than nonwhites and males. The gap between life expectancy and adjusted life expectancy tended to be smaller for whites than for nonwhites. Therefore, life expectancy on its own does not provide a picture of the morbidity experience of a particular population cohort during its lifetime. By combining mortality experience with disability, Sullivan paved the way for the current notions of "years of healthy life" and "active life expectancy." Based on Sullivan's approach, estimates of disability-free life years have been made for France and Canada (Wilkins and Adams, 1983; Colvez and Robine, 1986).

Chen and Bush (1979) criticized the crude mortality and morbidity indexes proposed by Sanders and Sullivan on the grounds that these indexes assume that disability states are equally undesirable. Chen and Bush maintained that the indexes lacked sufficient discriminatory power, policy relevance, explicit value weights, and the ability to incorporate transition probabilities among states other than death. For example, limitation in amount or kind of major activity—work, school, or play—is considered to have the same value of dysfunction as being unable to perform that same activity. Disability-free life years do not take into account preferences for different states of health-related quality of life. These indexes remain important, however, because they adjust survival time for the "quality" of that survival time in the most complete specification of health-related quality of life.

The four classifications and resulting measures that make the Health Resource Allocation Strategy operational are indexes that combine duration of survival as modified by other domains of health-related quality of life. The Disability/Distress Index, Health Utilities Index, Quality of Well-Being Index/General Health Policy Model, and EuroQol Instrument produce a single index score that summarizes different health status and quality of life domains. The summary score is obtained by applying preference weighting strategies to each item or domain contained in the index. These preference-weighting strategies are described in Chapter 6.

Profiles

Not all developers or consumers of health and quality of life data accept the need for or desirability of summarizing health into a single index number. Like the gross national product, a single health index cannot be a wholly comprehensive measure. Unless the analyst can ascertain the relative contribution of different domains to the overall index score, changes or trends in the index value are difficult to interpret.

For some purposes decision makers may need specific social indicators of different domains of health and quality of life to characterize individuals and populations. For example, decision makers may be interested in evaluating the relative impact of a treatment or intervention on different domains of health and quality of life. They can use a battery or profile of different health measures or a profile of interrelated components as an alternative to the aggregated index.

Several health profiles have been developed to cover many of the domains of health-related quality of life in a systematic and unified manner. The Sickness Impact Profile (SIP) assesses sickness-related dysfunction in 12 different areas of activity, as shown in Table 5.3. The SIP was developed to provide a measure of perceived health status sensitive enough to detect changes or differences in health status that occur over time or between groups (Bergner et al., 1981). The SIP was designed to be broadly applicable across types and severities of medical conditions and across demographic and cultural subgroups. The measure can be administered by an interviewer in 20 to 30 minutes, or it can be self-administered.

Table 5.3 also contains selected statements or items from the SIP. These items were derived from open-ended descriptions of behavioral dysfunction given by patients, health care professionals, individuals caring for patients, and people who considered themselves "healthy" (Gilson et al., 1975; Bergner, Bobbitt, Kressel, et al., 1976). In completing the SIP, respondents are asked to endorse or check only those statements that describe them and are related to their health. A preference-weighting technique from psychology (category scaling as described in Chapter 6) was applied to develop a scoring method that assigns scale values to each item.

Responses to the 136 items are used to produce a percentage score for each of the 12 categories. In addition to a profile of the 12 scores, the SIP produces a physical dimension score combining body care and movement, ambulation, and mobility; a psychosocial dimension score combining emotional behavior, affective behavior, social interaction, and communication; and an index score across all 12 categories. Percent-

Table 5.3 The Sickness Impact Profile: Categories, dimensions, and selected statements

Dimension	Category	Items describing behavior related to	Selected statements
Independent	SR	Sleep and rest	I sit during much of the day.
			I sleep or nap during the day.
	E	Eating	I am eating no food at all, nutrition is taken through tubes or intravenous fluids.
			I am eating special or different food.
	W	Work	I am not working at all.
			I often act irritable toward my work associates.
	HM	Home management	I am not doing any of the maintenance or repair work around the house that I usually do.
			I am not doing heavy work around the house.
	RP	Recreation and pastimes	I am going out for entertainment less.
			I am not doing any of my usual physical recreation or activities.
Physical	A	Ambulation	I walk shorter distances or stop to rest often.
			I do not walk at all.
	M	Mobility	I stay within one room.
			I stay away from home only for brief periods of time.
	BCM	Body care and movement	I do not bathe myself at all but am bathed by someone else.
			I am very clumsy in body movements.
Psychosocial	SI	Social interaction	I am doing fewer social activities with groups of people.
			I isolate myself as much as I can from the rest of the family.
	AB	Alertness behavior	I have difficulty reasoning and solving problems, for example, making plans, making decisions, learning new things.
			I sometimes behave as if I were confused or disoriented in place or time, for example, where I am, who is around, directions, what day it is.
	EB	Emotional behavior	I laugh or cry suddenly.
			I act irritable and impatient with myself, for example, talk badly about myself, swear at myself, blame myself for things that happen.
	C	Communication	I am having trouble writing or typing.
			I do not speak clearly when I am under stress.

Source: Bergner et al., 1981.

age scores can be obtained for each of these components—categories, dimensions, or the overall measure—by summing the scale values endorsed in each component, dividing by the sum of the values of all items in the component, and multiplying by 100.

A major strength of the Sickness Impact Profile is its broad coverage of health-related quality of life domains and its sensitivity to a wide variety of health conditions. A British-English version of the Sickness Impact Profile, renamed the Functional Limitations Profile, is available (Patrick, 1979; Charlton et al., 1983; Patrick and Peach, 1989). The Functional Limitations Profile (FLP) includes preference weights for the 136 items obtained from a British population (Patrick et al., 1985). Similar dimension scores and overall score can also be computed for this British version.

The Nottingham Health Profile (NHP), patterned originally after the SIP, is a two-part instrument. Part I contains 38 items that cover six domains of experience: pain, physical mobility, sleep, emotional reactions, energy, and social isolation. Items were weighted using the preference-weighting technique of paired comparisons (see Chapter 6). Scores can be calculated for each of these domains, although no overall index score can be obtained since preference weighting was applied within domains but not across domains. Part II of this profile includes perceived problems in seven areas of life: paid employment, jobs around the house, personal relationships, social life, sex life, hobbies, and holidays (Hunt et al., 1980).

The Nottingham Health Profile has been used widely in evaluating health interventions and in clinical studies, primarily in Britain and Western Europe. The measure has been used, among other applications, to study quality of life following myocardial infarction (Wiklund et al., 1989), combined heart and lung transplantation (O'Brien et al., 1988), hyperbaric oxygen therapy for multiple sclerosis (Monks, 1988), onset of arthritis of the hip joint (Wiklund et al., 1988), migraine headaches (Jenkinson, 1990), joint pain (Parr et al., 1989), stroke (Ebrahim et al., 1986), and irritable urethral syndrome (O'Dowd et al., 1986). Other studies have shown that the Nottingham Health Profile is sensitive in determining variations within and between illness groups (Jenkinson et al., 1988). The NHP has been translated into many different languages, some versions of which have undergone extensive cultural changes and validation (Alonso et al., 1990).

Another well-known and widely used health profile is the short-form health survey (SF-36) developed from measures used in the Health Insurance Experiment (Brook et al., 1979) and applied in the Medical Outcomes Study (MOS) to investigate the outcomes of medical care for different conditions (Stewart et al., 1989). Table 5.4 lists the concepts and domains included in the revised 36-item MOS short-form health survey along with sample questions.

Physical, social, and role functioning scales measure behavioral dysfunction caused by health problems. Subjective measures of well-being include mental health, energy/fatigue, and bodily pain. Overall evaluation of health is captured in the six-question general health perceptions scale. The short-form health survey can be self-administered in approximately three minutes. A new version of the instrument can be administered and scored using an optical character reader. This scanner is connected to a small computer that computes the profile of scores and compares the current scores with previously obtained scores. Population norms can also be included in the computer data base for comparison with individual scores (Ware, personal communication).

These questions and scales in the short-form health survey are scored in two steps: (1) questionnaire items are recoded, if necessary, and (2) items in the same scale are combined to score that scale. Unlike the Sickness Impact Profile and Nottingham Health Profile, all items in the current version of the Medical Outcomes Study short-form health survey are weighted equally using the simple sum of recoded item scores. All seven short-form health survey measures produce profile scores ranging from 0 to 100, with higher scores indicating better health. A physical and psychosocial dimension score can be computed. Studies to supply preference weights for these 36 items are under way.

Table 5.4 Concepts and questions from the Medical Outcomes Study 36-Item
Short-Form Health Survey (SF-36)

Health-related quality of life concepts	Number of items	Selected questions
Physical functioning	10	Does *your health* limit you in these activities? If so, how much?
		vigorous activities, such as running, lifting heavy objects, participating in strenuous sports
		walking *more than a mile*
		bathing or dressing yourself
Role limitations	7	During the *past 4 weeks,* have you had any of the following problems with your work or other daily activities as a result of your physical health? . . . as a result of any emotional problems?
		cut down the *amount of time* you spent on work or other activities
		accomplished less than you would like
		had *difficulty* performing the work or other activities (for example, it took extra effort)
Social functioning	2	How much of the time, during the past month, has your *health limited your social activities* (like visiting friends or close relatives)?
Bodily pain	2	How much *bodily* pain have you had during the *past 4 weeks?*

Concepts and domains of health-related quality of life	Number of items	Selected items
General mental health	5	How much of the time during the *past month*
		have you been a very nervous person?
		have you been a happy person?
		have you felt downhearted and blue?
Vitality	4	did you feel full of pep?
		did you feel tired?
General health perceptions	6	In general, would you say your health is "excellent," "very good," "good," "fair," or "poor?"
		Please choose the answer that best describes how *true* or *false* each of the following statements is for you.
		I seem to get sick a little easier than other people.
		I am as healthy as anybody I know.
		My health is excellent.

Source: Ware, 1992.

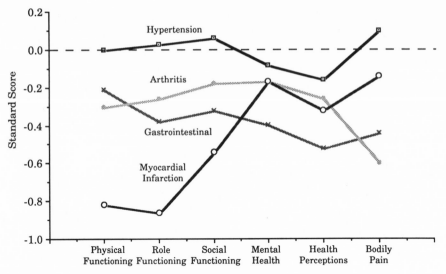

Figure 5.2   Health profiles for patients with four common conditions from Medical Outcomes Study. The mean health scores for each chronic condition group and for the group with no chronic conditions are standardized. The difference between each chronic condition group and patients with no chronic conditions (deviation score) was divided by the standard deviation for the total sample for each health measure. *Source*: Stewart et al., 1989.

Figure 5.2 shows the standardized scores from a 20-item version of the short-form health survey for four common conditions from the Medical Outcomes Study in contrast to each other and in relation to the group with no chronic conditions. These conditions are hypertension, myocardial infarction, gastrointestinal problems, and arthritis. The mean on each health measure for patients with no chronic conditions is set at 0.

Standardized scores are plotted in Figure 5.2 in terms of their difference from the group with no chronic conditions, controlling for the effects of other chronic conditions and sociodemographics. Physical functioning was worst for patients who had a myocardial infarction and best for hypertensive patients. Health perceptions were poorest for patients with gastrointestinal disorders and best for patients with hypertension. Role functioning varies greatly across these four chronic conditions. Bodily pain was worst for patients with arthritis and best for hypertensive patients. These findings emphasize the usefulness of comparing different conditions using a profile of health status scores based on a common metric. Analyses and implications of MOS baseline data are available in Stewart and Ware (1992).

A number of investigators have adopted an alternative, circular format for presenting profile data on health-related quality of life (Ware, personal communication; Tibblin et al., 1990; Gundarov, 1991). This circular presentation is sometimes referred to as the "rose of quality of life." With this rose, each domain of health-related quality of life is depicted as a radius of a circle. The lowest values of each scale, usually scored as zero, are placed at the center of the circle; the highest values, usually scored as 100, are placed on the circle.

Scores for each domain are plotted on their respective radii and the points connected to form an inner geometric figure that represents health-related quality of life. If all of the scores to the individual domains represented in the rose are equal, then the inner figure will be another circle. More likely, the scores will vary, forming an irregularly shaped figure. The larger the inner figure, the higher the quality of life of either the individual or group of individuals being assessed. This graphical summary of the multiple domains included in a health profile is a succinct and intuitively appealing way of representing health-related quality of life.

Batteries

The battery approach refers to collections of specific measures that are scored independently and reported as individual scores (Patrick and Erickson, 1988). Batteries are common in clinical trials and epidemiologic investigations. Entire scales, subscales, or individual items from the best available instruments are administered and effects are tested for each measure in the battery.

Major examples of the battery approach are the health status measures contained in the national surveys conducted by the National Center for Health Statistics (NCHS). Table 5.5 lists the concepts, domains, and measures of health-related quality of life included in various sections of recent NCHS surveys organized according to our schema of concepts, domains, and indicators. Supplements to the National Health Interview Survey (NHIS) have included an even broader array of concepts and measures. Recent supplements have addressed child health (1988); health insurance, immunizations, mental health, dental health, diabetes, orofacial pain, and digestive disorders (1989); health promotion and disease prevention, podiatry, hearing, assistive devices, income, and AIDS knowledge and attitudes (1990) (National Center for Health Statistics, 1989–1991). Supplement topics for 1991 were objectives for the year 2000: hearing, drugs (marijuana and cocaine), immunization and infectious diseases, nutrition, tobacco and alcohol use, environmental health, unintentional injuries, heart disease and stroke, pregnancy and smoking, child health, AIDS knowledge and attitudes, and income. Topics for 1992 are cancer control and epidemiology, family resources, childhood immunization, AIDS knowledge and attitudes.

The NHIS has contained primarily self-reported measures of impairment and functional status, but the National Health and Nutrition Examination Surveys (NHANES) have covered a broad range of concepts using measures obtained both from health examination and interview-administered questionnaires. Early NHANES surveys focused on estimates of disease incidence and prevalence in the United States; later surveys include data on functional status, perceptions, and opportunity. Questions in the current NHANES (1987–93) include a wide range of concepts and domains of health-related quality of life. The emerging focus on psychological and social function indicates recognition by NCHS that these domains are important to include in combination with the more traditional domains of physical function and impairment.

The battery approach, as illustrated by these national survey measures, does not yield an overall score for summarizing overall effects or provide any indication of the relative importance of each domain of health-related quality of life, which would permit intermeasure comparisons. To overcome these problems, data from batteries of independent measures can be used to develop profiles with all domains being measured

Table 5.5 Concepts, domains, and measures of health-related quality of life included in previous National Center for Health Statistics surveys

Concepts and domains	NHIS, 1991[a]	NHANES, 1988–94[b]	NHEFS, 1987[c]
Opportunity			
Social or cultural disadvantage			
Resilience		+	+
Health perceptions			
General health perceptions	+	+	+
Satisfaction with health			
Functional status			
Social function			
Limitations in usual social roles	+	+	+
Integration		+	
Contact		+	
Intimacy and sexual function		+	
Psychological function			
Affective	+	+	
Cognitive		+	
Physical function			
Activity restrictions	+	+	+
Fitness	+	+	+
Impairment			
Symptom/subjective complaints	+	+	+
Signs	+	+	+
Self-reported disease	+	+	+
Physiologic measures	+	+	
Tissue alterations			
Diagnoses			
Death and duration of life			+

[a] National Health Interview Survey.
[b] National Health and Nutrition Examination Survey–III.
[c] National Health and Nutrition Examination Survey–1 Epidemiologic Follow-Up Study.

on the same scale. In one example, Testa and colleagues (1989) developed a profile measure from the battery of measures used in the original evaluation of antihypertensive agents reported by Croog et al. (1986). Testa and colleagues selected 10 of the 20 scales contained in the original quality of life assessment and used statistical techniques to produce a shortened version with all measures on the same scale or metric.

Composite measures, whether combining mortality with other domains or aggregating negative and positive domains, can play an important role in allocating resources and evaluating treatments. Cost–effectiveness analyses require some index or overall outcome measure for calculation of the cost–effectiveness ratio. Cost–utility analyses require an index that incorporates utilities or preference weights.

At the practical level, single indicators, profiles, and batteries may permit analysis of individual domains of health-related quality of life, both as independent and dependent variables in causal structures, for example, the relative impact of a lack of social resources on physical, psychological, or social functioning. Composite measures are most useful for comparing the outputs of different treatments and for comparing the results of health interventions on different populations. Users should be able to analyze all composite measures of health or quality of life by their constituent domains to consider the contribution of each concept or domain to any overall score that is created.

GENERIC AND SPECIFIC MEASURES

A second way to classify health-related quality of life measures is by the range of populations to which the measures are applied and the range of concepts and domains included in the measure. Increasing knowledge and use of health status and quality of life assessments have spawned a debate over the relative merit of generic versus disease-specific measures. *Generic health status measures* are designed to be broadly applicable across types and severities of disease, across different medical treatments or health interventions, and across demographic and cultural subgroups. These measures are also designed to summarize a spectrum of core concepts of health and quality of life that apply to many different diseases, impairments, conditions, patients, and populations.

Specific health status measures are those designed to assess specific patient populations or diagnostic groups or individual concepts and domains. *Disease-specific measures* are applied to specific diseases or health conditions, such as arthritis, chronic obstructive pulmonary disease, or inflammatory bowel disease. Disease-specific measures are often developed with the goal of detecting minimally important changes in condition-specific health-related quality of life in longitudinal studies or clinical trials. *Minimally important changes* are changes in health or quality of life that clinicians and patients think are discernible and important, or that have been detected with an intervention of known efficacy, or are related to well-established physiological measures (e.g., grip strength for arthritis patients or spirometry for those with chronic obstructive lung disease).

Not all specific measures are disease-related. *Domain-specific measures* may be designed to assess a specific condition or symptom (e.g., back pain or dyspnea) or specific domains (e.g., sexual or emotional function, general health perceptions). *Population-specific measures* address special populations usually defined by age or the combination of age and medical condition (e.g., older adults or developmentally disabled children).

Domain-specific measures of single concepts or conditions are the most numerous of all within the health status field. These single-concept measures range from the assessment of specific symptoms such as nausea and vomiting (Morrow, 1984) to more global concepts of life satisfaction (Patrick, Danis et al., 1988). Mental health measures of depression, anxiety, and other emotional states are frequently used in population-based surveys as well as clinical research for assessing individual concepts of psychological status.

Investigator preference for generic or disease-specific measures depends on the purpose and period of assessment. Investigators involved in clinical trials or clinical practice need outcome measures specifically tailored to the intervention under investigation or related to major clinical outcomes. The primary goal of these studies is to assess *within-subject* change in health status over two or more points in time. The ability to detect small changes is important in determining the statistical power of a trial and the sample size needed to detect a difference between the experimental and control groups.

Investigators conducting epidemiologic investigations or population-based studies may be primarily interested in *between-subject* or *group* differences, particularly in cross-sectional studies. Health-related quality of life measures may then be used as covariates in the analysis or as indicators of health risks. Discrimination between groups of respondents is therefore important.

Policy analysts involved in health services evaluation, resource allocation, or population comparisons over time may also be interested in health status change across large samples of different diagnostic groups. Comparisons across different diseases, populations, and interventions require uniform criteria for classifying populations into health states at a point in time. For policy studies, it is often important to distinguish differences between subjects; for clinical trials, it is important to note within-person changes. In epidemiologic investigations, it may be important to both discriminate between groups and assess changes over time in cohort studies or repeated cross-sectional investigations.

Generic Measures

Generic measures may provide operational definitions of several concepts summarized by a single index value or in a profile of interrelated scores. The Quality of Well-Being Scale (QWB), for example, has been applied to groups of patients with AIDS, cystic fibrosis, and arthritis (Kaplan et al., 1989) and population groups with different self-reported health conditions (Erickson et al., 1989). The Sickness Impact Profile has been used in the United States and abroad with a large number of different populations.

Figure 5.3 shows overall SIP percentage scores as reported in 27 different studies on population or patient groups with different medical conditions. These studies are arranged according to the overall SIP score plotted from minimal to maximal dysfunction (low to high scores). Most of the scores shown in Figure 5.3 are not standardized for age or sex, although all studies reported here were conducted with adults. Most obtained data from both men and women. The scores in Figure 5.3 obtained from clinical studies of treatment effectiveness are for patient or treatment groups *before* treatment.

Overall SIP scores for general populations of primarily well adults or those who have survived myocardial infarction or cardiac arrest are at the low end of the dysfunction continuum. Scores for patients with chronic debilitating illnesses such as rheumatoid arthritis, chronic pain, oxygen-dependent chronic obstructive pulmonary disease, or amyotrophic lateral sclerosis are considerably higher. When these cross-sectional samples are compared, the SIP appears to discriminate in expected directions among different populations and degrees of disease severity. The SIP has also been shown to be responsive to changes in functional status posttreatment.

The overall scores shown in Figure 5.3 summarize all 12 SIP categories. The profile of category scores is considerably different for different conditions. For example, the psychosocial categories contributed more to the overall score for ulcerative colitis and chronic pain, physical categories for rheumatoid arthritis, and eating behavior for moderately obese patients. The scores in Figure 5.3 are point-in-time samples.

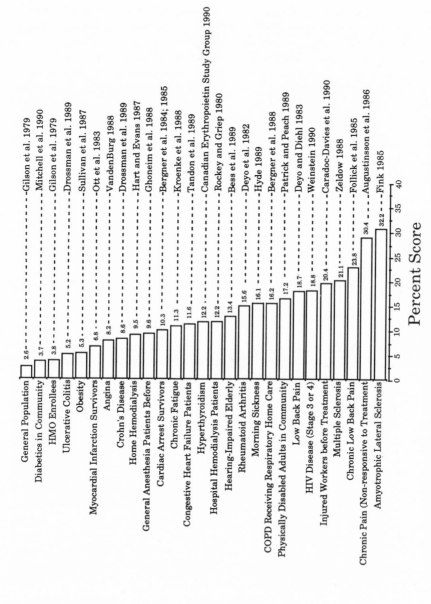

Figure 5.3 Applications of Sickness Impact Profile to different populations and medical conditions. See specific studies for estimates of confidence intervals.

Table 5.6 Major concepts of health-related quality of life contained in selected generic measures

Concept dimension	Generic measure					
	Disability/ Distress Index	Health Utilities Index	Nottingham Health Profile	Quality of Well-Being Scale	Short Form Health Survey (SF-36)	Sickness Impact Profile
Opportunity			+			
Health perceptions			+		+	+
Functional status						
Social		+	+	+	+	+
Psychological	+	+	+		+	+
Physical	+	+	+	+	+	+
Impairment		+		+	+	+
Death and duration of life	+	+		+		

Although the SIP has been used to assess change in many of these studies, SIP items do not measure prognosis for survival. Thus, patients with non–life threatening conditions such as moderate obesity or chronic pain may be more dysfunctional than survivors of myocardial infarction, even though their prognosis for survival may be higher.

Table 5.6 shows the five core concepts of health-related quality of life contained in six well-known generic measures. The functional status domains of physical, psychological, and social are also included, since these are central domains for most generic measures. The six measures listed in Table 5.6 cover different domains. All measures include physical function. Only the Nottingham Health Profile contains a measure of opportunity. The Quality of Well-Being Scale, the Health Utilities Index, and the Disability/Distress Index combine duration of life with specific domains of impairment, as well as physical, psychological, and social function. No measure contains all seven concepts of health-related quality of life.

Few measures combine the most negative domain (e.g., death) *and* the most positive domains and indicators at the upper end of the health-related quality of life continuum. Measures containing more positive or perceptual domains incorporate a time or a prognostic dimension because survival is not usually at stake with positive well-being.

Specific Measures

Disease-specific measures, such as the Karnofsky Performance Status Scale for cancer (Karnofsky et al., 1948; Karnofsky and Burchenal, 1949), the American Rheumatism Association (ARA) functional classification for arthritis (Steinbrocker et al., 1949), and the New York Heart Association Functional Classification (Criteria Committee, 1964) have been used extensively for several decades. These measures were developed to meet the need for rapid classification of patients and not necessarily to evaluate changes in functional status or other domains of health-related quality of life. Hence, the responsiveness or ability to detect small but minimally important changes is limited. The ARA classification, for example, may detect large changes such as those following hip replacement but miss smaller changes following drug therapy judged successful by other criteria (Deyo, 1984).

The popularity of disease-specific measures arises primarily from the need of researchers and decision makers to use scales that are most responsive to clinical changes over time (Deyo, 1984; Kirschner and Guyatt, 1985; Guyatt, Walter et al., 1987). For clinical research and practice, it is particularly important to discriminate between improved and unimproved patients and to measure accurately even minimally important changes.

Table 5.7 lists selected disease- or condition-specific measures and references for their development or application to each condition. We selected the most frequently referenced measures for areas where many alternatives exist, such as arthritis and cancer. Although sexually transmitted diseases were included in our review, we found few published references to disease-specific health-related quality of life measures for these conditions. Several measures for AIDS are under development.

Some measures shown in Table 5.7 cover specific conditions or impairments such as the Dyspnea Index (Mahler et al., 1984) and the Chest Pain Questionnaire (Rose, 1965). The Dyspnea Index includes a baseline measure and transition index for functional impairment as well as magnitude of task and effort needed to evoke breathlessness. The Rose Chest Pain Questionnaire was first developed as a diagnostic test to identify anginal pain with acceptable specificity and repeatability, although it has been used in trials of antianginal treatment (Bulpitt and Fletcher, 1987). Other disease-specific measures, such as the Health Assessment Questionnaire for arthritis (Fries et al., 1980) and the Quality of Life Index for cancer (Spitzer et al., 1981), are more "general." They include broader aspects of functional status with specific reference to states or changes of particular concern to patient populations. Generic measures and these disease-specific measures overlap considerably. The Arthritis Impact Measurement Scales (Meenan et al., 1980, 1982), for example, were adapted from early work on the Quality of Well-Being Scale (Patrick et al., 1973a) and the Health Insurance Experiment (Brook et al., 1979).

Although items concerning pain, discomfort, and functional status are often part of generic measures, disease-specific measures tend to use different wording for items and instructions tailored to the diagnostic group, condition, or population under investigation. Items in arthritis-specific measures, for example, may include the phrase "due to my arthritis." Cancer-specific measures include items on nausea and vomiting, common side effects of chemotherapy. Disease-specific measures may also have greater detail or more items concerning specific functions (e.g., fine hand manipulation in arthritis).

As mentioned previously in this chapter, not all specific measures are disease- or condition-specific. Some health status and quality of life measures apply to specific population groups. Two population groups—children/adolescents and older adults—deserve particular attention.

Child Health Status Measures

Much attention in the assessment of child health has focused on infant mortality and on birth weight. These two indicators are the only continuous source of information on

Table 5.7   Selected disease-specific measures of health status and quality of life

Diagnosis/condition	Measure	Reference
Alzheimer/dementia	Blessed Information-Memory-Concentration Score	Katzman et al., 1988
	Brief Cognitive Rating Scale	Reisberg et al., 1983
	Clinical Dementia Rating Scale	Hughes et al., 1982
	Dementia Mood Assessment Scale	Sunderland et al., 1988
	Dementia Rating Scale	Blessed et al., 1968
	Global Deterioration Scale	Reisberg et al., 1982
	Gottfries, Brane, and Steen Scale	Olafsson et al., 1989
	Mini-Mental State Examination	Folstein et al., 1975
	Progressive Deterioration Scale	DeJong et al., 1989
	Sandoz Clinical Assessment–Geriatric	Shader et al., 1974
	Short Portable Mental Status Questionnaire	Pfeiffer, 1975
Arthritis	American Rheumatism Association Classification	Steinbrocker et al., 1949
	Arthritis Impact Measurement Scales (AIMS)	Meenan, 1982; Meenan et al., 1992
	Functional Capacity Questionnaire	Helewa et al., 1982
	Health Assessment Questionnaire (HAQ)	Fries et al., 1982
	McMaster-Toronto Arthritis Patient Preference Disability Questionnaire (MACTAR)	Tugwell et al., 1987
	WOMAC (Western Ontario and McMaster universities)	Bellamy et al., 1990 Bellamy et al., 1988
Asthma	Asthma Symptoms Checklist	Brooks et al., 1989
	Living with Asthma Questionnaire	Hyland et al., 1991
	Quality of Life Questionnaire for Asthma	Townsend et al., 1991
	Simple Asthma Scales	Richards et al., 1988
Back pain	Manchester Back Pain	Million et al., 1982
	Oswestry Low Back Pain Disability Questionnaire	Fairbank et al., 1980
	Roland Scale	Roland and Morris, 1983
	Waddell Disability Index	Waddell and Main, 1984
Cancer	Breast Cancer	Coates et al., 1987
	Breast Cancer Chemotherapy Questionnaire	Levine et al., 1988
	CARES	Ganz et al., 1990
	EORTC—Quality-of-Life Questionnaire	Aaronson et al., 1991
	Functional Living Index: Cancer	Schipper et al., 1984
	Karnofsky Performance Status Measure (KPS)	Karnofsky et al., 1948, 1949
	Quality of Life Index (QL-Index)	Spitzer et al., 1981
	Questionnaire for Patient Self-administration—Lung Cancer	Kaasa et al., 1988
	Rotterdam Symptom Checklist	De Haes et al., 1990
Diabetes	DCCT Questionnaire (DQOL)	DCCT Research Group, 1987
Digestive diseases	Ostomy Adjustment Scale	Burckhardt et al., 1989
	Rating Form of IBD Patient Concerns (RFIPC)	Drossman et al., 1989
	Inflammatory Bowel Disease Questionnaire (IBDQ)	Guyatt et al., 1989a
Heart	Cardiac Follow-up Questionnaire	Wiklund et al., 1989
	Chest Pain Questionnaire	Rose, 1965

(continued)

Table 5.7 *(Continued)*

Diagnosis/condition	Measure	Reference
	Chronic Heart Failure Questionnaire	Guyatt et al., 1989b
	Karolinska-Erasmus Classification	Olsson et al., 1986
	Minnesota Living with Heart Failure Questionnaire	Rector et al., 1987a
		Rector et al., 1987b
	New York Heart Association Functional Classification (NYHA)	The Criteria Committee of the New York Heart Association, 1964
		Goldman et al., 1982
	QOL and Severe Heart Failure Questionnaire	Ringsberg et al., 1990
	Quality of Life Myocardial Infarction	Oldridge et al., 1991
	Specific Activity Scale (SAS)	Goldman et al., 1981
	Summary Index for Angina	Wilson et al., 1991
Neurological		
Head injury	Glasgow Outcome Scale	Jennet and Bond, 1975
	Modified Sickness Impact Profile	Temkin et al., 1989
Multiple sclerosis	Expanded Disability Status Scale (EDSS)	Kurtzke, 1983
	Minimal Record of Disability	Slater et al., 1984
Psychological/psychiatric	Beck Anxiety Inventory	Beck et al., 1988
	Beck Depression Inventory	Beck et al., 1961
	Center for Epidemiological Studies Depression Scale	Radloff, 1977
	General Health Questionnaire	Goldberg, 1972
	Geriatric Depression Scale	Yesavage et al., 1983
	Hamilton Rating Scale of Anxiety	Hamilton, 1959
	Hamilton Rating Scale of Depression	Hamilton, 1960
	Hospital Anxiety and Depression Scale	Zigmond and Snaith, 1983
	Montgomery-Asberg Depression Rating Scale	Dratcu et al., 1987
	Profile of Mood States	McNair et al., 1981
	Psychosocial Adjustment to Illness Scale	Derogatis, 1986
	Rosenberg Self-Esteem Scale	Rosenberg, 1965
	Self-Rating Anxiety Scale	Zung, 1971
	Self-Rating Depression Scale	Zung, 1965
	State Trait Anxiety Inventory	Speilberger et al., 1970
	Symptom Checklist (SCL-90)	Derogatis et al., 1973
Rehabilitation	Edinburgh Rehabilitation Status Scale	Affleck et al., 1988
	Level of Rehabilitation Scale	Carey et al., 1977
Respiratory	Bronchitis-Emphysema Symptom Checklist	Traver, 1988
	Chronic Respiratory Disease Questionnaire	Guyatt et al., 1987a; Guyatt et al. 1987b
	Dyspnea Index	Mahler et al., 1984
	MRC Chronic Bronchitis Questionnaire	Britten et al., 1987
Urological	Benign Prostatic Hyperplasia: Symptoms, Bothersomeness, and Activities	Epstein et al., 1991
	American Urological Association Symptom Index	Barry et al. (forthcoming)

child health status available across a wide geographical area and for different ethnic groups. Thus, they will continue to be important in assessing disparities in health status in different geographic regions and in different population groups.

Few measures have been designed to provide a generic profile or index of child health status. Rather, researchers and clinicians have developed a large number of measures that assess specific domains, diagnostic groups, or stages of development. The plethora of specific measures suggests that a single measure or group of measures may not satisfy all the purposes to which child health status assessment are put.

Developmental-specific instruments, such as the Denver Developmental Screening Test (Frankenburg and Dodds, 1967; Frankenburg and Camp, 1975) and Gesell Developmental and Neurologic Examination (Knoblock et al., 1980), assess the stages and progress of development of children in order to detect developmental disorders or delay. Specific developmental milestones are available for children ranging from one month to six years, while school performance, assumption of responsibilities, and physical maturation provide landmarks from age six. Measures based on these milestones are widely applied.

Domain-specific instruments measure particular aspects of child health. An example from the cognitive domain is the Stanford-Binet Intelligence Scale (Goldman et al., 1983) that is applied to individuals from two years through adulthood to evaluate general intelligence. It presents the individual a variety of tasks of known increasing difficulty. In the social and behavioral domains, researchers use the Child Behavior Checklist and Behavioral Profile developed by Achenbach and colleagues (Achenbach and Edelbrock, 1983) to detect mental health or behavioral problems. A large number of disorder-specific measures are available, such as those used for children with asthma, cerebral palsy, and cystic fibrosis. Again, these measures are applied widely to evaluate selected child populations.

Three measures are notable for being applicable to all children. They are the battery of scales put together for the 1988 Child Health Supplement of the National Health Interview Survey (U.S. Department of Commerce, Bureau of the Census, 1988), the Health Insurance Study child health measures developed by the Rand Corporation (Eisen et al., 1980), and the Functional Status II-R measure developed by Stein, Jessop, and colleagues (Lewis et al., 1989; Stein and Jessop, 1990). These instruments measure child functional status to assess the global impact of any disease, injury, or impairment.

The Child Health Supplement, for example, included the following questions specific to growth and development in all children ("Has _____ ever had a delay in _____'s growth or development?"), learning disability for children three years and above ("Has _____ ever had a learning disability?") and emotional and behavioral problems for children three years and above ("Has _____ ever had an emotional or behavioral problem that lasted three months or more?").

According to their parents, 4.0 percent of U.S. children (17 and older) have had a delay in growth or development, 6.5 percent (3–17) have had a learning disability, and 13.4 percent (3–17) have had an emotional problem that lasted three months or more or required psychological treatment (Zill and Schoenborn, 1990). Developmental, learning, and behavioral disorders are among the most prevalent chronic conditions of childhood and adolescence. Nearly 20 percent of young people ages 3–17 years were reported to have one or more of these conditions, and these conditions are associated with family disruption.

Most measures of child health capture domains defined by adults or practitioners, particularly those that use parents or teachers as respondents (Patrick and Bergner, 1990). Information on health status tends to fall into four major types: reports of specific health conditions, reports on symptoms whether or not associated with specific health conditions; reports on restricted life activities associated with health problems; and general and subjective measures of health (Fink, 1989). Not surprisingly, these domains are similar to those incorporated into adult health status measures.

Researchers have yet to test the content validity of a measure with children and adolescents, particularly young people from minority groups. Child health status measures, like all other measures of health-related quality of life, have to face the ultimate test of acceptability and usefulness to the major stakeholders: children, adolescents, parents, professionals, researchers, and decision makers.

Older Adults

Table 5.8 lists selected measures specific to older adults. Some measures, such as the Multidimensional Functional Assessment Questionnaire used in the Older Americans Resources and Services battery, are comprehensive and include most domains of health-related quality of life. Others, such as the often-used Index of Activities of Daily Living, cover the single domain of physical function, since these activities are central to the well-being of older adults. Life satisfaction is another concept developed originally with older adult populations because of the importance of this domain in later years of life.

Kane and Kane (1981) provide a comprehensive discussion of health and quality of life measures developed for older adults. They distinguish between instruments developed and used to provide a comprehensive assessment of clients for clinical decision makers and those applied in research and evaluations. In their words, "An all-purpose instrument can rarely be produced" (Kane and Kane, 1981, p. 248). Measures used in clinical settings with older adults need to be flexible, allowing practitioners to pursue in-depth domains of particular relevance to particular older patients. Ideal instruments show sensitivity to change, comprehensive coverage of both abilities and actual performance of behaviors, and acceptability to clients and providers. Furthermore, ideal measures provide for branching, that is, the use of short, portable screening questions that detect dysfunction that requires full-scale assessment. For example, a single question might be used to screen for the presence or absence of sleep problems in older adults. Respondents who indicate they have a sleep problem on this item would then complete a larger battery of items concerning different aspects of sleep dysfunction.

Measures applied in research and evaluation with older adults must emphasize data-collection modes that provide consistency in approaching respondents, in coding data, and in analyzing and interpreting results. Objective indicators of functional status, such as those provided by performance-based measures, are prized. Minimizing interviewer effects and respondent bias is essential. Discrimination among the subject population and the ability of the measure to assess stability over time are important features. Although the distinctions between client assessment and research applications may blur in actual use of instruments, selection of appropriate measures depends on the relative

Table 5.8   Selected measures of health-related quality of life specific to older adults

Measure	Reference
Comprehensive (include impairments)	
Comprehensive Assessment and Referral Evaluation	Gurland et al., 1977
Multidimensional Functional Assessment Questionnaire (MFAQ)	Pfeiffer, 1975
Multidimensional Observation Scale for Elderly Subjects (MOSES)	Helmes et al., 1988
Older Americans Resources and Services (OARS)	George and Fillenbaum, 1985
Physical function	
Activities of Daily Living (ADL) Scales	
Barthel Index	Mahoney and Barthel, 1965
Index of ADL	Katz and Apkom, 1976
Index of Activities of Daily Living Scale	
Functional Status Index	Jette and Deniston, 1978
Philadelphia Geriatric Center Instrumental Activities of Daily Living (PGC-IADL)	Lawton and Brody, 1969
Physical Self-Maintenance Scale (PSMS)	Lawton and Brody, 1969
Emotional function	
Memorial University to Newfoundland Scale of Happiness (MUNSH)	Kozma and Stones, 1980
Philadelphia Geriatric Center Morale Scale	Lawton, 1972
Social function	
Social Disability Questionnaire	Branch and Jette, 1981
Life satisfaction (perceptions)	
Life Satisfaction Index	Neugarten et al., 1961
Perceived Quality of Life Scale	Patrick et al., 1988

emphasis of different types of measures and their ability to meet the major objectives of the user.

Generic and Specific Measures

Four different approaches to the use of generic and disease-specific measures seem relevant: (1) use of both generic and disease-specific measures with overlapping concepts and domains in the same study; (2) comparison of a generic instrument to a generic instrument modified for a specific population; (3) addition of a condition-specific supplement to a generic instrument; or (4) use of a battery of specific measures and reports of individual scores.

The first approach is to include both generic and disease-specific measures within the same investigation, *even if the concepts and domains assessed are similar.* An example of this approach is the six-month, randomized, double-blind study of auranofin therapy for treating patients with rheumatoid arthritis (Bombardier et al., 1986). The arthritis-specific measure used in the trial was the Health Assessment Questionnaire (HAQ), which specifies eight areas of daily function (e.g., hygiene), each with two to three activities (e.g., take a tub bath) (Fries et al., 1982). Patients report difficulty in performing each activity during the past week with scores from 3 ("unable to do") to 0 ("without any difficulty"). Lower (better) values are raised if aids, devices, or help from another is needed.

This trial also incorporated the generic Quality of Well-Being Scale (Bush, 1984a; Kaplan and Anderson, 1988), which classifies patients into one of four or five given categories of performance (e.g., "had help with self-care activities") and the least desirable symptom or problem for each day. The HAQ and the QWB showed comparable sensitivity to treatment, although the instruments have different content, length, mode of administration, and method of scoring. Previous clinical findings of the efficacy of auranofin were corroborated in the trial. Measures from both the HAQ and the QWB Scale were consistent with more traditional clinical measures such as the number of tender joints, grip strength, and erythrocyte sedimentation rate.

Interpretation of the benefit associated with auranofin proved similarly difficult with the HAQ or QWB Scale (Thompson et al., 1988). On the HAQ, patients receiving auranofin reduced their disability by an average of 0.31 point. The authors concluded that 0.17 points of the 0.31-point improvement would have been achieved by placebo alone, and the net effect was equivalent to all auranofin patients improving from being able to walk outdoors on level ground "with much difficulty" to "with some difficulty." Similarly, the 0.020 overall gain on the QWB was judged equivalent to all auranofin patients improving on the physical activity scale from "moving one's own wheelchair without help" to "walking with physical limitations," a gain of 0.017 point. In contrast to the HAQ, the QWB did not detect any placebo effects, possibly because of the generic nature of the instrument.

The authors of this study concluded that the advantages for the HAQ were ease of administration, extensive validation, and proven sensitivity to therapeutic efficacy. The QWB required more care in administration and was not explicitly concerned with rheumatoid arthritis patients. The value weights assigned to the QWB, however, permitted the examination of adverse clinical effects of therapy that could be compared directly. Clearly, a tradeoff is involved between the detection and weighting of different intervention effects when using generic and specific measures.

The second approach to examining the relative strengths of generic and disease-specific measures is to compare a generic instrument and a generic instrument modified for the specific population of interest. This approach has been used to study head injury (McLean et al., 1984; Temkin et al., 1988) and to assess back pain (Roland and Morris, 1983). Both investigations modified the Sickness Impact Profile to improve its sensitivity to the clinical condition being evaluated. The study of head injury (Temkin et al., 1989) added items to the SIP to capture head injury sequelae and behaviors typical of young adults, who experience head injury most frequently. These items were reweighted to be included in the overall as well as the psychosocial, physical, and independent category scores derived from the SIP. No improvements were found in the ability of the modified SIP to classify patients into subgroups. Temkin and her colleagues (1989) concluded that the modifications failed to make improvements sufficiently large or consistent to provide a practical advantage over the original SIP.

In a study of back pain, Roland and Morris (1983) selected 24 of 136 items that they felt were most appropriate for back pain from 8 of the 12 different Sickness Impact Profile categories. Each item was scored as a 0/1 variable. The phrase "because of my back" was added to each statement to distinguish dysfunction attributed to back pain from that due to other causes. Scores on this scale ranged from 0 to 24 with higher scores representing worse dysfunction. Overall Sickness Impact Profile scores, on the other hand, include a 45-item physical dimension, 48-item psychosocial dimension, and 43 items in independent categories of eating, work, sleep and rest, household management, and recreation and pastimes.

A separate study (Deyo and Centor, 1986) compared the complete Sickness Impact Profile with the version modified for back pain (Roland Scale) in a clinical trial with 203 subjects, most of whom (79 percent) had acute back pain. Both the overall SIP and the Roland Scale showed significant correlations between change scores and changes in self-rated improvement, clinician-rated improvement, spine flexion, and resumption of full activities. The Roland Scale showed slightly better discrimination between improvers and nonimprovers than either the overall SIP or its Physical Dimension score. The "pruned", condition-specific Roland Scale was at least as responsive as the lengthier SIP in both discrimination and in the quantification of changes. Furthermore, reliability and construct validity of the shorter scale were comparable to those of the complete SIP (Deyo, 1986).

Modifying generic instruments for use with specific populations or with persons having a specific medical condition is appealing. Many generic instruments have demonstrated reliability and validity during a long history of use. The danger, however, is that selecting relevant items and/or modifying wording to existing instruments, changes the measure substantially. The psychometric properties of the revised instrument should be evaluated for the population in which it is intended for use. The conceptual domains contained in generic instruments may also not cover all the domains of importance to persons with the condition, their families, and their providers. Persons with the condition should be asked whether the modified generic measure covers their health-related concerns, and qualitative probing should be used to elicit new domains. Without this conceptual and methodological check, investigators seldom learn just how different medical conditions affect the lives of our patients and their families.

The third approach uses a generic health status instrument with a disease-specific supplement. This is similar to the first approach except that the disease- or condition-specific measure is constructed to have a different conceptual basis and minimal overlap with the generic measure. The intention is *not* to measure the same concepts as a generic measure with specific reference to a medical condition but to capture the additional, specific concerns of patients with the condition that are not contained in generic measures.

Researchers have used this approach to study patients with inflammatory bowel disease (IBD) (Drossman et al., 1989). In a study of 150 patients with Crohn's disease and ulcerative colitis, the SIP was used to measure functional status. A 21-item Rating Form of IBD Patient Concerns (RFIPC) was constructed by eliciting items through semistructured interviews concerning the worries, fears, or concerns that IBD patients might have. Although these concerns were IBD-specific, four items—bowel control, pain, sexual performance, and feelings of aloneness—are also measured in terms of behavioral dysfunction in the Sickness Impact Profile. Patients rated items on the Rating Form of IBD Patient Concerns from 0 to 100 (0 = not at all concerned to 100 = a great deal concerned) using a visual analogue scale. Researchers calculated an average score of all concerns (sumscore).

In cross-sectional comparisons, both the SIP and the RFIPC proved to be discriminating measures of health-related quality of life in patients with inflammatory bowel disease. The SIP was sensitive to different disease populations; patients with Crohn's reported more dysfunction (overall SIP = 8.6) than patients with ulcerative colitis (overall SIP = 5.2). The RFIPC showed a similar pattern of concerns between the two patient groups, although inpatients as compared to outpatients reported considerably higher concerns with dying, intimacy, body image, being a burden, and finances. This pattern of concerns is consistent with the greater severity of disease among inpatients. The correlation between the overall RFIPC score and the overall SIP score was 0.46 (p = 0.0002). This moderate correlation indicates a strong but not predictive relationship between behavioral dysfunction and worries and concerns in this patient population. Including the SIP in this study permits analysts to compare this population with other healthy and condition-specific populations (see Figure 5.3). Comparisons show that inflammatory bowel disease patients report moderate overall dysfunction comparable to adult patients with rheumatoid arthritis (unstandardized for age and sex). Inflammatory bowel disease patients, however, appear to report somewhat higher (worse) psychosocial dimension scores.

One problem that may arise with this approach is that the generic and specific measures may have different metrics, or scoring systems. The generic measure, for example, might be preference-weighted and provide a profile and overall score for different dimensions, whereas the specific measure is weighted statistically with an overall score developed through item-reduction and simple averaging of different item responses. Analysts would not be able to compare on the same metric the scores produced by the generic measure with those produced by the specific measure. Thus, rather than a profile of generic and specific measures, this approach may yield a battery of independent scores that must be analyzed separately.

A preferred strategy would be to develop disease-specific supplements that use the same metric as the generic measures being applied in the population under investigation. An example are the TyPE questionnaires developed by Paul Ellwood and colleagues at InterStudy to complement the Short Form–36 Survey instrument (Ellwood, personal communication). These questionnaires are being developed by clinicians who treat patients with back pain, diabetes, gastrointestinal disorders, and other conditions.

The fourth approach uses a battery of specific measures scored independently and reported as individual scores. These batteries are common in clinical trials and epidemiologic investigations, where entire scales, subscales, or individual items from the best available instruments are administered and effects tested for each measure in the battery.

Although generic instruments may be included in health status batteries, collections of specific measures are more often used. Batteries of specific measures can be used to address a broad range of outcomes, but comparisons between different independent scores may be difficult.

Summary Recommendation

Using short, generic measures with disease-specific supplements is the most desirable course in assessing health-related quality of life. The relative weighting of generic and specific outcomes may prove difficult, however, unless both types of outcomes are based on a common metric. Monitoring and evaluating health outcomes on a routine basis will undoubtedly rely, in part, on a common definition of health-related quality of life. Although payers are more interested in generic outcome assessment on a relative value scale, patients and providers are concerned with outcomes of specific treatment decisions.

Selecting the most appropriate measurement strategy to achieve the user's objectives involves more than identifying the type of measure needed. Many different combinations exist of (1) indicators, indexes, profiles, and batteries, (2) generic and specific measures, and (3) preference-weighted and statistically weighted instruments.

The last section of Table 5.1 refers to the metric or weighting system used to produce scores for each domain of health-related quality of life and/or an index score. Chapter 6 describes the methods by which items and domains are weighted to produce health indexes, profiles, or batteries. Chapters 7 and 8 then provide a guide to users for selecting measures for primary data collection and secondary analyses.

6

Assigning Values to Health States

This chapter defines the basic notion of health state preferences and how to measure them. Step 3 of the Health Resource Allocation Strategy involves assigning values to health *states* to create *levels* of health-related quality of life. These values, referred to as *health state preferences*, or *utilities*, reflect the perceived "quality" or "desirability" of a health state.

Preference or utility assessment provides the means of integrating values attributed to the worth of life at given points in time (health states) with the quantity of life (weeks, months, years) spent in various states. Thus, assigning preferences to health states permits different domains of health-related quality of life to be combined into a single index (e.g., combinations of different levels of functional status and perceptions).

Health state preferences also provide the means for assessing tradeoffs in health-related quality of life over time. Changes in one domain, such as physical function, can be related to changes in another domain, such as emotional function. For example, physical function might improve and emotional function deteriorate between two points in time. Preference weights for both physical and emotional function permit calculation of average improvement or average deterioration, depending on the weights assigned. The calculation of years of healthy life relies heavily on health state preferences.

Composite measures of health-related quality of life consist of two or more health descriptions aggregated to provide a summary score for each domain in a profile or battery as well as an overall index score. Aggregation of different health status and quality of life items, states, or domains into summary measures requires that items be weighted by some method. Two basic strategies are frequently used to combine components of health-related quality of life measures: statistical weighting and utility or relative preference weighting (Kaplan et al., 1976; Bush, 1984b).

In this chapter, we describe statistical weighting methods and preference weighting methods. Statistical methods are used most commonly to develop health status measures in which all items or attributes are considered equal. Preference weighting methods assign different weights to items or attributes. Preference weights can be derived by methods other than primary data collection or they can be explicitly measured. The final section of this chapter addresses the theoretical, methodological, and practical differences between preference- and non–preference-weighted measures.

Bush (1984b) suggested that these two strategies reflect separate measurement traditions; however, the wording of questions and method of administration may be similar. Regardless of the weighting method, many of the same conceptual and practical issues arise in development or application of a health-related quality of life assessment.

STATISTICAL WEIGHTING

Summated Ratings

The method of summated ratings from the psychometric tradition in psychology provides the basis for the most commonly used statistical method of weighting. Summative models underlie most efforts to scale people with respect to different types of judgments and sentiments (Nunnally, 1978). The *summative model* assumes that individual items in a measure are monotonically related to underlying attributes and that a summation of item scores is approximately linearly related to the attribute. In health-related quality of life measures, the term "attributes" is used to describe the behaviors or health perceptions included in an operational definition, and all domains may be considered as possible attributes for the purposes of weighting to create a composite measure.

The summative scale in Table 6.1 consists of the five mental health items and scoring information for the Mental Health Index from the Medical Outcomes Study Short-Form Health Survey. An investigator obtains a total mental health score by adding positive scores on individual items. Scoring is reversed for negative attitudes or perceptions; this step is commonly called item recoding. After item recoding and handling of any missing data, a raw score is computed for the scale. This score is the simple algebraic sum of responses for all items, recoded and original, on a scale ranging from 5 to 30. If the respondent answers at least half of the items on this or other multi-item scales (or half plus one in the case of scales with an odd number of items), scores should be calculated. Some investigators may take a more conservative approach and require a higher percentage of item responses before calculating a scale score.

Raw scores can be transformed into a 0-100 scale as shown in Table 6.1. This transformation converts the lowest and highest possible scores to zero and 100, respectively. Scores in between these values represent the percentage of the total possible score achieved. Raw scores and transformed scores can be compared with population data, either available in published form, or obtained from scale developers. Users of health status instruments are advised to register their use of an instrument with the developer in order to be kept informed about potential advances in scoring and use of a particular instrument.

Summative scales are sometimes referred to as *Likert* scales because of the contribution of the psychometrician, Rensis Likert, to their popularity and use (Likert, 1932). Summative scales have five attractive advantages: they "(1) follow from an appealing model, (2) are rather easy to construct, (3) usually are highly reliable, (4) can be adapted to the measurement of many different kinds of attitudes, and (5) have produced meaningful results in many studies to date" (Nunnally, 1978, p. 604).

An alternative to Likert scales is the visual analogue scale (VAS) that has been widely used by investigators because of its simplicity and promise in detecting very small changes in health-related quality of life (Freyd, 1923; Scott and Huskisson, 1977). Visual analogue scales are lines anchored at either end by the extremes of the domain being measured, for example, from no pain to unbearable pain. Respondents are asked to place a mark on the line, often 10 centimeters in length, to indicate their status on the particular domain. Investigators then measure the distance from the zero

Table 6.1 Mental health items and scoring information for scale construction: MOS Short-Form Health Survey

These questions are about how you feel and how things have been with you *during the past 4 weeks*. For each question, please give the one answer that comes closest to the way you have been feeling. How much of the time during the *past 4 weeks* . . . (Mark one on each line.)	All of the time	Most of the time	A Good bit of the time	Some of the time	A Little of the time	None of the time
1. Have you been a very nervous person?	1	2	3	4	5	6
2. Have you felt so down in the dumps nothing could cheer you up?	1	2	3	4	5	6
3. Have you felt calm and peaceful?	1	2	3	4	5	6
4. Have you felt downhearted and blue?	1	2	3	4	5	6
5. Have you been a happy person?	1	2	3	4	5	6

Item Scoring:

Items 1, 2, and 4 are scored according to the precoded values ranging from 1 to 6.

Items 3 and 5 are recoded as follows:

Precoded value	Final scoring
1	6
2	5
3	4
4	3
5	2
6	1

Scale scoring

Compute the simple algebraic sum of the final item values for mental health items 1, 2, 3, 4 and 5. The lowest and highest possible raw scores for this scale range from 5 to 30 with a possible range of 25.

Formula and example for transformation of raw mental health scale scores

$$\text{Transformed scale} = \left[\frac{(\text{Actual raw score} - \text{lowest } \textit{possible} \text{ raw score})}{\textit{Possible} \text{ raw score range}} \right] \cdot 100$$

Example: A mental health score of 21 would be transformed as follows:

$$[(21 - 5)/25] \times 100 = 64$$

Where lowest possible score = 5 and possible raw score range = 25

Source: International Resource Center for Health Care Assessment, 1991.

point (no pain) to the marked line (some fraction of 10 centimeters) and use the physical representation as the measure of health-related quality of life.

Guyatt, Townsend, Berman et al. (1977) compared a seven-point Likert (summated rating) scale with a VAS scale in measuring quality of life in chronic lung disease. These investigators found that both showed improvement, but that the variability of the improvement was greater using the VAS. The two methods showed comparable responsiveness; the ease and interpretation of the seven-point scale made it the recommended approach in clinical trials.

Visual analogue scales require that respondents have the dexterity and fine motor movements to place a mark on a line that accurately represents their perception or behavior. Older respondents may have difficulty with this task. The VAS also implies a continuous level of measurement using the precise length of a line that may not match the perceptual discrimination between different levels of health-related quality of life. Because seven-point summated ratings scales produce similar results and permit verbal descriptors that precisely identify what is intended by the measurement, they are preferred over the VAS for most applications.

In constructing a summative model for health-related quality of life, the analyst creates a pool of items related to one domain or attribute of health. Each item is assumed to measure part of the same underlying continuum. Using a Likert-type scale, often five points ranging from "all of the time" to "none of the time" or "strongly agree" to "strongly disagree," these items are administered to groups of respondents.

Analysts correlate item scores with total scale scores and compute the coefficient alpha for the total item pool to evaluate the internal consistency of the scale. Total scores are reached by summing all items. Each item is weighted equally, although theoretically it is possible to apply differential weights to items on a summative scale.

Factor analysis is then used to explore the homogeneity of different scales and to look at the underlying factor structure. In factor analysis, statistical procedures produce coefficients for each item. Applying either component analysis or common factor analysis, factors are estimated from the correlations among responses to items obtained from all respondents. The items or variables within each factor are highly correlated, and the usual factor-analytic model expresses each item as a function of factors common to several items and a factor unique to the item. Factor loadings, the relationship of the original items to each factor, are expressed as coefficients for each item on each factor.

Factors are labeled subjectively according to the analyst's interpretation of the properties of closely associated items. The loading of an item on a given factor is the "weight" of that item, and the percentage of variation explained by a particular factor and its items provides weights for the factor itself. As a consequence, items that are infrequently answered or that correlate poorly receive low weights, regardless of how important these items (behaviors or states) may be in social terms (Kaplan et al., 1976). For example, low levels of functioning such as unconsciousness or intravenous feeding are uncommon in community surveys of health status and might well receive low weight or yield a low-weighted independent factor. These items might then be dropped from a health status measure because they do not contribute to the overall variance among respondents. These states of health, however, may be important or highly undesirable to many persons in the population to be assessed.

Developing a generic health status measure for resource allocation using statistical weighting can be enhanced by applying item analysis to large and varied populations. Large and diverse samples increase the likelihood that rare health states or events will be included in the measure. Making health status measures comprehensive, however, can lead to lengthy questionnaires with items that do not apply to many respondents.

Infrequently answered items also detract from a measure's responsiveness in detecting health status change (Deyo and Patrick, 1989).

Cumulative Scales

Another type of statistical weighting is based on the principle of cumulative scaling. Guttman scalogram analysis is the most commonly used cumulative technique (Guttman, 1944). Guttman scalogram analysis, or *cumulative scaling*, is a means of determining if the interrelationships among three or more items meet several special properties which define a Guttman scale. First, cumulative scales must be unidimensional so that the component items measure movement toward or away from the same single underlying attribute, in our case "health." Second, Guttman scales must be cumulative so that component items can be ordered by degree of difficulty. The cumulative nature of the scale implies that respondents who reply positively to a difficult item will always respond positively to less difficult items and vice versa (Goodenough, 1944). Cumulative scaling thus tests the extent to which activities, behaviors, or attitudes are ordered in a sequence.

For example, respondents in a health status assessment might be asked if, during the last week, they (1) were confined to bed, (2) were confined to the house, (3) traveled outside the house with difficulty, or (4) traveled outside the house without difficulty. These behaviors can be ordered or weighted on an ordinal scale of mobility according to their location in the sequence. If one represents the presence of a disabled activity, "dysfunction in mobility," and zero represents the presence of a nondisabled activity, "functional in mobility," then it is logically intuitive that these descriptions of mobility and other activities of daily living may fall into sequences as shown in Table 6.2. If a person is able to travel outside the house without difficulty, he or she is assumed to be nondisabled in the other three mobility categories. Similarly, if the person is confined to bed, we can assume that the person cannot move freely about the house or in the street. If such patterns exist, weights can be applied to the patterns from "no dysfunction" to "severe dysfunction."

If the four items under analysis formed a perfect Guttman scale, all responses would conform to the ideal pattern shown in Table 6.2. Rarely, however, do the data fit the ideal pattern expected by the researcher; people may be inconsistent in their behavior or

Table 6.2 Typical Cumulative or Guttman Scale Based on Mobility

| | Mobility status | | | |
Person	Confined to bed	Confined to house	Traveled outside house with difficulty	Traveled outside house without difficulty
1	0	0	0	0
2	0	0	0	1
3	0	0	1	1
4	0	1	1	1
5	1	1	1	1

the survey question may elicit inconsistent answers. The scalability of items is evaluated by the *coefficient of reproducibility*, a measure of the extent to which a respondent's scale score is a predictor of a response pattern (1 minus the result of dividing the total number of errors by the total number of responses). Coefficients of reproducibility higher than 0.9 are considered to indicate a valid scale. The *coefficient of scalability* is used to evaluate the unidimensionality of the scale. It also varies from 0 to 1. The result should be well above 0.6 if the scale is truly unidimensional and cumulative.

Guttman or cumulative scaling in health status assessment can be traced to the work of Katz and his colleagues (1963) using daily living activities such as bathing, dressing, eating, and transferring. Since then, researchers have used these techniques to reduce items on health status measures or to determine whether a given set of disabilities forms a sequence (Skinner and Yett, 1973; Williams et al., 1976; Bebbington, 1977; Stewart et al., 1982).

Williams (1983), in reviewing the use of cumulative scaling for health indicators, pointed out the crucial importance of the theoretical assumptions behind a single cumulative phenomenon. He observed that (1) a scale is not a conclusive demonstration that one concept is present; (2) numerous cases not conforming to the cumulative scale still have to be assigned; (3) cumulative scaling depends on the population in which it is tested, and results vary for different populations; (4) a very large population is necessary to obtain a representative sample of possible sequences; (5) the meaning of resulting scales is problematic; and (6) cumulative scaling is not only a technique but also a theory. The theoretical assumptions of cumulative scaling require rigorous testing before being applied to health status index development. The evidence to date would suggest this method is inappropriate for generic measures applied to populations of varied age, gender, and level of disability.

PREFERENCE WEIGHTING

Expected utility theory distinguishes among four measurement concepts (Bush, 1984b): *occurrence* of an event or attribute such as symptoms or behaviors, the relative *desirability* of the attributes, the *probability* that the attribute will occur at some later time, and the expected *utility* or desirability of the attribute, given its probability. All these concepts are involved in some health-related quality of life assessments. However, the most commonly understood use of the term "utility" is preference, or the relative desirability people associate with health-related quality of life states or descriptions.

Methods for assigning weights to health-related quality of life items have been reviewed repeatedly (Patrick, 1976; Rosser, 1983b; Torrance, 1986; Hollandsworth, 1988). Froberg and Kane (1989a–d) published a four-part series of papers that analyze and critique state-of-the-art methods of measuring health state preferences. These methods derive from utility theory in economics, psychological scaling methods developed from philosophy and physics, and decision-analytic methods emerging from the discipline of decision sciences.

Assigning preferences to health states involves four steps: (1) identify the population of judges who will assign preferences; (2) sample and describe health states from the classification system in order to assign preference weights; (3) select a preference measurement method; and (4) collect preference judgments, analyze the data, and assign preference weights to health states. The next four sections cover these steps in the preference-weighting process. As an example, we use the preference measurement methods, data collection procedures, and results from a recent Institute of Medicine study of the National Heart, Lung, and Blood Institute Artificial Heart Program (Hogness and Van Antwerp, 1991).

Identifying a Population of Judges

The first major decision in generating and applying preference weights to health states is the selection of judges to assign preferences. Potential judges could be patients, family members, respondents living in the community, health professionals, or any other persons who agree to participate in the study. Patients are commonly used to obtain preference weights in studies of individual treatment decisions or patient utilities for different medical care outcomes (Mulley, 1989). In this case, patients are asked to weight their own state of health and the potential outcomes of treatments such as surgical interventions, "watchful waiting," or nontreatment. Patients are "ideal" respondents in that they are actually experiencing the states of health being weighted.

In social preference studies, groups of respondents who are interested in the health outcomes are used to assign preferences. These respondents may be asked to weight health states as though they were experiencing them or to assign preferences according to the desirability of the state to a hypothetical person. In either case, the question arises of whether a judge can truly understand what a health state is like unless he or she has experienced it. Judges in hypothetical scaling studies are given descriptions of the health states. From these descriptions, they state their preferences for the various states using one of the methods described below. Often the characteristics of health states are familiar to judges through personal experience or association with a relative or individual who has been in one of the health states described. Previous experience with the health state description can and should be assessed in social preference studies, particularly when comparing preferences obtained from patients, physicians, and the general public.

To adequately represent society's preference for well-being in a measure applied across populations, researchers should obtain probability samples of community preferences for different health states (Patrick, 1979). These probability samples should be representative of the community, including socioeconomic status, color/ethnicity, age, geographic region, gender, and disability status. These characteristics ensure adequate representation of the community, including groups that may experience inequalities in access to health care and in health-related quality of life. Such broad value preferences will be necessary for a national index of health-related quality of life.

As a general rule, policy analysts and researchers should elicit preferences from judges who represent the population for which the measure will be applied. Patients are appropriate judges to assign preferences to health outcomes evaluated in clinical trials or medical decision-making studies. Policy studies will require social preferences from community samples. For example, the State of Oregon used a random sample of state residents to assign preference weights to health states used in the priority assignment to different health care procedures (see Chapter 14).

Health state preferences are remarkably stable across different populations. Most investigators have found few, if any, differences among groups defined by age, gender, socioeconomic status, ethnic background, religious affiliation, professional back-ground, or patient status (Kaplan and Bush, 1982; Sackett and Torrance, 1978; Wolf-son et al., 1982; Balaban et al., 1986).

Our example of health state preference measurement comes from the recent report of the Institute of Medicine Committee to Evaluate the National Heart, Lung, and Blood Institute (NHLBI) Artificial Heart Program (Hogness and Van Antwerp, 1991). This committee was charged with advising the NHLBI on identifying priorities for allo-cation of its research resources for the development of total artificial hearts (TAHs) and other mechanical circulatory support systems (MCSSs). In estimating the cost-effectiveness of total artificial heart implantation, the committee needed to assign preferences to health state descriptions of end-stage heart disease to form the basis for calculating years of healthy life.

Potential judges for assigning preferences included patients with end-stage heart disease, their families, cardiologists and cardiac surgeons, patients with heart trans-plants, patients on the waiting list for heart transplants, or a representative sample of the general population. Because of limited resources and time, the committee itself provided the relative weights assigned to each health state included in the cost–effectiveness model. Available resources thus drove the selection of judges, even though this public policy decision was being conducted from the societal viewpoint. On the other hand, the committee received a large amount of information about end-stage heart disease and possible treatments, listened to patients and practitioners de-scribe their experience of the health states, and discussed the health states among themselves. Therefore, the judges were well informed about the decision context and health states involved in the preference measurement.

Sampling and Describing Health States

The number of possible health and illness states may approach infinity because of the very large number of domains or attributes that could describe an individual's health and quality of life. In this sense, every person has a unique description of health-related quality of life. The definition of health states for preference assignment most often uses a health state classification system that describes all states of interest.

A classification system might be based on the five domains (attributes) of survival, impairment, functional status, perceptions, and opportunity. By using such a classifica-tion system, health states can be formed that are (1) *holistic*, in which combinations of levels from each attribute are treated as a unit—travels freely, performs self-care activities, and works with some limitations are judged together; or (2) *decomposed* or single attribute, in which the level of each attribute is treated as a separate health state—travels freely, performs self-care activities, and works with some limitations are judged separately.

Each possible combination of levels of health-related quality of life attributes repre-sents a unique health state. In a classification system involving 5 levels of mobility, 3 of physical activity, and 4 of emotional function, there would be $5 \times 3 \times 4 = 60$ potential combinations of levels. If all combinations were possible, there would be 60 potential health states as well. Some combinations might not be logically possible. For example, in creating the Quality of Well-Being Scale, Patrick et al. (1973a) developed a matrix of 100 potential combinations or health states using 5 levels of mobility, 4 of physical activity, and 5 of social and role activity. Only 29 of these combinations were originally thought possible. For example, it was considered unlikely that a person could walk freely, be confined to a special unit of a hospital, and perform work without any difficulty. Later field work indicated that some combinations originally thought impossible—like traveling freely while confined to a bed or chair—were indeed possible in practice.

Health state classification systems can therefore involve a large number of different potential states, as illustrated by the Quality of Well-Being Scale, Health Utilities Index, Disabilities/Distress Index, and EuroQol Instrument. Investigators must decide whether judges will (1) rate each level of an attribute separately in decomposed states using multiattribute utility methods, or (2) judge holistic health states composed of different combinations of attributes and levels (Fischer, 1979; Veit and Ware, 1982; Froberg and Kane, 1989a). Regardless of whether holistic or decomposed states are used, similar methods of assigning preference values are employed.

The purpose and application of the health-related quality of life will determine the number of different attributes and health states needed and the measurement strategy to be used. For some purposes, such as clinical studies with limited and defined populations as in kidney dialysis or cardiac transplantation, a more restricted set of attributes will suffice to describe the health states. In other applications, such as resource allocation across different treatments or procedures, a comprehensive set of attributes and levels is required. For example, in a double-blind randomized clinical trial of an oral gold pharmacologic agent for treating arthritis, investigators measured the utility of only two states per patient—the health state at baseline and at follow-up (Torrance and Feeny, 1989). In a cost–utility assessment of neonatal intensive care for very low birth weight infants, investigators needed to measure the utilities for 960 different health states using 6 (physical function) × 5 (role function) × 4 (socioemotional function) × 8 (health problems) (Torrance et al., 1982; Boyle et al., 1983).

Measures applied in the Health Resource Allocation Strategy generally involve the most common domains and levels of health, including symptoms such as pain (impairment), physical and emotional function such as ambulation and depressed mood, role function such as ability to work (functional status), and general perceptions of health such as distress or satisfaction (perceptions). In assigning preferences to holistic descriptions, no more than seven to nine attributes, preferably fewer, should be used because judges cannot process simultaneously more than five to nine pieces of information (Miller, 1956). When a larger number of attributes is needed, the decomposed approach is preferable.

Holistic health state descriptions, whether derived from a classification system or defined according to the purpose of an individual study, can be written in narrative or taxonomic form. *Narrative* descriptions, often referred to as "scenarios," describe the health state using complete sentences and paragraphs. *Taxonomic* descriptions are "classifications" in that concepts and domains are written in phrases that describe the level of the attribute being weighted.

A sample health state description written in narrative form to describe an actual patient with cancer would read as follows:

> I am in the age range 40–64 years. I live alone and am confined to my home. During the past 6 months I have lost 35 pounds in weight. I am able to eat only small amounts of food at present and I vomit occasionally. I am tired and weak and walk with the aid of a walker. I require assistance to get into and out of the bathtub. Social contact with my friends and family is infrequent. (Llewellyn-Thomas et al., 1984)

This same health state description written in taxonomic form would read as follows:

Age:	40- to 64-year-old employee/housekeeper
Mobility:	In house
Physical activity:	Walks with limitations
Social activity:	Does not perform major but performs self-care activities
Symptom/problem:	Sick or upset stomach, vomiting, or diarrhea (watery bowel movements)

As shown in this example, the narrative format was written in first-person singular and listed all symptoms or problems associated with the state, whereas the taxonomic description included only the most severe ones. Llewellyn-Thomas and her colleagues (1984) studied the preferences assigned to these two types of health state descriptions. Sixty-four patients assigned weights using the standard gamble technique and category rating methods. The format of the health state description had a major influence on the results, and significant differences were observed in the preference weights assigned.

Unfortunately the two sets of descriptions used in this study differed not only in format but also in content. A greater number of symptoms were included in the narrative descriptions and the narrative descriptions used capacity wording ("I am able or unable to . . ."), whereas the taxonomic descriptions were written in performance mode ("I do or do not do . . .").

Regardless of these problems, this study illustrates that the way health states are described and presented can influence results. Tversky and Kahneman (1974) found that judges rely on information processing "heuristics" to help them make decisions or judgments. For example, a judge may view each attribute in a health state description in the set, select one of particular significance, and then use it as a guide to choosing among alternatives. Cognitive processes differ, therefore, depending on the type of descriptive format used.

Because of the large number of health states used in many preference studies, researchers most often take the taxonomic approach. It reduces the respondent burden in reading the descriptions and the derivation of each description from a health state classification system is more obvious. In fact, teaching judges how the health state descriptions have been derived from the classification system is desirable. Better understanding of the health state description permits considered judgment and attention to the preference measurement task.

Computer-based interactive video programs are being developed to help describe different health states and treatment outcomes to aid physicians and patients in jointly making decisions on different courses of treatment (Mulley, 1990). These video programs provide "rich" information, and both the narrative presentation and the outcome probabilities can be tailored to the circumstances of the individual patient. In exploratory studies of this approach, patients specify treatment preferences, such as surgery or "watchful waiting," before and after viewing the video. This technology might well be adapted for eliciting health state preferences. Cognitive burden might be lessened using interactive video programming, and respondents might prefer such procedures to written descriptions. Future research will test the effect of visual presentation of health states on the preference values obtained.

In assigning preferences to health states describing end-stage heart disease patients under different treatment options, the Committee to Evaluate the NHLBI Artificial Heart Program chose to use holistic descriptions written in taxonomic form. Table 6.3 contains health state descriptions for four permanent or chronic states for end-stage heart disease patients who continue to receive conventional medical or surgical treatment. The table also describes two states for patients who have received a long-term fully implantable artificial heart or a heart.

Table 6.3 also indicates the classification system used to describe these states. The system uses attributes from the domains of physical, mental, social, and role functioning; self-care activities; general health perceptions; and survival expectancy. These attributes were chosen as the most important ones for end-stage heart disease. Groups 1–4 roughly correspond to the New York Heart Association Classification System of Class I–IV end-stage heart disease. (Group 1 deviates slightly from the NYHA Class I in which patients are asymptomatic.) This correspondence to an existing classification system provided further grounding to the health state descriptions.

The health states in Table 6.3 are described by functional status (physical, mental social, role, self-care) and perceptions (current health and discomfort) rather than by clinical terms. The emphasis is on how functional or dysfunctional a person in this health state is rather than on clinical diagnosis or the pathological process. The description also includes survival expectancy or prognosis. Health states should also describe any states that may or may not follow the one under consideration (Torrance, 1986). Most often prognosis is held constant in the measurement process or in the health state description. In this case, however, survival expectancy was part of the health state description and also of the preference measurement exercise, as described later.

In addition to the six states shown in Table 6.3, the committee received similar descriptions of the six states describing these same persons as hospital patients. Patients were first described as being in an acute care hospital in the intensive or cardiac care unit. Second, hospitalized patients were described as receiving regular care in a hospital medical or surgical unit.

Preference Measurement Strategies

Five broad approaches to measuring or estimating health state preferences have been used:

1. Arbitrary weights can be assigned by investigators.
2. Preference weights can be estimated using investigator judgment.
3. Weights can be derived from published values in the literature.
4. Weights can be measured through primary data collection efforts.
5. Weights can be revealed by administrative or social decisions.

These methods divide into those that involve weights derived by methods other than primary data collection and weights obtained from primary data collection. The next two sections discuss these different approaches to preference weighting in detail.

DERIVED PREFERENCE-WEIGHTING METHODS

Arbitrary Weighting

Perhaps the simplest method of preference weighting is to assign higher scores to items that reflect what the investigator defines as a higher level of health-related quality of life. These assigned weights are an extension of the 0/1 assumed value weight of

Table 6.3 Long-term health states used to describe end-stage heart disease patients under different modes of treatment

Domain/concept	Patients who continue to receive only conventional medical or surgical treatment (no MCSS or Tx)[a]				Patients who have received	
	1. Mildly impaired, NYHA Class I	2. Symptomatic, NYHA Class II	3. Seriously impaired, NYHA Class III/IV	4. Moribund, NYHA Class IV	5. Long-term fully implanted artificial heart	6. Heart transplant
Physical						
Vitality/energy	Considerable	Moderate	Limited	Very little	Premorbid normal	Premorbid normal
Maximum physical activity/limitation	Able to walk 5 mph, shovel snow, carry 20 pounds up 8 stairs	Able to walk 4 mph, rake garden, engage in intercourse	Able to walk 2.5 mph, change bedsheets, push power mower	Sedentary only (e.g., TV, reading); no physical activity	Able to return to pre-illness activity, except for strenuous physical activities	Able to return to pre-illness activity
Percentage of time in bed during daytime	None	None	Very little	Almost all in either bed or chair	None	None except during acute rejection
Mental						
Anxiety/depression	Seldom depressed or anxious	Occasionally depressed or anxious	Depressed and anxious about half of typical day	Depressed most of time; very anxious	Some anxiety about MCSS failure risk; not depressed	Much anxiety about possible rejection in first year only; some anxiety about effects of long-term immunosuppression
Affect or mood	Generally positive; some concern about future health	Concerned about risk of sudden death	Same as Group 2; hopeful about future illness course	Same as Group 2; despondent about chance of transplant	Generally positive, with realistic concern about device or battery failure	Generally positive with realistic concern about rejection

Social						
Interpersonal contacts	Same as premorbid state	Normal social contacts but mostly at home	Enjoys visits from numerous friends	Only sees relatives and close friends	Same as premorbid state	Same as premorbid state
Role						
Role functioning	Premorbid normal; able to work at job not requiring physical exertion	Performs work or major activity with some limitations	Unable to work or perform major activity	Unable to work or perform major activity	Premorbid normal, except for constant availability of backup energy source	Premorbid normal, except during rejection or infection episodes
Self-care (bathing, dressing, etc.)	Able to perform all	Able to perform all	Limited in one or more activities	Severely limited	Able to perform all	Limited in self-care during rejection episodes
General health perceptions						
Current health	Good	Moderately good	Poor	Very poor	Good; accepts battery recharging need; realization of total dependence on a mechanical device	Good except during acute rejection or infection
Discomfort (shortness of breath)	Breathlessness only with exertion	Only if patient overexerts	Periodic, especially with exertion	Periodic *without* exertion	None	None except during acute rejection
Survival expectancy	Small risk of sudden death; life expectancy 15–20 years	Risk of sudden death or disability; life expectancy about 5 years	Risk of sudden death; life expectancy is about 2 years	Life expectancy is maximum of 6 months	Some risk of MCSS failure: 80% probability of life expectancy >5 years	Some rejection risk; 70–85% probability of life expectancy >5 years

Source: Hogness and Van Antwerp, 1991.

[a]MCSS stands for mechanical circulatory support system, a generic term referring to a device used to supplement or take over the pumping function of the heart or one of its ventricles.

mortality indicators; that is, it is worse to be dead than alive (Patrick, 1976). For example, the following numbers might be assigned to a classification of mobility:

1. Are you able to use public transportation?
2. When you travel around your community, does someone have to assist you because of your health?
3. Do you have to stay indoors most or all of the day because of your health?
4. Are you in bed or chair for most or all of the day because of your health?

In this example, the ability to use public transportation is assigned 1, which equals better health; confinement to bed or chair is assigned 4, which equals worse health. These ordinal numbers do not reflect distance between the ranks. Therefore, they are not useful in statistical procedures requiring an interval level of measurement.

Such ad hoc numerical scales have intuitive appeal because they are straightforward and appear to reflect the social consensus that being confined to a bed or chair is worse than traveling freely around the community. The difficulty arises in combining arbitrary weights from different dimensions of health-related quality of life, such as mobility and emotional functioning. Does one prefer being confined to a bed or chair with a happy outlook and no psychological distress as compared to traveling freely in the community with significant depression? What is the strength of the preference?

Tradeoffs between different domains of health-related quality of life provide the primary reason for explicitly assigning preference weights to health states using primary data collection. Paterson (1984) gives the following example: "What if a patient at baseline could lift a jar down from a cupboard but not dress herself? Two months later she cannot lift the jar but can dress herself. Is she better or not?" The answer requires that a preference weight be applied to the physical functions of lifting and dressing. Which physical function represents more severe dysfunction to the patient herself and to society?

Another reason for assigning explicit preference weights is to investigate the degree of consensus on the desirability of health states relative to death. People consider some chronic health conditions to be worse than death (Rosser and Kind, 1978; Pauker et al., 1981; Torrance, 1986); conditions so identified include coma, chronic pain, and severe dysfunction. Various social and functional states, such as institutionalization and social isolation, may also be considered worse than death.

The system of using investigator-assigned weights to define metric values for measures breaks down when patients rate combinations of attributes. Measures defined, valued, applied, and interpreted by the investigator are also not the most socially relevant or meaningful indicators (Patrick, 1976).

Early investigators frequently used ad hoc numerical scales to quantify health states. Examples of this approach include the Karnofsky index (Karnofsky and Burchenal, 1949), the Grogono-Woodgate index (Grogono and Woodgate, 1971), and Spitzer's QL index (Spitzer et al., 1981). Although these measures have been widely used in clinical investigations, their use in economic and policy studies has been limited, primarily because of the arbitrary way these concepts were combined and weighted.

Investigator Judgment

Another simple approach to obtaining health state preferences is to estimate the weights or a range of plausible values. Judgments can be made by the analysts or by a panel of expert judges, usually physicians or health professionals. A range of values is then investigated through sensitivity analysis to determine the effect of different weightings on the study conclusions (Torrance et al., 1973; Weinstein, 1981). Investigator judgments are used extensively in cost–effectiveness studies because they are easy to obtain at little cost (Weinstein, 1981). Furthermore, sensitivity analyses may show that the study conclusions are relatively insensitive to changes in the preference weights. Investigator judgments, however, tend to be confined to the single investigation or investigator. This specificity makes comparisons across different studies difficult, if not impossible. Comparisons between investigator-estimated and empirically derived weights, however, would make this approach more credible.

Published Literature

A related approach is to refine investigator judgments with evidence found in the literature. The body of studies in which health state preferences have been measured is increasing (Mulley, 1989). Sometimes this literature can be used to derive an estimate of preference weights for a particular study. For example, a recent study used cost–effectiveness analysis to estimate the health and economic implications of exercise in preventing coronary heart disease (CHD) (Hatziandreu et al., 1988). To measure the health effects of exercise programs, the investigators calculated the expected number of CHD events and the gain in years of life saved. This analysis allowed comparisons with other preventive measures. Gains in life expectancy were adjusted for changes in health-related quality of life due to decreased morbidity from nonfatal CHD. The investigators calculated quality-adjusted life expectancy by assuming that each year following the onset of a nonfatal form of CHD was equal to 0.8 of a health year. This preference weight was derived from previous studies of the cost effectiveness of interventions to prevent or treat coronary heart disease (Weinstein and Stason, 1985).

Using published values simplifies the preference-weighting task. However, researchers need to answer these questions before using published values in current studies:

1. Were the judgments made by people and instruments appropriate to the study?
2. Were health states in published studies similar to those in the current study?

Table 6.4 contains sample utilities, or preferences, for selected health states found in the literature. The health states shown in Table 6.4 range from healthy (1.00) to unconscious (less than 0.00). These utilities indicate that most states are considered to be better than death, although some are considered worse than death. The utilities were obtained from different populations using different methods of preference weighting. Therefore, the utilities are not strictly comparable. Preference weights assigned to health states used in the Disability/Distress Index, Health Utilities Index, Quality of Well-Being Scale, and EuroQol Instrument are listed in Appendix I. For each measure, preference weights were derived using a single method with one or more populations.

Weights Revealed by Administrative or Social Decisions

Another approach to deriving preference weights for states of health is the revealed preference, or *social decision*, valuation approach (Rosser and Watts, 1972; Patrick, 1976; Hurst and Mooney, 1983). In this approach, preferences are revealed by a wide

Table 6.4 Sample utilities for selected health states

Health state	Utility
Healthy (reference state)	1.00
Life with menopausal symptoms (judgment)	0.99
Side effects of hypertension treatment (judgment)	0.95–0.99
Mild angina (judgment)	0.90
Kidney transplant (TTO,[a] Hamilton, patients with transplants)	0.84
Moderate angina (judgment)	0.70
Some physical and role limitation with occasional pain (TTO)	0.67
Hospital dialysis (TTO, Hamilton, dialysis patients)	0.59
Hospital dialysis (TTO, St. John's, dialysis patients)	0.57
Hospital dialysis (TTO, general public)	0.56
Severe angina (judgment)	0.50
Anxious/depressed and lonely much of the time (TTO)	0.45
Being blind or deaf or dumb (TTO)	0.39
Hospital confinement (TTO)	0.33
Mechanical aids to walk and learning disabled (TTO)	0.31
Dead (reference state)	0.00
Quadriplegic, blind, and depressed (TTO)	<0.00
Confined to bed with severe pain (ratio)	<0.00
Unconscious (ratio)	<0.00

Source: Torrance, 1987, p. 595.
[a]TTO = time tradeoff.

variety of social decisions. Health programs with alternative objectives and targets, populations, and goals are allocated different amounts and types of resources by political leaders, health professionals, and program administrators. The health budget of the United States, for example, is distributed among competing agencies, disease categories, target populations, and health activities. The courts compensate disability, disfigurement, and abuse at different levels. Life insurance companies and other risk agents use economic factors to assign values to different dysfunctions and disabilities. These same values might be used to construct broad social preference weights.

Economists have long used human capital valuation to estimate the cost–benefit ratio of social arrangements or the compensation of death and disability (Dublin and Lotka, 1930). Estimates of the value of human livelihood are usually based on future earnings or some other measure of economic value, such as willingness to pay. Rosser and Watts (1972) analyzed 500 compensation awards made by British courts to derive relative values for various health conditions. Disability and distress define eight levels, the lowest or least dysfunctional being slight social disability and slight distress. Persons confined to bed with severe distress were awarded 158 times as much as those at the least severe level of disability/distress.

Human capital valuation methods are often criticized for treating life or livelihood as a market item. Exchanging livelihood is qualitatively different from exchanging goods. For the most part, measures based on earnings place positive value on the productive individual with earning power, denying value to the nonproducer or those who do not trade a product in the market—homemakers or retirees, for instance. Furthermore, such measures maintain the status quo by failing to recognize the extent to which health care increases life satisfaction, equity, and quality regardless of the individual's productivity. Thus, the human capital approach violates the principle of quality by denying value to those outside the market. This problem has been mitigated by "shadow pricing," imputing economic values to the nonmarket section; for example, housework is assigned the monetary value of maid's work.

The disability/distress awards by the courts may overcome the market criticism because the courts are arenas for both sympathy and monetary exchange. However, the courts are not often a social device for redistribution of wealth, and they tend to lean heavily in favor of the status quo. Another major disadvantage with the court award approach is the unlikelihood that such awards will ever be available in sizable numbers to construct categories with a high level of disability without distress. The courts, perhaps as a reflection of social values, presume that sick or disabled persons must suffer distress. A host of practical problems arise when attempts are made to construct social metrics from court awards or other social decisions. Substantial inconsistencies arise in placing values on livelihood, and these inconsistencies make the construction of standardized measures difficult, if not impossible.

Serious efforts should be made in this direction, however, because such decisions represent actual social behavior, eliminate the distance between theoretical construct and empirical measure, and increase validity. The relationship between explicit value scaling and implicit social decision evaluation should be explored as a means of validation.

EXPLICIT WEIGHTING BY PRIMARY DATA COLLECTION

Table 6.5 lists the most commonly used methods of explicit preference weighting developed by psychologists, economists, and decision theorists. These methods differ according to their incorporation of risk and the level at which various health states are aggregated or decomposed in the preference measurement task.

The first way in which these methods differ is the incorporation of risky or riskless choices. *Risk aversion* refers to an individual's reluctance or unwillingness to select an option with an uncertain outcome in favor of one with a certain outcome, even though the long-term expected payoff associated with the risky choice may be higher. A person with end-stage heart disease, for example, may wish to follow a medication regimen

Table 6.5 Methods of explicit preference weighting

Psychophysical
    Paired comparisons
    Category scaling
    Magnitude estimation

Utility
    Standard gamble
    Time tradeoff

Multidimensional
    Multiattribute
    Analytic hierarchy process

rather than have a heart transplant, given that the medication regimen does not involve the risk of death, but the heart transplant promises a higher level of physical and emotional function. Risk aversion may lead individuals to be more inconsistent in their choices, because of their discomfort in valuing choices with risk involved.

Time preferences may also vary. Some people may wish to take a risk for a specific period of time—to stay alive in order to see a grandchild born, for example. These people are not necessarily risk averse, but they place a higher value on immediate and short-term survival. Others may place a higher value on length of life and be willing to experience an immediate decrement in quality of life, for example, in pursuing preventive behaviors, to live a longer and perhaps higher quality of life later.

The methods in Table 6.5 also differ in the level of aggregation resulting from the preference measurement task. As described earlier, two basic approaches to defining health state descriptions for preference measurement are (1) holistic states, in which various health status descriptors are presented together as combinations of levels of functioning on various specific domains, and (2) decomposed states, in which each health state is separated into a level relative to a specific domain. Holistic scaling procedures require judges to assign utility values directly to comprehensive outcomes using psychophysical or utility scaling methods. The major advantage is that values are obtained for the different combinations of outcomes as a whole, mirroring what actually happens when people evaluate their overall state. The major disadvantage is the large amount of information judges must assimilate before assigning preferences to a comprehensive description.

Decomposed procedures, often referred to as multiattribute utility (MAU) methods, were devised to overcome the major shortcoming of judging comprehensive descriptions using holistic scaling methods. The major advantage of decomposed methods is that they focus on one attribute at a time and reduce the number of subjective judgments required to assign preferences to a complete set of outcomes. Judges using the decomposed scaling approach follow these two steps: (1) they assess one conditional utility function over each attribute; and (2) they make a small number of judgments to establish functional form and scaling parameters of the composition rules used to aggregate across attributes (Fischer, 1979). Decomposed methods, therefore, require estimation of the conditional utility functions and some rule by which the utilities for individual attributes can be combined. Composition rules can be obtained two ways— from statistically inferred models where the investigator develops an algebraic model of preference decisions or from explicitly decomposed models where the overall evaluation process is broken into a set of simpler subtasks (Froberg and Kane, 1989a).

The statistically inferred models require that judges assign preferences to a sample of holistic health states. Thus, the attributes in the states can be separated and their individual effects analyzed. The explicitly decomposed models require that judges evaluate each level of a particular attribute assuming all other attributes are held constant. Although many explicitly decomposed models have been used, the conditional utility function-based procedure described by Fischer (1979) is most commonly used.

Regardless of the decision to use holistic or decomposed states, a scaling method must be used to elicit preference weights. These methods can be grouped into three different types: psychophysical methods, utility methods, and multidimensional methods, which may involve either psychophysical or utility methods.

Psychophysical Methods

Analysts have a number of indirect and direct methods to elicit preferences when they use psychophysical scaling methods. Respondents are asked to indicate the intensity of their preferences by a numerical response. The designation "direct" versus "indirect" depends on whether subjects make numerical or nonnumerical responses. *Direct scaling models* assume that judges are capable of directly generating an interval or ratio scale and that errors in judgment are reduced by averaging judgments over subjects. *Indirect scaling models* require judges to choose between alternatives. The data are later converted to an ordinal, interval, or ratio level of measurement. The distinction between "direct" and "indirect" may be inappropriate. There is no evidence that numerical responses are more "direct" than nonnumerical responses. Nevertheless, a large number of *subjective numerical estimate* models are in use. Their most ardent proponents are followers of S. S. Stevens (1960), who pioneered these techniques.

Numerical models are available for constructing ordinal, interval, or ratio scales. Kendall's coefficient of concordance, used to evaluate the degree of agreement among ranks, provides one numerical model for constructing ordinal scales. This model can be used with any single set of stimuli rank-ordered by subjects who are assumed to replicate each other. Indirect methods involve comparisons of alternatives or discrimination between two states or conditions with a scaling model derived from laws of comparative judgment (Torgerson, 1958). *Paired-comparisons* methods take alternatives in pairs with one statement compared to the other. In the tradition of Thurstonian scaling, Fanshel and Bush (1970) advocated paired-comparison techniques to calculate weights for 11 health states.

The number and complexity of case descriptions needed to describe levels of function make Thurstonian techniques of paired comparisons difficult to use. Thurstone (1927) developed five cases of the "law of comparative judgment," which is a model for constructing an interval scale to measure the property of a set of imperfectly discriminable stimuli. A great body of research has resulted from this approach, one major advancement being the extension of these methods to ratio scales (Bock and Jones, 1968).

The general problem with paired-comparison techniques is the excessive number of pairs required in designs using the $n(n - 1)/2$ possible pairs. Ordinarily, in a complete judgment design, the stimuli cannot exceed nine or ten. Many applications of paired comparisons also require multiple presentations of pairs. In studies involving a large number of pairs, the method is impractical. Incomplete designs where certain pairs are omitted entirely can be used, although few studies using this approach have dealt with complex stimuli or stimuli with no underlying physical continuum.

Various procedures have been created for adapting Thurstonian models to data derived from sorting stimuli into a set of ordered categories. These procedures— variously named the method of successive categories, method of successive intervals, or method of graded dichotomies—all relate to Torgerson's (1958) general model known as the "law of categorical judgment." This model assumes that (1) the discriminable dispersions of all stimuli are the same, (2) the discriminable dispersions of all category boundaries are the same, and (3) all the coefficients of correlation between stimuli and category boundaries are the same. Scales constructed under the law of categorical judgment closely approximate those constructed for the same stimuli under the Thurstonian law of comparative judgment (Saffir, 1937). Thus, it is possible to compare one model with another on the basis of empirical criteria if the experimental conditions are the same.

Direct psychophysical scaling models elicit numerical estimates of preference without requiring judges to choose between alternatives. The simplest method for attaching quantitative values to health states is equal-appearing intervals, or category scaling. Figure 6.1 illustrates a category scale for judging the relative desirability of health states. The category scale is a visual analogue scale where each step is considered to be an equal interval: the distance from 0 to 5 is the same as the distance from 20 to 25, 35 to 40, and so forth. Other methods, such as a sorting board with slots at equal intervals or booklets with the visual analogue scale on each page, can be used with the method of equal-appearing intervals. The most desirable health state is placed at one end of the scale and the least desirable at the other end. The remaining health states are placed on the line or in the slots between these two anchors in their order of desirability or preference.

Category scaling methods thus require a judge to assign each health state (stimulus) to one of several categories (usually between 3 and 11). They include the instructions that all categories are to be interpreted as psychologically equal between designated anchor points such as perfect health and death. The physical categories presented to the judges are usually equally spaced. Judges are requested to make relative placements along the scale according to their feelings about the relative desirability of the health

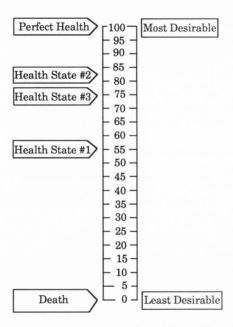

Figure 6.1 Category scale for judging relative desirability of health states. Judges place health states 1–3 on this category scale, or feeling thermometer, with anchors at 0 (death is least desirable) and 100 (perfect health is most desirable). Each scale step represents an equal interval from 0 to 100, indicating judgments are made on an interval scale, although judges may be indicating only ordinal preferences. *Source*: Furlong et al., 1990.

states. In Figure 6.1, health state 1 placed at 55 would be considered 20 units less desirable than health state 3 placed at 75.

Most category judgments are converted onto a 0–1 scale with death as the least desirable anchor state equal to 0 and perfect health as the most desirable anchor state at 1. In this case, the preference value for each of the other states is simply the scale value associated with its placement. If death is not considered to be the least desirable state and is placed at some intermediate point on the scale, say d, the preference values for the states are derived from the formula $(x - d)/(1 - d)$, where x is the scale placement of the health state (Torrance, 1986).

Some investigators consider that category scales can only provide ordinal rankings, not interval or ratio values (Parducci, 1974). Whether the scale values resulting from the method of equal-appearing intervals are actually at the interval level of measurement can and should be evaluated (Blischke et al., 1975). The most common analytic approach is to average the numerical assignments for each stimulus across judges to obtain an interval scale. Numerous studies have shown the rating scale methods to be convenient and easily understood by respondents. These methods also possess comparatively high reproducibility (Patrick, 1972; Patrick et al., 1973a, 1973b; Carter et al., 1976; Torrance, 1976a). Despite the use of anchors, however, individual judges may be biased toward the middle of the scale, making it difficult to separate real differences.

The third psychophysical method of preference weighting is magnitude estimation. *Magnitude estimation methods* require judges to compare each state to a selected standard and then report how much "better" or "worse" it is (Patrick, 1972; Patrick et al., 1973b; Rosser and Kind, 1978; Kaplan et al., 1979). Researchers develop numerical models for ratio scales by having subjects estimate the magnitude of the variable property for each stimulus in the set. The crux of these methods—magnitude or ratio estimation—is the assumption that respondents can assess their experience and assign numerical values with ratio meaning. Like other numerical models, ratio scales using these procedures are based on the assumption that each subject or judge is like every other one, that is, they differ only because of random errors. This assumption allows averaging of these subjective estimates.

The method of equivalence devised by Patrick (1972; Patrick et al., 1973b) requires judges to make decisions between alternative courses of action. These decisions reflect a preference for different levels of health. In the *equivalence method*, health states are judged as outcomes of a health program according to the number of people affected by the program. Stated briefly, the method consists of the following question:

> Suppose there exist scarce resources that must be allocated briefly to one of two groups of people, the first at a level of maximum function F_i and the other at a lower level F_j. If prognosis were held constant for both groups, how many people in F_j would you consider equivalent to the standard population F_i?

Each judgment, then, can be treated as a ratio of the standard. The ratios can then be averaged to obtain a preference scale for the case descriptions. This method is analogous to indifference curve analysis in economics, where, stated in numbers of people, the question asks for the point of equivalency or indifference between two descriptions of function.

Although the equivalence method does not furnish a theoretically related measure, it does provide a different measurement context from the numerical scaling models. This method is more closely related to the way in which the value scale is interpreted and put to use in the Health Resource Allocation Strategy. Utility methods, described next, are also based on treatment decisions using chance or time as the metric rather than number of persons affected by a health program.

Utility Methods

As noted in Chapter 3, modern interest in utility measurement by economists, decision theorists, and operations researchers follows from the classic study by von Neumann and Morgenstern, *The Theory of Games and Economic Behavior*, published in 1944. Earlier attempts to measure utility were based on indifference curve analysis or other methods that yielded an ordinal scale or mere ordering of outcomes. For some time, ordinal utility measures were accepted as the foundation of the microeconomic theory of consumer behavior.

Von Neumann and Morgenstern's mathematical theory of games demonstrated the possibility of obtaining cardinal or numerical scales of utility under conditions similar to indifference curve analysis. Since that time, a large body of new research has involved the measurement of cardinal utility under different conditions. Health utility modeling has led to the use of a number of other scaling techniques, most notably the von Neumann–Morgenstern standard gamble. In this technique, judges must choose between an uncertain or risky alternative with specified probabilities of good and bad outcome and a certain, nonrisky alternative intermediate outcome (Torrance et al., 1972, 1973; Vertinsky and Wong, 1975; Torrance, 1976a). Utility-based methods provide an indirect means for preference measurement. Values are based on the subject's responses to decision situations.

The *standard gamble method*, based on the axioms of expected utility theory, has been widely used to measure health state utilities (Torrance, 1986). Figure 6.2 illustrates the standard gamble for a chronic health state considered better than death. In this approach, judges are asked to consider the choice between options. Choice A is treatment with two possible outcomes: either return to usual health (probability p) or immediate death (probability $1 - p$). Choice B has the certain outcome of the chronic health state B_i for life. In another example, the certain outcome may be "remains at current level of health." In this instance, the gamble outcomes may consist of immediate death or complete recovery, corresponding to an idealized treatment decision.

The respondent is asked to indicate the value of p at which point she or he would be indifferent about the certain outcome and the gamble. This value is used to calculate the relative utility of the certain outcome. Several good descriptions of the standard gamble method are available, and a guide on the design and development of health state utility instrumentation is available from McMaster University (Furlong et al., 1990).

The probability wheel and chance board are visual aids that help judges assign preferences to health states when using the standard gamble method. The terms "probability" and "chance" indicate that risk is involved in the choice. Figure 6.3 illustrates a chance board similar to that suggested by Furlong et al. (1990). The top of the board is labelled Choice A and the bottom part Choice B. Judges are generally asked to decide between A or B, accepting or not accepting a treatment. In assigning preferences to

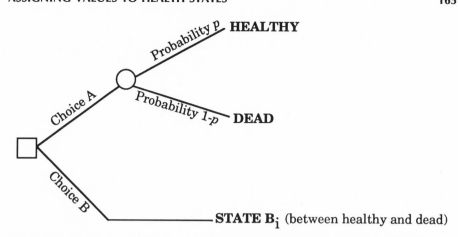

Figure 6.2   Standard gamble decision tree for a chronic health state considered better than death. This decision tree has one choice node (square between *A* and *B*) and one chance node (circle between healthy and dead). The judge assigns utility values to consequences associated with paths through the tree. Choice *A* involves uncertainty or some probability *p* of being healthy and probability 1 − *p* of death. The utility value is the probability *p* at which the judge is indifferent between the certain outcome (Choice *B*) and the gamble (Choice *A*). *Source*: Torrance, 1986. p. 20.

health states considered better than death, Choice *B* is fairly straightforward because it describes only one health state with a 100 percent chance of occurrence. This state describes communication, cognition, mobility, self-care, and pain. If a judge prefers this option, then he or she will be certain of living in this health state for the rest of life.

Choice *A* is more complex because there are two possible results. The chances of each of these results occurring are shown by the numbers in the boxes appearing above each description and the size of the matching area in the circle between the numbers. These circles are pies that represent the probability of the person being in the health state. In Figure 6.3, there is a 90 percent chance of perfect health and a 10 percent chance of death, most likely associated with surgical or medical treatment. Judges are asked which choice they would prefer, *A* or *B*.

In the standard gamble method, the sequence of probability values are varied in a converging Ping-Pong fashion by alternating between high and low values: 10/90, 90/10, 20/80, 80/20, and so forth. This convergent cascading addresses the concerns of Tversky and Kahneman (1981), who pointed out the need to reduce the possibility of an anchoring bias where a strategy of constantly increasing/decreasing encourages respondents to overestimate or underestimate their indifference point. This strategy also reduces a framing effect associated with consistently increasing or decreasing probabilities, which are often interpreted by judges as gains or losses relative to a point of reference.

Calculation of the utility values associated with a chronic health state considered better than death is straightforward. The probability *p* of Choice *A* is varied until the judge is indifferent between the two alternatives, at which point the preference value for the health state is simply *p*. In the example seen in Figure 6.3, if the judge considered Choice *A* to be equal to Choice *B*, the utility for the health state shown would be 0.90.

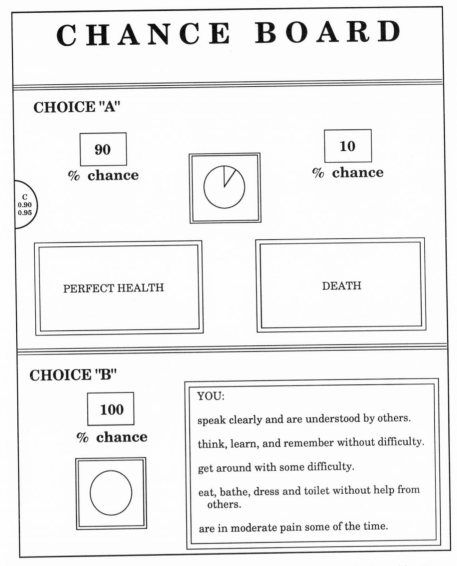

Figure 6.3 Chance board for assigning preferences using the standard gamble. *Source:* Adapted from Furlong et al., 1990.

Figure 6.4 shows the logic of the standard gamble method applied to health states considered worse than death. In this case, the choice presented to judges is between Choice *A*, an uncertain alternative between healthy (probability *p*) or state W_i (probability $1 - p$), or Choice *B*, the certain outcome of death. Judges are commonly asked to imagine they have a terminal disease, which will lead to death if untreated. If treated, there are two probabilities: probability *p*, the disease will be eliminated with a return to health; and probability $1 - p$, treatment will result in state W_i, considered worse than death. In calculating a utility value for states considered worse than death, probability *p* is varied until the judge is indifferent between the two alternatives. At this point, the

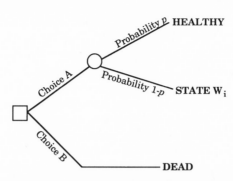

Figure 6.4 Standard gamble decision tree for a chronic health state considered worse than death. For this decision tree, the judge chooses between Choice A, a choice with uncertainty or some probability p of being in perfect health and probability $1 - p$ of being in a state that is considered worse than death, and Choice B, a choice with the certain outcome of death. Probability p is varied until the judge is indifferent between Choice A and B. The utility value is negative, as defined by $-p/(1 - p)$. *Source*: Torrance, 1986, p. 22.

preference value for state W_i is $-p/(1 - p)$. If the state is considered much worse than death, such as persistent coma or unconsciousness, then judges are unlikely to choose the gamble (Choice A) unless the probability of returning to a healthy state is high. All utilities elicited in this standard gamble result in negative values.

As Torrance (1986) illustrates, the standard gamble method can also be applied to temporary states where the choice is not always between health and death, as seen in Figure 6.5. In this case, the temporary intermediate state i, the one being evaluated, is the choice with certain outcome. State i is evaluated in relation to the most desirable state (health) and the worst temporary state j. To calculate the utilities for temporary

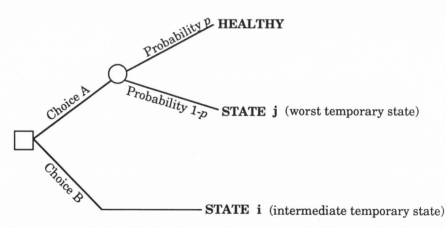

Figure 6.5 Standard gamble decision tree for a temporary health state. The judge in this decision analysis chooses between Choice A, which involves uncertainty or some probability p of being healthy and probability $1 - p$ of being in the worst temporary state, such as the health state following a severe myocardial infarction, and Choice B, which is the certain outcome of a temporary intermediate state, such as undergoing treatment for an attack of angina. The utility value for the intermediate temporary state S_i is $p + (1 - p)S_j$ or the worst temporary state. Source: Torrance, 1986, p. 22.

states, the formula $S_i = p + (1 - p)S_j$ is used, with i the state being measured and j the worst state.

Interviewers and judges often report that the standard gamble is difficult to administer and to understand. This method is preferred by many investigators, however, because of its use of expected utility theory and the economic theory supporting it. Once judges have learned what is expected of them, most are comfortable with the judgment tasks involved in the standard gamble. The relative health state utilities may vary as function of the gamble outcomes considered, however (Llewellyn-Thomas et al., 1982). Responses derived from the standard gamble approach incorporate risk preferences; they do not distinguish between the values people attach to various health states and their willingness or reluctance to accept risk.

Another utility technique similar to equivalence methods is *time tradeoff*. In this technique, judges choose between two health states with different lengths of time (Torrance et al., 1973; Torrance, 1976b; Sackett and Torrance, 1978; Wolfson et al., 1982). This is a paired-comparison technique in which the subject chooses between two alternatives. Figure 6.6 applies a time tradeoff to chronic health states considered *better* than death. The subject is offered two choices: Choice A, state i for time t (life expectancy of an individual with the condition) followed by death; and Choice B, healthy for time $x < t$ followed by death. Time x is varied until the respondent is indifferent between the two alternatives. At this point the required preference value for state i is given by $h_i = x/t$.

The time tradeoff technique can also be used to measure preference for health states considered worse than death, as illustrated in Figure 6.7. The judge is again offered two choices: A, health for time $x < t$ followed by state i until time t, followed by death; and B, immediate death. Time x is varied until the respondent is indifferent between the two alternatives, at which point the required preference value for state i is given by $h_i = x/(x - t)$. The equation is derived by equating the two alternatives, $1.0x + h_i (t - x) = 0$, and solving for h_i.

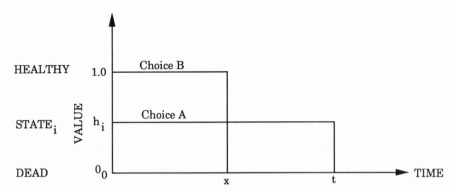

Figure 6.6 Time tradeoff decision diagram for a chronic health state preferred to death. This decision diagram involves tradeoffs under certainty. The judge has two choices: A, being in some state of health between perfect health and death (State i) for time t or the remaining years of life of the judge (or a hypothetical individual), or B, being in a state of perfect health for a shorter period of time ($x < t$) followed by death. The utility value for State i is x/t at the point when the judge is indifferent between Choice A and Choice B. *Source*: Torrance, 1986, p. 23.

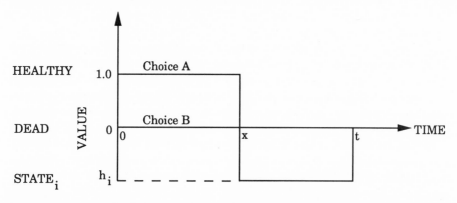

Figure 6.7 Time tradeoff decision diagram for a chronic health state considered worse than death. This decision diagram involves tradeoffs under certainty. The judge again has two choices: A, being in perfect health for a time ($x < t$) followed by a state worse than death (h_i) for the remaining period of life, followed by death; or B, immediate death. The utility value for State i is negative and is the point at which the judge is indifferent between Choice A and B or $x(x - t)$. *Source:* Torrance, 1986, p. 24.

The time tradeoff method can also be applied to temporary health states. As in the standard gamble application, state i (the health state being evaluated) is compared to other states j where state j is the worse state. Judges are offered two choices: A, temporary state i for time t (the time spent in the temporary state), followed by health; and B, temporary state j for time $x < t$, followed by health. Time x is varied starting at the extremes and converging toward the middle until the judge is indifferent between the two choices. At the indifference point, the preference value for state $i = 1 - (1 - h_j)x/t$. If $h_j = 0$, then $h_i = 1 - x/t$.

A time tradeoff board can be used as a visual aid to help make the judgment. Furlong et al. (1990) provide instructions for constructing a laminated board with sliders, and changeable scales and health states, parallel to the apparatus used in the standard gamble. These visual aids help instruct judges and elicit preferences during face-to-face interviews. As discussed later, careful administration of scaling instructions and procedures is necessary to obtain reliable preference judgments.

In two instances, group administration of preference measurement techniques is desirable: (1) a particular group of experts is assembled; (2) utilities need to be estimated in the most convenient and efficient manner possible. Group administration of utility methods is possible using variants of the standard gamble and time tradeoff methods. The utility assessment procedures used by the Committee to Evaluate the NHLBI Artificial Heart Program provide such an example.

The committee was presented with the six health state descriptions listed in Table 6.3 and the following assumptions:

1. The patients have end-stage heart disease on the basis of physiological data—left ventricular ejection fraction < 20 percent.
2. The family situation and supports are constant and consistent with the needs of someone in that state—spouse and other relatives are present, helpful, and supportive where needed and appropriate.

3. These patients had full third-party coverage of health care costs with no limits or substantial copayments.

Figure 6.8 represents the time tradeoff board illustrated to permit assignment of preferences. The top part of the board is labeled Life *A* and the bottom half, Life *B*. In each case, the preference assignment task is to compare Life *A* and Life *B* with different amounts of time spent in each state. Life *A* in this example is perfect health, or "healthy as can possibly be," the duration of life in the perfect health state, the time of death, and the duration of life lost due to premature death. Life *B* is a less desirable health status lasting the maximum duration under consideration. In this example, Life *B* is health state 1 for Group *W* of end-stage heart disease, patients with only mild impairment. The survival expectancy of this group is 20 years, so the time tradeoff board allows for 20 years of remaining life. In Figure 6.8, the white space in Life *A* indicates years of life spent in perfect health. The shaded space indicates premature death or the number of years lost through an early death, here in year 16 of survival, meaning 4 years lost through early death. The shaded area in Life *B* represents the amount of time spent in the Group *W*, mildly impaired state, for the 20-year duration of survival expectancy.

Figure 6.9 is a time tradeoff answer sheet with various choice options and utility values assigned to the different choices (in parentheses). Preference judgments can be elicited from a group by projecting such an answer sheet on a screen or printing it in an answer booklet. As in the standard gamble method, the converging, or Ping-Pong, approach is used. It begins with a comparison of Life *A* and Life *B*, both set at 20 years (20/20). Respondents who prefer Life *B* in this choice may have misunderstood the task, because Life *B* is usually less desirable than perfect health. In such cases, the choices are repeated.

The second choice (0/20) is presented to check on whether the judge might consider the state being evaluated as worse than death. The choice is between Life *A*, 0 years of remaining life due to immediate death, and Life *B*, 20 remaining years of life. If Life *A* is chosen, the state being judged is considered worse than death, and a different procedure must be used to elicit preferences. Judges are asked to continue with each choice if their preference is marked in a diamond ("go" sign) and to stop if their preference is marked in a hexagon ("stop" sign). All choices are presented until all judges have reached a stop sign.

The configuration of the time tradeoff board changes when judging states considered worse than death. (See Figure 6.10.) For these states, the time scale for Life *A* is set at immediate death with 0 amount of remaining life left; the time scale for Life *B* is the only thing that changes. In this example, health state 4 for group *Z* (Moribund) of end-stage heart disease patients is used. The survival expectancy of this group is 6 months, or 24 weeks. Because the time intervals must be consistent across groups, the survival expectancy for the time tradeoff exercise was set at 30 weeks of remaining life. In this illustration, Life *A* is immediate death, while Life *B* is 27 weeks in perfect health, followed by 3 weeks in the group *Z* health state. Judges who preferred Life *A* to Life *B* would be indicating their unwillingness to spend even 3 weeks as a severe end-stage heart disease patient described in group *Z*.

Table 6.6 shows the mean utility scores and standard deviations for the six patient groups and health states collected by the time tradeoff method. The mildly impaired

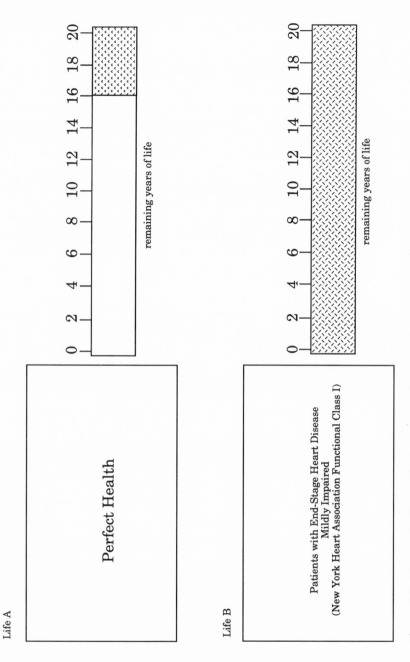

Figure 6.8 Time tradeoff board for assigning preferences to health states considered better than death. *Source:* Adapted from Furlong et al., 1990.

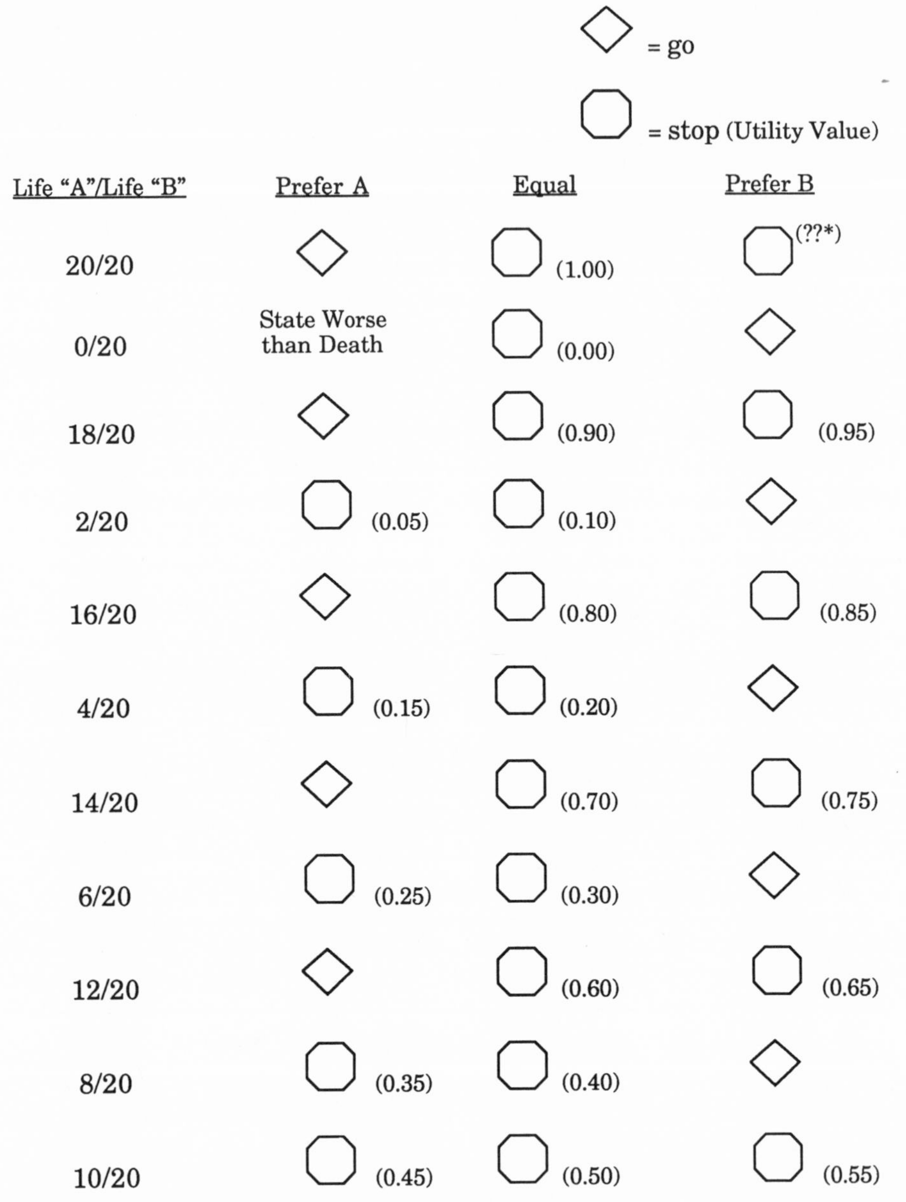

Figure 6.9 Answer sheet and utilities for time tradeoff for states considered better than death.

Group 1 was assigned a utility of 0.82, and the symptomatic Group 2 and Group 3 were assigned lower utilities. The Moribund Group 4, with a life expectancy of 6 months, was assigned a very low utility (0.08), indicating that the committee as a whole considered this health state to be near death. The two major groups of interest, Group 5 with the total artificial heart and group 6 with a heart transplant, were assigned utilities between Group 3 and Group 1. The committee considered heart

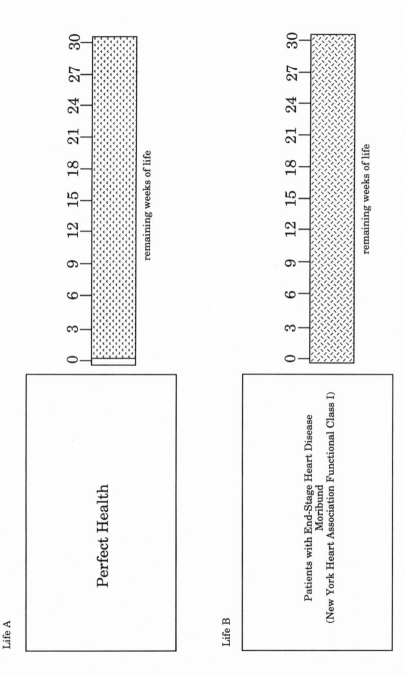

Figure 6.10 Time tradeoff board for assigning preferences to health states considered worse than death. *Source:* Adapted from Furlong et al., 1990.

Table 6.6 Mean utilities and standard deviations for end-stage heart disease states: Results of the time tradeoff method from Committee to Evaluate the NHLBI Artificial Heart Program

Patient group/health state	Utility for long-term health states	Utility in regular hospital (med/surg)	Utility in ICU/CCU
1. Mildly impaired	0.82 (0.09)	0.70 (0.19)	0.55 (0.27)
2. Symptomatic	0.70 (0.12)	0.57 (0.18)	0.45 (0.24)
3. Seriously impaired	0.52 (0.22)	0.10 (0.22)	−0.01 (0.24)
4. Moribund	0.08 (0.20)	0.01 (0.26)	−0.11 (0.22)
5. Long-term fully implanted artificial heart	0.66 (0.12)	0.52 (0.16)	0.40 (0.22)
6. Heart transplant	0.75 (0.18)	0.55 (0.22)	0.42 (0.26)

transplant patients to have a higher utility score (0.75) than patients with a total artificial heart (0.66).

Utility scores for hospital patients in regular medical or surgical wards and those in intensive care or coronary care units (ICU/CCU) were generally lower than those for long-term health states. Because these utility scores were obtained by directly "adjusting" those derived for the long-term health states, this declining pattern was expected. These utility scores provided the preference weights for the cost–utility analyses of the artificial heart program. Incorporation of preference weights into the calculation of years of healthy life is described and discussed in Chapter 9.

One potential limitation of the time tradeoff technique is that it does not directly account for nonlinearities in the time–utility function in which a person places a much higher premium on immediate rather than long-term survival. Another criticism is that time tradeoff does not realistically reflect treatment decisions that people are faced with. Nevertheless, the technique has appeal, because the tradeoff of time spent in different health states is very important to those receiving treatment.

Multidimensional Methods

The major set of multidimensional methods is based on *multiattribute utility theory*, widely used in the decision sciences. These multidimensional, or decomposed, approaches to health state preference measurement have one advantage: they require judges to focus individually on each component of a health outcome. Judges rate only a subset of the health states rather than the entire universe of combinations. These methods require use of an explicit model combining the dimension-specific utilities. The model forms the overall characterizations of the preferences associated with health states.

Multiattribute utility theory establishes an axiomatic basis for the various models used. The following are most common: additive, quasi-additive, and multilinear (Fischer, 1979). Three utility independence conditions underlie these models: utility independence, mutual utility independence, and additive utility independence (Keeney and Raiffa, 1976). Figure 6.11 illustrates these assumptions and model forms.

Using multiattribute utility theory, the investigator searches for the best mathe-

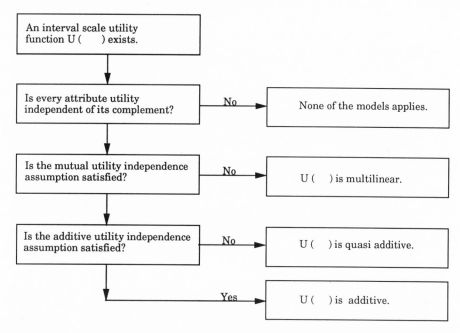

Figure 6.11   Utility independence assumptions and utility model forms. *Source*: Fischer, 1979.

matical model for estimating the values of unmeasured health states. Each model can be tested for *validity*, the number of health states required to estimate the "weights." The best-fitting model represents a tradeoff between validity and efficiency.

These mathematical models are built from the single-attribute preference functions for each attribute. Each single-attribute preference function is defined over all levels of a particular attribute. The resulting models differ in the way the preference functions are combined to form the overall health index and in the weights for each attribute. Torrance et al. (1982) and Keeney and Raiffa (1976) describe these methods in detail. The mathematical models developed through these procedures should be replicated on a new set of raters to determine if similar results are observed. Once a valid model and an appropriate subset of health states are identified, final weights for the model can be obtained.

Another variant of the multidimensional approach is the Analytic Hierarchy Process (AHP) developed by Saaty (1980). The AHP is a decision and planning tool that can be used with individuals or groups. Researchers analyze a problem in a hierarchical structure and develop paired comparisons between alternatives. Then judges use the nonnumerical paired comparisons to rate the relative importance of each health dimension. For each pair of dimensions, ratings of importance are obtained. For example, a five-point verbal descriptive scale may be used:

Equal in importance	scored as 1
Slightly more important	scored as 3
More important	scored as 5
Substantially more important	scored as 7
Overwhelmingly more important	scored as 9

Respondents may compromise between labels. These compromises are scored as the even number between the indicated scores. The comparisons are put into a matrix with reciprocals in corresponding off-diagonal elements. If dimension A is rated by a judge as more important than B (score = 5), then dimension B is considered less important than A (score = 1/5). The disadvantage to the AHP method, like other paired-comparison methods, is the large number of judgments required.

COMPARISON OF HEALTH STATE PREFERENCE MEASUREMENTS

Reliability, Stability, and Validity

The reliability and validity of health state preference measurements have been addressed by numerous investigators and reviewed by Froberg and Kane (1989b), who discuss three types of reliability. *Intrarater reliability* is a single judge's consistency when a health state is presented more than once. *Reproducibility*, sometimes referred to as test–retest reliability, is the consistency of results obtained from scaling methods across repeated administrations over short time periods. *Interrater reliability*, or precision, is the consistency among judges regarding scale values. Data are available on all three types of reliability only for category scaling method applications.

In their review, Froberg and Kane (1989b) conclude that intrarater reliability and reproducibility are acceptable for category scaling, standard gamble, and time tradeoff. In general, the Pearson's product-moment or intraclass correlations range from 0.70 to 0.90, with the exception of the six-week test–retest correlation reported by Torrance (1987) for the time tradeoff procedure. Compared to other measures of sentiment and opinion, these coefficients indicate a high degree of reliability.

Few data exist on the stability of health state preferences over long periods of time. This is particularly true for health states near the extremes of the continuum of health-related quality of life, for example, perfect health and death or states of health considered worse than death. Torrance (1976c) used three methods to study preference values obtained one year apart. He found the following product–moment correlations: category scaling (0.49), time tradeoff (0.62), and standard gamble (0.53). These coefficients indicate that health state preferences may change over time, although few studies are available to interpret the direction or predictors of change. Clear candidates for study would include (1) significant deterioration or improvement in medical status, (2) change in survival expectancy, (3) treatments like chemotherapy, (4) aging, and (5) significant life events such as loss of loved ones or severe marital discord.

Evaluating the validity of health state preferences poses a formidable challenge. Since no criterion exists by which to evaluate results, the construct must be validated to determine the extent to which hypothesized relationships among health state preference methods are supported by empirical data. These theoretical relationships may concern (1) the convergence or discrimination of results obtained from different preference measurement methods, or (2) the degree to which preference measurements predict other variables or vice versa in a hypothesized model. Most often, the convergence of results among methods is used to evaluate validity, sometimes with one method considered to be the criterion. Torrance (1987) evaluated category scaling and time tradeoff using the standard gamble as the criterion. He concluded that time tradeoff methods had acceptable validity. Category scaling methods produced values that may be interval or cardinal, but these values, obtained under conditions of certainty without taking risk into account, required transformation, usually a power function, before adequate correlations were obtained with judgments from the standard gamble.

Few theoretical guides help predict relationships among methods or among preference values and external variables. Cumulative evidence from existing scaling studies suggests that different techniques can lead to different results, although the origin of the difference may not always be obvious. A high correlation among scaling methods will not guarantee that different methods will produce equivalent results (Read et al., 1984).

Category scaling and magnitude estimation have been compared using the psychophysical laws of judgment (Patrick, 1972; Patrick et al., 1973b; Kaplan et al., 1976). Kaplan and colleagues found category scaling preferable to magnitude estimation, because magnitude estimates were compressed at the death or zero end of the hypothesized health–death continuum. Haig et al. (1986) suggest that using death as the zero point contributes to a floor effect whereby judges cannot rate states of health as worse than death. In general, category scaling and magnitude estimation methods have produced results comparable to or consistent with psychophysical laws.

Stevens rejected category scaling because he believed the method biased judges to use each category of the scale the same number of times (Stevens and Gallanter, 1957). He registered this opinion again in a comparison of category scaling and magnitude estimation of the values assigned to health states (Stevens, 1971). In a more recent study, Anderson (1976) showed that category scaling can yield interval-level measures. The experiments of Kaplan and Ernst (1983) support this view: the ease of the task and the well-defined response scale of category scaling lends support to its continued development and testing.

Few causal modeling studies have been conducted to predict health state preferences or to use preferences to predict other constructs. Churchill et al. (1987) predicted that mean scores from end-stage renal disease patients rating their own health would be highest for transplant patients, lowest for hospital hemodialysis patients, and intermediate for home/self-care hemodialysis and continuous ambulatory peritoneal dialysis patients. Study results corroborated these predictions with the mean time tradeoff utilities ranging from 0.43 for hospital dialysis to 0.84 for transplant patients. Kind et al. (1982) found that magnitude estimation methods produced values significantly correlated (0.82) with British court awards for damages in personal injury claims. In general, published studies support the contention that scaling methods produce results consistent with hypothesized directions in severity of illness, different treatment conditions, and treatment decisions.

Unfortunately, few of these studies have been replicated by different investigators, making it difficult to conclude the clear superiority of one method over another. Although methodological work is needed, particularly with multidimensional aspects (Veit and Ware, 1982), adequate scaling methods already exist for obtaining social metrics for health states.

Practical Considerations

Assigning preferences to health states can involve considerable investment of time, energy, and resources, particularly if investigators are not experienced in different measurement techniques. Respondent burden is also a consideration. Experience shows that some people resist judgment tasks. They find probabilities or time difficult to work with. Other people find it offensive to assign numbers to quality of life.

Other practical considerations concern the need to develop extensive instrumentation means—visual aids, trained interviewers, interviewer manuals, and response recording forms. Data, sometimes requiring statistical transformation, must be entered and analyzed. Measurement must be standardized in scaling studies to ensure precision, to help interviewers administer the preference assignment task, and to increase confidence in study results.

Rapid progress is being made in designing methods for collecting preference data using standardized instrumentation, interview procedures, and data analytic techniques (Furlong et al., 1990). Computer-assisted personal interview methods will undoubtedly appear when the required investment in hardware and software becomes more reasonable. Interactive videodisc presentations and computer preference choices will help to make judges more familiar with the health states being evaluated and ease the response burden.

Response rates in preference assignment studies conducted in patient and general populations are high with all methods, ranging from 50 to 100 percent. Little work has been done, however, on the cognitive burden—the effort required to perceive, think, and remember—associated with different scaling methods. More must be done to locate groups in the population who simply cannot perform the judgment tasks reliably. Young children, persons with severe cognitive impairment and emotional or physical illness, and persons with hearing or visual impairments will require simple methods of value assignment. These simple methods are necessary if these groups are to participate and understand the decision-making process or the choices being presented. Few barriers may exist, however, in eliciting preferences from a wide range of persons, because choices among alternative courses of action are made frequently by all persons.

Selecting a Preference-Weighting Strategy

Deciding between different preference measurement methods is no simple task. No single "best" method exists on which to base estimates of criterion validity or practicality. Decision theorists and economists have long favored the standard gamble method because it uses a set of axioms based on the theory of expected utility. The standard gamble also mirrors many clinical decisions because it requires judges to make preference choices under conditions of uncertainty; that is, outcomes of clinical treatments are seldom known with certainty in advance. Because expected utility theory also involves an assumption of cardinality, or the achievement of at least an interval scale, the standard gamble is also purported to yield the most accurate level of measurement in the scaling of opinions.

The cognitive burden of the standard gamble procedure, the possibility that utilities derived from this procedure may be affected or biased by risk aversion, and some judges' inherent dislike of "gambling" contribute to skepticism about its use. In addition, evidence suggests that people make choices inconsistent with the expected utility theory on which the standard gamble and time tradeoff methods are based

(Shoemaker, 1982). Thus, theories of rational choice help but do not *answer* the question of accuracy in preference measurement.

The need to obtain preference values for a large number of health state descriptions in a relatively economical and timely fashion will lead to increased use of the psychophysical methods of direct scaling, particularly category scaling and magnitude or ratio estimation. The extent to which these methods yield preference values that are more or less valid than the utility methods is unclear, because few comparisons among methods have been made by investigators using different health states.

The choice of preference measurement method should be based on the decision or problem to be solved and the use to which the data will be put. Decisions that involve uncertainty, as in most clinical applications, are suited best to the standard gamble method. Population studies requiring telephone interviews or a large number of health states require one or more of the less complex methods such as category scaling or magnitude estimation. Clinicians and other health professionals familiar with the decision context are able to perform difficult judgment tasks using the standard gamble or time tradeoff.

Progress in health state preference measurement will be enhanced by increased use of simple response formats such as category scaling, group administration of preference measures, and repeated administrations on different population and patient groups. Simple methods might be used and compared to the more complex utility and psychophysical methods. The cognitive processes and burdens associated with preference assignment tasks should also be carefully evaluated. Finally, more research is needed on the reproducibility and stability of preferences in different population groups and on the determinants of preferences. These studies should be based on theoretical ideas about expected differences or similarities between results, similar to the construct validation processes applied to health status and quality of life instruments discussed in Chapter 7.

Although statistical weighting and relative preferences methods have been compared on theoretical grounds (Bush, 1984b), no data have been published comparing the results of these two methods for combining health-related quality of life variables or descriptions. Even if argued on the grounds of social justice, the contribution of social preference weights to a composite index of health-related quality of life should be examined. The two techniques should be compared to determine the extent to which explicit preference weighting increases the discrimination, sensitivity, and validity of the overall measure of health-related quality of life. Torrance et al. (1982) describe 960 possible states using 6 (physical function) × 5 (role function) × 4 (socioemotional function) × 8 (health problems). Theoretically, each possible state could be valued. Nonetheless, there are practical limits to the number of combinations that can be scaled, even though millions of different states of well-being would exist in the population if the list of categories and concepts contained in Table 4.1 were all used in the description.

There are many other issues involved in applying the relative preference approach, including the stability of the judgments and the zero origin of the well-being continuum (Patrick, 1979; Boyle and Torrance, 1984). Two additional issues, however, require closer examination. The first concerns factors that significantly influence the preference judgments people make about health and quality of life or the context-independence of direct scaling efforts. The content of the description (Sackett and Torrance, 1978), the mode of presentation (Llewellyn-Thomas et al., 1984), the explanation of the scaling task (Rosser and Kind, 1978), the age of the judge (Sackett and Torrance, 1978), and the medical experience of raters (Carter et al., 1976; Rosser and Kind, 1978) have all been found to be significant influences on the utility values obtained in one study or another. Results are not consistent, however, from the few systematic attempts to investigate the effects of rater characteristics as age, sex, income, marital status, or cultural group) (Kaplan et al., 1978; Rosser and Kind, 1978; Patrick et al., 1985). The large standard deviations or wide dispersion in scale judgments observed may lead to greater social consensus than actually exists (Rosser and Kind, 1978; Boyle and Torrance, 1984). This possibility should be investigated more thoroughly to better define which factors or rater characteristics significantly influence preference judgments.

COMPARING STATISTICAL AND PREFERENCE WEIGHTING

Preference-weighted measures of health-related quality of life are necessary for cost–effectiveness calculations involving quality of life adjustment. Years of healthy life, discussed in Chapter 9, integrate quantity and quality of life into a single combined measure. The Health Resource Allocation Strategy, therefore, requires health-related quality of life measures that are preference weighted.

Not all uses of health status and quality of life measures, however, may require or benefit from preference weighting. In a study of patients with back pain, Deyo and Centor (1986) compared the preference-weighted Sickness Impact Profile (SIP) with a version modified for back pain (Roland Scale) in which 24 SIP items were selected as relevant to back pain. The phrase "because of my back" was added to each statement, and each item was scored as a 0–1 variable. Scores on the Roland Scale ranged from 0 to 24, with higher scores representing worse dysfunction. Both the overall SIP and Roland Scale showed significant correlations between change scores and changes in self-rated improvement, clinician-rated improvement, spine, flexion, and resumption of full activities. This "pruned," condition-specific scale was at least as responsive as the lengthier SIP in both discrimination and quantification of changes. Reliability and validity of the two scales were also similar (Deyo, 1986).

Measures of social preference also may not correspond to measures of individual preference that are increasingly used in clinical investigations to help decide between treatment alternatives. Currently available studies suggest there is wide social consensus on the preferences assigned to health states. Weights from a general population sample on the Quality of Well-Being Scale agreed closely with those from a sample of rheumatoid arthritic patients (Balaban et al., 1986). Patrick et al. (1985) found similar agreement on SIP preference weights obtained from general population samples in Seattle and London.

Methodological studies will not address the desirability or possibility of using health state preferences to design a normative theory of health. Values are the metric for the social sciences. Regardless of their potential application in the weighting of health-related quality of life measures, health state utilities will continue to be examined to understand how individuals and social groups make decisions about their well-being.

7

Selecting an Instrument for Primary Data Collection

Developing a new measure of health status or quality of life for collecting data requires considerable resources as well as months or years of investment. Designing the questionnaire, conducting studies of reliability, validity, and responsiveness, and gaining experience in different populations can take five to ten years from inception to publication. Many of the generic measures discussed in Chapters 4 and 5 took decades to develop and millions of dollars from public and private sources. The newer disease-specific measures, used most often in combination with generic ones, can also take years to develop and test. Thus, most investigators do and *should* choose to use existing measures rather than embark on the development of new ones.

In previous chapters we provided guidelines for selecting one of the existing primary data collection instruments to implement the Health Resource Allocation Strategy. In this chapter we review additional criteria for selecting and using existing instruments in collecting, analyzing, and interpreting health-related quality of life data. We present ten steps for investigators to follow in collecting health-related quality of life data. These steps apply to health-related quality of life assessments other than resource allocation, including population monitoring and clinical evaluations.

Three major types of guidelines can be used in selecting measures and instruments: (1) type of application and objectives of measurement; (2) methodological concerns: reliability, validity, stability, and responsiveness; and (3) practical concerns: resources, time, method of administration, and acceptability to respondents and investigators. We review the ten steps and discuss these guidelines to assist in the selection of instruments for assessing health-related quality of life. We also propose a set of questions that investigators should ask in evaluating health-related quality of life instruments.

The term *instrument* is used in this chapter to define questionnaire content, method of administration, scoring algorithm, and interpretation of scores obtained from one or more measures of health-related quality of life. In other words, the apparatus, its application, its resulting numbers, and its interpretation can be viewed as a "package" analogous to a mercury gravity or aneroid-manometer type of blood pressure apparatus or forced expiratory volume for assessing respiratory function.

Selection of measures is *context-specific*. No single formula will identify the "best" measure or measures to use. However, the guidelines presented here can be used to do the following: devise an optimal measurement strategy, select existing measures, develop new measures where appropriate, and construct questionnaires or interview schedules.

STEPS IN COLLECTING HEALTH-RELATED QUALITY OF LIFE DATA

Figure 7.1 outlines ten major steps investigators usually follow in selecting instruments and in collecting primary data on health-related quality of life. The assessment strategy can be viewed as a circular flow from specifying the problem to analyzing, interpreting, and presenting findings. One study does not necessarily provide an unambiguous answer to a problem. The flow is circular in that the final step returns to problem definition, indicating that several assessments may be necessary to answer a particular health decision or problem. For example, both primary and secondary data may be used to evaluate the effects of a particular health insurance program on health-related quality of life outcomes with repeated application of the measurement steps. Investigators may also spend decades on one health policy area, such as environmental regulation or technology assessment, repeating the basic steps of primary data collection two or more times.

The ten steps shown in Figure 7.1 generally follow a sequential pattern, although several steps may occur concurrently. Revisions to each step may also occur throughout the study whenever changes occur in the environment of the investigation—in funding, study objectives, field conditions, or other aspects. In a full-scale investigation including health-related quality of life assessment, investigators should:

1. Define the application and purpose of data collection by describing the decision and problem to be addressed, specifying the objectives of assessment, and assigning priorities to these objectives if there are more than one.
2. Specify available resources including time, money, personnel, and the projected burden on respondents, interviewers, data analysts, and investigators.
3. Describe known characteristics of the population to be assessed.
4. Identify all domains of health-related quality of life relevant to the decision and all parties interested in the decision.
5. Assess the methodological characteristics of potential measures of domains through literature reviews, compendiums of measures, and contacts with developers. Calculate sample size requirements based on means, sample variances, and known effect sizes published in the literature or obtained from developers and other users.
6. Assess practical considerations and choose instruments that are appropriate to the application and objectives of measurement; contain relevant concepts; have known reliability, validity, and responsiveness; are acceptable to respondents and personnel; and conform with resources available for conducting the study.
7. Conduct a pretest or pilot study that includes, if possible, experience in collecting data under exact conditions of the full study and in analyzing results.
8. Prepare plans for collecting, editing, scoring, and analyzing data, including example table shells and a statistical model of health-related quality of life and its determinants in the investigation.
9. Collect data using standardized procedures and continuously monitoring the quality of data collection and incoming data.
10. Consider how findings can be presented in a clear, concise format, addressing the decision as precisely as possible.

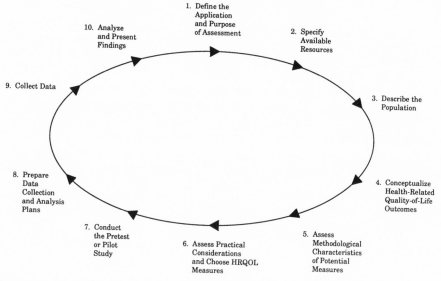

Figure 7.1 Ten steps in a health-related quality of life (HRQOL) assessment. *Source*: Patrick and Erickson, 1992.

STEP 1. DEFINE THE OBJECTIVES OF ASSESSMENT

In Chapter 2, we discussed how to specify a health policy decision. For most decisions, investigators should list causal hypotheses concerning all relevant determinants of health-related quality of life, the method of socioeconomic evaluation being used, and all components of the policy problem. Health decisions are specified by identifying (1) alternative courses of action under consideration; (2) all the groups interested in the decision, including when and why they are interested; and (3) the possible values associated with the outcomes of each alternative.

For example, an investigator might be interested in the appropriate treatment for patients with angina. Possible actions include no surgical procedure, angioplasty, and coronary artery bypass surgery. Clinicians, patients, families, and administrators involved in reimbursement might be interested in these alternatives for different reasons. The interested parties also may value outcomes for the three courses of action differently. In this example, the investigator is interested in the effects of interventions, so the primary purpose of assessment is to evaluate change over time.

Kirshner and Guyatt (1985) identified three major objectives for measuring health status: (1) discriminating among persons at a single point in time, similar to psychological measures of traits such as intelligence and personality; (2) predicting some future outcome or the results of a more intrusive or costly criterion measure, commonly referred to as the "gold standard"; and (3) measuring changes over time, as in the typical design of a cohort study or randomized controlled trial. Methodological and practical considerations are different according to the purpose of assessment, and these considerations may be competing.

For example, a health-related quality of life measure may discriminate adequately between well and ill individuals by using lengthy questionnaires investigating relatively fixed traits. In contrast, a measure used to evaluate change over time would not benefit substantially from including fixed characteristics. It would be more efficient if it tapped only behaviors or abilities susceptible to change in response to the intervention under study (Kirshner and Guyatt, 1985).

Many quality-of-life measures have been designed and tested primarily in cross-sectional investigations to discriminate among different population groups. Such measures may discriminate well at a single time, but this does not ensure that the measures will be responsive to detecting changes over time (Deyo and Patrick, 1989).

As noted in Chapter 5, the choice of a disease-specific or a generic measure may also depend upon the objective of assessment. Disease-specific instruments often have greater relevance for clinicians and patients, better focus on the functional areas of particular concern, and perhaps greater responsiveness to disease-specific interventions. Generic measures, on the other hand, permit comparisons across interventions and diagnostic groups and typically cover a more comprehensive range of function and well-being than disease-specific measures. For most policy applications, generic measures are necessary and should be supplemented with items or measures addressing condition-specific concerns of particular population groups.

Practical considerations also follow from the primary objective of assessment. Measures designed to capture change over time may require transition questions, items written specifically to measure change. For example, respondents can be asked to rate how their quality of life has changed on a seven-point scale ranging from "much better" to "much worse." The seven-point scale can then be used for comparison with difference scores obtained from health status measures to compare these differences with respondents' overall ratings of change. However, for discrimination between different groups of persons based on gender, age, or other characteristics, items measuring change may be inappropriate and unacceptable to investigators and respondents.

STEP 2. SPECIFY AVAILABLE RESOURCES

The major practical consideration involved before selecting an assessment strategy for measuring health-related quality of life is the amount of resources to be devoted to the assessment. These resources include time, money, and personnel. Identifying resources at this stage not only helps in selection, but also uncovers the interested parties' expectations for the relevance and usefulness of the assessment.

All aspects of an assessment—selecting measures, collecting and editing data, analyzing data, and presenting findings—are time-consuming. Researchers can spend weeks or months constructing a comprehensive *and* targeted questionnaire or interview schedule. They must survey the literature, specify the problem, and conceptualize the outcomes. Designing an efficient data collection instrument is only the first step to implementation. Even a simple questionnaire may be prepared in 10 to 20 versions before it is ready for pretesting.

The entire time frame for the assessment, analysis, and presentation should be estimated in advance and revised, if necessary, to meet the deadlines often presented by those sponsoring the research. Developing a timeline, along with a detailed plan outlining all the tasks to be accomplished and the personnel needed for each phase, is recommended. This timeline also helps in budgeting for the assessment. Figure 7.2 illustrates an implementation timeline for a health-related quality of life assessment by telephone in a three-year investigation of the effectiveness of preventive services. Recruitment, assessment, intervention, computer tasks, and analysis and report production are distributed across the timeline. The personnel, equipment, supplies, data

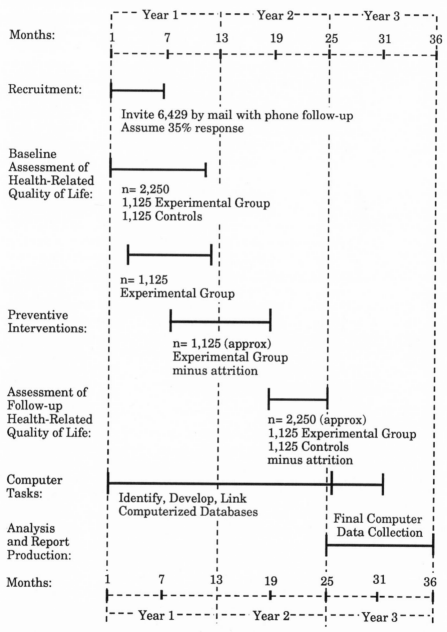

Figure 7.2 Implementation schedule for health-related quality of life (HRQOL) assessment (year 1 begins May 1, 1992).

collection instruments, computer time, and associated expenses can be estimated for each category and adjusted for final funding.

Novice investigators seldom allocate sufficient time, money, and personnel for health-related quality of life assessments. Experienced primary data collectors allow for additional resources to handle unexpected problems in design and implementation. Known resource constraints on time and money provide boundaries for most investigators. Funding agencies also examine budgets in detail for proportion of resources allocated to specific project tasks in relation to project objectives and project design.

STEP 3. IDENTIFY THE POPULATION TO BE STUDIED

At a minimum, four major characteristics of populations and potential respondents should be considered in selecting measures of health-related quality of life: (1) level of symptoms and disability (well versus ill); (2) age (younger versus older); (3) level of cognitive ability (able to provide reasonably accurate information versus disoriented or cognitively impaired); and (4) ethnic or cultural identity.

Level of Disability

Well populations require an assessment strategy and measures different from populations with significant symptoms and disability. Concepts and measures from the positive end of the health-related quality of life continuum are needed to assess healthy populations (Stewart and Ware, 1992). Nearly 70 percent of the general population reports their health as excellent or very good. Items concerning need for assistance with activities of daily living would, therefore, not be discriminating or responsive measures for such well populations.

Several core domains of health-related quality of life, such as role functioning, physical functioning (ambulation, mobility, etc.), and self-care may have little relevance to well populations where dysfunction is rare in work activities, in mobility, and in carrying out the usual activities of daily living. Health status measures based exclusively on these domains may be too narrow to provide an assessment of well persons on the continuum of health-related quality of life. If the measure does not "register" for a large percentage of respondents, the content validity of the measure is low for the population under study.

Furthermore, detecting improving health among persons who are already quite well may prove difficult because of the "ceiling" effect: if you start out at the top, there is no place to go "up." Measures that do not contain items pertaining to minor or common symptoms and signs, health perceptions, and psychological well-being generally are not responsive to improvement, because there is nowhere to go at the top of the scale. Inclusion of emotional well-being, positive affect, vitality, and health perceptions aids in discriminating and measuring change in well populations.

As health providers and society in general place more emphasis on health promotion and disease prevention, there is increasing need for measures that incorporate the positive benefits that may result from health-promoting environments or behaviors and preventive interventions. These "positive" measures are especially relevant for assessing changes in relatively well individuals that may result from health-promoting influences and activities. At present, the main approach to assessing the effects of health promotion is to measure subsequent reduction in disease incidence or lengthening of life. Yet these two outcomes may not be the only outcomes or the most important ones. Even if morbidity and longevity are unaffected, health promotion may enhance health by increasing energy, stamina, feelings of well-being, resilience, autonomy, and productivity. These are outcomes potentially related to behavior change.

Detecting worsening health among people who are already ill presents a different challenge. Bindman and colleagues (1990) studied severely ill patients at two points in time using the Medical Outcomes Study Short Form (MOS-20). Baseline MOS-20 scores for these hospitalized patients were low. While many patients reported worsening health at follow-up, their low baseline scores made it difficult to detect health status decline.

Researchers need more comprehensive generic measures with multiple domains and multiple items to detect subtle changes in both well and severely ill populations. Besides such generic measures, they should include disease-specific measures to assess ill respondents. To assess well respondents, they should use specific measures of health perceptions (general and satisfaction with health), resilience, and positive affect. Generic measures usually provide the basis for population comparisons as well as the assessment of floor and ceiling effects. Specific measures provide the basis for detecting changes at the two ends of the health-related quality of life continuum.

Age

Chapter 5 described measures developed specifically for children and for older adults. While progress is being made in applying existing measures and developing new ones for these two populations, considerable challenges remain to collecting health-related quality of life data on children and older adults. In both age groups, data collection procedures include health examinations and health interviews. Many health examination procedures were developed primarily in the field of medicine. These often include performance-based measures in which respondents are asked to do specific tasks. Their performance on these tasks is evaluated and scored according to stage of development, speed at which the task is performed, or other criteria. Direct measures of older adults' functional status, such as ability to walk, hold objects, open doors, or perform other behaviors, are common in geriatric evaluation. The 50-foot walk time, Performance Activities of Daily Living (Kuriansky and Gurland, 1976), and functional vital signs (Williams et al., 1982) are examples of such direct measures of performance. Health examination data provide the means for obtaining unrecognized and undiagnosed conditions, including nonsymptomatic conditions. Recognizing and listing health conditions, however, is less useful in classifying or measuring level of health-related quality of life of children and older adults.

Measures developed primarily from the social sciences include questionnaires, interviewing procedures, and techniques of scale development, including scoring and analysis. Mothers and teachers provide most information about the health status of children, although reliable reports of behavior have been obtained from children over 12 years of age (Fienberg et al., 1985). Problems exist in obtaining information that is reliable from child to child, given the changes in questionnaire content needed for different age groups. Fink (1989) points out the serious limitations to using reported diagnoses, symptoms, impairments, and general measures as reported by parents. The validity of these reports can be questioned along with the difficulties in combining these different reports into a profile of child health status.

The problems are different with older adults. Most well older adults complete self-administered or interviewer-administered health status questionnaires with relative ease, possibly because they have the time and interest to participate in studies. A problem that commonly arises in assessing seniors is asking them to rate their current health in comparison to "usual" health or asking if reported changes are "due to health" or "due to age." Changes in health status may be attributed by older adults to age and not to health-related conditions. Some measures ask seniors to compare their health to others their own age. Well older adults do not consider their age peers the most appropriate reference group, since a wide spectrum of abilities can be observed at any age, including our "oldest old" or those 85 years and above.

Cognitive Function

Cognitive functioning or mental incapacity is of major concern when assessing the health-related quality of life of older or severely impaired adults. With such populations, interviewer-administered questionnaires are recommended to reach a representative sample of the population. If only self-administered questionnaires are used, the resulting sample will include only those capable of completing the instrument on their own or with help from others.

Mental status evaluations are routinely administered at the beginning of interviews with older or disabled adults. Commonly used examples include the Folstein Mini-Mental State (Folstein et al., 1975) and the Short Portable Mental Status Questionnaire (Pfeiffer, 1975). New cognitive screening tests have also been developed for administration over the telephone (Brandt et al., 1988). These instruments are short measures of symptoms used to screen for cognitive difficulties. They are not diagnostic tests for dementia or the etiology of organic diseases such as Alzheimer's disease. Respondents who score below defined cutoff points are generally not interviewed. Instead, a proxy respondent, usually a caregiver, is requested to complete the interview.

The correspondence between respondent and proxy response to health-related quality of life measures varies depending on the domain assessed and the choice of proxy. As might be expected, proxy reports of more observable domains such as physical functioning, activities of daily living, cognition, and social activity are highly correlated with reports from the respondents themselves (Magaziner et al., 1988; Epstein et al., 1989; Rothman et al., 1991). Reports of psychological functioning and satisfaction with health, less observable domains of health-related quality of life, are more moderately correlated.

Proxy respondents tend to consider patients more impaired, that is, overestimate patient dysfunction, relative to the respondents themselves. Overestimation of disability is particularly characteristic of those proxies with the greatest contact with the respondent. The psychological distress and burden perceived by the proxy respondent can affect their assessments of patients' own psychosocial functioning (Rothman et al., 1991).

Age can also influence the direction of proxy evaluations of health. As seen in Figure 7.3, proxy respondents in the National Health Interview Survey were more

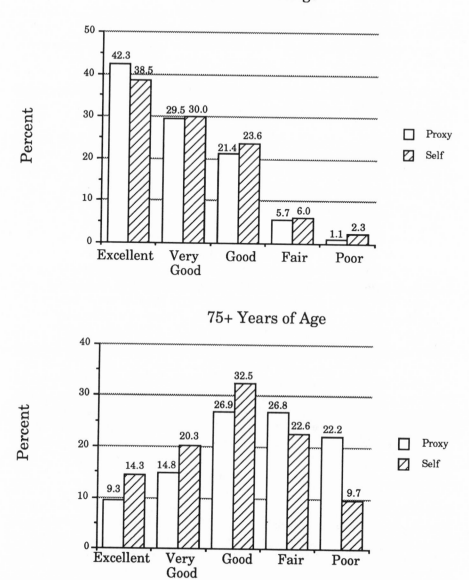

Figure 7.3 Self versus proxy ratings of health status for two age groups, NHIS, 1985. *Source*: National Center for Health Statistics, Current Estimates from the *National Health Interview Survey, United States, Vital and Health Statistics*. Unpublished data.

likely to rate persons 35–44 years of age in excellent health than the persons themselves. For persons 75 years of age and over, however, proxy respondents were more likely to give ratings of "fair" or "poor" than the persons themselves.

These studies indicate that care must be taken in combining proxy-generated with patient-generated scores in assessing particular domains of health-related quality of life. Out of necessity, investigators will continue to rely on proxy data when individual respondents are unable to participate. Most proxy respondents are willing and able to cooperate with interviewers.

Two strategies can be employed to improve proxy reporting. First, respondents can nominate their own proxies; in fact, they tend to select proxies who are able to respond reliably (Clipp and Elder, 1987; Bassett et al., 1990). Second, investigators can reduce the ambiguity in instructions to proxy respondents, ask proxies to rate their perceived accuracy of the information provided, and use one or more proxies to obtain convergent views of patient status. Perhaps most important, investigators should avoid proxy reports of highly subjective domains, because only the person affected can truly communicate their affective feelings and cognitive evaluations of their health and quality of life.

Ethnic Identity

As cultural anthropologists demonstrate repeatedly, a person's conception of what constitutes "disease" or "health" can depend on his or her cultural traditions, language, and group mores as well as more individual characteristics such as age, educational level, and income (Fabrega, 1974; Kleinman et al., 1978). Thus, comparisons between different ethnic groups and across different cultures cannot be made without considering cultural variables. The cross-cultural content of measures, the cultural meaning of different domains, and the translation of measures from one language or culture to another are important considerations in assessing health-related quality of life.

The cross-cultural content of health status measures is relevant to both generic and condition, or domain-specific, measures. Cross-cultural studies of preference weighting using the Sickness Impact Profile (Patrick et al., 1985), the Nottingham Health Profile (Hunt and Wiklund, 1987), and the EuroQol Instrument (Brooks et al., 1991; Nord, 1991) suggest a universal ranking or rating of health states. For example, most people consider that it is better to walk *without* limitations than to walk *with* limitations.

The suggestion that health-related quality of life domains can be generalized across different cultures is not surprising. Activities and behaviors related to walking, mobility, sleep, eating, household management, work, and recreation are clearly found in almost every, if not all, cultures. At the most disabling levels of physical activities necessary for human survival, there may be near-universal agreement on what is "bad" and "good" health.

Although the domains and relative preference for health states may hold for different cultures, the meaning and interpretation of different health states may well vary among these different populations. Symptoms such as bleeding or vomiting, considered undesirable in many Western cultures, may be signs of religious inspiration to others. Persons exhibiting these "symptoms" under certain conditions may be venerated and held in high esteem. Good and Good (1980) provide a "cultural hermeneutic" model for translating illness realities and decoding a person's symptoms by grounding reports of symptoms in the cultural context of the person rather than using only somatic referents.

In one sense, disease-specific measures are translations of generic health status concepts into the cultural categories, vocabularies, and perspectives of different groups. For example, patients with chronic back pain who attend back pain clinics are a "subculture"; they communicate with symptoms of back pain, and they evaluate the effectiveness of treatments in unique terms.

Increasingly, instruments created for use in one language are being translated for use in other cultures and with persons of different ethnic identity. Protocols and techniques for obtaining an accurate and culturally valid second-language translation of health status measures are available (Brislin et al., 1973; Gilson et al., 1980). For example, many instruments that were originally developed in English are now available in French, German, Spanish, Japanese, and Swedish (Sullivan, 1985; Hunt, 1986; Hendricson et al., 1989; Alonso et al., 1990). Empirical evidence indicates that it is possible to apply instruments developed for use in one culture in a different setting (Patrick, 1985).

Investigators still report problems finding technically adequate translations of health status measures (Aday et al., 1980; Geronimus et al., 1990). These problems stem from the fact that a health status measure developed in one culture and then translated to another can impose the concepts and language of the originating culture onto the receiving culture. There are many conceptual and linguistic problems to be overcome before a translated version can be used to assess health-related quality of life with confidence. Different dialects and regional, idiomatic language abound within many countries. Hendricson et al. (1989) conclude that diligent translation may not, by itself, be the key factor. Rather, using a dual-language format and idiomatic language style are crucial factors. Certain aspects of acculturation, particularly familiarity with questionnaire research, may critically affect the validity of the health status data obtained from different cultures (Deyo, 1984).

Extreme care must be taken with both generic and disease-specific measures developed in the United States and Europe when applied to populations whose native language is not American or British English, German, or French. The construct validity of the Mexican Spanish version of the Sickness Impact Profile (SIP) was lower, for example, among patients using this version than among those using the American English version (Deyo, 1984). It is important that people in the community to be investigated translate and format questionnaires. Four major phases may occur: preliminary translation, evaluation of preliminary translation, ascertainment of cross-language equivalence, and assessment of validity, reliability, and responsiveness (Del Greco et al., 1987). Preliminary forward translation provides a questionnaire as near as possible in meaning to the original; this is best done by someone familiar with the objectives of the measurement instrument and expert in both the original language and the language into which the translation is being made.

Having the preliminary translation translated back into the original language by someone not familiar with the original-language version, called backward translation, provides one evaluation of the translated questionnaire. The backtranslated questionnaire can be compared with the original version, and items that have changed meaning can be retranslated. Bilingual experts may also look at both versions of the questionnaire to assist in translating each question in terms of its content, meaning, clarity of expression, and comparability to the original question.

Cross-language equivalence can be assessed by administering both the original and translated versions of the questionnaire to bilingual subjects in random order of presentation and comparing their responses to each. A high correlation between responses is an indication of cross-language equivalence. Translations consistent with local dialects and the total "instrument in translation" should be investigated for reliability and validity before assuming a high correlation with the original-language version. Investigators are also advised to proceed cautiously in the interpretation of similarities and differences in the reported behavior of people belonging to different cultures (Lonner and Berry, 1986).

STEP 4. CONCEPTUALIZE RELEVANT OUTCOMES

Using the concepts and domains that define health-related quality of life, outcomes to be used for discriminating between different groups, predicting future health status, or detecting change over time can be identified by answering three questions:

1. What are the potential differences between groups or the main effects of the intervention?
2. What are the potential side effects or unintended consequences of the intervention?
3. What are all the outcomes of interest to consumers/patients, families, clinicians, decision makers, and society at large?

The main, intended effects of proposed interventions are generally known in advance of the actual intervention. For example, several different treatment options exist for patients with a fractured hip. They include bed rest with traction, cast immobilization, and surgery. Open reduction and fixation of the hip fracture fragments is the most common surgical treatment for intertrochanteric and subtrochanteric fractures. An Institute of Medicine Committee has addressed these treatment options and the health and functional status outcomes involved in hip fracture effectiveness research (Heithoff and Lohr, 1990). For all patients, survival, morbidity (including pain and other symptoms), functional status (including physical capacity and ability to function in daily life), emotional well-being, social functioning, and general outlook on health are important. Hip replacement may improve physical gait and balance, improve physical activity, reduce pain, and improve affective behavior. In addition to the generic domains of health-related quality of life, assessment of hip replacement outcomes might concentrate on pains and specific activities such as walking, dressing, climbing stairs or inclines, sitting, transferring, getting out of a chair, and engaging in vigorous physical activity.

Listing the proposed effects of an intervention uncovers the assumptions of program design and the model of change adopted by the investigators or funding agents. Outcomes may be competing, and a main endpoint must be chosen for a clinical trial or a policy change. In most clinical trials, health-related quality of life measures are not the major endpoints of the trial, although increasingly these outcomes are arrayed in combination with the major endpoint, which is most often a measure of disease or impairment. Including the entire spectrum of outcomes in the conceptualization and selection process also helps to develop a priori hypotheses concerning expected relationships among different outcomes.

Listing the potential side effects or unintended outcomes is not a straightforward task. For interventions with a biological or medical model, such as pharmaceutical agents, side effects may be suspected or already recognized. In other cases, there may be little basis for predicting unintended outcomes. Such outcomes may be desirable or undesirable, although most "side effects" are considered unwanted consequences of an otherwise desirable intervention. In hip replacement surgery, patients might get wound infections, such as staphylococcus, in the hospital. Such infections can lead to reduced muscle tone and changed physical balance and ambulation. Unexpected desirable consequences might also be uncovered. In a study of hip fracture using the Sickness Impact Profile, investigators found that high levels of dysfunction in sleep and rest were improved dramatically following surgical treatment on the hip (Bergner et al., 1981).

Unintended outcomes may also be uncovered through qualitative interviews with all the parties interested in the decision or problem. Focus groups with different patient and family groups and interviews with clinicians can bring out many previously unrecognized or unmeasured concerns. Such a strategy was used with patients with inflammatory bowel disease (IBD). Investigators wanted to develop a condition-specific supplement for use in evaluating the impact of the disease and different treatment alternatives (Drossman et al., 1989). Videotaped, qualitative interviews with IBD patients and their families indicated that generic health status measures did not adequately address many of the perceptions and quality of life concerns of these patients and families. Additional domains concerning fear of cancer and other complications, of the loss of bowel control, of feeling dirty and smelly, and of intimate relations were also important to persons with the condition. These videotaped interviews permitted investigators to evaluate the language used to describe different concepts and domains by patients and their families.

INFORMATION ON MEASURES OF HEALTH-RELATED QUALITY OF LIFE

An important aspect of selecting an instrument for primary data collection is a review of the literature to determine the availability of measures and relevant empirical experience with each measure. Appendix II lists major sources of information about measures of health-related quality of life. The information is organized according to its format, whether a book, journal article, special journal issue, or reference center.

Books included in this appendix review health-related quality of life assessments; see the books by Frank-Stromborg (1988), Kane and Kane (1981), and McDowell and Newell (1987). Other books are included because they describe various applications of a single instrument of health-related quality of life; see Stewart and Ware (1992). The books by Smith (1988), Spilker (1990), Walker and Rosser (1987), and Wenger et al. (1984) all describe different applications of various measures, principally in the context of clinical trials. The book by Drummond et al. (1987) discusses application of health-related quality of life assessments for program evaluation and policy analysis.

Section B, Recent Journal Issues, identifies conference proceedings and supplemental volumes devoted entirely to the issue of assessing health-related quality of life. The two supplements edited by Lohr and Ware (1987) and Lohr (1989) address issues for a broad range of applications, from clinical practice to population monitoring. The volumes edited by Katz (1987) and by Feeny et al. (1991) are more relevant to applications in clinical trial settings. The Spilker and Tilson (1990) supplement reviews the recent literature and categorizes it according to disease-specific applications and assessments used.

In addition to these books and special journal issues, a number of professional journals routinely publish articles on the development and application of measures of health-related quality of life. The list of journals in Appendix II is not intended to be exhaustive. Rather, the journals listed are those most likely to publish relevant articles on an ongoing basis. By regularly scanning these journals, the quality of life scientist is likely to remain current with new developments in the field, particularly with generic measures.

In addition to these publications, four reference services are available. The United States government operates two centers that provide information on measures of health-related quality of life. The Clearinghouse on Health Indexes prepares a quarterly, annotated bibliography on current applications that have appeared in either published or unpublished format. The National Library of Medicine maintains several data bases that can be accessed through commercial time-sharing networks. The most useful data base for identifying what has been done in the area of assessing health-related quality of life is MEDLINE. A list of keywords, or mesh terms, for searching this data base is given in Appendix II, Section E.

Two services have been developed for the specific purpose of helping investigators identify relevant assessments. One is the On-Line Guide to Quality-of-Life Assessment (OLGA). This system, which operates on personal computers, helps the researcher identify potential assessments. It then links the assessment to recent empirical studies in which it has been used. The other service is the Health and Psychosocial Instruments data base maintained by Behavioral Retrieval System. This mainframe data base contains references to almost 2,000 assessments that have been developed for medical and nursing care as well as health services research.

In addition to these information sources, others that discuss philosophical and ethical dimensions in assessing health-related quality of life are beginning to appear. Reviewing this literature periodically will help guide the practicing researcher in the interpretation of health-related quality of life data.

STEP 5. ASSESS METHODOLOGICAL CHARACTERISTICS OF POTENTIAL MEASURES

In assessing a complex concept, such as health-related quality of life, many methodological and practical issues of measurement need to be considered. Major methodological issues are summarized in Table 7.1. The first two issues, weighting and level of aggregation, have been discussed at length in Chapters 5 and 6. The measurement properties of reliability, responsiveness, and validity are discussed in the next three sections of this chapter. All five are important considerations to the selection decision.

Reliability

Perhaps no principles of science are more often used and more often misunderstood than "reliability" and "validity." In the past, the social and health sciences have

Table 7.1 Methodological considerations in health-related quality of life assessment

Weighting
  Statistical
  Relative preference

Level of aggregation
  Combining two or more concepts into a summary score
  Measuring a general concept

Reliability
  Internal consistency
  Test–retest reproducibility
  Interrater reliability

Responsiveness
  Change over time
  Pace of change

Validity
  Content validity
  Criterion validity
  Construct validity

depended on systematic application of data collection procedures to obtain higher-quality data and answer problems with confidence. Questions of how reliable and valid the operations or data collection procedures are deserve continued serious attention.

Reliability is a generic term that refers to the stability and equivalence of repeated measures of the same concept. One must be careful in using this term, since there are different types of reliability, although reliability most often refers to how well a measurement can be replicated on the same persons. Variability in measures occurs over time or across different methods of gathering data. *Stability* refers to whether people give consistent responses to the same health-related quality of life questions at different points in time. Responses to many questions, such as self-rating of health or role functioning, are assumed to be consistent if no changes occur that cause people to respond differently to the same question. *Equivalence* concerns whether consistent responses occur when different data collection personnel use the same instrument or when more than one item or instrument is used to measure the same respondents at a single point in time (Nunnally, 1978).

Reliability coefficients estimate the proportion of observed variation in a score that can be considered true as opposed to random error (Nunnally, 1978). *Internal consistency* is the correlation among items in an instrument, using statistics such as split-half comparisons or the more general alpha coefficient. Measures of internal consistency assess the inconsistency or nonequivalence of responses to different questions constructed to measure the same concept.

Split-half reliability reflects the correlation between responses to two subsets of items measuring the same concept (such as cognitive function) when items are split in half. *Coefficient alpha*, the most commonly used method, is the correlation coefficient used to estimate the degree of equivalence between responses to sets of items or questions tapping the same concept (Cronbach, 1951). Coefficient alpha will be higher (1) the more items are included in the measure of a particular conceptual domain and

(2) the higher the average intercorrelation between responses to all possible combinations of items in the domain.

The minimum level of internal consistency required differs according to the type of analysis. According to Nunnally (1978), internal consistency reliability above 0.90 is desirable when making comparisons between individuals; for group comparisons, on another hand, reliabilities above 0.70 are acceptable. Values lower than these indicate that some items in a measure do not tap the domain in the same way as others or they tap different domains. Analysts can obtain a point-in-time estimate of reliability of a health-related quality of life instrument by using internal consistency analysis.

For discriminating between persons in cross-sectional studies, internal consistency reliability is important. For longitudinal investigations where change over time is assessed, reproducibility, stability, and responsiveness are important to distinguish between those who remain stable and those who experience change.

Reproducibility, or test–retest reliability, refers to the correlation between responses to the same items administered to the same respondents at different times. A measure administered two or more times to the same group of individuals that results in high intercorrelations among scores would have high reproducibility. Time introduces an interesting paradox with respect to the concept of reproducibility. If something is highly variable by nature (blood pressure or a mood), it is difficult to observe whether differences in repeated measurements are caused by a change in the observed phenomenon or by irreproducible observations. In other words, what proportion of the measured variable is "true" variation? Reproducibility estimates may differ because of *actual* changes in health-related quality of life or because of randomly occurring changes. With health status measures, reproducibility is measured using the Pearson's correlation or kappa statistic (intraclass correlation), depending on the measurement characteristic of interest (Deyo et al., 1991).

In the health sciences, the quest for "true" variation has led to experiments with simultaneous observation of a given phenomenon by multiple observers. In such instances, the observers become an integral part of the measuring process. It becomes difficult, if not impossible, to separate the unreliability of the measuring instrument (such as the stethoscope) from that of the observer.

Interobserver or interrater reliability refers to the correlation between responses to the same items obtained by different observers, raters, or interviewers. Interobserver reliability is particularly important for administering and interpreting scores obtained from disease-specific measures such as the Karnofsky Scale, New York Heart Association Functional Classification, American Rheumatism Classification, and the numerous psychiatric measures like the Brief Psychiatric Rating Scale. Clinicians rate patients using these classification systems. Interrater reliability coefficients reflect the level of agreement between observers. Pearson product moment, kappa, or Spearman rank order coefficients are used to measure agreement. Correlations of 0.80 or higher among observers are desirable. Correlations are even higher between observers using psychiatric rating scales such as the Brief Psychiatric Rating Scale and the Hamilton Rating Scale for depression (Hamilton, 1960; Overall and Gorham, 1962).

Before constructing an instrument from available measures, analysts should find the levels of reliability for each measure and on what populations reliability studies have been conducted. Ideally reliability studies should be available on a random sample of those in the population under investigation, that is, persons or patients with or without medical conditions, to permit generalizability of previous reliability findings. Analysts should also study research reports describing how reliability coefficients were obtained so they can detect possible sources of bias. For example, in evaluating the test–retest reliability of a measure, the interval between administrations can be too short. The respondent may remember previous responses and thus upwardly bias the estimate. On the other hand, if the interval is too long, then the respondents' health status may have deteriorated, resulting in a downward bias. The period between two testings for short questionnaires may need to be a month at minimum to avoid subject recall of earlier responses. For longer questionnaires, a two-week period is usually sufficient.

Test–retest reliability indicates the extent to which measurements are repeatable over a short time period; measures of stability are applied to see if any fluctuations in scores occur over longer intervals, usually six months or more (Nunnally, 1978). Because many health status concepts tend to be stable over time, assessment at the beginning of a clinical trial can be used to predict the status of either an individual or a group at the end of a trial. This prediction increases the power of hypothesis testing by reducing the associated error. The consequence for clinical trials is that the increased power associated with intertemporal stability can reduce the requisite sample size (Ware, 1984c; Rogers et al., 1979).

Researchers rarely obtain perfect reliability estimates. There is a danger of permitting the perfect to become the enemy of the good, or of committing the error of errorlessness; some investigators give up measurement of a phenomenon for scientific studies when they find any degree of unreliability. On the other hand, highly reliable data may have low validity. The important question should be, How reliable is this measure in relation to the purpose of the research? Global measures created from generic health status measures often have high reproducibility and internal consistency reliability, although individual items or subscales can have markedly reduced reliability coefficients.

Responsiveness

Responsiveness is the ability of an instrument to detect small but important changes (Guyatt, Walter et al., 1987). These are changes that clinicians, patients, families, or others think are discernible and important, have been detected with an intervention of known efficacy, or are related to well-established physiologic measures (e.g., grip strength for patients with rheumatoid arthritis or spirometry for those with obstructive lung disease).

The measurement of change in health-related quality of life is particularly important where subjective reports constitute one of the primary endpoints of a trial or study. Advance knowledge of instrument responsiveness aids in selecting measures, permits accurate estimation of sample size to assure adequate statistical power, and assists in prioritizing (and reducing the number of) endpoints to be assessed (Deyo et al., 1991).

As noted in Chapter 5, disease-specific measures with items selected to assess particular concerns or worded to attribute change to the condition of interest (e.g., back pain in the modified SIP) may be particularly sensitive to within-subject changes and thus more responsive than generic measures that contain items unrelated to change. For a measure to detect subtle but important changes, scores must be stable among persons who are stable (reproducible) and changing among persons who experience actual change. This is necessary because the observer wishes to detect changes above and beyond the variability in persons who do not receive an experimental intervention. In addition, a measure must be valid to reflect true change.

There is uncertainty about how to quantify responsiveness. Perhaps the most common method of evaluating responsiveness is to compare instrument scores before and after a treatment of known efficacy. An improvement in scores would be evidence of responsiveness as evaluated using the paired t test statistic for within-subject changes. Liang et al. (1985) used this method to judge five questionnaires simultaneously employed in a group of arthritis patients before and after major joint replacement surgery.

A second method for comparing responsiveness is to calculate effect size or the changes in mean score (from baseline to follow-up) to the standard deviation of baseline scores (Kazis et al., 1989). Guyatt, Walter, and Normal (1987) suggest a variant of effect size using a different denominator: the standard deviation of score changes among stable subjects. If one knows the smallest score difference that would be minimally important, then this could be used in the numerator to provide a responsiveness coefficient analogous to a reliability or validity coefficient.

A third method for evaluating responsiveness is based on the receiver operating characteristic (ROC) curve most commonly applied to diagnostic tests. Changes on a health status instrument are viewed as diagnostic tests for patient improvement, and the investigator seeks to distinguish those who improve from those who do not. Any change in health status scores will include some true positives and some false positives; the ROC curve is constructed by plotting the sensitivity (true-positive rate) against one minus specificity (false-positive rate). The area under the ROC curve then indicates the ability of the health status measure to discriminate improved from unimproved subjects, that is, it reflects the probability of correctly identifying the improved patient from randomly selected pairs of improved and unimproved patients (Deyo and Centor, 1986; Deyo et al., 1991).

Because of increasing use of health-related quality of life measures in longitudinal investigations, researchers are giving more attention to responsiveness. When responsiveness is important but suboptimal, several methods are available for improving it. Some proposals include using finer response categories, disaggregating scores, using specific transition questions ("much better" to "much worse"), and showing respondents their previous responses (Guyatt et al., 1989; MacKenzie et al., 1986; Tugwell et al., 1983). Transition indexes consisting of five to seven categories are simple to construct and measure change directly, an advantage to both respondent and investigator. As Feinstein et al. (1986) point out, clinicians constantly employ transition questions informally in asking patients "Do you feel better today?" or "Is your appetite improved?"

Validity

Techniques are available for estimating the internal consistency, reproducibility, and responsiveness of health-related quality of life measures. No such precision in techniques and their application exists for validity. Validity is a more emotionally charged term than reliability or responsiveness because conceptions vary widely about how analysts might be led astray in drawing conclusions from the data.

The term *validity* refers to both the validity of *findings* and validity of *measurements*. The first type is based on the design of the study and methods used, and the second refers to the measurements themselves. In this chapter, we are concerned primarily with measurement validity. The American Psychological Association (1974) identifies three major categories that subsume most types of validity proposed: content, criterion, and construct validity.

Content validity refers to whether a particular measure adequately represents the domain or universe of content it is supposed to measure. Items of a measure must be judged for their presumed representativeness of the universe defined by the theoretical constructs chosen for investigation. Ware (1987) recommends including physical, mental, social, and perceptual health as a minimum standard for content in comprehensive generic measures. For the Health Resource Allocation Strategy, measures of health-related quality of life must include health states defined by this same minimum standard of content, incorporation of death or duration of survival, and preference weights that permit tradeoff between quantity and quality of life and between different health-related quality of life domains.

As noted, additional domains may be important to persons with a specific condition. Generic measures may contain items of little or no relevance to respondents. For example, items concerning incontinence or eating behavior may not concern persons with arthritis. Questions concerning bladder and eating habits would add to respondent burden and might irritate persons for whom they are not relevant. Condition- or population-specific measures add content validity to an assessment and increase interest in the assessment.

It is not always possible to specify in advance, however, which domains and items are relevant to a particular population or investigation. This is particularly true when testing a new treatment or attempting to affect a broad aspect of quality of life such as social function or satisfaction. For example, the Quality of Well-Being Scale was sensitive to unexpected outcomes in a controlled trial evaluation of auranofin therapy for patients with rheumatoid arthritis (Bombardier et al., 1986). In a study of patients with hyperthyroidism using the Sickness Impact Profile, the sleep and rest category suggested worse dysfunction than any other category, and these difficulties are highly responsive to therapy (Canadian Erythropoietin Study Group, 1990). Although this phenomenon was reasonable in retrospect, it had not been anticipated and, indeed, is not a type of dysfunction emphasized in medical textbooks.

Criterion validity is the correspondence between a proposed measure and another measure of some variable taken to be a more accurate, or criterion, variable. When a future value of the criterion is selected for matching with the proposed measure, *predictive* validity is achieved.

Criterion validity is the most prized type of validity because the consistency notion behind it can often be used efficiently. Having a criterion, or "gold standard," is familiar logic to clinicians, who regularly use diagnostic tests that have been examined for criterion validity (sensitivity, specificity, predictive value) against an accepted gold standard.

No gold standard exists, however, for most behavioral and perceptual health-related quality of life measures. Thus, which measures an operationalized concept of health-related quality of life should correlate with is open to question. Two measures might be highly correlated and still be invalid. Some investigators suggest adopting an existing measure as a gold standard against which to compare other measures. There is no basis, however, for identifying a single measure that can serve as such a criterion. In this field, like most areas of social science, construct validation is necessary.

Construct validation involves specifying the factors, or constructs, that account for variance in the proposed measures as well as the hypothesized relations among them. The analyst seeks empirical evidence according to the logic of scientific inquiry to give meaning to a particular measure. To determine construct validity, the analyst should specify a theory expressing how components of a measure are expected to relate to each other and to other measures. Hypotheses are stated regarding the direction and, if possible, the strength of relationships that might be expected. Validity is supported when the associations are consistent with the hypotheses. If different measures of the same construct are logically related and highly correlated, then *convergent* validity has been achieved; if a logically different measure is not as highly correlated as a more logically related measure, then *discriminant* validity is evident.

Construct validity of a health-related quality of life measure depends upon the two related concepts of convergent and discriminant validity. Kaplan et al. (1976) produced evidence for the construct validity of the Quality of Well-Being Scale by showing that scores increased with age, number of chronic conditions, number of symptoms, and number of physician contacts. As predicted, time (day-specific) scores correlated more highly with self-ratings of current well-being than with self-ratings of overall health status containing prognostic outlook, suggesting that the measure has discriminant validity.

Campbell and Fiske (1959) proposed the multitrait–multimethod procedure for evaluating the convergent and discriminant validity of measures. This approach uses a matrix of intercorrelations among measures that involve two or more traits, each measured by two or more methods. Different measures of the same trait should correlate more highly with each other (convergent) than with different measures of different traits. At the same time, both of these intercorrelations should be higher than the correlations among different traits measured by the same method (discriminant validity).

Developers of the Dartmouth COOP Charts, nine pictorial charts measuring patient function, used the multitrait–multimethod approach to construct validity in assessing convergent and discriminant validity of the Charts (Nelson et al., 1990). The analysis involved comparing the COOP Charts with the RAND health status measures, a set of measures using multi-item scales that correspond to the COOP charts. If the COOP charts are valid, the investigators hypothesized they would observe moderate to strong associations with corresponding paired measures. In addition, correlations between different measures of the same concept, for example, COOP physical function with RAND physical function, should exceed correlations between different concepts measured by different methods, for example, COOP physical function compared to mental function, or by the same method, for example, COOP Physical with COOP mental.

Table 7.2 shows a multitrait–multimethod correlation matrix for 1,007 chronic disease patients participating in the Medical Outcomes Study. The average convergent validity correlation was 0.62, indicating good agreement between different measures of the same dimension of function. The average off-diagonal correlation was 0.39, somewhat smaller than the average convergent validity correlation, supporting the validity of the measures.

Table 7.2 Multitrait–multimethod matrix from the Medical Outcomes Study sample (N = 1,007)

Functional measures	COOP charts							RAND scales[a]						
	Physical Function	Emotional Status	Role Function	Social Function	Pain	Overall Health	Social Support	Physical Function	Emotional Status	Role Function	Social Function	Pain	Overall Health	Social Support
COOP charts														
Physical Function	1.00													
Emotional Status	0.02	1.00												
Role Function	0.35	0.39	1.00											
Social Function	0.23	0.53	0.59	1.00										
Pain	0.25	0.26	0.44	0.36	1.00									
Overall Health	0.36	0.48	0.57	0.50	0.38	1.00								
Social Support	0.08	0.38	0.27	0.40	0.22	0.36	1.00							
RAND scales														
Physical Function	0.59[b]	0.12	0.52	0.34	0.36	0.43	0.15	1.00						
Emotional Status	0.01	0.69[b]	0.41	0.53	0.25	0.48	0.44	0.15	1.00					
Role Function	0.40	0.29	0.60[b]	0.47	0.40	0.50	0.27	0.65	0.61	1.00				
Social Function	0.20	0.44	0.53	0.62[b]	0.33	0.52	0.36	0.41	0.64	0.58	1.00			
Pain	0.28	0.30	0.50	0.43	0.60[b]	0.41	0.27	0.53	0.38	0.60	0.50	1.00		
Overall Health	0.37	0.33	0.51	0.44	0.38	0.61[b]	0.30	0.60	0.45	0.62	0.58	0.54	1.00	
Social Support	0.05	0.41	0.24	0.34	0.17	0.32	0.61[b]	0.16	0.48	0.27	0.38	0.22	0.29	1.00

Source: Nelson et al., 1990.

[a]RAND Scales: Physical Function (K = 10), Emotional Function (K = 32), Role Function (K = 13), Social Function (K = 4), Pain (K = 12), Overall Health (K = 7), Social Support (K = 19). K indicates the number of individual items included in the scale. Average convergent validity correlation equals 0.62; average of correlations is 0.39; Hays–Hayashi MTMM Quality Index equals 0.89 of off-diagonal.

[b]Indicates convergent correlations.

The construct validity of some generic health status measures has been established (Kaplan et al., 1976; Brook et al., 1979; Bergner et al., 1981; Stewart et al., 1988), although no general theory of expected differences has emerged. The construct validity of disease-specific measures is less well established, despite recent attempts to correlate disease-specific measures with patient and clinician global ratings and with disease-activity indexes (Guyatt et al., 1991). Comparisons among biological disease markers and scores obtained from three arthritis-specific instruments (Fries et al., 1980; Jette, 1980; Meenan et al., 1980) and one generic instrument (Bergner et al., 1981) on rheumatoid arthritis patients showed that the generic measure performed as well as the disease-specific assessments (Deyo, 1988).

The concepts of reliability, responsiveness, and validity often lead to the notion that the goal of measurement is to determine the "real" value of the concept or domain under investigation. Kaplan (1964) called this conception the "fiction of the true measure." Measurement is always concerned with approximation, because error and exception are always present. It is futile to conceive of the "real measure" in relation to possible measures. Errors can be reduced and measurements sharpened, but the standard of comparison should be the *first* approximation in a series of measurements, not the "real value," which will never be tapped.

For each approximation, measures should get better than before—the only "certainty" that science can claim. In no way does this strict empiricism depreciate the value of the measurement enterprise. Health services researchers seldom have direct measures of what they wish to measure; they have to use some indicator or index. Researchers must distinguish between the situation in which close approximation is possible and those in which they imagine they might find a reality that could be directly measured and correlated with indirect measures.

As Hans Reichenbach noted in his discussion of the unreliability of knowledge: "Empirical science, in the modern sense of the phrase, is a successful combination of mathematical with observational method. Its results are regarded, not as absolutely certain, but as highly probable and sufficiently reliable for all practical purposes" (1963, p. 30).

STEP 6. ASSESS PRACTICAL CONSIDERATIONS

The art of selecting and applying health-related quality of life measures does not depend only on methodological expertise and skill. Even the "best" measures can be defeated by insufficient resources, lack of commitment on the part of investigators, negative reactions of respondents, and complexity in scoring and interpreting. Practical considerations often dictate which measures get chosen and applied. Our advice, however, is to construct a mental scale that weighs different methodological and practical considerations against the objectives of assessment. By trading off the different inputs into the assessment process, investigators can improve decision making and select assessment approaches that are more likely to succeed.

In addition to specifying resources near the beginning of the investigation, there are other practical considerations in selecting health-related quality of life measures. These include acceptability to respondents, method of administration, length and cost of

Table 7.3 Practical considerations in health-related quality
of life assessment

Standardized or nonstandardized assessment strategy
    Identification and explanation of real differences among selected clinical populations
    Resource requirements—time and effort

Acceptability
    Previous experiences in clinical applications
    Respondent burden—the "unhealthy" respondent
    Interviewer burden

Method of administration
    Direct observation
    Face-to-face interview
    Telephone interview
    Self-administered questionnaire
    Proxy respondents

Length and cost of administration
    Other components of interview schedule or questionnaire
    Completion rates and quality of data

Method of analysis and complexity of scoring
    Availability of computer scoring
    Aggregation or disaggregation into component parts

Presentation of data and usefulness to decision makers
    Degree of certainty on value
    Numbers, graphs, and interpretation of data

---

administration, method of analysis, and presentation of data. Table 7.3 lists the major practical issues, many of which concern the final steps in collecting, analyzing, and presenting findings.

Standardized or Nonstandardized?

In deciding which instrument to use to answer a specific problem, the choice often is between developing a new assessment strategy or using an existing, standardized instrument. An instrument developed for a specific application—a nonstandardized instrument—is initially attractive because of the apparent uniqueness or complexity of the clinical situation. A problem-specific instrument may seem to maximize the potential for discovering and explaining differences among selected treatment groups. However, to the extent that the instrument is specific to disease, treatment, and sociodemographic characteristics of individuals participating in a given clinical trial, it will be difficult to assess whether the findings are due to the treatments or whether there is some confounding with regard to patient selection. And when a nonstandardized instrument is used, results cannot be generalized beyond the specific application.

In addition, experience with developing new instruments to assess health-related quality of life has shown that substantial amounts of time, effort, and money are required, almost always more than anticipated. The reason for the great expenditure of resources has been the need to conceptualize the problem, taking into account all the important methodological issues.

An alternative to developing a completely new instrument is to use a battery of standardized questionnaires. Such an approach can include a generic measure of health-related quality of life as well as measures of specific health concepts such as mood, satisfaction, or general health perceptions likely to be affected by the chosen treatment. Sugarbaker et al. (1982) did this in their study of patients of soft tissue sarcoma. They used the Sickness Impact Profile and complemented this global measure of health status with the Katz Activities of Daily Living Index, Psychosocial Adjustment to Illness Scale, and the Barthel function scale. The Nocturnal Oxygen Therapy Trial investigation (1980) also used the Sickness Impact Profile to assess overall health status and included Halsted impairment index, Minnesota Multiple Personality Index, and Profile of Mood States as other standardized instruments in the total quality of life battery which was fielded in a clinical trial designed to study the efficacy of nocturnal oxygen therapy.

Acceptability, Length, and Cost of Administration

The basic notion of acceptability refers to the ease with which an instrument can be used in a particular setting. One set of issues concerns how well a given instrument satisfies the research needs and resource constraints of the investigator. Among these concerns are (1) the length of the instrument and how this affects other assessments in the study; (2) the cost of including a particular instrument in a study in terms of the resources required, for example, whether interviewers are required, the detail of the data collected with the instrument, and the need for complex computer programs for analysis; and (3) the extent of previous experience with the instrument, for example, whether it has been used in the same type of application. The investigator also needs to be aware of completion rates, prevalence of missing responses, or other experiences that will influence the study outcome.

A second set of issues is associated with respondent burden and includes both the time and amount of psychological stress required to complete a questionnaire (Ware, 1984c). The length of response time may differ by complexity of the questionnaire and by personal characteristics of the respondent such as age, education, and health status. Longer response times have been observed among the elderly and the dysfunctional (Bush, 1984a; Ware, 1984c). Also, persons who are taking medications that affect memory or cognition may have difficulty complying with instructions from either an interviewer or a self-administered questionnaire.

Third are a number of acceptability issues associated with the impact of a given instrument on an interviewer. One questionnaire characteristic that can burden the interviewer is the amount and type of training required. For some instruments, the training is minimal; for others, such as the Quality of Well-Being Scale and the Sickness Impact Profile, the developers recommend careful instruction and practice for the interviewers (Bergner, 1984; Bush, 1984a). Training for the Quality of Well-Being Scale may take several days for interviewers to learn the concept, administration techniques, and pitfalls. Once training is completed, however, fieldwork is simplified because of the tightly constructed procedures surrounding data collection.

Method of Administration

The five most commonly used methods for obtaining information on health status and health-related quality of life are listed in Table 7.3. The methods differ in costs to administer, amount and type of interviewer training, and respondent burden (Ware, 1984c). Some instruments have been developed so they can be administered by more than one of these methods. Another important issue for questionnaires that may be included as part of a household survey study is whether proxy respondents can be used.

Telephone and personal interviews have advantages over self-administered questionnaires, because response rates are higher and the level of missing data is lower, particularly when self-administration is by mail (Aday, 1989). Self-administered questionnaires, on the other hand, have a distinct advantage in terms of lower survey costs and the promise of anonymity to respondents. A hybrid method consisting of the interviewer-supervised, self-administered questionnaire is becoming increasingly popular in health status studies. Minimally trained interviewers are present to control the circumstances of administration, answer procedural questions, and check for missing data before the respondent leaves.

The price tag of different methods will often determine the choice. In weighing the relative advantages and disadvantages of each method, investigators should pay particular attention to the human resources required in the use of alternative methods and the level of accuracy needed in answering the particular research question at hand.

Methods of Analysis and Complexity of Scoring

When a composite health status or health-related quality of life measure is used, one practical consideration concerns the availability of algorithms for assigning weights to individuals in given health states. In some cases, these may be simple procedures that can be done by hand. In others, the logic is sufficiently complex to warrant use of a computer scoring system to assure accuracy. In this situation, a key consideration is whether the needed computer programs already exist or will have to be written. Even if the programs exist, the computer language or other machine configuration patterns may be incompatible between different computer centers.

THE SELECTION DECISION: WHAT QUESTIONS SHOULD I ASK?

Table 7.4 is a guide for investigators to use in evaluating health-related quality of life measures; it offers an assessment strategy that will address the objectives of measurement and the conceptual, methodological, and practical considerations involved in any assessment. For each step in the selection process, questions are posed to help investigators choose among the many alternative measures of generic and specific health-related quality of life. The questions are arranged according to the ten steps of health-related quality of life assessment. The selection decision and design of the assessment strategy will involve context-specific consideration of all questions.

In choosing health-related quality of life measures, tradeoffs are most often necessary among competing goals of inquiry. The decision or problem being addressed, the objectives of measurement, and conceptual, methodological, and practical considerations all need to be weighed in making choices. Often less than optimal choices are

Table 7.4 Guide to evaluating health-related quality of life (HRQOL) measures

Step	*What questions should I ask?*

1. **Application and purpose of assessment:** *Does this measure fit the application and primary objectives of measurement? Will this measure permit testing of hypotheses concerning the determinants of health-related quality of life?*

   To select treatment and monitor patient outcomes (clinical practice): *Will this measure detect changes in HRQOL domains of primary interest to individual patients and their families?*

   To identify determinants of health, investigate course of disease and illness, and test efficacy of treatments (clinical and epidemiologic investigations): *Will this measure discriminate, predict, or measure important changes in groups under investigation?*

   To establish priorities, examine effectiveness of health policies and programs, and allocate resources (program evaluation and policy analysis): *Will this measure permit comparisons in HRQOL outcomes across competing interventions?*

   To track trends in levels of health, risk factors, and use of services (population monitoring): *Will this measure detect trends in repeated cross-sectional or cohort measures of HRQOL?*

2. **Specifying available resources:** *How much time, money, and personnel are available for the HRQOL assessment?*

   To select an existing measure or develop a new one: *Is there an existing measure containing relevant domains appropriate to the measurement objectives and population to be assessed? If not, do I have the resources and time to develop a new measure?*

   To identify the characteristics of an instrument for use in a particular setting and application: *Can this measure be self-administered by mail or in person and/or interviewer-administered by telephone or in person? How much time does it take to train interviewers or data collection personnel? Are instructions, guides, or manuals available to help in training interviewers and administering the instrument? Do interviewers like administering the instrument? What is the average length of time it takes to complete the assessment? Does the time vary by method of administration? Can respondents complete the assessment in the time allowed? Does the measure contain items that respondents might find offensive or consider irrelevant?*

   To obtain the instrument for use: *Is the measure copyrighted? If so, who owns the copyright and how do I get copies and permission to use it? How much, if any, does the measure cost per respondent?*

   To assess investigator willingness to incorporate HRQOL in the study: *How much time and resources are allocated to HRQOL assessment?*

3. **Description of population:** *What is the level of disability, age, cognitive ability, and ethnic or cultural identity of the target population?*

   To match the disability level of population with the domains of HRQOL in the measure: *Does this measure contain domains of positive and/or negative HRQOL suitable for the health or illness status of the population and measurement objectives (discrimination, prediction, evaluation)?*

   To match the function levels and domains of interest to the age of the population: *Does this measure contain the domains of HRQOL most relevant to infants, young children, adolescents, working adults, or older adults?*

   To match the respondent burden and domains of HRQOL to the cognitive ability of the population: *Can this measure be answered by a cognitively impaired respondent or will proxy respondents be needed?*

   To assess the cultural sensitivity of the measure to the target population: *Does this measure contain domains of interest, language, and instrumentation that are culturally appropriate to the groups being assessed? Has this measure been used in this population before?*

(continued)

Table 7.4 *(Continued)*

Step	What questions should I ask?

4. **Conceptualization of HRQOL outcomes:** *What domains of HRQOL should be measured in the assessment? How short or long should the assessment be?*

To identify the main and potential unintended outcomes of interest to consumers/patients, families, clinicians, decision makers, and society at large: *Does this measure or battery of measures contain the generic and condition-specific domains of survival, impairment, functional status, perceptions, and opportunity of main interest to the population?*

To assess the minimum and maximum content of the instrument: *Does this measure or battery cover the essential domains necessary for discriminating populations, predicting future status, or evaluating change? What is the minimum number of items necessary to assess each domain and relative number of necessary items across domains to achieve measurement objectives?*

5. **Assessment of methodological characteristics:** *What type of measure is appropriate to the assessment? What weighting system is used? What is known about the reliability, validity, and responsiveness of potential measures?*

To match the type of measure and weighting system to the application and primary objectives of measurement: *Is a single indicator, index, profile, or battery most appropriate to the application and primary measurement objectives? Is a single index needed for cost–effectiveness analysis? Are the items and domains in the measure weighted using statistical or utility systems? For which populations are preference weights available?*

To assess the known reliability of measures in relation to purpose of measurement: *What is the internal consistency, reproducibility, and/or interrater reliabilities or potential measures? Can this measure discriminate among different levels of HRQOL in the target populations?*

To assess responsiveness: *Can this measure detect minimally important diferences in repeated evaluations of HRQOL of respondents in the target populations? Does this measure contain items or questions that directly assess change, e.g., transition questions?*

To assess construct validity: *What is the strength of association between this potential measure and other measures hypothesized to be conceptually similar or different?*

6. **Choice of HRQOL measures:** *What tradeoffs need to be made between content, population, methodological concerns, investigator support, and resources involved in the assessment?*

7. **Conduct of pretest or pilot study:** *How well will the selected measures perform in the full study?*

To decide between a pretest or pilot: *Has this measure or battery been applied in this population and setting previously? Is it necessary to obtain validity or reliability data in this application of the measure(s)?*

8. **Preparation of data collection and analysis plans:** *What resources are needed to prepare the data for analysis? How should the HRQOL data be analyzed?*

To develop an implementation plan: *What coding, editing, and rescoring are involved in data collection and preparation of data files for analysis? Are scoring instructions or computer scoring programs available? Can scoring programs be purchased from the developers?*

To develop a data analysis plan: *What tables, descriptive data, and analyses are necessary to test the hypotheses in the investigation?*

9. **Collect data:** *How can the quality of the HRQOL data being collected be improved?*

To standardize data collection procedures: *Have experienced interviewers been selected and has sufficient training taken place? Are interviewers or data collection personnel all receiving the same instructions and training?*

(continued)

Table 7.4   *(Continued)*

Step	*What questions should I ask?*
	To monitor quality of data being collected: *Are interviewers reading questions as written, using common probes, providing uniform answers? How much missing data are there in completed interviews or self-administered questionnaires?*
10.	**Preparation of findings:** *How can the results best be presented to the intended audience?* To select a method for presenting findings: *Are methods available for presenting and interpreting findings to patients, clinicians, policymakers, other investigators, or the public?* To design tables, figures, and other means of presentation: *Do the illustrations follow the logic of the investigation? Do the illustrations contain too much information? How can the amount of information in any one illustration be reduced?*

made, because one or more considerations are neglected. For example, a measure with demonstrated reliability and validity, with comprehensive content, and with a long tradition of application may simply not fit into the practical constraints of resources and investigator willingness to adopt.

Many uses of health-related quality of life measures require brief, well-defined instruments that can be applied and interpreted easily. There is an increasing need for standardization of instruments or the use of standardized, generic measures in combination with newly developed specific ones. The use of these measures for health decision making will be increased by incorporating overall scores as well as scores for each component of the instrument.

Short, generic health-related quality of life measures (1–60 items) have been developed from longer versions based on minimal psychometric criteria for content validity, internal consistency reliability, and validity. However, "short" and "comprehensive" can be conflicting goals for some applications and populations. The full domain of health-related quality of life outcomes of interest to patients, providers, and payers simply cannot be represented in short measures. Some concepts—cognitive function, sleep and rest behaviors, recreation, and satisfaction with health, for instance—are seldom represented in short, generic measures. These omissions may not seriously compromise the usefulness of short-form measures in relatively well populations, but outcome assessment in specific populations such as older adults, persons with mental illness and physical disability, and institutionalized persons may require long-form assessments. How well short-form measures will detect subtle changes in behavioral and subjective health status also requires testing and comparison with clinical measures.

Not only technical knowledge but also creativity and conceptual skill are essential in selecting an appropriate assessment strategy. A catholicity of outlook, combined with scientific rigor, aids in selecting measures that will identify interventions that enhance health-related quality of life.

STEP 7. CONDUCT PRETEST AND PILOT STUDIES

Pretest or pilot studies are necessary aids to help investigators address the methodological and practical considerations involved in health-related quality of life assessment. *Pretests* are generally small investigations involving 5–25 administrations of a measure or battery of measures. This helps investigators estimate the length of time the assessment takes to complete, respondent reactions to different measures, completeness of instructions and other instrumentation, format and flow of the questionnaire, and other considerations in health survey research (Aday, 1989). Investigators should debrief both respondents and interviewers to learn how to improve plans for formatting questionnaires and monitoring and carrying out the assessment. Debriefing involves going over the data collection instrument step by step, asking respondents to repeat their understanding of the instructions and the items contained in the questionnaire. Pretests should be conducted using respondents from the population to be assessed and the actual interviewers involved in the study.

Pilot studies, large pretests involving 25 or more respondents, are complete studies, including data collection, scoring, and analysis, which are often small investigations in their own right, published separately. Pilot studies are advisable if an investigator wishes (1) to test specific hypotheses before the main study; (2) to test several different measures or methods of administration; (3) to collect data on the reliability, validity, and responsiveness of a measure in a particular application; or (4) to "practice" the assessment on a small number of persons before a large-scale investigation. Pilot studies are often methodological in focus, helping the investigators select among different measures or assessment strategies. Such studies can be particularly useful in learning how to analyze and present health-related quality of life data. Often pretests and pilot studies uncover unanticipated problems in conceptualization, methodology, and practical administration of measures, thereby avoiding problems in the main investigation.

STEP 8. PREPARE DATA COLLECTION AND ANALYSIS PLANS

Experiences from pretest and pilot studies can guide the development of data collection and analysis plans for the full-scale investigation. One area requiring detailed planning is the scheduling of data collection. Ideally studies should begin formally only after adjustments from the pretest or pilot study have been made. For example, if the pilot study indicated that data collection forms need revision, then these changes should be made before data collection is started on the main study. Often, however, the schedule for data collection does not permit full consideration of the pretest findings. Adequate time needs to be given to analysis of pretest/pilot data and revision of plans.

Data analysis plans should describe how each of the hypotheses in the investigation is to be tested. Included in the information specified by the plans are the dependent and independent variables, the cutoff points for the health-related quality of life measures in the analysis, and the statistical tests to be used in hypothesis testing.

STEP 9. COLLECT DATA

The major consideration in this step of an investigation is how to improve the quality of the health-related quality of life data being collected by interview or by self-administration. Carefully done pretest and pilot studies help to anticipate or eliminate many problems, but many sources of error may lower the quality of health-related quality of life data. Fowler and Mangione (1990) identify four major sources of error: (1) sampling error whereby a sample may not be exactly the same as the population from which it was drawn; (2) the questions themselves when they are misunderstood or answered inaccurately; (3) the interviewers and data collection procedures, which may bias answers; and (4) the coding, editing, and data entry process, which introduce errors into the data.

Standardization of procedures and monitoring of data collection are the major means by which to address survey errors. *Standardization* means applying the same procedure across a set of respondents and situations so that any differences can be compared and interpreted as indicating real differences in what is being measured. Standardized interviewing techniques, for example, reading questions as written, using common probes, and providing uniform answers to the most commonly asked questions, help to minimize errors from interviewers and data collection procedures.

In health-related quality of life assessments, terms such as "more than usual," "worse than before," "in general," and "ever been told" may be difficult for respondents to evaluate. Changing reference periods from question to question, say from "last two weeks" to "in the last year," may also confuse respondents. Respondents may also find it difficult to attribute changes in health to specific functional areas such as physical or emotional functioning or to identify the most undesirable symptom or condition from a long list of medical conditions and symptom complexes. Investigators should identify these problems in pretest studies and develop standardized responses for interviewers to use in reply to questions from respondents.

Among the increasingly available computer-assisted data collection techniques are computer-assisted interviews in person (CAPI) or by telephone (CATI), as well as computer-assisted self-administration (CASA) (Jette et al., 1986, Roizen et al., 1991; Ware, 1990). Proponents of these methods suggest that computers standardize administration and possible responses to a greater extent than do traditional methods of data collection. Also, computers can be programmed to screen for invalid responses as data are collected, for example, out-of-range responses or inconsistencies in answering questionnaire items. Editing data as they are collected may reduce the amount of missing data available for analysis. "Skip patterns" may also be programmed, helping to assist the respondent in completing the questionnaire. Respondents unfamiliar with or resistant to computers, however, may require special assistance or encouragement.

Interviewer selection and interviewer error are also major concerns. Often nurses and other health professionals are asked to act as data collectors for health-related quality of life assessments. The role of interviewer and data collector as neutral, unbiased "measurer" may be unfamiliar to persons used to relating to persons and patients as clinicians. The caring and data-collecting objectives may not always be consistent.

To some extent, rigorous interviewer training can aid in standardizing health-related quality of life survey procedures (Weinberg, 1983). Spending time on the rationale for measurement, the importance of data quality, how and when to probe, and the role of the interviewer in the survey helps to orient interviewers and improve data quality. Practice interviews, particularly with respondents similar to those in the main study, are valuable training aids.

Supervising fieldwork and monitoring incoming data and data entry are also important survey management tasks (Aday, 1989). For telephone surveys, a consistent program of monitoring, evaluation, and feedback is important (Fowler and Mangione, 1990). For personal interviews, tape-recording, evaluation, and feedback procedures are necessary. For self-administered questionnaires, monitoring for completion of answers and follow-up to obtain missing data are necessary concerns, particularly for respondents in ill health. Double entry of survey data, feedback to data entry personnel on error rates, and range and consistency checks on computerized data are commonly used to improve the quality of data for analysis.

Considering all facets of data collection and their inter-relationships is often a demanding and daunting task to investigators. Attention to the details of data collection, however, tends to result in higher response rates and higher quality of data for analysis. If health-related quality of life data are important to the conclusions of the investigation and therefore to the investigator, then quality control of data collection is likely to be implemented. The data can only be as good as the attention paid to collecting and analyzing them.

STEP 10. ANALYZE AND PRESENT FINDINGS

The final practical issue concerns presentation of health-related quality of life findings. In most ways, presentation does not differ from other kinds of clinical or policy data (Spilker and Schoenfelder, 1990). The results of analyses including means, standard errors, and change scores should be presented in tabular or graphic form and should not contain too many data points (e.g., no more than five rows and four columns in tables). Both tables and figures should be simple to understand with clear titles, legends, and footnotes.

Presentation of findings may also vary according to the intended audience for the findings. Busy politicians and administrators often require presentations that reveal the "bottom line" in the simplest fashion possible, most often in the form of graphs and simply stated conclusions. Analysts and researchers, on the other hand, tend to desire data presented more completely and without interpretations and conclusions. The presentation of findings can bias interpretation and conclusions, a fact well-known and well-used by many investigators and analysts.

Decision makers and other readers find data more comprehensible when they are presented as closely as possible to the logic of a particular investigation. For example, comparing a population's health-related quality of life before and after treatment in the same table reporting the results of a controlled trial is desirable. Subjective data may also be graphed along with objective data from physiological records to provide evidence of the consistency or inconsistency of results. Reporting effect sizes as they have appeared in previous publications using a particular measure is recommended to permit cumulative knowledge of measured effects using the same instrument.

Whenever possible, raw data should be reported before they are converted to percentage improved, unchanged, or deteriorated or transformed mathematically. Such manipulation of data may make the nature of the measured effects less clear and possibly contribute to an over- or underinterpretation of findings. For example, different measures with different response categories and different scores are often converted into broad categories of change in reporting the findings of controlled trials or cohort studies. Interpretation of the actual change scores using the original units of the measure may be obscured in combining the results of different studies.

Graphical presentations are often easier to understand than tabular presentations of complex data. Histograms with shading and line graphs with data points are commonly used. Putting the actual data on the histogram and designing line graphs to permit estimation of data points are aids to the reader that may counteract unintended visual effects in data presentation.

Some health-related quality of life instruments yield an overall or summary score as well as component scores. Investigators should present both the overall score and its component parts to help in understanding the contribution of different components to the overall score. The profile scores might, for example, be illustrated in graphical form with the overall score in the graph or in the text.

The presentation of health-related quality of life data, like efficacy data of any kind, is an art. Data can be reported in subtle ways that suggest the conclusions investigators desire to communicate rather than in a more neutral form. A recommended procedure is to prepare data for presentation using several alternative formats and selecting the one that is most "truthful" to the data and results of the study and most understandable to readers unfamiliar with the investigation. An old but wise rule for analysts is to present data in such a way that the reader or decision maker could replicate the study and the findings as originally presented.

Primary data collection is not the only method for assessing health-related quality of life. Increasing use is being made of secondary data sources from national or large population surveys to estimate the health-related quality of life of whole communities or of special populations. Many of the conceptual, methodological, and practical considerations involved in secondary analysis of health-related quality of life data are similar to those presented in this chapter. The techniques of analysis, however, may be considerably different, as described in the next chapter.

8

Developing a Strategy for Secondary Data Analysis

In addition to using information available from primary data collection, health-related quality of life can be measured using existing data. In secondary analyses, data collected for one purpose are reanalyzed for an alternative use. To fit data to the different purpose of measurement, the analyst must make various assumptions. As a result, information obtained from secondary analyses is generally less precise than that obtained by primary data collection.

Secondary data may be useful when looking for differences in health-related quality of life that can be measured in terms of order of magnitude, for example, a twofold or fourfold difference. Existing data may also be used to test out hypotheses as part of the process of designing primary data collection. For example, existing data collected in the National Health Interview Survey were analyzed as if they had been collected in the form of a preference-weighted health-related quality of life measure to determine whether or not such data could be collected in national surveys.

Availability of data is another important reason for considering use of secondary data analysis. In the case of some health decisions, the reanalysis of existing data may be the only available course of action. For example, national data may be the only source of information available for identified minority populations, including children living in poverty, people with disabilities, and persons without health insurance.

This chapter is based on research conducted at the National Center for Health Statistics for the purpose of developing measures of health-related quality of life using data from the National Health Interview Survey. In conducting these analyses, Erickson and colleagues (1988, 1989) identified seven steps for developing a measure of health-related quality of life based on existing data: (1) identify a classification system, or other measure, to use as the standard; (2) review existing data sets and identify the health-related concepts included in each; (3) compare the existing data with those required by the classification system or measure of health-related quality of life; (4) specify all assumptions necessary for obtaining comparability between the classification system and the existing data; (5) calculate health-related quality of life scores using the classification system's preference weights and computational formula; (6) validate the health-related quality of life scores by estimating their relationship with other health and sociodemographic variables; and (7) conduct sensitivity analyses to determine the effect of the assumptions on the computed scores.

These steps are used to develop a strategy for analyzing secondary data along with health-related quality of life measures in the Health Resource Allocation Strategy.

Thus, the focus of this chapter is on matching a classification system, the Quality of Well-Being Scale in particular, to data from the National Health Interview Survey to calculate years of healthy life. The same steps and procedures can be used, however, to construct other measures of health-related quality of life using existing data.

The next section discusses conceptual and methodological considerations in identifying a measure of health-related quality of life that will be sensitive to the policy options being considered (Step 1). The second section describes some of the major sources of data, including the ongoing National Health Interview Survey. Other sources include registration systems and administrative records. These data sources can be used for identifying concepts of health-related quality of life (Step 2). In the third section we describe considerations for matching the measure with the data and for validating the constructed measure (Steps 3–7). The last section provides insights into interpreting these constructed scores for health decision making.

SELECTING AN ASSESSMENT STRATEGY

In selecting a particular classification system or measure to use with existing data, the analyst considers issues similar to those used in developing and implementing a primary data collection strategy. The analysis must be related to the causal hypotheses of relevant determinants of health-related quality of life, to policy options, and to stakeholders. Once these concerns have been identified, an appropriate classification system can be selected. For example, if the analysis is to evaluate the use of neonatal intensive care units (NICUs), the health status measure needs to assess physical function and independence, two health status characteristics that NICUs have been designed to improve. If the target population is one of older adults, as in an evaluation of nursing homes, the concepts need to be sensitive to changes in physical, social, and mental functioning suitable for older persons with restricted activity.

Secondary analysis of data collected in the National Health Interview Survey (NHIS) was undertaken to evaluate the potential of assessing health-related quality of life in the general population of the United States. NHIS data are used for monitoring health levels to detect change over time, for investigating determinants of health-related quality of life, and for identifying gaps in health levels between different population groups. Thus, measures that included concepts of health-related quality of life and their operational definitions that were suitable for use in the general population were considered for use in this research project.

To identify measures that might be used with NHIS data, researchers reviewed the literature of health-related quality of life measures developed since 1965 (Clearinghouse on Health Indexes, 1973–1991). Within the list of measures that were suitable for use with the general population, only those measures that had been applied in several studies and involved subjects with sociodemographic characteristics similar to the noninstitutionalized United States population were included in the final phase of this research project.

Documentation is very important in determining whether an existing data set and a classification system are sufficiently well matched to conduct secondary data analysis. Information needs to be available, either in the literature or from researchers, to explain the underlying conceptual framework and the data collection methods for each measure. The more detailed the information about the selected measure, the better will be the comparison with the existing data.

As a result of the literature review, three measures of health-related quality of life were identified for further consideration. Two of these were the Health Utilities Index and the Quality of Well-Being Scale. The third was the Health Profile that was included in the Health Insurance Experiment (Brook et al., 1979) and was developed for use with persons in the general population who were between 14 and 65 years of age. This profile was a major source of information about the contribution of alternative national health insurance plans to changing health status outcomes.

Other widely used measures, for example, the Sickness Impact Profile (SIP) and Nottingham Health Profile (NHP), were excluded from the analysis (Bergner et al., 1981; Hunt et al., 1986). Because the SIP was developed to assess the level of disease impact on an individual's level of functioning, it would have insufficient relevance and variability in a predominantly healthy population such as that of the United States where 85 percent of the civilian noninstitutionalized population reports no limitation in activity. Items in the SIP questionnaire are also conceptually different from those in general national surveys, particularly the National Health Interview Survey. Thus, there would be little opportunity for matching items in the NHIS with those in the SIP.

The NHP was originally based on the same principles of item construction and instrument development as the SIP. In addition, the NHP was developed in the United Kingdom with preference weights obtained from British respondents. Using the NHP would require the assumption that British and American values assigned to health states are the same. Although Patrick et al. (1985) demonstrated that British and American subjects weighted the SIP similarly, no such work has yet been done for the NHP. For these reasons, the NHP was also considered inappropriate for the National Health Interview Survey research.

In addition to identifying measures that were conceptually similar to the data collected in the NHIS, the literature review focused on only those measures with demonstrated reliability and validity. Just as with primary data collection, measurement properties are important in selecting an assessment for use in secondary analysis. For example, the analyst needs to determine whether reliability and validity have been established for each classification system that is being considered for use. Special attention should be given to those studies of reliability and validity that have been done in a population similar to the proposed study group.

By selecting only those classification systems or measures for use with existing data that have well-established measurement properties, the secondary data analyst incorporates the science behind these measures into the analysis. In this way the attention given to the development of the conceptual and measurement frameworks in each assessment is carried through to the secondary analysis.

After classification systems that are relevant to the health problem or decision under consideration and the stakeholders in the decision have been selected, existing sources of data are reviewed to identify those that best match the concepts of health-related quality of life that are included in the classification system. The next section describes the major national data sets that can be used for secondary analysis in the context of the Health Resource Allocation Strategy.

MAJOR SOURCES OF EXISTING DATA

This section summarizes national data sets that contain person-based information on concepts of health-related quality of life. We excluded data sets in which health care facilities, rather than individuals, were the units of analysis and those in which the variables of interest are based on events. In addition, we further selected data sets that have information about not only health-related quality of life but also its determinants—sociodemographic characteristics, health behaviors, and health insurance coverage. The data we discuss are national in focus and readily available for reanalysis; thus, we have omitted proprietary data sets such as the Medical Outcomes Study (MOS) and those developed for public opinion polling.

Health Surveys

Table 8.1 summarizes information on selected population-based health surveys conducted by the National Center for Health Statistics (NCHS) and the Agency for Health Care Policy and Research (AHCPR). Although each of these surveys was designed by drawing on the experience of the others, no organized plan is followed for deciding which measures to include in the various surveys. Rather, each survey is designed to maximize the information collected to meet the purpose of the particular survey. The periodicity, populations covered, data collection methodologies, and sample designs are described in Table 8.1 for four major surveys.

The National Center for Health Statistics, which operates with legislative authorization from the U.S. Congress, is the major statistical organization concerned with generating health statistics to reflect the health status of the U.S. population. The NCHS data systems collect statistics on a wide range of health data, including illness and disability and their impact on the economy, mortality, life expectancy, environmental hazards, determinants of health, health resources, utilization of health care, health care costs and financing, and family formation and growth (Pearce, 1989). Many of these programs collect indicators of health status and quality of life ranging from mortality and life expectancy to the incidence or prevalence of specific diseases. They also include such indicators of disability as restricted activity days as well as health-related quality of life issues like self-perceived health status.

The Agency for Health Care Policy and Research, previously known as the National Center for Health Services Research until 1990, is the major government agency concerned with the funding the development and the application of health services research. Its extramural programs have supported the development of many of the indexes and profiles currently available for the measurement of health-related quality of life, including the General Health Perceptions Scale, the Quality of Well-Being Scale, and the Sickness Impact Profile. The primary responsibility of the intramural program of AHCPR is the design, implementation, and analysis of data from national panel surveys of medical care expenditures and their relationship health status.

The National Health Interview Survey, one of the principal population-based health surveys conducted by NCHS, has collected data on the civilian noninstitutionalized of the United States continuously since 1957. A major component of this survey is the collection of information about the prevalence of approximately 100 chronic conditions and impairments (Adams and Benson, 1990). Chronic conditions are also used to

Table 8.1 Summary description of national health surveys in the United States

Periodicity	Population covered	Data collection methodology	Sample design
		National Health Interview Survey (NHIS)	
Continuous since 1957; supplements to core questionnaire change each year or more frequently	Civilian noninstitutionalized population of the 50 states and District of Columbia	Initial household interview conducted face to face with an adult household respondent; supplements may require self-response (face to face or by telephone) from a sample person	Multistage probability sample; each week's sample is broadly representative of the target population and weekly samples are additive over time 1973–84: 376 primary sampling units; based on 1970 census registers plus area segments and permit segments (using building permits issued since 1970); 42,000 households containing 110,000 persons 1985–present: 201 primary sampling units; based completely on independent listing of areas in the survey sample; 50,000 households containing approximately 135,000 persons; because of budget constraints, only a 3/4 sample was implemented for 1985
		National Health and Nutrition Examination Survey (NHANES)	
New cycle begins approximately every four years; Cycle I, 1971–75; Cycle II, 1976–80; Cycle III, 1988–94	Civilian noninstitutionalized population of the coterminous United States in Cycle I; expanded to cover all 50 states in 1976 Cycle I—persons ages 1–74 years; Cycle II—persons ages 6 months–74 years; Cycle III—persons aged 2 months and older	Face-to-face interview with an adult household respondent to determine household membership, obtain background information, and select sample person(s); face-to-face household interview with sample person; detailed tests, examinations, and dietary interview for sample person in survey's mobile examination center	Multistage probability sample; Cycle I used 100 primary sampling units and examined approximately 21,000 persons in the detailed nutrition components; Cycle II used 64 primary sampling units and examined approximately 21,000 persons; Cycle III will examine approximately 40,000 persons

(continued)

Table 8.1 *(continued)*

Periodicity	Population covered	Data collection methodology	Sample design
		NHANES I Epidemiologic Follow-up Survey (NHEFS)	
Initial follow-up in 1982–84 recontacted in two-year intervals since initial follow-up	All 14,407 persons who were ages 25–74 at time of examination in NHANES-1	Initial follow-up was face-to-face interview plus blood pressure and weight measurements; proxy interview for those who had died or were incapacitated; continued follow-up for 1985–86 by telephone; signed authorizations obtained at each contact to permit obtaining information from hospital and nursing home records	Efforts were made to trace all 14,407 persons in the universe; more than 92 percent were located; effort continues to locate persons lost to follow-up
		National Medical Expenditures Survey (NMES)	
First conducted in 1977; next cycle in 1980; most recent cycle, 1987	1980: Civilian noninstitutionalized population of the 50 states and District of Columbia in national sample; Medicaid-eligible households in New York, California, Texas, and Michigan 1987: Civilian noninstitutionalized population of the U.S.; American Indians and Alaskan Natives; institutional population	1980: three face-to-face and two telephone interviews with an adult household respondent; review of administrative eligibility and claims records for persons reported to be covered by Medicare and Medicaid 1987: Face-to-face interviews and self-administered questionnaires; review of claims records for health care expenditures data	1980: Multistage area probability sample drawn from 106 primary sampling units for national sample of 10,000 households; probability samples of about 1,000 households from state Medicaid eligibility lists in each of the four states 1987: Multistage probability sample for a national sample of 14,000 households plus 2,000 households representing American Indians and Alaskan Natives; and 10,500 persons in the institutional sample

Source: Adapted from Pearce, 1991.

define limitations of usual social role. The NHIS also collects information on the incidence of acute conditions, that is, reported conditions that had their onset within the two weeks prior to the interview (with the exception of certain conditions defined as chronic regardless of onset) and resulted in either medical attention or one or more days of restricted activity. Information is collected on all illnesses or injuries, including conditions that are considered to be chronic by definition or those that lasted at least three months over the past year and caused respondents (1) to restrict their usual activity for at least a day (by staying in bed, staying home from work or school, or cutting down on usual activities); (2) to seek medical attention during the two weeks prior to the interview; (3) to be hospitalized during the past year; or (4) to experience a long-term limitation of activity. All conditions are coded to a modified version of the most recent International Classification of Diseases (ICD).

The National Health and Nutrition Examination Survey (NHANES) has collected information cyclically since 1971. Each "cycle" of NHANES has been conducted over a four- to six-year period. This survey of the civilian noninstitutionalized population collects data that are best obtained by direct physical examination, clinical and laboratory tests, and related measurement procedures (McDowell et al., 1981). Examinations take place in specially constructed mobile examination centers consisting of truck-drawn trailers; these centers provide a standardized environment for precise measurements. Condition data are obtained in two ways. The medical history component of the survey has a checklist of chronic conditions; the examination part of the survey provides diagnostic information for selected diseases. Data collected as a result of physical examination, for example, blood pressure readings, visual acuity, and serum cholesterol, can be used to develop normative distributions for the U.S. population.

The NHANES-I Epidemiologic Follow-Up Survey (NHEFS) is a longitudinal survey which follows 14,407 people from age 25 to 74 who were examined in the first cycle of the NHANES (Cohen et al., 1987). The major purpose of NHEFS is to examine the relationships between risk factors measured in the first NHANES and subsequent morbidity and mortality. The follow-up information is obtained through a household interview with the original respondents or their proxies. The detailed questionnaire for the 1982–84 survey includes items derived from existing instruments that have been designed to measure specific concepts of health-related quality of life. For example, the Center for Epidemiologic Studies Depression Scale (CES-D) is included in its entirety (Radloff, 1977); selected items from the General Well-Being (GWB) schedule are also included (Fazio, 1977). The functional limitations section consists of items selected, and sometimes modified, from the Functional Disability Scale for arthritis (Fries et al., 1980), the Rosow-Breslau Scale (Rosow and Breslau, 1966), and the Index of Activities of Daily Living (Katz et al., 1963).

Also included in this comprehensive questionnaire are checklists to obtain information on specific health conditions, items on sleeping problems and change in sleep patterns, scales to measure personality traits, and questions to determine health habits such as smoking and alcohol consumption and physical activity. In the NHEFS, physical examinations have been limited; at the end of the interview the respondent has his or her pulse taken, blood pressure read, and weight measured.

The 1987 National Medical Expenditure Survey (NMES), conducted by AHCPR, is a one-year panel survey of the U.S. population (Edwards and Berlin, 1989; Edwards and Edwards, 1989). One component is a household survey of the noninstitutionalized

population; another focuses on American Indians and Alaska Natives; the third component surveys residents of long-term care facilities. The NMES is the third in a series of
national surveys designed to collect information on both health status and personal
health expenditures.

The content of the National Medical Expenditure Survey health status questionnaire
reflects the research of the 1970s and early 1980s. In addition to questions about an
individual's limitations in physical and social activity that have been staples for health
surveys since the inception of the National Health Interview Survey in 1957, NMES
asks about affective well-being. These questions draw on items from the General Well-
Being Schedule. The NMES also asks about health perceptions, drawing on items from
the General Health Rating Index. Another difference between the health status content
of the NMES and many other health surveys is the extensive amount of information
that this survey collects on symptoms and health problems.

The National Medical Expenditures Survey and its forerunners, the National Medical
Care Expenditures Survey and the National Medical Care Utilization and Expenditures
Survey, are the major national surveys that collect information on personal health
expenditures and sources of payment. Thus, this data set has both the health-related
quality of life and health care costs components for applying the Health Resource
Allocation Strategy.

National survey data in general, and those summarized in Table 8.1 in particular, are
available for public use, usually in computer tape format, within one to two years after
the end of the data-collection period. The growing emphasis on making national data
files publicly available has resulted in improved documentation of sample design and
tape layout.

One standard item in the documentation package is a description of the survey
design, including the sampling plan. This is particularly important in complex survey
designs that yield samples that are representative of national populations. For example,
sampling weights must be used to analyze responses on data collected in all of the
surveys summarized in Table 8.1. Using unweighted data, especially when subgroups
of the population have been oversampled to assure that they are included in national
estimates, may lead to questionable findings and provide misleading information to
decision makers.

Another standard item of documentation is the questionnaire used to collect the data.
Reviewing the questionnaire is particularly important for understanding the context in
which each item on the data tape was collected. It is important to know (1) which
respondents were asked a given question or set of questions, that is, whether or not the
questions are asked of only a subset of the sample that had certain characteristics; (2)
how the questions were worded, for example, in terms of an individual's capacity or
performance; and (3) what period of recall was used for obtaining information about
health status and function level.

Recently, documentation that accompanies the data tapes has included tallies of the
responses to each question. These counts are valuable for checking one's own tabula-
tions to verify that the file is being used correctly; these marginals can also be used to
validate programming. In some cases, these counts are also valuable indicators of the
expected sample sizes available for analysis. Some variables represent such rare events
that the number of cases available is too small for detailed analysis. This can occur

even when the overall sample size exceeds 100,000, as it does in the National Health Interview Survey. Although a small sample size may be a problem for estimating the prevalence of a chronic condition or health-related dysfunction, it is generally not a problem in constructing a measure of health-related quality of life.

Most statistical agencies, such as the National Center for Health Statistics and Agency for Health Care Policy and Research, have individuals who can be consulted about the use of their data files. The availability of these experts is especially important when the data are from complex sample health surveys.

Registration Systems

In addition to health status data available from health surveys, health-related quality of life data as well as other types of health data are available from administrative records. A major source of health status data has been the vital statistics registration system, maintained in the United States by the National Center for Health Statistics. Mortality statistics that are published in annual volumes and summarized in the *Monthly Vital Statistics Report* (National Center for Health Statistics, 1988) are important principally for health policy decisions involving health status. In addition to showing overall mortality, these data are compiled by cause of death, by geographic location, and by sociodemographic variables. Life tables, including life expectancy at birth and other points in time, are calculated from the mortality data and published by NCHS at regular intervals. These tables provide one of the two types of data needed for calculating years of healthy life.

Disease-specific health status data are available from selected registration systems. For example, the Centers for Disease Control maintain registers on prevalence of tuberculosis and other reportable diseases. The National Cancer Institute maintains the Cancer Surveillance, Epidemiology and End Results Reporting (SEER) data base for selected cancer diagnoses. Medicare and Medicaid files maintained by the Health Care Financing Administration contain information about health condition and health care expenditures for selected groups, especially elderly, disabled and low-income persons in the U.S. population.

Although data from disease-reporting systems may be useful for assessing health-related quality of life, they have important limitations. These data are usually collected only about ill health rather than physical, social, or emotional functioning. The item on self-assessed health status, which is generally considered a good reflection of an individual's overall health status, is rarely included in registration systems. Another limitation is that the reported cases do not form a representative sample. If all cases are reported, there is no bias. Usually, however, bias is introduced because of incomplete registration or reporting.

This section has reviewed the major national surveys and registration systems that can be used for conducting secondary data analyses to assess health-related quality of life of the United States population. The next section describes procedures for matching the classification system and the existing data to develop and validate a measure of health-related quality of life. These steps are illustrated using the classification system of the Quality of Well-Being Scale and data from the National Health Interview Survey.

CONSTRUCTING AND TESTING MEASURES

After identifying the health-related quality of life measure and the corresponding data set, the questionnaires used for collecting the data need to be compared item by item to identify the information in the existing data that corresponds to that in the classification system. When there is less than perfect agreement between the questionnaires, assumptions for dealing with missing or incomplete data or any other difference between the classification system and the existing data need to be stated. For example, if a small number of persons have failed to respond to one or two items in the questionnaire or a large number of items are missing, most likely because they were not asked in the questionnaire used for collecting the existing data, the analyst may choose to fill in the missing responses with plausible and consistent data. The process of estimating missing data in health surveys is referred to as imputation.

In recent years a number of imputation methods have been developed, ranging from the simple to the complicated (Sande, 1982). The simplest rule is to assume that all missing values take on the same value. In a secondary analysis of health-related quality of life data, the analyst may choose to assume that the missing responses indicate no dysfunction. A more involved method is to use a mean or other typical value to represent the missing data. Alternatively, the missing data can be modeled using regression techniques. Although modeling can reduce bias in the estimated means and other sample statistics, achieving a good fit to the data can require a great deal of effort. The current survey can also be used to form complete responses through the use of nearest neighbor procedures.

External data sources that have equivalent items to the missing data can also be used as sources for developing complete responses. These methods of imputation, including sequential hot deck, and random choice procedure, may require statistical matching on classification fields such as age, gender, and color. In practice, most imputation problems are handled by a combination of these methods.

Once these assumptions have been stated and any necessary imputations completed, the measure of health-related quality of life can be constructed and scored. The resultant measure needs to be validated; this can be done by using an external data source as a criterion or by testing hypotheses about the relationship of the constructed measure with other health variables. The final step is to conduct sensitivity analyses. These five steps are described in greater detail next.

Comparability

In matching the two questionnaires, the analyst needs to evaluate each question in terms of item content, question framing, recall period, and respondent characteristics (e.g., age and health conditions). *Item content*, which is the most important consideration in whether or not the classification and existing data agree, refers to whether an item in the questionnaire that was used to collect the data assesses the same health characteristic or concept as in the classification system. For example, the Quality of Well-Being (QWB) Scale asks whether the respondent "limped, used cane, crutches, or walker." The 1979–80 NHIS asked similar questions about using crutches, cane, or walker but did not ask about limping. This comparison, as well as others for the Physical Activity Scale of the QWB, is shown in Table 8.2.

Table 8.2 Comparison of physical activity questions asked in the Quality of Well-Being and in the National Health Interview Survey, 1979–80

	Quality of Well-Being		National Health Interview Survey	
Agreement	Item number[a]	Contents/recall/mode and respondent type	Item number[b]	Contents/recall/mode and respondent type
Yes?	PAC1	Confined to wheelchair most or all of the day/last four days/performance. Respondents: all	HCS 8a (7)	Use of wheelchair/ now/performance. Respondents: all
Yes	PAC1A	Cannot control wheelchair without help/last four days/performance. Respondents: all	HCS 1–2 (a)	Assistance in ADL-type[c] activities/now/ performance. Respondents: all
Yes	PAC2, PAC2A	Most all of day in bed health-related/last four days/performance. Respondents: all	HCS 5 (a–b)	Stay in bed most or all of day (due to illness or disability or health problem. How many days? /two weeks/performance. Respondents: all
No	PAC3, PAC3A	Most or all of day in chair or couch/last four days/performance. Respondents: all		No correspondence.
No	PAC4	Trouble with lifting, stooping, bending, or using stairs/last four days/performance. Respondents: all		No correspondence.
Yes?	PAC5	Limped, used cane, crutches, or walker/last four days/performance. Respondents: all	HCS 8a (4, 5, 8)	Crutches, cane, walker/now/performance
No	PAC6	Other physical limitation in walking/last four days/performance. Respondents: all		No correspondence.

Source: Erickson et al., 1988.

[a]PAC = Physical Activity.

[b]HCS = Home Care Supplement of the 1979–80 National Health Interview Survey.

[c]ADL = Activities of Daily Living.

As indicated by the left-hand column in this table, three levels of agreement between the QWB and the NHIS were identified. They were definite agreement (yes), question-able agreement (yes?), and no agreement (no). Items are classified as being in definite agreement when they agree on content, framing, recall period, and respondent charac-teristics. No agreement between items indicates that the NHIS did not collect any information about a health-related quality of life concept that is used in the QWB. For example, the 1979–80 NHIS did not collect any information about bending, stooping, or lifting. The questionable category is used for items for which there is some, but less than perfect, agreement. For example, agreement between the QWB item about limping, using a cane, crutches, or walker (PAC5) and the NHIS is considered to be questionable because of the lack of information in the NHIS on limping.

Question framing refers to the mode in which the item is asked. Two modes, performance and capacity, are most frequently used in assessing health-related quality of life. The *performance mode* asks what the respondent does: "Did you drive your car yesterday?" The *capacity mode* asks what the respondent says he or she is capable of doing: "Could you drive your car yesterday?" Anderson and colleagues (1977) found that respondents reported 15 percent less dysfunction when questions were asked in capacity rather than in performance mode. This difference is attributed to respondents' denial of dysfunction or limitation. As indicated in Table 8.2, all of the QWB Physical Activity Scale items are asked in the performance mode.

Recall period refers to the interval for which the information is collected. Most national surveys use two-week recall periods for counting events such as short-term disability days, usually those that are attributed to limitation in activity or role function. Items that are used to characterize individuals may have recall periods as long as one year. In designing a questionnaire, researchers determine the length of the recall period by the concept being assessed. For example, to estimate incidence of acute conditions, the NHIS asks about the presence of acute conditions that occurred during the two weeks prior to the day of interview. NHIS uses a one-year recall period to estimate prevalence of chronic conditions or to classify individuals, for example, those with a low, moderate, or high number of bed days.

Differences in length of recall period used in the classification system's questionnaire and the existing data base can affect the estimates of health-related quality of life obtained in a secondary data analysis. Two-week recall periods are likely to result in an overestimate of dysfunction due to the respondent's tendency to report events even though they may have occurred outside of the two-week period. This is called telescoping. One-year recall periods may result in underestimates of dysfunction due to the increased likelihood of forgetting (Cohen et al., 1984). In some cases, underreporting associated with forgetting may be balanced by the overreporting due to telescoping.

The QWB and 1979–80 NHIS differ in the length of recall period used. The QWB asks about functioning on a day-by-day basis over the past four, six, or eight days, depending on the QWB version. The NHIS uses a two-week reference period to collect information about conditions or events. This latter method, although simpler, may miss two or more health-related dysfunctions that occur on the same day. If items are treated equally, then recall period does not matter. On the other hand, when preference weights are used in the measure of health-related quality of life, a different score may result when two or more dysfunctions occur on the same day. Thus, the recall period is an important consideration in the case of preference-weighted health-related quality of life scores.

The analyst also needs to watch for other differences between the two questionnaires that may bias the calculated estimates of health-related quality of life in one direction or another. For example, the questionnaire used to collect the existing data may incorporate skip patterns or complex questions, which may preclude a large segment of the sample from answering selected items. Questionnaires that use either or both of these design features may result in a high percentage of nonresponse. In such cases the resulting scores may be biased.

One possible source of bias attributable to skip patterns is the use of special topic supplements. The 1979–80 National Health Interview Survey, for example, added items designed to assess use of home care aids and services among the disabled and elderly. In this survey, people were asked about mobility in the community only if they reported limitation either in daily living activities—for example, bathing, dressing, or eating—or in instrumental activities—for example, preparing meals, shopping for personal items, or doing routine household chores. Thus, the number of people with health-related limitations in either driving a car or using public transportation is underestimated due to the design of the special topic supplement.

More commonly, responses may be obtained on selected groups of the populations through screener questions and skip patterns. Some questions may be asked only of women of childbearing age. Or survey designers who wish to obtain detailed information about joint pain for only those persons with arthritis might design the questionnaire to collect detailed information about pain for only those persons in the total study population who report having arthritis. These selection patterns are important as potential sources of bias in the final constructed scores of health-related quality of life when using existing data.

The comparison process may also indicate that the method of administration differs between that used with the classification system and with the existing data. For example, data for the classification system may be collected by means of a self-administered questionnaire, although the existing data were collected using household interviewers. In the comparison between the Quality of Well-Being Scale and the National Health Interview Survey, this was not a problem. Both questionnaires were interviewer-administered.

Another practical consideration is the use of proxy respondents. Data from the National Health Interview Survey indicate a differential response rate in perceived health status by age and proxy or self-responses. Among younger people, proxy respondents rate a higher proportion in excellent or very good health than do self-respondents; for older persons, proxy respondents rate a higher proportion in fair or poor health than do self-respondents. This interaction between age and proxy response is generally explained as young people are healthy and away from home at the time of the interview, whereas older respondents are too sick to participate in the interview, whether they are at home or in the hospital. Some health status assessments, such as the Quality of Well-Being Scale, have been designed to take self- and proxy, or surrogate, response into consideration.

The purpose of the comparison step is to identify the similarities and differences between the classification system and the questionnaire used to collect data in the existing database. Items for which there is agreement between the two data-collection procedures can be used directly in computing estimates of health-related quality of life (Step 5). Items that differ in content, response mode, or recall period, or in practical considerations, such as skip patterns or proxy response, generally require the analyst to make certain assumptions before the items can be used to construct health-related quality of life scores.

Assumptions

For items for which there is no agreement—those items in the classification system that have not been obtained for the existing data set—or for which there is questionable agreement, the analyst must either impute the information or make an assumption about the impact of the missing data on the health status of the individual or group. Table 8.2 shows examples of both types of disagreement.

For assessments that assign scores to dysfunction, ignoring an item has the effect of assuming that missing information indicates no dysfunction. This assumption biases the score toward the healthy end of the scale; the population will appear healthier than it really is. On the other hand, the analyst can assume that missing data represent health-related dysfunction. This assumption biases the score toward the unhealthy end of the scale, making the population appear less healthy than it is. The true score will lie between these extremes.

The decision to ignore missing data may be acceptable if it has minimal impact on the resultant score. For example, the lack of information on lifting, bending, and stooping in the NHIS could be ignored in constructing the NHIS-QWB because this dysfunction has a small preference weight (0.06) (Appendix I). If missing data make substantial contributions to the health-related quality of life scores such as with the symptom–problem list of the QWB, however, imputation must be considered.

A number of imputation procedures, including hot and cold deck, distance function matching, and random imputation within classes, are available (Kalton and Kasprzyk, 1982; Sande, 1982). In working with complex sample surveys like the NHIS, imputations need to consider the sample design. For example, some health surveys oversample for race and age. If this oversampling is overlooked in the imputation procedures, using sampling weights may result in national estimates that are no longer representative of the total population. One assumption that is usually made when imputing missing health data is that persons in the same age-race-gender categories have the same health characteristics. This assumption is one way of accounting for the complex survey design.

Another set of assumptions is associated with the use of an external data source. Imputation methods frequently require an independent data source for supplying missing information. For example, in imputing symptoms to calculate the NHIS-QWB analysts needed a data base that could provide a link between the condition data collected in the NHIS and the symptom data needed to calculate a QWB score. Both types of data are collected in the National Ambulatory Medical Care Survey (NAMCS) (Tenney et al., 1974). NAMCS data are collected in physicians' offices from patients seen during a randomly selected week of practice. In using the NAMCS data base to impute symptoms based on self-reported health conditions in the NHIS, the analyst makes the assumption that people who go to the doctor have the same symptom–health profile as does the general population. The impact of this assumption on the calculated health-related quality of life scores can be assessed by conducting a sensitivity analysis on the final scores.

Once assumptions are made about discrepancies in the information required for the classification system and those in the existing data base, the analyst is ready to calculate health-related quality of life scores. This is essentially a two-step procedure in which the first step is to validate the components of the overall score; the second step is to validate the overall score itself.

Scoring and Validation

Calculation of health-related quality of life scores starts with grouping individual items in the existing data set into concepts measured by the classification system. For example, in constructing Quality of Well-Being scores for the National Health Interview Survey, Physical Activity items in Table 8.2 (bending, stooping, lifting, or using stairs) had to be combined with limped, used a cane, crutches, or walker, or had other physical limitations, to form the second level of the Physical Activity Scale (Appendix I).

Once all items in the existing data have been grouped according to their use in the classification system, individual components and subscale scores are validated before the overall score is computed. In developing QWB subscale scores for NHIS data, analysts compared original QWB scores that were obtained from a household survey of residents of San Diego, California, to the NHIS constructed scores. This comparison of the NHIS-QWB components against subscale scores obtained from primary data collection provides a type of criterion-related validity.

In the absence of a standard data set to serve as a criterion, external data sets can be used to compare the prevalence of dysfunction in different groups. For example, National Health and Nutrition Examination Survey data might be used to confirm the prevalence of dysfunction obtained from National Health Interview Survey data. This comparison makes sense as long as the items in the two data sets represent the same concept and the samples have similar gender-race-age distributions.

Subscale scores can also be correlated with other health data to test their validity. For example, the Social Activity subscale of the Quality of Well-Being Scale might be compared to self-reported health status. The hypothesis would be that self-reported health and Social Activity scores are positively related: people reporting themselves in excellent health would have higher levels of social functioning than those reporting themselves in poor health. This type of comparison with a hypothesized relationship between a component of health-related quality of life and another health variable provides a measure of construct validity.

Some of the assumptions in the secondary analysis may have to be adjusted and the scores recalculated in order to improve the correspondence between the scores from primary data collection and secondary data analysis. Validity of the adjusted scores can then be reassessed using the procedures described here. This process should be continued until the scores from primary and secondary analysis agree to the maximum extent possible.

After all of the component and subscale scores have been validated, the overall score can be computed using the formula associated with the classification system (Appendix I). One way of checking the validity of the overall score is to compare the scores against those obtained in a primary data set, the criterion approach discussed previously. If a primary data set is unavailable, construct validation can be used. With this approach, hypotheses about the relationship of the overall score to other health variables are formed and tested. For example, the NHIS-QWB score might be hypothesized to be negatively related to number of self-reported health conditions. People reporting more health conditions would have lower NHIS-QWB scores than those reporting fewer conditions.

The process for developing a valid overall, or total, score for each individual is the same as for the subscale scores. Fewer adjustments and repeated calculations of the overall score should be needed, however, because the validity of the subscale components has already been determined.

Sensitivity Analysis

After scores are validated, they must be checked for sensitivity, that is, to determine how responsive the overall constructed score is to variations in the underlying assumptions. For example, in the construction of NHIS-QWB scores, analysts ignored information about spending most or all of a day in a chair or couch for health-related reasons. The assumption behind this omission is that everyone in the general population is fully functional for this health state. As a result, the constructed score will be higher than if the NHIS had collected the necessary data. A more extreme assumption would be that everyone spends most or all of the day in a chair or couch. This assumption, which on face value seems unreasonably restrictive, sets a lower bound on the overall score when fully accounting for level of physical activity.

A sensitivity analysis might be made when information about spending most or all of the day in a chair or couch is taken from an external data source. The scores would then be reconstructed. Scores with and without imputation would be compared to determine the effect of the missing data on the overall score.

The research project to develop the NHIS-QWB indicated that a preference-based measure of health-related quality of life that is suitable for use in the Health Resource Allocation Strategy can be constructed using national data. Frequently, however, numerous assumptions are required to fit existing data to a classification system. As discussed in the next section, the use of health-related quality of life scores developed from secondary data analysis is more limited than are those developed from primary data collection.

INTERPRETATION FOR HEALTH DECISION MAKING

Interpretation of the health-related quality of life measure that results from the use of existing data is essentially the same as for the standard assessment on which it is based. That is, if a rising score means improving health with the original classification system, it has the same meaning with the score constructed from secondary data analysis. The main difference between scores based on primary and secondary data is the use of assumptions in deriving the constructed score. Because assumptions introduce variability and possibly bias from the true population level of health-related quality of life, they need to be carefully considered in drawing conclusions from the constructed scores. For example, applying symptom data from people who sought care in a physician's office to the general population assumes that the two populations have the same health and socioeconomic status and the same attitude toward using health services. The constructed scores will show bias if the two groups differ in any of these characteristics. As a result of the variability and possible bias introduced by the assumptions, information from secondary data analyses is most useful when looking for large differences between groups.

Use of existing data, however, has several important advantages. First, data have already been collected, edited, and prepared in machine-readable format; thus the analysis can be completed more quickly. Second, secondary analyses are usually less costly, because data are available. Third, it may be possible to test hypotheses using existing data that are (1) beyond the scope of primary data collection activities, (2) not part of the design of the primary data-collection activities, or (3) not part of the original purpose in collecting the data. This last advantage is particularly significant if the sample size of the data base is large, as is the case with many national surveys. The National Health Interview Survey routinely samples over 40,000 households in the United States annually, yielding over 100,000 respondents.

Confidence in constructed measures of health-related quality of life based on secondary data analysis depends on the soundness of the assumptions and the results of the sensitivity analysis. Even if health-related quality of life scores based on existing data have considerable variability, constructing such measures may give useful insight to the interactions of different health indicators. The process may also produce recommendations for additions to primary data collection activities. For example, the NHIS research may be used to guide the development of questionnaires for collecting data on health-related quality of life, especially for use in measuring years of healthy life, in national data sets.

Construction of health-related quality of life measures based on cross-sectional data that change from year to year, such as those mentioned previously, will not help with the need for data for trend analysis. Because specific data items collected in the currently available data files change each year, it is unlikely that measures based on secondary data analysis can be used to assess changes in health over time. Such measures, however, may prove useful in indicating whether the level of health of a population is rising or falling. In the future, more information on different concepts of health-related quality of life will be collected and available to help monitor changes in health status.

In addition to being of limited use for trend analysis, health-related quality of life scores based on existing data are restricted to including only those concepts that were collected initially. In contrast to primary data collection where the analyst may select the specific concepts to be included in the questionnaire, the secondary data analyst must accept the given conceptual framework. Also, the secondary data analyst has less influence over method of administration and acceptance of proxy respondents. This lack of control may affect the reliability and validity of the existing data. Both the conceptual and practical limitations may result in a relatively large amount of missing data, which, in turn, may require imputation to maintain the sample size.

In spite of the restrictions imposed on the interpretation of health-related quality of life scores based on secondary data analyses of national data, such analyses clearly have a role to play in guiding health decision making. One contribution of health survey data is their use of large samples that are representative of the total U.S. population. The impact of health interventions that are policy options for only a small subset of the overall population may be missed, however, with large-scale population surveys. Thus, data from large, nationally representative data bases may need to be supplemented with special population surveys for designing health policies that reach all persons in the population.

National registration data, especially those from the vital statistics system, are also important in health decision making. In addition to their traditional use as health indicators, mortality data can be used to represent the notion of moving between different levels of health-related quality of life over time. Years of healthy life, the measure used to compare relative costs and outcomes in the Health Resource Allocation Strategy, is computed by combining mortality with measures of health-related quality of life.

9

Estimating Prognosis and Years of Healthy Life

In the practice of medicine, prognosis is foretelling the course of a disease after a diagnosis has been made. Prognosis includes the prospect of survival, recovery, or deterioration attributed to a diagnosed condition. Information for determining a patient's prognosis is drawn from knowledge about the natural history of the disease in question, the usual course of the condition, or from special features of the individual case (Fletcher et al., 1982). The medical concept of *prognosis* can be generalized to health status measurement as the foretelling of the course of health status when an original health state has been determined. In this case, survival and deterioration or improvement in health for each individual are measured from the initial health state. Prognosis differentiates persons who appear to be in the same health state at one point in time but who will have very different outcomes. For example, one person with influenza and another with emphysema may both be bedridden on a given day but the health status of the person with influenza will improve in a short period of time, whereas the status of the person with emphysema will deteriorate over time.

When studying the health of a defined group or population, the common practice has been to express prognosis in terms of prospective change in the average level of health-related quality of life. Improvement or deterioration of the health status of the group is an aggregation of the prognoses for the individuals in the group and is a function of the health status of individuals in the group. With the Health Resource Allocation Strategy, we are interested in prognosis in an aggregate sense for allocating health care resources.

In this chapter we first define approaches for developing an operational definition of prognosis. Several studies and mathematical approaches for estimating prognosis are discussed. In the second section, we discuss incorporating prognosis into health status measurement through the years of healthy life measure. The third section describes three methods of calculating years of healthy life. We conclude by discussing major advantages of years of healthy life compared to other health indicators, especially for use in health decision making.

MODELING AND ESTIMATING PROGNOSIS

Figure 9.1 illustrates the basic notion of prognosis for a group of individuals. At a specific point in time t_0, a group will be in a given state of health-related quality of life S_0, one of the many possible states along the continuum of health-related quality of

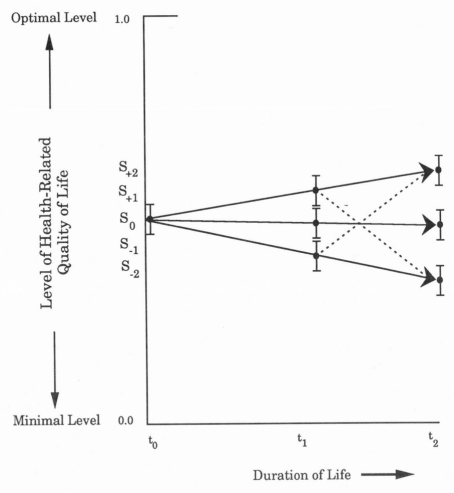

Figure 9.1 Prognosis for a prototype group of individuals:

⊥̄ represents average age health-related quality of life with confidence intervals
S_0 is the level of health-related quality of life at time of first measurement (t_0)
S_{+1}, S_{+2} are states of health-related quality of life that represent better health than S_0
S_{-1}, S_{-2} are states of health-related quality of life that represent worse health than S_0

⋯▶} represent movement between states through time (e.g., t_0, t_1, t_2)

Note that prognostic patterns include steady improvement, steady worsening, constant, and variable across three or more time points.

life. The "arms" extending above and below each point S on the vertical axis represent the confidence intervals around the estimate of health-related quality of life for the group. Between two points in time t_0 to t_1, there are three alternatives for the state of health-related quality of life of the group:

1. It can *improve* if the group moves to state S_{+1} at time t_1.
2. It can *deteriorate* if the group moves to state S_{-1} at time t_1.
3. It can *stay the same* if the group stays at state S_0 at time t_1.

States at time t_1 are also subject to variation as represented by the vertical arms. With three or more points in time, for example, t_0 to t_1 to t_2, the state of health-related quality of life of the group can be *variable*—the group can move to state S_{+1} at time t_1 and to state S_{-2} at time t_2, move to state S_{-1} at time t_1 and to state S_{+2} at time t_2, or follow some other pattern of change. For some applications, such as evaluation studies or population monitoring, it may be adequate to describe prognosis in qualitative terms, as improvement, deterioration, no change, or variable change. In other uses, especially where quantitative results are required, change in health status can be expressed numerically as either a difference score or a probability.

Figure 9.1 relates prognosis to change as follows. At t_0 looking forward, we project the different patterns shown in this figure based on information that is available at that time. For example, if we know the age and medical history of members of the group, then we can hypothesize whether the health status of the group improves, stays the same, or deteriorates over a given time interval. Change, on the other hand, is determined by being at t_2 and looking backward. In this case, we have actual data that we use to determine whether or not change has occurred; we can also plot the four patterns of change shown Figure 9.1.

Different approaches for estimating movement between health states have been proposed. The three most commonly used approaches for determining prognosis are (1) self-rating of change, (2) cohort studies, and (3) transition probabilities of movement among health states.

Self-Rating of Change

Self-ratings generally give information about prognosis in qualitative, rather than quantitative, form. The General Health Rating Index (GHRI), which was developed for use in the Health Insurance Experiment, is one example of the use of self-ratings to learn about respondents' perceptions of future health (Ware, 1984b). The following questions from the GHRI illustrate one way in which information about prognosis can be obtained by self-rating:

1. I will probably be sick a lot in the future.
2. In the future, I expect to have better health than other people I know.
3. I think my health will be worse in the future than it is now.
4. I expect to have a very healthy life.

For each of these questions the possible responses are definitely true, mostly true, don't know, mostly false, and definitely false.

Such qualitative information can be used to study the relationships between current and perceived future health status. The amount of information available for differentiating between persons in the same state and future outcomes will depend on the number of future states included in the questionnaire. Further, self-ratings of change in health are better suited to descriptive and analytic techniques based on qualitative data than on those methods of analysis that require continuous variables.

Cohort Studies

Cohort studies start with an assessment of health at some specific point and then follow the study participants for a designated period. The same measure of health status is used repeatedly over the time interval. Although clinical experiments such as clinical trials have used these longitudinal study designs for a long time, cohort studies for community-level decision making have only recently been designed and implemented.

In a community-based cohort study, Patrick (1984) and colleagues conducted a six-year study in the London Borough of Lambeth, England, for the purpose of guiding social policy for people with physical disability. Members of a sample of 630 adults with disability and 230 without disability were measured three times during the study using the Functional Limitations Profile (FLP), a British adaptation of the Sickness Impact Profile. Persons were classified into one of four change categories based on a five-point change in FLP score: steady deteriorators, steady improvers, negligible changers, and ambiguous changers. Among the persons with disability, deterioration was associated with age, initial level of health, and number of social contacts (Charlton, 1989).

This type of information can be used to estimate prognosis for people with disabilities in qualitative terms. For example, if a person's age, Functional Limitations Profile score, and social functioning are known, then he or she can be classified into one of the four change categories identified in the Lambeth study.

Transition Probabilities

Including prognosis in the Health Resource Allocation Strategy means that one must obtain numerical estimates of the likelihood that people will move from one state to another over time. In 1970, Fanshel and Bush first proposed modeling prognosis in terms of transition probabilities between states of health-related quality of life. In this approach, an individual has some probability of moving to a different state at time t_{+1}, given that he or she is in a specified state at time t_0. The simplest case is a two-state mortality analysis in which a person is either alive (State 1) or dead (State 0); then the transition probability of moving from State 1 to State 0 can be estimated from standard life table analysis. For a group of individuals, the proportion of persons alive at the beginning of an age interval and dying during that interval or any of the succeeding intervals would be the vector of probabilities. The number of elements in the vector will depend on the number of age groups used in the analysis.

Figure 9.2 illustrates a transition matrix that might be used in a multistate analysis. This matrix includes an entry for each age group by health state $S_1 \ldots S_I$, at baseline t_0 and for a change in state at some future point in time t_1. The general format for this matrix allows for n age groups and I states of health-related quality of life. For example, with two age groups, one under 65 years and one 65 years and over, and two health states, alive and dead, the matrix would have four cells (two states at t_0, for two age groups, and one state at t_1). The shaded areas in Figure 9.2 represents the matrix and cells that correspond to this example.

In practice, this matrix can become very large depending on the particular point-in-time health classification system being used. Suppose that an individual could be classified into 1 of 12 different health states ($I = 12$) and that the analysis is with 12 specific age groups ($n = 12$); then there would be 1,584 possible entries in the transition matrix (Berry and Bush, 1978).

Two ways to obtain estimates of transition probabilities are by expert judgment and by sample survey data. Chen and Bush (1976) used a modified Delphi technique to

$$t_1 \cdots t_K$$

Age Group	t_0	S_1	S_2	$\bullet\bullet\bullet$	S_I
1 e.g., <65 years of age	S_1 e.g., alive S_2 e.g., dead $\vdots$ S_I	p_{111} p_{121}	p_{112} p_{122}		
2 e.g., ≥65 years of age	S_1 e.g., alive S_2 e.g., dead $\vdots$ S_I	p_{211} p_{221} $\vdots$	p_{212} p_{222} $\vdots$		
$\vdots$					
N	S_1 S_2 $\vdots$ S_I	$\vdots$ p_{NI1}	$\vdots$ p_{NI2}		

Figure 9.2 Schematic representation of the transition probabilities associated with moving between states of health-related quality of life:

$S_1 \ldots S_I$ indicate states of health-related quality of life
$t_1 \ldots t_K$ indicate time of observation
$p_n|_K$ indicate transition probabilities for each age group in a given state of health-related quality of life at a given point in time

obtain preliminary estimates of moving between health states defined by the Quality of Well-Being Scale. Burton et al. (1975) used a Bayesian model to combine expert judgment along with actual observations to estimate transition probabilities for older persons enrolled in a health services research project.

Berry and Bush (1978) were among the first to conduct health surveys that could be used for estimating transition probabilities. These investigators collected data twice, approximately one year apart, in a household survey of 1,063 respondents. The data were used to estimate probabilities of moving between four states: asymptomatic, symptomatic but function not limited, symptomatic with limited function, and dead. The first three of these states are based on data obtained from the Quality of Well-Being Scale and the fourth from vital statistics. This analysis limited the number of states to four because of the small sample sizes in the transition matrix cells if more states were used. Three estimates of transition probabilities were made: one from observed relative frequencies, one on a linear logistic model, and one on a linear logistic model modified to account for variations in the lengths of the interval between household interviews. There was general agreement among the three methods in the estimates for the 12 different states of health-related quality of life for all ages, from 0 to 89 years. This suggests that linear logistic models can be used to estimate transition probabilities.

Recently, a number of different approaches have been used to estimate transition probabilities. For example, Manton (1987, 1988, 1989) used stochastic compartment methods to model movement between health states associated with progressive chronic disease. These methods, borrowed from pharmaceutical research, allow researchers to follow a cohort of individuals through healthy and unhealthy states. These transitions are based on available data from clinical studies, epidemiologic data cases, and expert information about disease processes. Using standard demographic methods with these data, future distributions of disease within a population can be projected.

As another example, Weinstein and colleagues (1987) used population estimates of transitions for forecasting coronary heart disease (CHD). These computer simulations project incidence, prevalence, and mortality of CHD. Data from the Framingham Study, a longitudinal study of residents of a small community in Massachusetts, were used to estimate the risk of developing heart disease (Department of Health, Education and Welfare, 1973). Estimates of mortality were based on data from the United States vital statistics registration system.

Increasingly, national data sets are being designed to follow cohorts of individuals over time. The National Health and Nutrition Examination Survey (NHANES) Epidemiologic Follow-Up Study (Madans et al., 1986; Cornoni-Huntley et al., 1990), the Longitudinal Survey on Aging (Kovar, 1989) and the Long-Term Care Survey (Liu and Manton, 1989) are three national surveys that are collecting information about health status over repeated time intervals. These surveys provide data from which to develop estimates of prognosis. The populations in these national surveys are representative of the total United States and the sample sizes are relatively large; thus they overcome a potential source of bias in the Framingham Study. They share a limitation of the Framingham Study, however, in that the repeated health status measures are collected at a broad time interval. The major problem with intervals of more than one year is that we do not know the pattern of movement between health states. That is, we do not know if a deterioration in health represents steady deterioration or a temporary decline as part of a variable pattern.

Several national health panel surveys, including the National Medical Expenditures Survey (Edwards and Berlin, 1989; Edwards and Edwards, 1989) and the National Medical Care Utilization and Expenditure Survey (Bonham, 1983), collect information on respondents every two to three months. In both of these surveys, however, the health status data collected were too limited to permit the calculation of transition probabilities. Although national probability samples have the advantages of being representative of the total population and of having large sample sizes, these surveys are complex and time-consuming to design and implement. Therefore, it is unlikely that we will have a single set of estimates of the probability of moving between states of health-related quality of life over intervals that are relatively short, for example, less than three months.

Instead, special studies, such as clinical trials and health surveys conducted for evaluative purposes, are more likely to provide the needed data. Verbrugge and Balaban (1989) used a longitudinal observational study to assess changes in disability status. In this study, 165 persons at least 55 years old were followed for 12 months or more. Respondents kept a health diary to report their health and activity levels each day during the study. In addition to showing that individuals can supply information about change in health status on a regular, self-report basis, this study provides detailed daily information about changes in health status. The authors reviewed the time flows (trajectories) for each of the 117 respondents who supplied complete data for analysis. The following six patterns emerged from this review:

1. Stability versus dynamism: patients' health status and activity were either very stable or dynamic over the period.
2. Large declines and improvements: large declines tend to be abrupt, whereas improvements tend to be gradual.
3. Parallel shifts versus lagged shifts: shifts in health status and activity occur together rather than lagging behind one another.
4. Optimism/improvement or pessimism/worsening: respondents tend to specialize in either improvement or worsening health.
5. Adjustment to disability: respondents adapt to situations of permanent disability, thus not seeing themselves as disabled.
6. Dynamics at the start and end of the diary: hospitalization tends to increase well-being, whereas increased dysfunction leads people to discontinue making entries in their diaries.

This study is an example of data with the potential for supplying estimates of transition probabilities over short intervals.

Modeling Prognosis

Another aspect of developing an operational definition of prognosis is selecting a mathematical model that represents movement between states. Movement can be modeled as continuous or discrete and as independent or dependent of previously occupied health states. Different mathematical approaches for calculating movement between health states have been proposed. One of the earliest efforts to incorporate transition probabilities into the measurement of health status was the adoption of the Markov process.

Markov models are stochastic processes with a transition matrix (sometimes called a technology matrix) in which the elements are the probabilities of moving from one state to another at a later point in time (Hillier and Lieberman, 1986). In health care applications, the probabilities have traditionally been chosen to reflect the impact of a health policy. For example, using the Older American Resources and Services method for assigning patients to point-in-time health states, Burton and colleagues (1975) estimated the effect of alternative forms of assistance provided to members of an elderly population on patient outcomes using the following Markov model:

$$X^k T^k = M^k$$

where

X^k is a vector with each element representing the number of people assigned to a given treatment program;

T^k is a matrix of probabilities of moving between states for each treatment;

M^k is a vector where each element represents the expected number of people who received a given service package and who end in a particular state; and

k represents health service assistance programs.

The impact of the various assistance programs being evaluated is determined by calculating two versions of the vector M^k. In one case assistance is provided; in the other it is not. The difference between the two estimates can be considered a measure of the effectiveness of the different service packages (Burton et al., 1975).

The Markov chain has a number of limitations in representing the multidimensional concept of health-related quality of life. One is that it is essentially a two-stage process. To overcome this shortcoming, investigators have looked at dynamic mathematical programming. For example, Chen and Bush (1976) used an approach known as "dichotomous integer programming" to assess the optimal program mix across health screening programs for phenylketonuria (PKU) and tuberculin testing; this application used the Quality of Well-Being scale as the point-in-time health-related quality of life measure.

These attempts to estimate and model transition probabilities indicate that prognosis can be incorporated into a comprehensive, operational definition of health-related quality of life. The methods proposed to date have received only limited acceptance for two reasons. First, relatively few data exist to estimate transition probabilities between health states. Second, mathematical-computing capability restricts the size of the transition matrix that can be processed. As an alternative, researchers have focused on combining life expectancy with health-related quality of life data to calculate years of healthy life. The next section describes recent research to develop the methodology for computing this summary statistic.

YEARS OF HEALTHY LIFE

Given the lack of estimates of transition probabilities between states of health-related quality of life, researchers currently use mortality data to incorporate prognosis into the operational definition of health-related quality of life (Chen et al., 1975; Department of Health and Human Services, 1991b; Hatziandreu et al., 1988; Kaplan et al., 1984; Torrance, 1986; Williams, 1985). Using this approximation, the proportion of those in a population who die is assumed to represent the probability of a target group moving from a given state of health-related quality of life to death. Life table models, which incorporate death as the standard endpoint, comprise the most frequently used approaches to make this combination of quantity and quality of life.

The life table summarizes the mortality experience of a population and supplies information about transitions by including a column showing the number of persons in a given population that will survive to some specified age. Of the different ways of constructing a life table, the current, or period, life table is the most relevant for calculating years of healthy life. The current life table, which represents the mortality experience of a given population, usually observed over a one- to three-year period, can be interpreted as tracing a cohort of newborn infants through their lifetime. The underlying assumption is that the mortality rates used in the table apply to the cohort.

Generally, the abridged form of life table, using five-year age groupings, is used (Shryock et al., 1975; National Center for Health Statistics, 1991b). Table 9.1 is an abridged life table for the total U.S. population for 1988. The column headings introduce life table notation and describe its meaning. Of particular relevance in interpreting years of healthy life are column 5, $_nL_x$, and column 6, T_x, both of which represent

Table 9.1 Abridged life table for the total population, United States, 1988

Age Interval	Proportion dying	of 100,000 born alive		Stationary population		Average remaining lifetime
	Proportion of persons alive at beginning of age interval dying during interval	Number living at beginning of age interval	Number dying during age interval	In the age interval	In this and all subsequent age intervals	Average number of years of life remaining at beginning of age interval
Period of life between two exact ages stated in years (1)	(2)	(3)	(4)	(5)	(6)	(7)
x to $x + n$	$_nq_x$	l_x	$_nd_x$	$_nL_x$	T_x	$\overset{\circ}{e}_x$
0–1	0.0100	100,000	999	99,147	7,494,642	74.9
1–5	0.0020	99,001	198	395,540	7,395,495	74.7
5–10	0.0012	98,803	120	493,688	6,999,955	70.8
10–15	0.0014	98,683	134	493,155	6,506,267	65.9
15–20	0.0044	98,549	431	491,767	6,013,112	61.0
20–25	0.0058	98,118	565	489,206	5,521,345	56.3
25–30	0.0061	97,553	596	486,274	5,032,139	51.6
30–35	0.0074	96,957	717	483,035	4,545,865	46.9
35–40	0.0096	96,240	924	479,021	4,062,830	42.2
40–45	0.0126	95,316	1,204	473,785	3,583,809	37.6
45–50	0.0189	94,112	1,777	466,443	3,110,024	33.0
50–55	0.0300	92,335	2,766	455,194	2,643,581	28.6
55–60	0.0473	89,569	4,238	437,859	2,188,387	24.4
60–65	0.0728	85,331	6,208	411,976	1,750,528	20.5
65–70	0.1055	79,123	8,344	375,656	1,338,552	16.9
70–75	0.1568	70,779	11,096	327,120	962,896	13.6
75–80	0.2288	59,683	13,654	265,113	635,776	10.7
80–85	0.3445	46,029	15,858	190,715	370,663	8.1
85 and over	1.0000	30,171	30,171	179,948	179,948	6.0

Source: National Center for Health Statistics. *Vital Statistics of the United States. Volume II—Mortality, Part A*, 1991.

number of persons in the stationary population. This population is called stationary because of the assumption made in developing the life table that there is no migration in the population and that births are evenly distributed over the calendar year.

The number of persons in the stationary population in any age interval on any date is given by $_nL_x$. For example, using data in Table 9.1, there were 455,194 persons in the age interval 50–55 years. This means that in a stationary population supported by 100,000 annual births, with the proportions dying in each age interval given by $_nq_x$, column 2, a census taken on any date would show 455,194 persons between the exact ages of 50 and 55 years. The total number of persons in the stationary population in the indicated age interval and all subsequent ages is given by T_x, column 6. For example, there would be at any given moment 2,643,581 persons who had passed their fiftieth birthday.

The last column, $\mathring{e}_x$, gives the average number of years of life remaining at the beginning of the interval. This is usually referred to as life expectancy. To relate the interpretation of number of life years remaining to other data in the life table, we note that the $_nL_x$ column can also be interpreted as the number of years lived in the interval for the persons in the stationary population who survive to the beginning of the interval. For example, the 92,335 persons alive at the beginning of the age interval 50–55, column 3, lived 455,194 person years. The number 2,643,581 in the T_x column is the sum of entries in the $_nL_x$ column from age 50 on and represents the total number of years lived by persons after reaching age 50.

Life expectancy is calculated by dividing the total number of years after a given age, column 6, by the number of persons alive at the beginning of the age interval. The expectation of life for the total population of the United States in 1988 was 74.9 years (top row, column 7). For persons reaching the age of 50, the number of average life years remaining is 28.6; this is found by dividing the entry in column 6 by that in column 3 (2,643,581/92,335).

Life tables can also be developed for single years of age rather than for five-year age intervals as shown in Table 9.1. When single years of age are used the table is referred to as a complete life table. In the United States, life tables, both complete and abridged, are computed and published annually in *Vital Statistics of the United States* (National Center for Health Statistics, 1988b). Complete life tables are available for the total population of the United States regardless of race, gender, and cause of death. Gender- and race-specific life tables and state-by-state life tables are also available (National Center for Health Statistics, 1991b). As of 1988, national life tables are unavailable for ethnic background, although ethnicity is collected on the death certificate. National life tables are not available for specific causes of death.

Annual tables, such as Table 9.1, are based on deaths reported in a single year and, except for census years, on population estimates rather than on census data. Complete life tables are based on census data and deaths from a three-year interval including the decennial census year.

One measure that includes both morbidity and mortality is Active Life Expectancy (Katz et al., 1983). Using data from 1,225 Massachusetts residents 65 years of age and over, a life table approach was used to calculate the number of person years adjusted for independence in activities of daily living over five-year age intervals. Independence in activities of daily living was defined as having no dysfunction in any of the six activities in the Index of Activities of Daily Living and living in the community during the 15-month study period. The proportions of the study group who were dependent in self-care, institutionalized, or who died were used to estimate $_nq_x$, which was redefined as the proportion losing independence in activities of daily living or dying during the age interval. Active Life Expectancy was determined by applying this proportion to a stationary population. According to this analysis, the average Active Life Expectancy declined steadily from 65 to 85 or more years of age. People in the 65- to 69-year age group had an average remaining Active Life Expectancy at age 65 of 10.0 years; for those 85 and older, the average remaining Active Life Expectancy was 2.9 years.

A major disadvantage of the initial approach to calculating Active Life Expectancy was that it ignored the possibility of improvements in health status, for example, moving from a state defined by dependence in one or more activities of daily living (ADL) to one defined by independence in ADL. This limitation stems from the unistate approach to developing a life table that was used to estimate the proportions dependent in ADL or dying during the interval ($_nq_x$). In the multistate life table version of the Active Life Expectancy, people are no longer assumed to stay in a dysfunctional state once they have been so classified. If a person moves from a state of complete independence or well-being to one of dependence or dysfunction, the multistate approach allows for the possibility of that individual recovering (Rogers et al., 1989).

Figure 9.3 shows regular and Active Life Expectancy (based on the multistate, increment–decrement life table method) for elderly people in Massachusetts. For persons 65 years of age, the regular life expectancy is 16.5 years and the Active Life Expectancy is 14.7 years; this can be interpreted to mean that approximately 90 percent

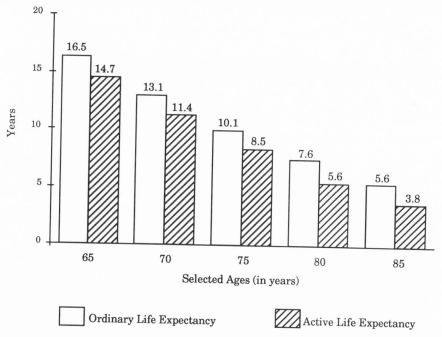

Figure 9.3 Remaining years of life measured in terms of ordinary and active life expectancies for persons in an independent functional state, selected ages. *Source*: Adopted from Rogers et al., 1989.

of the remaining life years will be with minimal dysfunction. The percentage of active life years remaining decreases steadily with age. For persons 85 years and older, 68 percent of the remaining life years, or 3.8 years, will be with minimal dysfunction.

The main disadvantage of the Active Life Expectancy approach is that various activities of daily living are considered to have the same impact, that is, that all forms of disability or dysfunction are considered to be equivalent. For example, dependence in ability to eat is considered to have the same value of dysfunction as does being dependent in ability to dress oneself. That is, Active Life Expectancy does not take into account the values that people place on different states of health-related quality of life. The preference method of combining morbidity and mortality overcomes this problem. The measure that results from using a preference-weighted health-related quality of life measure is called years of healthy life.

A year of healthy life is one year of life adjusted by some fraction between 0 and 1 that estimates quality of life during the year. If duration of life is one year and the health-related quality of life adjustment factor for a given health state is 0.5, then this translates to one-half year of healthy life. This is interpreted as equivalent to being alive for half a year in perfect health and spending the other half year with dysfunction. Or, if duration of life is five years and the quality adjustment factor is 0.80, then this translates to four years of healthy life and one year of life with dysfunction, which could result from either chronic or acute conditions; the interpretation is similar to the previous example. Note that the terms "well years," "well life expectancy," "healthy life years," and "quality-adjusted life years" are synonyms for years of healthy life.

Figure 9.4 shows examples of years of healthy life based on the Disability Distress Index (DDI), the Health Utilities Index (HUI), and the Quality of Well-Being (QWB) scale for different target populations. Since the health-related quality of life for a specific target population has not yet been evaluated using all three measures, we present data from different groups. For the DDI, estimates of the unadjusted, or ordinary, life expectancy and years of healthy life are for British patients with cystic fibrosis. For this group, the ordinary life expectancy and the years of healthy life were calculated to be 22 and 20 years, respectively (Gudex, 1986).

For the HUI, both the ordinary and quality-adjusted life expectancies are projections to death of a group of low birth weight infants (Boyle et al., 1983). Ordinary life expectancy is projected to be 47.7 years, with 36 years of healthy life. For the general population surveyed in 1974–75 using the QWB Scale, ordinary life expectancy was 73.5 years. This population was estimated to have 60.4 years of healthy life (Berry and Bush, 1978).

Although the years of healthy life calculated using the three different classification systems are not strictly comparable due to both their different operational definitions of health and their preference weights, the data indicate that children with cystic fibrosis have fewer years of healthy life than either the general population or low birth weight infants. To avoid misinterpretation of findings due to noncomparability of the different approaches to measuring years of healthy life, we recommend that a single classification system and its weights be used to develop years of healthy life within a single analysis.

This section introduced life table methodology as a way of including prognosis in a measure of health-related quality of life when transition probabilities between states are unavailable. When preference weights are used to adjust life years for the time spent in less than perfect health the measure is called years of healthy life. As indicated by the

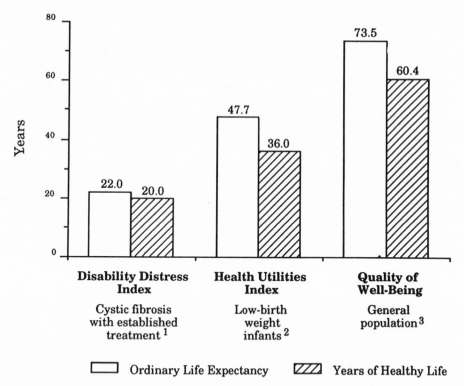

Figure 9.4   Comparison of years of healthy life using three different health-related quality of life measures.

[1] The life expectancy of 22 years for British patients with cystic fibrosis was estimated in 1983. Using this data and a quality of life estimate of 0.91 for patients receiving standard treatment, patients with cystic fibrosis can expect to have 20 years of healthy life.

[2] Infants weighing 1000–1499g and born from 1973 to 1977 in Hamilton, Ontario, had a projected survival of 47.7 years and 36.0 projected years of healthy life.

[3] The general population estimates are based on a household survey of persons living in San Diego County, California. Based on this survey and the corresponding life expectancy for 1974–1975, the estimated population can expect 73.5 life years and 60.4 years of healthy life.

Sources: Gudex, 1986; Boyle et al., 1983; Berry and Bush, 1978.

data in Figure 9.4, years of healthy life can be calculated for diverse population groups. The following section describes various methods for estimating years of healthy life, depending on the sample size and resources available for making the calculations.

CALCULATION OF YEARS OF HEALTHY LIFE

Methods for calculating years of healthy life can be grouped into three categories: life tables, cohort analysis, and simple estimation. In this section we describe how to use each of these methods to estimate years of healthy life and discuss some of the advantages and disadvantages of each.

Life Table Method

The simplest life table method is the ordinary life table approach used by Sullivan (1971). With this approach, calculating years of healthy life starts with two sets of data, either an abridged or complete life table and age-specific estimates of health-related quality of life. The life table must show the age intervals of a relevant population, the number of persons who are alive at the beginning of the age interval l_x and the number of people in the stationary population in each of the age intervals $_nL_x$.

The second data set, age-specific estimates of health-related quality of life, must be available for the same age intervals as the life table data. In addition, the estimates of health-related quality of life must be based on scaling methods that explicitly incorporate death as one of the states of health-related quality of life. The Disability Distress Index, the EuroQol, the Health Utility Index (four- and eight-attribute versions), and the Quality of Well-Being Scale health state classification systems satisfy this requirement.

For each age interval in the life table, there will be a corresponding average level of health-related quality of life H_x, which is obtained by the following formula:

$$H_x = \sum_{i=1}^{l_x} \frac{h_{x_i}}{n_x}$$

where

h_{x_i} = health-related quality of life of individual i in age interval x
n_x = number of people in age interval x
x = age interval

For example, the h_{x_i} would be the scores obtained from administering a classification system such as the DDI, EuroQol, HUI, or QWB to a sample of persons; these scores range from 0 to 1. The average health-related quality of life for persons in a given age interval, for example, 50–55 years, is found by summing the health-related quality of life scores for the individuals from the sample who are 50–55 years of age and then dividing by the number of persons in this age group.

Table 9.2 shows how life table and health status data are combined to calculate years of healthy life. The first four columns in this table are from the standard life table, Table 9.1. The average health-related quality of life scores for each age interval, column 5, are estimated from a curve fitted to Quality of Well-Being scores obtained from a general population survey (Kaplan et al., 1976). These average scores are multiplied by the number of person years in each age interval $_nL_x$, column 4. The adjusted person years are then summed from the bottom to the top of the table to obtain the number of quality-adjusted person years in the interval as well as in all subsequent intervals; this summing is the same procedure used to obtain the data in the T_x column in Table 9.1. Dividing the adjusted T'_x in each age interval by the number l_x living at the beginning of the interval results in the number of years of healthy life remaining. For example, for persons 50–55 years of age, the number of adjusted person years in this and subsequent intervals is 1,302,736. Dividing this by the number of persons alive at the beginning of the interval, 92,335, results in 14.1 years of healthy life remaining.

By using the estimates of health-related quality of life based on the formula by Kaplan and colleagues (1976), the years of healthy life at birth for the 1988 U.S.

Table 9.2 Calculation of years of healthy life for the total population, United States, 1988

Age interval — Period of life between two exact ages stated in years (1)	Proporation of persons alive at beginning of age interval who died during interval (2)	Number living at the beginning of the age interval (3)	(4)	Health-related quality of life adjustment factor (5)	Adjusted person years in this and all subsequent intervals (6)	(7)	Average remaining lifetime (8)
x to $x + n$	$_nq_x$	l_x	$_nL_x$	H^a	H_nL_x	T'_x	YHL
0–1	0.0100	100,000	99,147	0.88045	87,294	5,251,921	52.5
1–5	0.0020	99,001	395,540	0.86698	342,925	5,164,628	52.2
5–10	0.0012	98,803	493,688	0.84919	419,233	4,821,703	48.8
10–15	0.0014	98,683	493,155	0.83668	412,613	4,402,469	44.6
15–20	0.0044	98,549	491,767	0.82888	407,616	3,989,856	40.5
20–25	0.0058	98,118	489,206	0.82298	402,608	3,582,241	36.5
25–30	0.0061	97,553	486,274	0.81642	397,006	3,179,632	32.6
30–35	0.0074	96,957	483,035	0.80688	389,750	2,782,627	28.7
35–40	0.0096	96,240	479,021	0.79226	379,508	2,392,877	24.9
40–45	0.0126	95,316	473,785	0.77072	365,156	2,013,369	21.1
45–50	0.0189	94,112	466,443	0.74066	345,477	1,648,213	17.5
50–55	0.0300	92,335	455,194	0.70072	318,961	1,302,736	14.1
55–60	0.0473	89,569	437,859	0.64976	284,501	983,775	11.0
60–65	0.0728	85,331	411,976	0.58690	241,788	699,274	8.2
65–70	0.1055	79,123	375,656	0.51150	192,148	457,486	5.8
70–75	0.1568	70,779	327,120	0.42315	138,421	265,338	3.7
75–80	1.2288	59,683	265,113	0.32169	85,285	126,917	2.1
80–85	1.3445	46,029	190,715	0.20720	39,515	41,632	0.9
85 and over	1.0000	30,171	179,948	0.01176	2,116	2,116	0.1

$^aH = 0.8835 - 0.00623$ (age) $+ 0.000255$ (age)$^2 - 0.00000\ 47$ (age)$^3 + 0.0000000\ 16$ (age)^4. This formula is from Kaplan et al., 1976.

population was found to be 52.5 years (Table 9.2, top row, column 8). People 65 and older at the beginning of the interval had an average of 16.9 years remaining with 5.8 years of healthy life. Alternatively, persons in this age group were expected to experience an average of 11.1 years of ill health throughout their remaining lifetime. This dysfunction represents both acute and chronic as well as major and minor illnesses that occur throughout the remaining lifetime of this group of individuals.

Although this calculation is shown for the total population, the same methods can be applied for calculating years of healthy life according to various sociodemographic groups—people classified by color, ethnicity, or gender. When both the death rates and estimates of health-related quality of life have been collected for the same period and for comparable populations, the adjusted life table traces the total health experience of a single cohort that is subject to the age-specific mortality and well-being levels on which the table is based.

These methods also apply for different disease groups. When appropriate disease-specific or target-population-specific life tables are unavailable, assumptions about the mortality experiences of the study group may need to be made. For example, although arthritis is one of the most frequently reported conditions in the National Health Interview Survey (Collins, 1986), very few death certificates are recorded with arthritis as the primary cause of death. Thus, calculation of years of healthy life for people with arthritis may depend on the assumption that their mortality experience is the same as that of the general population.

For diseases that are common causes of death, "cause-eliminated life tables" provide an alternative to the use of the disease-specific life table for analyzing the mortality impact of specific diseases. In developing cause-eliminated life tables, deaths due to specific causes are assumed not to occur. Instead, persons who would die from a specific disease, such as tuberculosis, are assumed to return to a healthy state at the point of death (Curtin and Armstrong, 1988).

Cause-eliminated life tables can be used to estimate the impact that eliminating a specific disease may have on years of healthy life. For example, if we wanted to estimate the effect of eliminating cerebrovascular diseases from the U.S. population, the life table that has been calculated with cerebrovascular diseases eliminated can be used. In this case we would also want to have estimates of quality of life that were based on a population that was free of cerebrovascular disease. With these two sets of data, it is then possible to estimate years of healthy life as if cerebrovascular diseases had been eliminated. In general, using the cause-eliminated approach to estimating the impact of curing a specific disease or condition will underestimate the improvement in health. The underestimate will be higher if diseases are characterized by a number of complications and sequelae that either do not result in death or result in death from many causes. Arthritis, as noted, is an example of a disease that rarely causes death.

Diabetes mellitus, on the other hand, is one disease that causes death both directly and indirectly. A number of people with diabetes have vascular complications that result in death attributed to heart and cerebrovascular diseases. Using the life table with diabetes eliminated as a cause of death overlooks the contribution of diabetes to other causes of death. Thus, the number of years of healthy life gained by eliminating diabetes will be lower than if this measure were calculated from disease-specific life table data.

Initial use of the ordinary life table for calculating years of healthy life was motivated by practical rather than theoretical concerns. Recently this adjustment procedure was examined for mathematical rigor. Newman (1988) reformulated the original life table model into a multistate increment–decrement life table based on Markovian assumptions, thereby giving a theoretical basis for using morbidity to discount mortality. Assuming that the rate of recovery from illness is high and that most of the time a person is well, Newman shows that results from the standard life table approximate those from an increment–decrement life table. This finding adds theoretical rigor to the life table approach discussed previously.

Estimates of prognosis based on life table analysis rather than probabilities of transition between many different states of health-related quality of life are, at best, crude approximations. This is primarily because the life table approach reduces the number of possible states at time $t + 1$ to two states, alive or dead, rather than allowing for a symmetric transition matrix as shown schematically in Figure 9.2. That is, when life tables are used to estimate prognosis, there is no information about movement between different states of function over time for people who are alive.

Cohort Method

The second approach to calculating years of healthy life can be applied when working with cohort data for which the mortality experience of the study participants either is known or can be estimated. With this approach, the number of years survived by each member of the cohort is adjusted by the individual's health-related quality of life. Then the adjusted life years are summed to give an estimate of the years of healthy life for the group. The formula for this calculation when health-related quality of life data are collected more than once is

$$\text{YHL} = \sum_{i=1}^{I} \sum_{j=1}^{J} \frac{h_{ij} t_{ij}}{n_{ij}}$$

where

h_{ij} = health-related quality of life for the jth person measured the ith time
t_{ij} = duration of time spent by the jth individual in health state h_{ij} at time i
n_i = number of persons for whom health-related quality of life was measured at time i

When health status is measured at only one time for the cohort, the formula simplifies to

$$\text{YHL} = \sum_{i=1}^{N} \frac{h_i t_i}{N}$$

where

h_i = health-related quality of life for the ith person
t_i = duration of time spent in the health-related quality of life state for the ith person
N = total sample or population being studied

Table 9.3 presents a hypothetical data set to illustrate the calculation of years of healthy life using cohort data. Seven persons are enrolled in the study at period 1. Person 7 drops out of the study after the first period; person 6 drops out after the second period. In the first example, periods 1 through 3 are defined to be one year each. Thus, the duration of time spent in a given state of health-related quality of life is one year. This group of seven people experienced a total of 1.97 years of healthy life over the three-year study. This estimate of years of healthy life is based on the assumption that the two dropouts died and thus have a quality of life score of 0 for the periods after which they had actual health status scores. In the second example, the periods are defined to be 6 months duration, resulting in a total of 0.99 years of healthy life gained over the 18-month study period; again we assume that persons 6 and 7 dropped out of the study due to death.

Table 9.3 Two examples showing the calculation of years of healthy life using cohort data

Person	Period 1	Period 2	Period 3
1	0.77	0.77	0.79
2	0.75	0.78	0.81
3	0.80	0.78	0.82
4	0.73	0.78	0.80
5	0.68	0.73	0.78
6	0.77	0.78	—[a]
7	0.79	—[a]	—[a]

Example 1: If each of the periods of study represents one year, then $t = 1$. In this example, we assume that the persons who dropped out died and thus have a health-related quality of life score of 0 after dropping out. With these assumptions, the following results obtain:

$\sum \sum h_{ij} t_{ij} =$	5.29	4.51	4.00
$\sum \sum \dfrac{h_{ij} t_{ij}}{n_{ij}} =$	0.76	0.64	0.57
YHL = 1.97			

Example 2: If each of the periods of study represents some length of time other than one year, then $t \neq 1$. For example, the health-related quality of life might be measured every six months; then $t = 0.5$. Again, we assume that persons 6 and 7 died during the course of the study. The following results obtain:

$\sum \sum h_{ij} t_{ij} =$	2.645	2.255	2.00
$\sum \sum \dfrac{h_{ij} t_{ij}}{n_{ij}} =$	0.38	0.32	0.29
YHL = 0.99			

[a]The person dropped out during the course of the study.

If the persons who dropped out did not die but were lost to the study, for example, by moving from the area, then giving them a health-related quality of life score of 0 underestimates the years of healthy life for the group. One way of removing this bias is to remove the dropouts from the denominator at periods 2 and 3. Eliminating person 7 from period 2 calculations results in a mean health-related quality of life for this period of 0.75; removing persons 6 and 7 from period 3 calculations results in a mean of 0.80. Summing the mean health-related quality of life scores for the three periods gives a total of 2.31 years of healthy life for the group.

An alternative approach to dealing with dropouts is to impute scores by using either expert judgment or one of the available statistical methods, for example, hot deck, cold deck, distance function matching, and random imputation within classes (Kalton and Kasprzyk, 1982; Sande, 1982). Expert judgment hinges on the analyst or other some member of the research team making rules about how health status data for persons who drop out of the study will be handled on a systematic basis. An example of such a rule is that dropouts will be assigned the same health status score for the remaining periods of study. Under this assumption, person 7 would be assigned a score of 0.79 in periods 2 and 3; this value would be used in calculating years of healthy life.

Statistical methods of imputation involve assigning health status scores to persons who failed to complete the study according to some algorithm. This may involve a person with the same demographic characteristics serving as a "donor"; the health status score of the donor is assigned to the person with missing data. The underlying assumption here is that persons in the same demographic group will have similar health status scores. Other procedures involve the use of donors drawn from external data sets.

The choice of method for supplying missing information depends on the nature of the missing data. If expert judgment gives better estimates, for example, the study is such that you know a person's health status will behave in a particular way, or stay the same, as in the preceding example, then this is the preferred method. If, on the other hand, change in health status does not lend itself to expert prediction, then statistical methods are preferred. These methods are designed to introduce a level of variability and minimize bias in the imputation of missing information. Another consideration in selecting a method for imputation is the number of missing cases, or dropouts. If the number is too large to effectively adjudicate on an individual basis, then statistical methods are preferred. Caution is urged about using too many imputed values. If a large percentage of the sample has missing values, then it might be wise to do a sensitivity analysis in which years of healthy life are calculated with and without the imputed data to see if imputation makes a difference in the results.

The example in Table 9.3 is similar to community-based studies as well as national surveys that have been designed to assess health status and functional capacity of selected populations, particularly older adults. The Health Care Financing Administration is supporting six demonstration projects that are designed to demonstrate the costs and benefits of providing preventive services to the persons covered by the Medicare program. Each project is a cohort study in which participants receive preventive services for 2 years and are followed for an additional 18 months for evaluation. Health status is measured at selected intervals during the study period (Office of Technology Assessment, 1990).

Nationally, the Longitudinal Survey on Aging, which began as a supplement to the 1984 National Health Interview Survey (NHIS), is another example of cohort data that fits the design illustrated in Table 9.3. Subsamples of the original cohort of 16,148 persons are being selected for follow-up. For example, the 5,151 persons aged 70 years and older were first reinterviewed in 1986 to obtain information on activities of daily living, instrumental activities of daily living, and independent functioning. This same information was collected in 1988 and 1990. The National Death Index has been used to identify the date and the cause of death of persons who died (Kovar, 1989). Years of healthy life can be calculated for the cohort of individuals who participated in the 1984 supplement to NHIS and have been followed during subsequent years by combining these data on health-related quality of life and death along with an appropriate preference-weighting scheme.

Simple Estimation

One may want to estimate years of healthy life without going through the extensive calculations shown in Tables 9.2 and 9.3. Short cuts in the calculation may be required because there is insufficient time to calculate the average quality of life scores using either the life table or cohort method or because there is insufficient information to do so. Under these constraints, a crude estimate of years of healthy life might be developed if two pieces of information are available: an estimate of the average quality of life of the population based on a measure that includes mortality, and a relevant estimate of life expectancy. Multiplying these two estimates together will result in an approximation of the average years of healthy life for the population. The formula is

$$\text{YHL}_c = LY \times H$$

where

YHL_c = crude estimate of years of healthy life
LY = total number of life years remaining, for example, life expectancy at birth
H = average health-related quality of life score for the group; H will be a value between 0 and 1

Although this simple estimation of years of healthy life has advantages of being quick to calculate and not requiring extensive data manipulation, it is at best a rough approximation. This calculation assumes that H is either the same across the population age distribution or that average health-related quality of life scores for young persons balance those of older persons. We know from various studies (Kaplan et al., 1976; Erickson and Golden, 1991; Rodgers et al., 1989) that health-related quality of life scores decrease with age. Whether or not scores for the young balance those for the aged is a function of the age distribution. In most populations which have an unequal number of young and old persons, it is unreasonable to think that such balancing will occur.

In this section we introduced three different methods for calculating years of healthy life and discussed their advantages and disadvantages. The next section discusses the use of years of healthy life in the Health Resource Allocation Strategy, especially in comparison with other measures that might be used for allocate resources to health care such as life years and healthy year equivalents.

YEARS OF HEALTHY LIFE AND RESOURCE ALLOCATION

The three main approaches to estimating change in health status of groups over time—self-ratings of change, cohort studies, and transition probabilities—can be used in policy-making. The selection of a given approach depends on its use. Both self-ratings of change and cohort studies which give qualitative responses—for example, the same, better, or worse—are useful for population monitoring and for program evaluation, especially when a quantitative measure of prognosis is unnecessary. Self-ratings and cohort studies will be of limited use for allocation of resources and other applications where quantification of prognosis is required. Increasingly, methods such as cost–utility, cost–effectiveness, and cost–benefit ratios are being used to provide information for health decision making. Each of these ratios requires a numeric estimate of the health effect or benefit attributable to the health interventions being studied.

In addition to being the most appropriate measure of health-related quality of life for use in the Health Resource Allocation Strategy, years of healthy life has at least four advantages over other measures of quality of life. First, because it is based on life expectancy, a year of healthy life is an extension of a familiar concept; hence, it satisfies Moriyama's (1968) criterion that measures of health-related quality of life be easy to understand at both the group and individual level.

Second, at the policy level, the years of healthy life measure presents effects of different health programs or differences of population groups on a common unit of measurement that can be used in comparisons across health programs or target populations. As long as the same quality-adjustment factor is used across sociodemographic or disease-specific groups, the years of healthy life can be compared. This feature is especially important for the policy analyst who has to decide whether a maternal–child health program or a heart transplant program provides greater social benefit from the use of public funds.

In contrast, when outcomes are expressed in terms of the disease or health condition being studied, the units of measure are usually not commensurate. Success of an immunization program may be measured in terms of reduction in the number of measles cases; success of a prenatal care program in terms of infant deaths; success of a renal dialysis program in terms of return to work. Clearly these are disparate units of outcome, making comparison meaningless. Can we say that one fewer infant death is equivalent to one fewer case of measles? If not, then how many cases of measles do we need to avert in order to have equivalence? Without some sense of individual or societal tradeoffs between infant deaths and measles, such questions are impossible to answer.

Life years is another measure that is frequently used to compare outcomes across health interventions. Although this measure overcomes the problem of noncommensurate units that results from the use of disease-specific outcomes, it will underestimate the resources required for most, if not all, health interventions when compared to estimates based on years of healthy life. The cost per life year for an intervention will be lower than the cost per year of healthy life for the same intervention.

The lower cost–effectiveness ratio obtained when using life years results from adjusting life years by the proportion of time spent in good health. This adjustment results in a lower number of years of healthy life. The discrepancy between life years and years of healthy life will be larger or smaller depending on the cause of dysfunction. For example, for a person who lives a normal life and dies of a sudden myocardial infarction, the discrepancy between life years and years of healthy life will be small. A person with a chronic debilitating disease, on the other hand, may live a long time with limitations in physical and social function. In this case, the discrepancy between life years and years of healthy life will be large. Thus, when health interventions are designed for improving health among persons with chronic diseases, the use of life years to measure health effect will result in systematically lower cost–effectiveness ratios than will the use of years of healthy life.

Third, years of healthy life incorporates prevalence of the condition into the interpretation of the problem. By combining mortality and morbidity into a single index that expresses health-related quality of life in terms of time, years of healthy life allows the decision maker to consider programs on the basis of their impact on the population. A program that improves the health-related quality of life of several people by one year of healthy life can be weighed against an alternative program that improves the health-related quality of life by 0.1 year of healthy life for ten times as many people.

A fourth, important policy implication of years of healthy life is that the effects of mortality and health-related quality of life can be separated to determine which contributes more heavily to decrements in health status. Thus, the decision maker can determine whether interventions that lower mortality or those that raise health-related quality of life will be more helpful in increasing the number of years of healthy life of a target population.

Models of years of healthy life that permit the components of health-related quality of life to be analyzed separately, for example, the Health Utilities Index, are an additional benefit to the decision maker. With such models, the decision maker can choose not only between interventions that affect either mortality or health-related quality of life but also among those that have the most impact on a particular type of function. For example, an intervention to improve the health status of persons with arthritis may raise health-related quality of life by having a greater impact on improving ability to move about the community and perform self-care than on improving emotional well-being.

The ability to analyze the impact of specific health interventions on different components of years of healthy life stems from the inclusion of preferences in the measure. These preferences provide information about tradeoffs between the various components. Mehrez and Gafni (1989) argue that the years of healthy life measure does not fully represent an individual's preference for health. They propose the healthy-years equivalent measure as a more complete representation of the tradeoffs that individuals make about their health status. This measure differs from years of healthy life in that it includes individuals' preference for life years as well as for states of health-related quality of life.

That healthy-years equivalents include tradeoffs that individuals make between quality and quantity of life for alternative health interventions is important for measuring health-related quality of life. From a policy perspective, however, it is unlikely that this measure can be used in practice within the next decade for theoretical and practical reasons. Further theoretical development is needed to determine whether the measure is meaningful in a societal context. Mehrez and Gafni developed the measure in the context of medical decision making. Whether individuals' tradeoffs between quantity and quality of life can be aggregated to form a meaningful measure of health effect remains to be tested.

From a practical perspective, the healthy-years equivalent measure requires a more intensive data collection effort than does years of healthy life. For one reason, healthy-years equivalent requires that preferences data be collected to obtain von Neumann–Morgenstern utility functions. This means using either the standard gamble or time tradeoff technique, both of which require complicated cognitive processes on the part of the respondent. For another reason, two sets of preferences are needed, one for life years and another for states of health-related quality of life; years of healthy life requires only health state preferences. These additional data requirements translate into higher data collection costs.

Although current approaches to incorporating prognosis into the Health Resource Allocation Strategy provide useful information, modeling transitions between health states has had less attention than has either developing health state classification systems or estimating preferences. The delay in incorporating prognosis into a measure of health-related quality of life can be partly attributed to two factors: (1) the need to develop methods for defining health states and measuring preferences and (2) the time for these concepts and methods to gain acceptance. Another reason for slow development of methods for estimating prognosis is the lack of longitudinal data suitable for use in dynamic mathematical models. A final reason has been the burden of analysis imposed on computing capacity.

This chapter has focused on the development of years of healthy life as a measure of health-related quality of life that also includes mortality. Although different methods of calculation have been presented—methods that can be used for clinical studies and regional demonstration projects as well as community samples of the general population—the focus is on the use of national data for estimating years of healthy life. For the Health Resource Allocation Strategy, data that represent all persons in society are important for the equitable distribution of health care resources.

10

Costs in the Health Resource Allocation Strategy

To this point we have focused on the development of health outcomes, especially years of healthy life, for use in the Health Resource Allocation Strategy. Now we turn to Step 5 of the Strategy with a discussion of health care costs, basic definitions, and issues in cost estimation. As with concepts, domains, and indicators of health outcomes, the analyst must identify costs that are relevant to the policy decision. Since costs reflect the value of goods traded in the marketplace, the tradeoffs between goods and services are built into costs. This leads some people to think that costs are easier to measure than health outcomes. Although costs are self-weighting, the analyst must still exercise good judgment in choosing which health care costs to include in any analysis.

Accountants consider costs to be funds used to purchase goods and services. Economists, on the other hand, define costs as the value of a resource in an alternative use, that is, opportunity cost. Volunteer labor in a hospital serves as a good example of the different perspectives of the accountant and economist. To an accountant, volunteers' time is free. It does not appear in the wage bills of an organization and thus the accountant does not include this in the organization's accounts. Economists, however, maintain that volunteer labor is a real cost of running the hospital and contributes to its output. This labor would have value if donated to another organization or used for some other purpose or if the time had to be purchased at prevailing wage rates. Thus, economists argue that the opportunity of using this labor productively in other activities should be included in an assessment of costs (Warner and Luce, 1982). Economic costs are the relevant costs for use in the Health Resource Allocation Strategy, which incorporates principles of economic theory.

This chapter discusses conceptual issues in measuring health care costs. First, we define types of costs and discuss the importance of organizational context in deciding what to include as costs. We then describe some methods for estimating direct and indirect health care costs for use in the Health Resource Allocation Strategy. Not all costs have the same value; specifically, present costs are more highly valued than future costs. The economist's method for discounting future costs and the calculation of present values of future costs are illustrated. Finally, we discuss different national data sources that can be used to estimate costs in the Health Resource Allocation Strategy.

CONCEPTS AND DEFINITIONS OF HEALTH CARE COSTS

In health care, economic costs can be categorized into three broad categories: operating costs, personal costs, external costs. Table 10.1 gives examples of costs that may be

Table 10.1 Types of costs included in the economic evaluation of health interventions

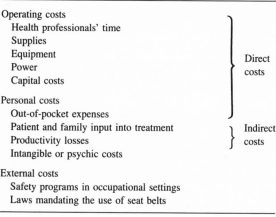

Source: Adapted from Drummond et al., 1987, p. 22.

included in each of these categories. *Direct costs*, that is, organizing and operating costs, are those associated with developing and operating a specific health care program. These include services of physicians and other health care providers (for example, nurses and pharmacists) as well as supplies and equipment (for example, solution, catheter, and tubing costs) needed for making diagnoses or providing rehabilitation services. All organizational costs are considered to be direct costs and usual involve monetary transactions (Drummond et al., 1987; Eisenberg et al., 1988).

Personal care costs are those that are borne by patients and their families and can be considered either direct or indirect costs. Direct personal medical costs include out-of-pocket medical expenses for items such as prescription and nonprescription medication, medical devices, and appliances. People can also incur direct nonmedical costs as a result of illness or as part of treatment. Such costs may include modification of a home to accommodate health care needs of the patient, care provided by relatives and friends, and transportation to obtain care (Eisenberg and Kitz, 1986; Eisenberg et al., 1988).

An example of the nature and scope of direct health care expenditures is shown in Figure 10.1. These data from the National Health Accounts illustrate how various sources of costs relate to overall expenditures in the United States. In 1988 some $539.9 billion, or over $2,000 per person, was spent on health care in the United States. The "Other Care" category shown in this figure includes dentists' services, other professional services, drugs and medical sundries, eyeglasses, and appliances. Program administration, government public health activities, and research and construction accounted for the remaining 12 percent.

Since 1960 the percentages of total expenditures representing hospital care and nursing home care have increased sharply, with the latter doubling during the past three decades. Expenditures for physician services and other spending remained constant while expenditures on other personal health care declined (Office of National Cost Estimates, 1990).

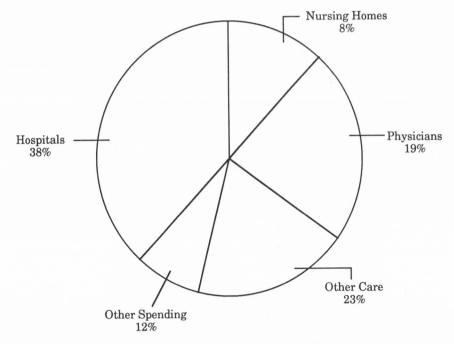

Figure 10.1 Direct health care costs, national health expenditures, 1990.

In addition to the direct costs of health care, patients and their families often incur indirect costs. The term *indirect costs* is used to indicate the value of resources lost. Indirect costs can be estimated by monetary transactions (Luce and Elixhauser, 1990b). In health care, such activities are usually described as changes in production due to health problems (see Table 10.1). Indirect costs of morbidity include reduced levels of work output, time spent to obtain health care, loss of productivity that results from a change of employment caused by illness, and lost leisure time.

Intangible, or psychic, costs include pain, anxiety, and loss of well-being associated with disfigurement, disability, and dependency (Luce and Elixhauser, 1990a). In addition to indirect costs of morbidity are those associated with mortality. In the case of death, the indirect costs result from a person leaving the labor force (Eisenberg et al., 1988).

For goods that are not traded in the market economists have methods for assigning monetary values. The result is sometimes referred to as shadow pricing (Rice and Hodgson, 1981). Shadow pricing may be used to estimate indirect and intangible costs. This technique involves approximating the value of the good as if it were traded in the market. For example, the market value of a housewife's time can be approximated by the wages or salary that she could command if she were to accept a comparable job in the labor market. Costs associated with pain and suffering are more difficult to approximate. For example, how does one estimate the cost associated with extreme pain due to pancreatic cancer? Although shadow pricing has been used, assigning monetary value to morbidity and mortality remains difficult and controversial.

One method frequently used for developing estimates of psychosocial costs is that of willingness to pay. This method is based on obtaining information about what individuals are willing to pay for certain goods and services. Information can be obtained through household surveys or other assessment methods, such as interviewing patients in a primary care setting. Two important assumptions underlie the notion of willingness to pay: (1) individuals can judge their own welfare better than someone else; and (2) the existing income distribution is acceptable. The latter is important since willingness to pay is a function of one's ability to pay (Drummond, 1980).

Even if one accepts these assumptions, valuation assigned to using the willingness-to-pay method is not without limitations. One is that it produces biased estimates based on the income distribution of the target population. Rich people are favored over middle-income and low-income populations. Another major problem with willingness to pay is the method used to collect data for estimating indirect costs. Analysts have questioned whether respondents can really assign a monetary value to small reductions in the probability of dying due to a disease or health condition (Rice and Hodgson, 1981; Thompson et al., 1984).

Another frequently used method for estimating indirect costs is the human capital approach. In human capital estimation, labor force earnings are used to estimate the changes in economic productivity that are attributable to morbidity and mortality (Hodgson and Meiners, 1982; Luce and Elixhauser, 1990b). Indirect costs of lost productivity based on marketplace estimates of earnings introduce certain biases into the resulting estimates. Since men generally make higher wages and salaries than women, men are more highly valued using this approach. Similarly, children, the elderly, and minority groups are less valued than middle-aged people and members of the majority (Rice and Hodgson, 1981).

Table 10.2 lists indirect costs associated with morbidity and mortality for fiscal year 1975. These data indicate the value of time lost from usual activity due to all diseases and to neoplasms. For each of the four types of activity—being employed, keeping house, being unable to work, and being institutionalized—costs attributable to health-related dysfunctions were measured with individual earnings used as the unit of measure for output loss (Paringer and Berk, 1977). The indirect cost for mortality was estimated by the value of expected future earnings for persons who died prematurely. These data suggest that the indirect morbidity costs of neoplasms are small relative to the indirect cost associated with all diseases. For example, for employed persons, the morbidity costs associated with all diseases were approximately 50 times that associated with neoplasms. Mortality costs for all diseases, however, were only five times

Table 10.2 Indirect costs for all diseases and neoplasms, United States, fiscal year 1975

Morbidity	All diseases	Neoplasms
Employed	$21,303	$422
Keeping house	$4,384	$194
Unable to work	$24,410	$440
Institutionalized	$7,750	$49
Mortality	$87,925	$17,079

Source: Paringer and Berk, 1977.

Note: All estimates are presented as percentage values that have been discounted at 6% per year.

the costs of neoplasms. This suggests that lost productivity for people with neoplasms is more likely to occur because of premature mortality than from lost time from usual activity.

Although the information on which these calculations are based is more than 15 years old, these data are presented here because they are based on regularly updated national sources. This information shows the types of indirect costs that can be calculated using national data and might be used in applying the Health Resource Allocation Strategy.

Some analysts also consider external costs borne by consumers (Table 10.1) as another classification of health care costs. The health intervention that generates the costs is designed to benefit other groups of individuals who may or may not be the direct beneficiaries of the output or intervention. For example, an occupational health and safety program may result in changes in the production process that may have economic benefit for the consumer. If a program improves safety in an automobile factory, the consumers are unlikely to be the same people that the program was designed and implemented to protect (Drummond et al., 1987).

Economic theory usually analyzes costs in terms of total, average, and marginal costs. Total costs consist of fixed and variable costs. Space and storage within a clinic are examples of fixed costs. Fixed costs do not depend on the quantity of output produced at any given point in time. If the clinic stays in business, these facilities do not change, that is, their size does not vary with the number of patient visits. Variable costs, on the other hand, are directly related to the quantity of output produced. Thus, these costs can fluctuate according to the amount of services, or output, produced. For example, if a clinic keeps longer hours to provide health care services, it will pay more for electricity and other utilities required over the extended hours. If a health care delivery system wants to reduce costs in a very short time yet still remain in business, it reduces its variable costs.

Average cost is the total cost divided by the amount of output produced. Thus, it consists of both fixed and variable costs. A simple example of estimating the average cost of a health care clinic might be to measure the total costs for a given time period, for example, one month, and divide this by the number of patients seen during the month. This would give the average cost of operating the clinic per person treated. Marginal cost is the additional cost per unit produced and reflects the rate of change in total cost as the quantity produced changes. In geometric terms, it is the slope of the total cost curve.

In cost–utility analysis, the average cost is used when the question is one of deciding *which* alternative health intervention to fund. For example, the decision maker may have to choose between surgical or medical treatment for angina. Marginal analysis is used when the decision focuses on *how much* of a program should be funded. For example, in deciding how much treatment for depression to fund, the alternatives might be one, two, or three visits to a therapist per week (Drummond, 1980; Kamlet, 1992).

In comparing health care costs and outcomes in cost–benefit, cost–effectiveness, and cost–utility analyses, total costs are comprised of the costs of the treatment, of side effects attributed to the treatment, and of associated morbidity. Some analysts add a fourth component to total costs, namely, those accrued for added years of life due to the success of the treatment.

In this analysis, the cost of treatment is expressed in terms of the change in costs for the new intervention when compared to an available alternative. Whether the change is expressed in average or marginal terms depends on the purpose of the analysis, that is, to decide whether to allocate resources to an intervention at all or to decide how much resources to allocate to a given intervention. We use the term net cost, or change in cost, to refer to both; whether average or marginal cost is appropriate will depend on the purpose of the analysis. The formula, given by Weinstein and Stason (1982), is

$$\Delta C = \Delta C_{Rx} + \Delta C_{SE} - \Delta C_{Morb} + \Delta C_{Rx} \Delta LE$$

where

ΔC_{Rx} = change in cost due to the treatment
ΔC_{SE} = change in costs due to side effects associated with the treatment
ΔC_{Morb} = change in costs due to morbidity
$\Delta C_{Rx} \Delta LE$ = change in costs over the individual's remaining lifetime due to the success of the treatment

The last component, which adds the medical expenditures that are accrued for added years of life, is controversial. For example, if antihypertensive medication prevents premature death due to heart attack, then this component adds future indirect costs of other illnesses that occur as a result of the person surviving the heart attack. Russell (1986) argues that these costs are no more relevant to deciding whether a program is a good use of resources than are expenditures for food, clothing, or housing. We agree with Russell that this last term should be omitted and recommend using only the first three terms to estimate net costs in the Health Resource Allocation Strategy.

Another feature of costs is that they are influenced by inflation. Economists use the term "nominal" to refer to costs incurred in the current period. Real costs, on the other hand, are those for which the inflationary component has been removed. Cost data from different years can be adjusted to current monetary units for comparison by using official price deflators, either for the gross national product or the gross domestic product, for each currency.

Standardization to current, or base year, dollars is accomplished by multiplying the ratio of the price deflators for the base year and past years by the cost estimate for the past year:

$$C_{bp} = \frac{D_{bp}}{D_{py}} \times C_{py}$$

where

C_{bp} = base year cost
D_{bp} = base year price deflator
D_{py} = past year price deflator
C_{py} = past year cost

For example, the cost per year of healthy life gained for scoliosis surgery was £2,600 in 1986 (Table 2.2). The deflators for 1987 (base year) and 1986 (past year) were 151.0

and 144.6, respectively. Using the formula, we find the cost per year of healthy life gained is £2,715.

As mentioned earlier in this chapter, health care costs are relevant for resource allocation. In practice it is often difficult to identify all sources of direct and indirect costs and obtain the data needed for calculating cost–effectiveness ratios. Information on charges is often more readily obtainable and thus frequently used as proxy estimates for costs. This practice, however, can lead to serious problems in interpreting the results of a cost analysis, since costs and charges are frequently very different (Finkler, 1982). In a competitive market, charges would reflect costs. The market for health care, however, departs from the competitive ideal. Hence, charges do not usually provide reliable information about costs.

Although this chapter focuses on the measurement of costs for use in the Health Resource Allocation Strategy, balancing costs with benefits is only one reason why organizations measure costs. Among the other reasons are direct payment for services, bad debt, and internal subsidization of one department by another. These data are used for price setting, reimbursement, and cash flow analyses. The perspective on costs and the data used to estimate them differ depending on the purpose of their use.

A cost to one person or organizational unit may not be a cost in a different context. For example, the cost a patient incurs for transportation to a health care provider is a cost to the patient and to society, but it is not a cost to health decision makers in the central government. In other words, different actors (patients, employers, funding agencies) have different perspectives as to what constitutes a cost (Drummond et al., 1987).

The appropriate perspective for use in the Health Resource Allocation Strategy is one that includes all medical and nonmedical costs as well as personal indirect costs regardless of who pays. This interpretation of costs is considered to be one that takes a societal viewpoint and thus enables the decision maker to choose among alternative, competing programs; analyses using more restrictive perspectives on cost are limited to drawing conclusions within the organizational context bounded by the choice of the cost data. For example, health insurers may try to determine the costs accruing to their companies. When interpreting the results of such studies, one should be clear about the objectives of the study and the perspective taken, since this will limit the inferences that can be drawn from the results, especially in regard to generalizing the results to society at large (Russell, 1986).

The next section describes the estimation of direct and indirect costs for use in the Health Resource Allocation Strategy in greater detail. Procedures for determining both operating and out-of-pocket costs are discussed and illustrated using examples from the literature. In addition, guidelines for reviewing and interpreting cost studies are presented.

ESTIMATING DIRECT AND INDIRECT HEALTH CARE COSTS

Three examples are used to illustrate the estimation of different types of costs: coronary artery bypass surgery compared to medical management; cholesterol screening for elderly persons; and pharmacologic treatment for arthritis. Whether the total cost formula contains three or four components, total costs or net total costs attributed to an intervention include some form of direct costs. Some direct costs are straightforward to estimate. For instance, the cost of prescription drugs is a direct cost with little variability. Other direct cost data may be subject to large variability. Arthritis patients may be hospitalized for other conditions besides arthritis and its treatment (Thompson et al., 1988).

Coronary Artery Bypass Surgery

In a comparison of coronary artery bypass surgery to medical management, the net costs consisted of the additional cost due to surgery, the difference in costs of medical management with and without surgery, savings from preventing adverse consequences of coronary artery disease, and difference in costs between medically and surgically treated patients in terms of subsequent heart operations (Weinstein and Stason, 1982). The treatment alternatives and their estimated average costs are presented in Table 10.3. The $17,500 estimate of the cost of surgery, which ranged from $15,000 to $25,000, was based on a review of the literature. The published data were adjusted into constant 1981 dollars to account for medical care inflation.

Costs of medical management include medications, office visits, and laboratory examinations. The price of standard medical treatment was determined by surveying local pharmacies and by using standard fees for physician office visits and laboratory tests. More treatment was allowed in the case of severe angina compared to mild angina. For example, costs for drugs and laboratory tests were assumed to be twice as high for people with severe angina as for people with mild angina. The figures for medical management in Table 10.3 represent the savings in medical services and treatments in the ten-year period following surgery. For people with severe angina, this is $2,290; for people with mild angina, it is $585.

Data to estimate the lower incidence of myocardial infarction (MI) following surgery were based on information obtained in two clinical trials. Over the ten-year period of this study, analysts made assumptions about the incidence of MI and the protective nature of coronary artery surgery. The result was an estimated saving of $1,275. The costs of repeated surgeries were assumed to be equal for both the medically and surgically treated patients; hence the expected difference in cost for the two groups is estimated to be 0.

The expected net cost for surgical treatment of severe angina is $14,000; this estimate ranged from $10,500 to $17,500. For people with mild angina, the expected net

Table 10.3 Expected resource costs and savings for coronary artery bypass surgery and medical management of severe and mild angina

Component	Severe angina average	Mild angina average
Surgery	$17,500	$17,500
Medical management	−2,290	−585
Myocardial infarctions	−1,275	−1,275
Subsequent surgery	0	0
Total	$14,000	$15,500

Source: Adapted from Weinstein and Stason, 1982.

Note: All estimates have been standardized to 1981 dollars and are presented as present values that have been discounted at 5% per year.

cost is $15,500, ranging from $12,000 to $19,000. Net costs are higher for people with mild angina because medical management savings are less, $585 compared to $2,290.

Cholesterol Screening

A recent cost–effectiveness study conducted by the U.S. Office of Technology Assessment (OTA) illustrates assumptions and sources of data necessary to estimate direct health care costs (Garber et al., 1989). This study assessed the impact on Medicare funds of the decision to include cholesterol screening and treatment for the elderly.

Total costs per year of treatment for the seven major medications for treating hypercholesterolemia were based on the following assumptions: (1) doctors prescribe the recommended dose; (2) patients comply with doctors' prescriptions; (3) doctors monitor patients regularly using recommended laboratory tests and procedures; and (4) doctors charge each patient $200 annually for this monitoring.

To estimate the retail charges for each prescription medication, analysts used the New Jersey list of allowable charges for the state pharmaceutical reimbursement program. Charges for over-the-counter medications were estimated based on data from a local drugstore chain. Analysts assumed these charges were representative and could be generalized to a broader population base. Although this study did not include direct personal costs in arriving at estimates of the total costs, other studies have included personal expenditures.

Pharmacologic Treatment for Arthritis

A study by Thompson and colleagues (1988) expanded the traditional definition of net costs to incorporate nonmedical economic impacts of arthritis. One of the impacts of treatment considered in this study was cost of transportation for outpatient visits. These costs were estimated at 20 cents a mile. A second nonmedical impact was the cost of home help. These costs were imputed for unpaid help by using the average hourly wage in private industry. A distinction was made between the aid provided by others to help the patient obtain treatment and help obtained for other purposes. This study also estimated the indirect costs of arthritis treatment by using change in income.

As the review of the cost data used in these three studies indicates, many of the concepts and definitions introduced in the first section may be difficult to include in empirical studies. Thus, it may be necessary for the analyst to compromise between the ideal and the practical.

Table 10.4 lists the major conceptual concerns in estimating costs and presents some acceptable practical responses that may be needed. The goal is to accept practical realities that will introduce the least amount of bias into the empirical estimates. The compromises must be clearly stated so that anyone reviewing the study will understand the analyst's decisions and how they may affect the study results.

Identifying all resources required for providing a health program or intervention may not be possible. The compromise is to include data that are readily available and to concentrate on obtaining costs that will differ between patients. Like all costs, it may be difficult to obtain data suitable for estimating marginal costs. Using average costs as an alternative may not be too serious a problem when previous studies indicate that marginal costs do not vary significantly.

Compromises on opportunity costs, indirect costs, and inclusion of overhead costs

Table 10.4 Selected compromises between conceptual definitions and empirical estimates of health care costs

Enumerate all resources involved in producing the program
  Include easily measurable costs and those that are expected to differ between patients
  State explicitly which costs are included and excluded in the cost analysis

Use marginal costs
  Average costs may be used if marginal costs are relatively constant or if capital costs are small

Use opportunity costs rather than charges
  Charges may be used if the cost–charge ratios across service categories are similar, when comparative rather than absolute costing is needed, and when charges are the value of interest

Include indirect cost
  Use when productivity gains or losses are expected
  Use market wage, i.e., the human capital approach, to estimate indirect costs
  Use the willingness-to-pay approach to estimate a broader range of costs than market productivity

Include overhead
  Overheads may be omitted if technology is marginal to the overall purpose of analysis

Account for future efficiencies, for inefficiencies of average operating conditions, and for changing technologies
  Estimate costs under average working conditions using sensitivity analysis

Include resources that are "free" from the perspective of the provider
  Use market wages
  For resources already owned by the provider, estimate their alternative use

Exclude transfer payments
  Transfer payments, e.g., taxes and disability payments, are not economic costs

Source: Adapted from Luce and Elixhauser, 1990b.

may be needed when exact data are unavailable or the effects of using alternative sources of data are anticipated to be small. Sensitivity analysis can be used to test the effect of compromises from the ideal in several cases: future efficiencies from learning or technological development; inefficiencies from using average rather than ideal conditions; inefficiencies from using overly skilled personnel to do tasks that could be done by people with less skill; and assessments of the impact of rapidly changing technologies.

As suggested by the analyses used in the three preceding examples, costs may be expended over a number of years. For example, costs for medical treatment for angina are incurred for the remainder of the patient's lifetime or until the symptom is relieved by surgery. Future costs need to be adjusted so that they are comparable with those that are expended in the present period. The next section introduces the procedure of discounting, the economic method for adjusting costs to account for intertemporal decision making.

DISCOUNTING HEALTH CARE COSTS

Generally, when economists describe streams of costs occurring over a period of time, they do so in terms of the present value or the net present value. From the perspective of investment, money is productive and can earn a positive rate of return if invested.

Money available today has a higher value than the same amount of money that is available at some time in the future. Thus, decision makers discount future dollars to present value terms before making allocations.

A second reason why costs are expressed in present value terms is that individuals are considered as having a positive time preference for an economic "good." Positive time preference is the notion that individuals prefer to consume a "good" today rather than delaying consumption to some time in the future (Olson and Bailey, 1981). For an economic "bad," the situation is reversed: individuals prefer to delay consumption until some time in the future (Lipscomb, 1989).

Discounting is the process used to convert future dollars to present values. The value of a future investment is usually converted to its present discounted value (PDV) using the following formula (Warner and Luce, 1982):

$$C_{PDV} = \sum \frac{C_1}{(1 + r)^1}$$

or

$$C_{PDV} = C_0 + \frac{C_1}{1 + r} + \frac{C_2}{(1 + r)^2} + \ldots + \frac{C_n}{(1 + r)^n}$$

where

C = costs

n = time period over which costs are to be discounted

r = rate of time preference, or discount rate

i = interval under study, ranging from the time of program initiation to the last year the program is expected to be operational

Table 10.5 presents an example of the effect of different discount rates, "r." If a health care program costs of $100,000 per year to initiate and is expected to incur costs and provide benefits over ten years at a discount rate of 5%, discounted costs are $872,174. That is, the present discounted value of the program that is estimated to cost $1,100,000 in undiscounted terms over the ten-year period is about $200,000 less in present value terms.

The remaining columns of Table 10.5 show the effect of different discount rates on the same cost flow over the same period. The smaller the discount rate, the higher the present value. For example, with a discount rate of 2.5 percent, the present value of a program is $975,207. The same program discounted at a rate of 10 percent has a present value of $714,456. This indicates that even seemingly small differences in the discount rate have large effects when the health programs are expected to be long-lived (Gramlich, 1981).

The choice of the discount rate is particularly important when gains from an intervention extend into the future. One example of a program with long-term benefits is a smoking cessation clinic. In this intervention, the benefits of not smoking will last well into the future through reduced rates of lung cancer, emphysema, and heart disease. In general, the longer the time interval over which benefits of an intervention will accrue, the more likely the discounted values will approach 0. The assumption behind this view is that money available well into the future—20 years, for example—has less

Table 10.5 Effect of different discount rates for health interventions costing $100,000 at start up and expected to last ten years

Years	Discount rate (r)			
	2.5%	5%	7.5%	10%
Start up of intervention	$100,000	$100,000	$100,000	$100,000
1	96,561	95,238	93,023	90,909
2	95,181	90,703	86,533	82,645
3	92,860	86,384	80,496	75,131
4	90,595	82,270	74,880	68,301
5	88,385	78,353	69,656	62,092
6	86,230	74,622	64,796	56,447
7	84,127	71,068	60,275	51,316
8	82,075	67,684	56,070	46,651
9	80,073	64,461	52,158	42,410
10	78,120	61,391	48,519	38,554
Present value[a]	$975,207	$872,174	$786,406	$714,456

[a]The present value is found by using the formula

$$C_{PDV} = C_0 + \frac{C_1}{1 + r} + \frac{C_2}{(1 + r)^2} + \ldots + \frac{C_n}{(1 + r)^n}$$

where C represents costs, PDV represents present discounted value, n is the time period over which costs are to be discounted, r is the rate of time preference, or discount factor, i ranges from 0 to n, or from the time of program initiation to the last year the program is expected to be operational.

value in the present. Thus, in studies that examine costs and benefits over a long interval, the analyst may want to use a lower discount rate rather than a higher one. For example, in a study of the lifetime costs of smoking, Hodgson (1992) used a 3 percent rate.

Although economic theory presents the notion of time preference and gives general formulas for calculating the net present value of costs, the theory gives little guidance about how to estimate the rate of time preference r. This rate should be the result of a balance between opportunity cost of capital (i.e., investment) and time preference. Economic theory does not tell us how to arrive at this balance (Rice and Hodgson, 1981).

Generally, analysts assume that a single rate applies to all members of society, but empirical evidence suggests that rates vary with age, income, sex, and race (Rice and Hodgson, 1981). In practice, however, analysts use one rate; that is, they assume that a uniform discount rate is appropriate for the study population. This simplified assumption is needed because of limitations in the data.

In short, which rate best represents any given population is unclear. The usual practice is to pick a range of rates to give an alternative understanding of the effect of discounting. Most analysts agree that a 10 percent discount rate is high and recommend 5 percent. Russell (1986) advocates that 5 percent be adopted as the standard for use in cost–utility analyses that are designed as inputs to the social decision process. If analysts need to use a second rate, Russell recommends using a rate of zero. As a result of comparing ratios obtained with a 5 percent discount rate to those obtained with no discounting, the analyst gains a good understanding of the effect of discounting.

We have now dealt with some of the technical issues of defining costs and have illustrated some of the approaches for using costs in economic analyses of health care. A central issue for applying the Strategy for improving equality of opportunity through the health care delivery system is the availability of national cost data.

NATIONAL COSTS DATA FOR THE HEALTH RESOURCE ALLOCATION STRATEGY

National data for assessing health care costs are needed as the other major source of information in the costs and outcomes comparison. These data can be used together with national data on health status and health-related quality of life in the application of the Strategy. Even if special studies are needed to supplement national cost data, the availability of national data may be especially valuable for estimating indirect costs of illness and for testing for bias introduced by using data derived from special, smaller-scale studies.

The United States National Health Accounts are one type of national data available on health care costs. These can be used to assess expenditures on diseases (coded according to the International Classification of Diseases) by the different types of services that are shown in Figure 10.1. Within specific categories, such as hospital services, costs in the National Health Accounts can be further disaggregated to indicate type of hospital. Generally, however, the groupings are too broad for widespread use in cost–utility analysis and the Health Resource Allocation Strategy.

More detailed information of the type that can be used for comparing costs and outcomes in the Strategy are available from national claims data bases and from health surveys. Table 10.6 summarizes data available from Medicare and Medicaid claims files and from three health surveys, the National Medical Expenditures Survey (NMES), the National Medical Care Utilization and Expenditure Survey (NMCUES), and the National Health Interview Survey (NHIS). The listing of types of costs, both direct and indirect, is adapted from Luce and Elixhauser (1990b).

The Medicare program is a federal insurance program that covers persons 65 years and over, permanently disabled workers and their dependents who are eligible for old age, survivors, and disability benefits, and persons with end-stage renal disease. The hospital insurance program of Medicare pays for institutional patient care, excluding nursing homes. The supplementary medical insurance program covers physician services, institutional outpatient care, and selected ancillary services.

Approximately 33 million persons were enrolled in the Medicare program in 1988. Of these, 30 million were 65 years of age and over; the other 3 million consisted of disabled persons. Medicare enrollees spent almost $90 billion dollars on health care in 1988 (Office of National Cost Estimates, 1990). The largest growth in Medicare spending over the previous five years was for physician services even though Medicare has closely monitored and controlled physician fees since 1985.

The Medicaid program is also a federally supported health insurance program. Unlike Medicare, which is federally administered, Medicaid is operated by the states. Persons are covered by Medicaid if they are eligible to receive benefits from the

Table 10.6 National sources of direct and indirect cost data

Type of costs	Medicare	Medicaid	NMES[a]	NMCUES[b]	NHIS[c]
Direct medical costs					
Institutional patient care	+	+	+	+	+
Institutional outpatient care	+	+	+	+	+
Home health care	+	+	+		
Physician services	+	+	+	+	+
Ancillary services					
Medications		+	+	+	
Devices and appliances			+	+	
Diagnostic tests		+	+	+	
Treatment services	+		+	+	+
Prevention services			+	+	+
Rehabilitation		+	+	+	
Direct nonmedical costs					
Care by family and friends			+		
Indirect costs in terms of wages/time					
Change in productivity			+	+	+
Absenteeism, etc.				+	+
Income lost by family members			+		
Time spent by patient seeking care			+		
Time spent by others attending patient			+		
Intangible costs					
Psychosocial costs			+	+	
Pain					+
Change in social function			+	+	+

[a] NMES = National Medical Expenditure Survey.
[b] NMCUES = National Medical Care Utilization and Expenditure Survey.
[c] NHIS = National Health Interview Survey.

Supplemental Security Income for the Aged, Blind, and Disabled program or from the Aid to Families with Dependent Children program. Individual states may also include persons who have incomes that are below a given level. The federal law that established the Medicaid program, Title XIX of the 1965 Social Security Act, requires that the states provide inpatient and outpatient institutional care, physician services, home health care, and diagnostic tests. States may also provide medications and rehabilitation services (Office of National Cost Estimates, 1990). In 1988, there were almost 23 million Medicaid recipients; these persons accounted for over $52 billion in personal health care expenditures.

As indicated in Table 10.6, the information contained in the Medicare and Medicaid files relates to direct medical care costs. These data bases collect no information on direct nonmedical costs and none on indirect costs or intangible costs. Owing to the limited types of services covered, certain types of direct medical costs cannot be estimated using data from these two federal insurance programs; these include devices and appliances and preventive services. The categories used in Table 10.6 represent broad classes of costs. Thus, within some of them, detailed data needed for presenting complete or nearly complete estimates of costs may not be available; for example, data on ancillary services, including psychologists, social workers, and nutritionists, are not likely to be available.

National survey data also collect information that can be used to estimate indirect as well as direct costs. The NMES and NMCUES collect a wide array of information on health care costs. Both surveys were designed to collect data on the civilian noninstitutionalized population. In addition, NMES collected data on institutionalized populations and Native Americans in 1987. Participants in the household interview survey components of both NMES and NMCUES were interviewed five times during the year, approximately every three months after the initial interview. Information was collected on access to and use of medical services and on associated charges and sources of payment, as well as on health status and health insurance. These surveys consisted of a standard set of questions, or core, asked at each interview and supplementary questionnaires that were used at different times during the year (Bonham, 1983; Edwards and Berlin, 1989; Edwards and Edwards, 1989).

As shown in Table 10.6 both the NMES and the NMCUES collect some information on all of the direct medical care cost listed in this table. Since NMES is more recent and thus builds upon the strengths and limitations of the two previous medical care surveys, it provides more complete coverage of health care expenditures. This can be seen by the fact that it includes some information on direct nonmedical costs, specifically, those associated with care by family and friends. Luce and Elixhauser (1990a) also include child care and housekeeping, home modification to accommodate illness, social services, repair of property, and law enforcement as part of direct nonmedical costs. Neither NMCUES or NMES collected data that can be used to estimate these costs.

As an example of the use of national data for estimating costs of illness, Harlan et al. (1986) estimated the total value of productivity lost to acute respiratory conditions was $8.4 billion based on data collected in NMCUES. This estimate of indirect costs combined the value of work-loss days for employed persons and the value of bed-disability days for homemakers. For homemakers, bed-disability or restricted-activity days that can be attributed to a disease or health condition are used to estimate time loss from usual activity. When restricted activity was substituted for bed disability as the measure of lost productivity for homemakers, the value of lost productivity was $9.1 billion.

These national estimates of indirect costs due to acute respiratory illnesses are more than four times greater than those associated with cardiovascular conditions. Again, using data from the National Medical Care Utilization and Expenditure Survey, Harlan and colleagues (1989) estimated that the value of productivity lost to cardiovascular conditions, using bed-disability days as a measure for homemakers, was $1.7 billion. When restricted-activity days were used as a measure for homemakers, the value of productivity lost increased to $2.1 billion.

In this approach to estimating indirect costs, illnesses experienced primarily by children are excluded from the calculations. For example, one of the acute respiratory conditions included by Harlan et al. (1986) was otitis media, a disorder that primarily affects young people. Since youths are rarely in the labor force, otitis media does not have a significant impact on the overall estimate of indirect costs.

Although both NMES and NMCUES collected data that can be used to estimate some indirect costs, these surveys did not collect information about forgone leisure time, which is generally considered to be an indirect costs. Both collected some data that fit into the category of psychosocial costs. Included in this category are things such as disfigurement, disability, and loss of well-being. Other psychosocial costs, for example, loss of opportunity and family contact, were not collected in either survey. Neither survey collected data on the value that others place on patients' health and well-being, although Luce and Elixhauser (1990a) list this among the intangible costs.

The NHIS is included in this table because, although not including economic cost information directly, it collects much information that can be used to gain information on both medical care and productivity losses that can be used in estimating costs. For example, Hodgson (1992) used data from the NHIS to estimate medical care costs to society that are associated with smoking.

These national survey data indicate the value of person-based rather than aggregate data from administrative records for understanding the relationship of health care expenditures to health-related quality of life. Such data can be used to identify utilization patterns, impacts of illness on productivity loss, and sources of costs, such as burden on families and friends, pain, and suffering, that impact on society's well-being. These indirect costs are important considerations in making health policy.

For allocating resources across society, the policymaker needs to consider these nonmedical direct costs and indirect costs. The Health Resource Allocation Strategy incorporates these costs in the cost–utility ratio that is the basic input to the decision process. Using the model with national cost data that are collected through probability samples will enhance the decision-making process since total population representation will help ensure that the allocation is not only efficient but also equitable.

11

Ranking Costs and Outcomes of Health Care Alternatives

In allocating resources to health care, the decision maker compares health care costs and outcomes for an array of interventions to identify those that result in the highest level of benefit within the given budget constraint. In applications of the Health Resource Allocation Strategy, the main estimate of interest is the ratio of incremental cost to year of healthy life gained from a program or set of programs.

In this chapter we discuss the analysis and interpretation of cost per year of healthy life gained. In the first section we discuss how to calculate the ratio of cost per year of healthy life gained associated with alternative courses of action. In the second section we apply the logic of meta-analysis as a framework for presenting and analyzing costs and outcomes data from different studies. In the third section, these meta-analytic techniques are used to compare costs and medical effectiveness of alternative health interventions. Allocating resources to a set of different health interventions under a budgetary constraint requires the ranking of cost–utility ratios usually for the purpose of rationing. Ideally these ratios are derived from a single source of data on costs and outcomes—costs, states, weights, or prognoses—so that meta-analytic techniques are unnecessary. The last section discusses Step 8 of the Health Resource Allocation Strategy, that is, procedures for reviewing the preliminary rankings and adjusting them to reflect stakeholder values.

CALCULATION OF COST–UTILITY RATIOS

Estimating Net Health Effects

In the cost–utility ratios used in the Health Resource Allocation Strategy, the denominator is the difference between benefits attributed to the alternatives being compared. This difference is referred to as the net benefit, or net effect. For example, for a given disease, the alternatives may be to treat or not to treat, either of which results in a number of years of healthy life. The difference between the treatment and no-treatment alternative is the *number of years of healthy life gained*. Figure 11.1 illustrates the years of healthy life gained for a typical individual in this treatment–no-treatment example. The lightly shaded area indicates the years of healthy life gained due to the treatment. The sum of the two shaded areas indicates the total years of healthy life experienced by this individual if the treatment is given.

Net effects can be calculated from three types of data: (1) cross-sectional data

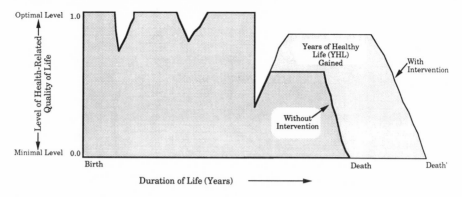

Figure 11.1 Years of healthy life added by intervention for a prototype individual. *Source:* Torrance and Feeny, 1989.

collected on a single sample at one point in time; (2) repeated cross-sectional data collected on different samples at two or more points in time; and (3) longitudinal data, also known as cohort or panel data, collected on the same group of people at two or more points in time.

Cross-sectional data can be used for comparing the health status of different population groups. For example, self-ratings of health by black and white persons in the United States can be compared. In 1990, a lower percentage of black persons than white persons reported themselves in excellent health—32.1 percent compared with 40.6 percent. The net effect is that 8.5 percent more of the white population reported themselves in excellent health than did the black population (Adams and Benson, 1991).

Repeated cross-sectional data are used to monitor the prevalence of health conditions such as hypertension and diabetes and to track population trends in functional status and perceptions of health. For example, the percentage of the total population reporting limitations in usual social role has been relatively constant from 1970 to 1988. For persons under 18, however, the percentage with a limitation in usual social role has been steadily increasing—a net increase of approximately 3 percent. Thus, single point-in-time and repeated cross-sectional studies are useful for detecting and then monitoring differences in levels of health of different population groups. Repeated cross-sectional data are useful for analyses of changes in population health levels across time.

In cohort studies the same measures are taken in the same individuals at various time intervals to detect change over time. Health effects are measured for each individual, rather than for groups of individuals. The net treatment effect for each individual is found by subtracting the baseline health status score from that obtained at selected intervals after the intervention has been administered. The difference score gives the change in health-related quality of life from baseline to the period of measurement. Health status at one point in time is related to that at a subsequent point in time. Working with individuals rather than groups takes into consideration the correlation between health status scores over time; there is also less variation in estimates when studying the same individuals over time. We therefore recommend using cohort data wherever possible to implement the Health Resource Allocation Strategy.

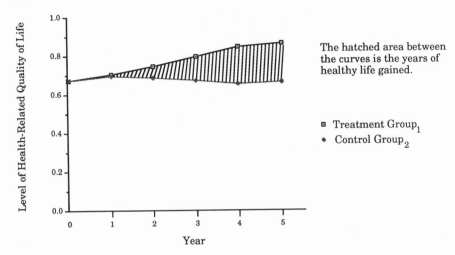

Figure 11.2 Calculation of additional years of healthy life gained. The hatched area between the curves is the years of healthy life gained.

The data in Figure 11.2 illustrate the calculation of the years of healthy life gained for a cohort of individuals receiving treatment. The treatment group is compared to a control group representing usual care or the status quo. Individuals have been randomly assigned to either the treatment or control group and followed for five years. For the control group, the average score represents the level of health-related quality of life for a one-year interval. Mean scores can be summed over the five-year period to calculate the number of years of healthy life during the interval.

Similarly, mean scores for the treatment group can be summed to yield the number of years of healthy life for this group. The area between the curve bounded on the bottom by the scores for the control group and on the top by the scores for the treatment group represents the years of healthy life gained by the treatment. This is analogous to the areas shown in Figure 11.1 for the prototypical individual.

In this example, the level of health-related quality of life for the control group remains fairly constant over the five-year period. For the treatment group, on the other hand, the level rises continuously. The gain in years of healthy life for the first year is the difference between the average scores at year 1. The number of people in the treatment group is used for averaging since this group is the one benefiting from the treatment. Summing the average number gained for all five years results in the total years of healthy life gained due to the treatment.

As indicated by this example, net effect is interpreted in terms of years of healthy life gained. This measure of net effect has the advantage of being expressed in units of measurement, namely, life years, that are biologically and intuitively meaningful.

Estimating and Interpreting Effect Size

Changes in health status, that is, mean difference scores obtained from a health-related quality of life measure other than years of healthy life, often lack biologic meaning or familiarity. Interpretation of effect size is therefore difficult in comparison to more commonly used measures such as blood pressure, cholesterol level, or other clinical indicators. Investigators have developed special analytical techniques to aid in the interpretation of health-related quality of life effects, frequently by relating changes in health status to changes in some clinically familiar measure.

One approach to forming these relationships is through statistical modeling in which health status measures are compared to clinical measures. Brook et al. (1983) used data from the Health Insurance Experiment (HIE) to interpret changes in five health status variables (Table 11.1). The HIE was funded by the Department of Health and Human Services, which contracted with the RAND Corporation to design and conduct a community-based study for assessing the impact of various health insurance options, including free care (Newhouse, 1974; Brook et al., 1979, 1983). RAND tracked participants over either a three- or five-year period and calibrated responses to an extensive battery of health status measures on scales ranging from 0 to 100.

In estimating changes in health-related quality of life over the course of the study, difference scores were first calculated for each concept that was measured. Then statistical regression techniques were used to help provide "clinical meaning" to the changes. For example, a 3-point change in general health perceptions was determined to have the same meaning as a 10-point change in blood pressure. A 10-point difference in physical health was found to have the same effect as chronic, mild osteoarthritis. A 3-point difference on the 38-item mental health scale had the same effect as being fired or laid off from a job.

Wells, Manning, and colleagues (1989) used a variance component model with the same data from the Health Insurance Experiment to interpret changes in mental health scores. This variance component model accounts the role of families in determining psychological well-being. Wells et al. found that a difference of 2.3 points on the mental health scale was the same as a person being fired or laid off during the last 12 months.

The difference in the two estimates for effect size interpretation is not surprising: they are based on different assumptions and different statistical methods. Furthermore, different variables were used in the specification of the two models. However, the fact that the same scale with the same respondents will give apparently different magnitudes

Table 11.1 Interpretation of effect size for five health status variables used in the health insurance experiment

Health status variable	Interpretation
Physical functioning	A 10-point difference = the effect of having chronic mild osteoarthritis
Role functioning	A 1-point difference = a probability 1 percentage point higher of being limited in the performance of one's principal role
Mental health	A 3-point difference = the impact of being fired or laid off from a job
Social contacts	A 10-point difference = an increase of 2 percentage points in the probability of being psychiatrically impaired
Health perceptions	A 5-point difference = the effect of having been diagnosed as having hypertension

Source: Brook et al., 1983.

of change for the same interpretation, for example, being fired or laid off from a job, points up some of the problem areas for modeling effect size. Until standardized procedures can be developed, investigators should present fundamental assumptions and variance estimates along with change scores.

A second approach for interpreting health status effects not expressed in person or time metrics is to ask people to assess change in their health status and then to calibrate this reported change. Self-assessed changes are usually obtained using self-administered or interviewer-administered questionnaires (Guyatt, Walter et al., 1987). Respondents are asked to make global ratings of changes in symptoms or functional status. For example, in a study of chronic respiratory disease, Jaeschke et al. (1989) asked patients to rate their changes in their shortness of breath on day-to-day activities. Patients were asked:

> Overall, has there been any change in your shortness of breath during your daily activities since the last time you saw us? Please indicate if there has been any change in your shortness of breath by choosing one of the following options. Has your shortness of breath been:
>
> 1. Worse
> 2. About the same
> 3. Better

If patients, using this transitional scale, stated they were worse, they were asked how much worse, and response options from the following seven-point scale were offered:

> 1. Almost the same, hardly any worse at all
> 2. A little worse
> 3. Somewhat worse
> 4. Moderately worse
> 5. A good deal worse
> 6. A great deal worse
> 7. A very great deal worse

If patients stated that they were better, they were asked how much better using a similar response option substituting the word "better" for "worse." Thus, a 15-point global ratings scale was created for changes in dyspnea, fatigue, and emotional function ranging from −7 (a great deal worse), through 0 (no change), to +7 (a great deal better). These global ratings provided a means for interpreting changes in scores obtained from the Chronic Respiratory Questionnaire and Chronic Heart Failure Questionnaire.

Using this rating system, Jaeschke and colleagues define the minimally important difference as the smallest difference in a health-related quality of life score that patients perceive as a change which would require a modification in their treatment (Jaeschke et al., 1991). In a study of patients with either chronic airflow limitation or congestive heart failure, global ratings of change for selected health characteristics resulted in a change score of 0.5 per question. This score represented the minimally important difference.

One problem that might be encountered in interpreting the net effects, regardless of the metric, is the presence of either floor or ceiling effects. *Floor effects* occur when respondents report very low scores for a given assessment at baseline. Bindman and colleagues (1990) found that low baseline scores prevented the identification of larger decreases in health over the six-month interval. A similar phenomenon may occur at the top of a health-related quality of life measure. When respondents are at the highest point of the measure, there is no room for improvement over time. This is referred to as the *ceiling effect*. With both effects, the net difference before and after treatment or between two treatment alternatives may be artificially low. In this case, the cost–effectiveness ratio reported as part of the Health Resource Allocation Strategy will be higher than expected. Distortion in the ratio due to ceiling and floor effects can be avoided by selecting a measure of health-related quality of life appropriate for the purpose of measurement and the population in which it is being used.

In addition to statistical models and direct assessment of change, a third interpretation of health effects is based on comparison with results from other studies in which the same instruments were used. This method of establishing meaning for different outcome measures is very similar to those used in calibrating various physiologic measuring devices commonly used in medicine today, such as the sphygmomanometer. This approach requires studying large data bases with information on diverse populations. The data bases must contain both health-related quality of life scores and clinically familiar measures. The National Health and Nutrition Examination Survey developed by the U.S. National Center for Health Statistics is one source of such information (Kovar, 1989).

Private data bases that assess health-related quality of life on a wide range of patients are now being developed. Paul Ellwood (1990) is spearheading the development of the Outcomes Management System. A similar data base was developed during the course of the Medical Outcomes Study (Tarlov et al., 1989). Both of these data bases, which are limited to primary care practices, may be made publicly available for purposes of conducting research and for interpreting health-related quality of life data. If they continue to grow and become widely available, these data bases promise to be useful in interpreting health status outcomes among selected segments of the U.S. population, that is, persons seeking medical care.

One method for improving the interpretation of health status outcomes is to standardize calculation of the effect size using a statistic proposed by Glass (1976). The resulting "scale-free index" is independent of the unit of measurement associated with particular measures or instruments used in different studies. Standardized effect size (ES) is based on the ratio of the difference between pre- and postintervention means and the preintervention standard error as follows:

$$ES = \frac{m_2 - m_1}{s}$$

where

m_1 = preintervention mean
m_2 = postintervention mean
s = preintervention standard error

Kazis and colleagues (1989) pooled data from several studies of arthritis patients and calculated effect size statistics. Following the advice of Cohen (1977), these investigators proposed the following benchmarks: an effect size of 0.20 or less would be considered small and one of 0.80, large. These guidelines were used to interpret changes in health status obtained from the components of the Arthritis Impact Measurement Scales and clinical measures, such as grip strength and platelet count.

Different methods can be used for determining the health effect due to a single intervention or to a set of different alternatives. Effect size statistics are particularly useful for understanding health status change that is measured in some unit that is not expressed in biologically meaningful terms. The standardized effect size statistic was developed to provide an index independent of the original unit of measurement, permitting analyses of results obtained from different studies. Standardized effect sizes, however, are unsuitable denominators in a cost–effectiveness ratio, because it is difficult to interpret the meaning of this unit of measurement.

For health status change that can be expressed in either life years or years of healthy life—that is, a measure that incorporates an intuitively meaningful unit such as duration of life—effect size interpretation using estimation procedures or global ratings of change is less necessary. The intuitively meaningful interpretation that can be given to such measures makes them very suitable for use in ratio comparisons of costs to outcomes.

Calculating the Cost–Utility Ratio

When calculating the cost–utility ratio for the Health Resource Allocation Strategy, net costs and net effects need to be determined for each alternative health intervention of interest. The cost–utility ratio is calculated by dividing the net costs by the net health effects. If the decision is to fund or not to fund a given health intervention, then average net costs and net effects are the data required for calculating the ratio. On the other hand, if the decision is how much a given intervention should be expanded or contracted, for example, by increasing or decreasing the number of individuals eligible to receive benefits, then the required data are the marginal health care costs and marginal health effects. Marginal costs and effects are also appropriate for use when deciding how to expand or contract health care coverage, for example, from one year to the next.

Regardless of whether the decision is based on average or on marginal data, the cost–utility ratio is calculated by dividing the relevant costs by the relevant effects. This ratio estimates the net costs of a given health intervention for a one-unit gain in health effect and can be expressed as follows:

$$R' = \frac{\sum c_i}{\sum e_i}$$

where

$\sum c_i$ = net costs
$\sum e_i$ = net effects

R' estimates the average net cost per gain in year of healthy life. The estimator

$$C'_R = RE = \frac{\sum c_i/n}{\sum e_i} E$$

gives the population total for costs when the total net effects for the population are known.

The large sample standard error for the cost–utility ratio, R', assuming simple random sampling, is then

$$se_R = N \left[\sum \frac{(c_i - Re_i)^2}{n(n-1)} \right]^{1/2} \times [1 - \Phi]^{1/2}$$

where

c_i	= costs for the ith individual
e_i	= effects for the ith individual
n	= number of individuals in the sample
N	= number of individuals in the population
Φ	= sampling fraction
$[1 - \Phi]^{1/2}$	= finite population correction term

In expressing the ratio estimator and its standard error in this form we assume that the ratio of health costs to health effects is relatively constant over the population of interest and that the total health effects for the population are known (Snedecor and Cochran, 1989).

The foregoing formulas for estimating the cost–utility ratio and its standard error are appropriate for evaluating alternative health care interventions in which both costs and benefits accrue over a short time period such as in the treatment of acute conditions. Acute bronchitis, common cold, dental conditions, nausea and vomiting, eye and ear infections, and other acute conditions, generally last three months or less. The use of antibiotics and decongestants to ameliorate symptoms and acute conditions result in both costs and health effects.

Costs and benefits that accrue over a longer time horizon need to be discounted to determine the present value. Although discounting costs has been a readily accepted practice in health services research, the validity of discounting health effects has been questioned. Some analysts argue that health effects are not subject to the same market forces as money. Berwick et al. (1980) showed that use of discounting is important in health decisions that involve time. In an analysis of a cholesterol screening program for children, these researchers found that programs will be judged more cost effective if they are postponed until the benefits are realized closer to the time of the intervention. Based on these results and those from similar studies, discounting of health effects is now accepted by most health services researchers.

With health interventions that are expected to last for a number of years the discounted net costs and discounted net effects are used in calculating the cost–utility ratio. That is, Σc_i and Σe_i represent discounted net costs and effects. Typical examples of interventions in which time is an important factor are those that have been developed for use with chronic conditions. In addition to the cholesterol screening program for children, another example of a health intervention with long-term costs and effects is the neonatal intensive care unit (NICU). Benefits are expected to accrue throughout the lifetime of the individual who received care in the NICU, perhaps 40 years or longer.

Interpreting the Cost–Utility Ratio

Because both the numerator and denominator of the cost–utility ratio are in net terms, the cost per year of healthy life indicates the cost per unit of health effect of switching from one alternative to another. A low ratio is considered more cost effective than a high ratio. A single ratio by itself, however, is not very helpful. It is the ranking of ratios for various health interventions in terms of cost per year of healthy life gained that gives the decision maker insight about how to best allocate resources to get the largest health benefit (Detsky and Naglie, 1990).

When net effects are expressed in terms of years of healthy life gained, three essential treatment impacts are included in the measure: (1) number of life years added by the intervention; (2) improvements in health status due to the intervention; and (3) any side effects attributable to the intervention. Net effects are the gains in life years and health improvements minus the side effects (Weinstein and Stason, 1977a; Russell, 1987). No health-related quality of life measure other than years of healthy life gained combines improvements due to the intervention, side effects, and life years gained.

To the extent that the health effects calculated for the sample on which the cost–utility ratio is based represent those of the total population of relevant stakeholders, the interpretation of the ratio is the incremental costs incurred for gaining an additional year of healthy life. When all relevant stakeholders are included in the estimate, the calculated ratio represents the best estimate for the population, absent any other source of bias. If, however, the estimate of health effects is based on data from a group unrepresentative of the population of interest, then the ratio can be either artificially high or low. For example, if the sample is healthier than most persons who would receive a given alternative, then the health effects may be relatively large, resulting in a smaller cost–utility ratio.

Clinical trials of pharmacologic agents are one source of data on health-related quality of life which may be based on unrepresentative samples of persons with a given health condition or disease. This bias toward healthier subjects stems from the strict inclusion and exclusion criteria which are used in such studies. For example, in studying the cost effectiveness of auranofin for the treatment of rheumatoid arthritis, Thompson and colleagues (1988) reported that persons over 66 years of age, with severe rheumatoid arthritis and/or serious concomitant disease along with various other abnormalities, were excluded from consideration in this study. That is, persons who were reasonably healthy were selected for the trial. Yet, following approval from the U.S. Food and Drug Administration for treatment of persons with rheumatoid arthritis, the drug may be prescribed for persons who would have been excluded from the trial. If the health effect obtained in a clinical trial sample, for example, is larger than would result from the general population, then the cost–utility ratio will be artificially low. That is, the treatment will appear to be more cost effective than it actually is.

Theoretically, the sample on which cost–utility estimates are made may have greater dysfunction than persons to which the treatment may be applied; this is the converse of the preceding case. For example, in a sample drawn from a nursing home or other residential health care facility, a cost–utility ratio may be artificially large when compared to the effects of treatment on a noninstitutionalized population. This distortion will result if the change in net effect is smaller than would be obtained from a more representative population.

In practice, most ratios are presented as comparisons between alternative health interventions derived from different studies and settings. Ratios for diverse interventions, perhaps calculated from diverse sources, require standardization of underlying assumptions and methods for accurate interpretation of the information presented. The next section presents a standardized format for comparing costs and outcomes from different studies based on techniques used in meta-analysis.

META-ANALYSIS AND THE COSTS AND OUTCOMES COMPARISON

Meta-analysis is a formal set of statistical techniques for combining results of previous research to test for treatment effects. This form of analysis has been proposed as a systematic and rigorous method of reviewing and summarizing the results of a body of scientific literature (Hedges and Olkin, 1985). The Health Resource Allocation Strategy with its standardized unit of measurement—incremental cost per year of healthy life gained—is amenable for use with two types of meta-analysis. The first is when a decision maker needs to know if cost–utility ratios in various studies using the same (or different) interventions to treat the same disease yield the same (or different) results.

For example, different researchers may compare medical and surgical interventions for treatment of mild and severe angina. The resulting cost–utility ratios may show that surgical treatment is more cost effective for severe rather than for mild coronary artery disease. If health effects have been measured using the same classification system and preferences, then the analyst can test the alternative of no difference between cost–utility ratios. Studies by Weinstein and Stason (1982) and Williams (1985) found coronary artery bypass surgery to be more cost effective for severe than for mild coronary artery disease. Ratios obtained in these studies, however, cannot be directly compared, because different classification systems and preference weights have been used to assess health effects.

Although the hypotheses and methods used for comparing costs and outcomes for the same intervention fit those of meta-analysis, lack of information from the original studies may make formal analyses difficult. Most meta-analyses require information about standard errors of the estimates and specific information about statistical tests performed, for example, *t* tests or *F* ratios (Mullen, 1989; Laird and Mosteller, 1990). To date, most of the studies that have calculated ratios of cost per year of healthy life gained have failed to include information about their statistical properties.

The second type of meta-analysis of cost–utility ratios involves the relative ranking of ratios across different interventions. This is an example of evaluating the relative effectiveness between alternatives for a diverse set of interventions. In this case, the analyst evaluates the ranking of the ratios rather than whether there is a difference between mean ratios for the same health problem or intervention. In these rankings, each estimate of cost per year of healthy life gained has been derived from separate studies. These studies may differ in target populations assessed, design and type of data, and purpose of assessment. For example, Torrance and Zipursky (1984) studied the cost effectiveness of antepartum treatment of primiparae and multiparae; Boyle and colleagues (1983) conducted a retrospective analysis of neonatal intensive care of low birth weight infants; and Churchill and colleagues (1984) studied hospital hemodialysis. Cost–utility ratios from these diverse studies can be used to form a cost and outcomes table. These studies are similar, however, in that each uses the same outcome measure, years of healthy life calculated with the same classification and preference weights, namely, the Health Utilities Index. That is, the years of healthy life measure used to calculate the cost–utility ratios is based on a single measurement system.

Years of healthy life that are obtained from different classification systems and preferences are not comparable. This lack of comparability can be illustrated by comparing the preference weights for similar function levels in the Disability/Distress Index (DDI) and Quality of Well-Being (QWB) Scale classification systems (Appendix II). For unable to perform major role activity in the DDI (level V-A), the weight is 0.946; for the QWB, assuming no other dysfunction, the weight is 0.894. If other dysfunctions were present, for example, limitation in physical activity and mobility, and if symptoms were also present, then the difference between the DDI and QWB scores would be even greater. Not only is it theoretically invalid to compare cost–utility ratios that are based on different approaches to calculating years of healthy life but also, as this example suggests, such comparison may lead to serious problems of interpretation.

The Oregon Plan (Kitzhaber, 1989; Hadorn, 1991) overcame this problem by using the same classification system and an associated set of preferences. In addition, this standard approach was applied across all interventions or treatment–condition pairs and across all age groups within the target population.

Light and Pillemer (1984) developed a three-step method that can be adapted for costs and outcomes analysis. The first step is to formulate the precise question being asked of the costs and outcomes table. In the context of the Health Resource Allocation Strategy, two broad aims of the costs and outcomes table are to evaluate existing programs and to allocate resources within a budget constraint for rationing. Within each use of the table, the purpose may be made more specific. For example, the analyst may wish to evaluate only those existing health interventions that use surgery or to ration resources selectively, for example, for elderly persons.

The second step is to select studies to include in the analysis. Studies can be selected from published or unpublished sources or both. Some analysts prefer to use only published sources, because these have been peer reviewed and are therefore presumed to be of higher quality. On the other hand, analysts using only published materials may suffer from publication bias, since there is a tendency for only those studies with favorable results or significant findings to be published (Mullen, 1989).

The third step is to generalize the results of the information. Two factors must be considered:

1. Were the study groups representative of the population of interest?
2. Did the study design include comparability of treatments and length of follow-up?

Although costs and outcomes studies usually contain sufficient information to compare ratios, the usual presentation of findings does not allow analysts to discuss or interpret the generalizability of findings.

To overcome this limitation, analysts need to expand the existing format to increase the amount of information presented in the costs and outcomes table. In addition to a description of the health intervention or program, the costs and outcomes table should specify the sociodemographic and health characteristics of the study population. Closely related is specification of the population that is *expected* to benefit from the program. Table 11.2 gives the format and recommended information to be included in the expanded costs and outcomes table.

Each row in this table identifies a major component of cost-effectiveness analysis

Table 11.2 Format and information for expanded costs and outcomes table

Intervention	Medical, surgical or other health service	Special features of the intervention	
Study group	Age, ethnicity, gender	Health status	Total number of persons affected by intervention
Design	Pre- or postcomparison	Clinical trial (randomized, double-blind)	Community-based intervention
Net effects	Method of measuring preferences	Source of preferences	Classification system used
Net costs	Source of cost data	Special assumptions or imputations	
Cost/years of healthy life gained	Discount rate used	Time period for discounting	Confidence intervals

that should be included in a costs and outcomes table; information in each row illustrates the type of detail that the analysts should consider supplying in the table. For example, in specifying the intervention the analyst should specify the type of intervention, whether surgical, medical or some other service, and special features that distinguish it from similar, and possibly competing, interventions. Specifying characteristics of the study design and of the study group—for example age, ethnicity, gender, health status, and total number of persons at risk—are important for determining the generalizability of the calculated costs and outcomes ratios. Preferably the detailed information will be displayed in the body of the table. For some purposes or in the case of very detailed information, however, it may be necessary to either use footnotes or include a technical appendix with the costs and outcomes table.

From this, the policy analyst can estimate not only the cost per year of healthy life gained but also the total cost of the program. If health effects for the population are known, then the decision maker can estimate the total costs from the relationship of $C'_R = RE$ given earlier. If population effects are estimated, then the analyst can do sensitivity analyses to assess the effect that different estimates for population health effects have on the total cost of each alternative.

Estimation of costs and outcomes often requires that the analyst make compromises. For example, direct costs for some resources may not be available. In a study designed to assess the costs of operating a rheumatology clinic in England, Thould (1985) reported that the costs of medical and surgical supplies in an outpatient department could not be determined because this clinic served both medical and rheumatology patients. In addition, indirect costs may also need to be approximated. In economic analysis of a program designed for early detection of prostatic cancer, Carlsson et al. (1990) derived estimates for travel costs to and from the health care center by assuming that study participants drove their own cars to the center; the cost for this travel was computed based on the reimbursement rate used for civil servants.

When important information on costs is unavailable, analysts may develop estimates based on assumptions. The study by Carlsson and colleagues (1990) illustrates the types of assumptions and imputation of information that may be used. In some cases the analyst may decide to omit selected cost data from the analysis. This is most likely when the missing information does not contribute significantly to the overall estimate of costs for the intervention. A technical note that accompanies the costs and outcomes table should be included with the analysis explaining about missing data and methods for dealing with them in the analysis.

The definition of health states and preferences used to estimate years of healthy life should also be clearly stated in any costs and outcomes table. This information may appear in the table title or as a technical footnote to the table. Specifying the definition of states and weights indicates whether measures of health effects used in constructing a costs and outcomes table are comparable.

Another technical point that affects the interpretation of the data in the costs and outcomes table is the discount rate, which affects the stream of costs and benefits. Thus, the discount rate should also be explicitly stated for both costs and benefits and separately for each program. Unfortunately, most published studies omit data needed to allow a meta-analyst to recalculate the costs and outcomes ratios using discount rates that differ from those in the original study.

The year that the data were collected should be noted in the costs and outcomes ranking. If the costs are adjusted to account for inflation, the year to which the adjustment is made should be clearly stated. Published data can be converted to constant monetary units with the information provided in the costs and outcomes study.

This discussion of technical requirement for the costs and outcomes table indicates that the analyst must pay attention to many details about the data and assumptions used. Meaningful interpretation of the data in the table hinges on a thorough understanding of the components used in developing the table. The presentation of the table also can also enhance the interpretation of results.

Presentation of Findings

In addition to representativeness of costs and outcomes data, presentation of the ratios is important to the overall acceptance of results. We recommend that the format of the costs and outcomes table include more than just the name of the intervention and the cost–utility ratio. Rather, the table contents should be expanded to include information that enhances the generalizability of results. The expanded table, like its abbreviated forerunners, must be clearly laid out and easy to read; the information can be readily interpreted; and the information is essential for decision making.

Although data on comparative health outcomes and costs is usually presented in tabular format, the information can be presented graphically as seen in Figure 11.3. Hypothetical estimates of confidence intervals have been added to indicate how variability in the cost per year of healthy life can be plotted. In Figure 11.3 confidence intervals for the ratios for coronary artery bypass graft (CABG) surgery of left main disease and treatment of severe hypertension overlap, indicating no statistical difference between the ratios for these two interventions.

Often, graphs such as Figure 11.3 are preferable to tables; they can convey more information in the same space and can be interpreted more easily. Figure 11.3 illustrates another important point about graphical presentation: to communicate effectively, a graph cannot be too cluttered or artistic. Graphic presentations are more likely suitable for presentation to groups of decision makers than are detailed tables. Thus, in

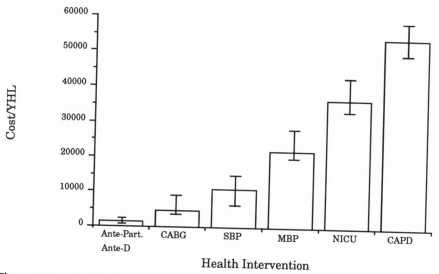

Figure 11.3 Graphical presentation of comparative health outcomes and costs:

Ante-Part.	= antepartum
Anti-D	= antibody in the blood
CABG	= coronary artery bypass graft left main disease
SBP	= severe hypertension
MBP	= mild hypertension
NICU	= neonatal intensive care unit
CAPD	= continuous ambulatory peritoneal dialysis

Note that confidence intervals are estimates. *Source:* Torrance, 1986.

presenting data from a costs and outcome table, the format needs to be appropriate for both the audience and the setting.

The next section translates these general principles of calculating, interpreting, and presenting cost–utility ratios into the two major applications of the Health Resource Allocation Strategy, medical effectiveness evaluations of existing programs and the rationing of health care resources.

COST PER YEAR OF HEALTHY LIFE FOR RESOURCE ALLOCATION

The cost per year of healthy life gained offers a powerful approach to address the main issues facing health care decision makers. By summarizing the tradeoffs between costs and health outcomes in a composite form, the ratio provides the decision maker with a statistic that addresses both. This summary allows the decision maker to simultaneously consider both costs and outcomes as he or she works to identify a set of interventions that will yield the socially optimal allocation.

Costs and Outcomes for Medical Effectiveness Evaluations

To develop a costs and outcomes table for identifying and eliminating ineffective health interventions, the decision maker must first decide the scope of the evaluation. Are all health interventions to be evaluated, or only those interventions that are related to a specific issue, such as health promotion or medical technology?

Once the purpose for doing a cost and outcomes analysis has been decided, the analyst selects the studies to incorporate in the costs and outcomes table. In choosing studies, the analyst needs to be cautious about using data collected from prior years that may not reflect current medical practice or costs. As a rule of thumb, any study over ten years old should be carefully scrutinized. The rapid change in medical technology since 1970 has affected both production costs and outcomes. Analysts need to account for innovation for each intervention analyzed. Technology transfer with associated cost reductions and other economies may result when a technology becomes more widely used.

The selected studies are then summarized using a standard format such as Table 11.2. During the process of compiling the costs and outcomes table, the analyst may identify additional concerns, for example, certain interventions may have been overlooked. If possible, missing information should be added before the summary is completed.

Also, the analyst needs to carefully review each study for comparability of assumptions and their impacts on costs and outcomes. For instance, what components were used to calculate costs? If the study includes social costs, the analyst should note whether shadow prices were used and whether they are based on the same wage rates. Similar attention to detail is needed to compare health effects. Assumptions about both costs and outcomes should be clearly stated as part of the analysis, that is, in the text that accompanies the costs and outcomes table.

Rank ordering of cost–utility ratios in the completed tables indicates the relative cost effectiveness of the interventions. Standard errors associated with the ratios indicate whether any two ratios are statistically different or whether any observed difference is due to chance alone. If the evaluation of medical effectiveness requires multiple comparisons between ratios within the same table, the significance level may need to be adjusted by the number of comparisons to be made (Snedecor and Cochran, 1989).

Analysis of existing studies designed to estimate the cost effectiveness of a variety of programs has been the most common use of the Health Resource Allocation Strategy to date. We advocate the use of meta-analytic techniques in compiling the costs and outcomes table. These methods will add rigor to the use of existing studies for evaluating existing health programs. Although lack of estimates of variability for performing statistical tests of significance may make it impossible to do meta-analyses of some costs and outcomes studies currently available, this limitation will be less restrictive in the future. The needed data are likely to be collected and reported in studies now under way.

Costs and Outcomes for Rationing Health Care

Another category of health policy options consists of making decisions as to which set of interventions will be funded on an annual basis. This type of option is most appropriate for health care systems that are characterized by a public decision-making unit with central authority over the delivery of health care services. In the United States, the Medicaid and Medicare programs are examples of centrally controlled health care delivery. In countries such as Great Britain, national health insurance systems provide this central decision-making body.

In centrally planned health insurance systems, a major focus of the decision process is whether to support all of a program or not. This fund–no-fund decision is based on the need to allocate scarce resources over a wide range of competing programs. Thus, data needed for allocating resources for the purpose of rationing health care require a broader coverage of health programs and population than do data used for evaluating existing programs.

Ratios for purposes of rationing must be based on national data collected in a population survey specifically designed for this purpose. This standardization will minimize inconsistencies between data collected on diverse populations, with different assumptions, and with different units of measurement. The study group and design, the classification system and source of preferences, and other methodologies would be the same for all health interventions.

With a standard data base, evaluations of costs and outcomes of various health interventions are bound to be easier to analyze and interpret than if a series of disparate studies are combined in a meta-analytic framework. The consistency of data is important when making major decisions such as determining which procedures will be supported and which will not be supported. Tough decisions involved in rationing health care demand the best data. The ideal situation is that a collection of ad hoc studies not be used to decide who shall live and who shall die.

In ranking the cost–utility ratios for rationing the important consideration is whether ratios are above or below a given budget threshold. The position of most ratios will be clear. For those near the budget line, however, it may be uncertain whether they are below the threshold and thus cost effective or above the threshold and thus are cost ineffective. For these borderline ratios, confidence limits can be used to indicate their position relative to the budget line.

For example, suppose the budget had been set at $5,500. Then, from an analysis without regard to the standard error, a ratio for heart transplantation of $5,200 would appear to be cost effective. However, by setting 95 percent confidence limits about this ratio using the appropriate standard error, we might see that costs per year of healthy life can range from $4,600 to $5,900. The upper range lies well above the designated budget constraint. This suggests that heart transplantation may not be cost effective, given a budget of $5,500. If the decision is made to include heart transplantation in the set of funded interventions without regard to variability in the ratio, then the decision could result in a cost overrun at the end of the budget cycle.

Whether the ranking of costs and outcomes is used for evaluation of medical effectiveness or for rationing, the analysis serves as input to the policy process. The ranking that results from applying Steps 2 through 7 of the Health Resource Allocation Strategy is not the final step. Rather, this ordering is submitted to the health decision makers for review and readjustment according to values of the stakeholders in the decision.

REVISING THE RANKING

The last step of the Health Resource Allocation Strategy consists of a sociopolitical assessment of the preliminary costs and outcomes rankings for all the interventions under consideration. Stakeholders may challenge these rankings based on either (1) the validity of the estimates contained in the cost–utility ratios; or (2) on conflict with what is known about prevailing community values. In this step decision makers gather information for use in the final ordering of health services priorities. This community review results in a reordering of the set of interventions to be supported within a given budget constraint that is more closely linked with community consensus on the values and goals of health care.

The hypothetical data in Table 11.3 illustrate readjustment of the rankings and determination of a final recommended order more in conformity with society's viewpoint. In this table, a set of health interventions has been ranked in ascending order according to costs per years of healthy life gained (column 3); the ratios have been calculated using the methods described in Steps 2–7 of the Health Resource Allocation Strategy. Additional costs and years of healthy life have been estimated for each intervention compared to the status quo, or "do nothing" alternative (columns 1 and 2). The lowest cost–utility ratios are those for preventive interventions such as immunizations and prenatal screening. The highest ratios are observed for surgeries associated with chronic diseases such as breast cancer and end-stage kidney and liver disease. With a budget of $2,600,000, interventions with costs per year of healthy life ratios of 50:50 or lower will be funded. Interventions with ratios higher than this are considered cost ineffective and will not receive support or be included in a basic package of health services benefits. This ranking yields a total of 649,100 years of healthy life gained (column 8).

Adjusting the Rankings

Using these data, we can examine the impact of adjusting the rankings according to stakeholder challenges to the costs and outcomes formula. Suppose that stakeholders concerned about the availability of neonatal intensive care units question the validity of the ranking shown in Table 11.3 on the basis of the costs of coronary artery bypass graft surgery relative to those for the NICU. These stakeholders argue that the average cost of CABG is too low and that the number of people at risk (column 4) is too high. Further, the NICU stakeholders argue that the average cost of NICU is too high and that the estimated number of persons needing this care is also too high.

These stakeholders submit new estimates (which should be supported by data) on both costs and numbers at risk for needing both procedures. The costs per year of healthy life are recalculated for these two procedures using the new information. This results in a second ranking, Table 11.4, in which NICU is determined to be cost effective. The new ratio for CABG, 125 instead of 18 (column 3), puts it below the budget constraint. The revised ranking, which is more socially acceptable than the original, results, however, in a slightly lower number of additional years of healthy life, 646,200 (column 8).

This same challenge to the preliminary ranking might be made on the basis that the prevailing community value is on the sanctity of life for newborns rather than on the extension and quality of life for adults needing bypass surgery. This controversial challenge, politically correct to some and not to others, is unlikely to be accompanied by data unless data on stakeholder and community values are available from Step 1 of the Strategy. The evidence that exists on community values and priorities for health services should be submitted with the challenge to the ranking based on cost–utility ratios. Without data on community priorities, the challenge should be treated as qualitative evidence, much like that of a legislative hearing that elicits the testimony of

Table 11.3 Preliminary ranking of costs and outcomes for evaluating existing health interventions

Intervention	Average costs (1)	Average years of healthy life gained (2)	Cost per year of healthy life gained (3)	Number at risk (4)	Total costs (in 1,000s) (5)	Years of healthy life gained (6)	Cumulative costs (in 1,000s) (7)	Cumulative years of healthy life gained (8)
Childhood immunization	100	50	2	2,000	200	100,000	200	100,000
Influenza immunization	100	40	3	7,300	730	292,000	930	392,000
Prenatal screening	200	40	5	3,100	620	124,000	1,550	516,000
Smoking cessation counselling	240	40	6	3,050	732	122,000	2,282	638,000
Rehabilitative exercise	120	12	10	150	18	1,800	2,300	639,800
Coronary artery bypass surgery	180	10	18	750	135	7,500	2,435	647,300
Breast cancer chemotherapy	400	10	40	50	20	500	2,455	647,800
Total hip replacement	1,000	10	100	100	100	1,000	2,555	648,800
Hospital hemodialysis	1,500	10	150	30	45	300	2,600	649,100
Corrective heart valve surgery	3,400	20	170	145	493	2,900	3,093	652,000
Neonatal intensive care	3,600	20	180	450	1,620	9,000	4,713	661,000
Liver transplant	4,000	10	200	15	60	150	4,773	661,150

Note: ——— indicates budget constraint.

Table 11.4 Final ranking of costs and outcomes for evaluating existing health interventions

Intervention	Average costs (1)	Average years of healthy life gained (2)	Cost per year of healthy life gained (3)	Number at risk (4)	Total costs (in 1,000s) (5)	Years of healthy life gained (6)	Cumulative costs (in 1,000s) (7)	Cumulative years of healthy life gained (8)
Childhood immunization	100	50	2	2,000	200	100,000	200	100,000
Influenza immunization	100	40	3	7,300	730	292,000	930	392,000
Prenatal screening	200	40	5	3,100	620	124,000	1,550	516,000
Smoking cessation counselling	240	40	6	3,050	732	122,000	2,282	638,000
Rehabilitative exercise	120	12	10	150	18	1,800	2,300	639,800
Breast cancer chemotherapy	400	10	40	50	20	500	2,320	640,300
Neonatal intensive care	900	20	45	150	135	3,000	2,455	643,300
Corrective heart valve surgery	1,000	20	50	145	145	2,900	2,600	646,200
-------	-------	-------	-------	-------	-------	-------	-------	-------
Total hip replacement	1,000	10	100	100	100	1,000	2,700	647,200
Coronary artery bypass surgery	1,000	8	125	500	500	4,000	3,200	651,200
Hospital hemodialysis	1,500	10	150	30	45	300	3,245	651,500
Liver transplant	2,000	10	200	15	30	150	3,275	651,650

Note: ------- indicates budget constraint.

different interested stakeholders. All challenges should be recorded and presented to the decision makers, who produce the final list of priority health services.

The Final Decision Process: A List of Priorities

Analysts and administrators involved in the allocation process recommend the revised set of cost–utility rankings to legislatively appointed policymakers or the legislators themselves, depending on the decision context. These legislated decision makers are the final arbitrators of the services to be included within the limits of available funding or in a benefit package of health services to be made available to stakeholders. In the final priority-setting process, decision makers should have the following information: (1) the revised ranking of cost-per-year-of-healthy-life-gained ratios for all the alternative courses of action in the decision process; (2) the total amount of outlays associated with each intervention based on numbers of persons at risk; (3) a record of stakeholder challenges to the cost–utility ranking; (4) information on community values and goals elicited in the initial step of the Strategy; and (5) a defined budget constraint.

The final decision makers, perhaps a standing congressional committee or a specially appointed body with legislative authority, use this information to produce the final list of health services included in the funding package. These decision makers will use the traditional methods of negotiation and bargaining in using the available information to assign priorities. Any revisions to the priority list based on the costs and outcomes comparisons, however, should be publicly identified to indicate any changes in the rank order made by these decision makers. Stakeholders should be able to compare any revisions to the ranking based on the judgment of decision makers with the ranking based on costs and outcomes data. In order to permit these comparisons, the final list of priorities should contain the same set of identifiable alternatives and specify their ranking from the cost and outcomes comparisons. The criteria used to make these judgmental revisions, ideally community values and goals, should also be specified with publication of the final list.

Effect of Allocating Resources across Special Populations

Thus far, we have been discussing the costs and outcomes comparison as if there is just one population to be served. Yet if one can identify subsets of the population, for example, on the basis of age or gender, then it is possible to develop a ranking of interventions for a selected group. One group which is singled out on the basis of age to receive special attention in the United States is the older adult population. The Medicare program provides health care coverage for almost all persons aged 65 years and over in the United States. In this case, the interventions included in the costs and outcomes table would change.

For example, from Table 11.3, the childhood vaccines, smoking cessation, liver transplantation, and neonatal intensive care programs can be considered inappropriate for an elderly population. The other interventions may be more or less relevant in terms of the population at risk. For example, among persons 65 years and over, fewer coronary artery bypass grafts would be expected than among younger adults. Yet among the fewer done, the average cost per year of healthy life would be expected to be higher due to possibilities for complications, longer lengths of stay, and fewer number of years of healthy life gained. Adding the same budget constraint would result in a different set of interventions being funded and a different number of years of healthy life provided.

Selected populations other than the elderly can also be identified, for example, women and children and people with disabilities. In the United States, these groups are targets for various income redistribution programs. Women and children who meet minimum income criteria are eligible to receive benefits in the Aid for Dependent Children Program (AFDC). People with disabilities may qualify for coverage under the Social Security Act and the Medicare program. These are examples of discrimination in the allocation of health care resources. If the interventions in Table 11.3 were singled out for women and children and people with disabilities, as we did for older adults, two different rankings of interventions and years of healthy life would result.

This differentiation stems from the fact that the costs and outcomes for each health intervention are influenced by the case mix of consumers who are eligible to receive the intervention. Using the data in Table 11.3, of the 2,000 persons who would benefit from childhood vaccines (column 4) almost all can be assumed to be children. With a homogeneous group, the additional costs and years of healthy life will not change appreciably from the information shown in this table if the resource allocation were restricted to a subpopulation that consisted of women and children.

On the other hand, corrective heart valve surgery would affect a wide range of individuals, children, people with disabilities, as well as the older adults. The severity of the problems to be corrected would vary within each group. Hence, the cost of the corrective surgery intervention as well as the additional years of healthy life are affected by the case mix. In general, the more severe the cases, the more costly they are, with a lower return in terms of years of healthy life gained.

The result is that when allocation is restricted to special target populations, for example, on the basis of age and gender, even if the budget constraint is not reduced, a set of interventions that is less cost effective than if done over the total population will be funded. Very often, the budget constraint will also be reduced. With fewer resources to allocate, even though the number of individuals in the selected, or target, population is smaller than the total population that might benefit from the allocation, the allocation will result in fewer years of healthy life gained at relatively higher costs.

Policy options can also be designed to identify ineffective or inefficient health care services. These options are of particular prominence in decentralized health care systems such as that in the United States. The major distinction for the policymaker between the centralized and decentralized health care systems is the type of option available. In a centralized health care system, as noted, the policymaker can decide which programs to fund. In the decentralized system, the option takes the form of recommendations and guidelines.

Use of the Health Resource Allocation Strategy to identify ineffective health programs proceeds as above. That is, the preliminary ranking programs are arrayed according to their cost–utility ratios from low to high. Stakeholders and policymakers review the ranking to identify those programs that might be replaced with more efficient ones. For example, one ratio might indicate that hospital hemodialysis is three times more costly per year of healthy life than is home dialysis. In this case, policymakers might recommend that home dialysis be the method of choice.

In this chapter we have discussed the last step of the Health Resource Allocation Strategy, namely, the calculation and ranking of cost–utility ratios and the adjustment of these rankings to meet social goals. This ratio along with meta-analytic techniques for summarizing information contained in various cost–effectiveness studies have been discussed in the context of two broad applications of the comparisons of costs and outcomes, evaluation and rationing. To assist the decision maker in using these data, we have proposed an expanded costs and outcomes table. With the Strategy fully developed and systematic methods for analysis described, we can now proceed to discuss the use of the Health Resource Allocation Strategy in the context of three policy applications that will be of major importance in the coming decades.

12

Preventing Disease and Promoting Health: Goals for the Nation

Federal initiatives in setting national health objectives were initially predicated on the notions that greater attention to known disease prevention practices (for example, controlling hypertension to prevent stroke) and to practices that showed promise for prevention (for example, dietary modification to reduce risk of heart disease) would result in a healthier population. In the short run, however, the effects of a prevention or promotion program may actually result in a worsened health-related quality of life. Kaplan et al. (1984) found that staying on a prescribed diet or taking medicine, in the absence of other health problems, reduces health-related quality of life by about 11 percent. Yet in the long run, following such a disease prevention program has been shown to lead to a greater quantity of life (Taylor et al., 1987). These examples illustrate the importance of considering quality and quantity of life together—years of healthy life—to evaluate interventions designed to promote health and prevent disease.

This chapter discusses the use of the Health Resource Allocation Strategy in setting prevention and promotion priorities. Many of the examples focus on elderly persons because the percentage of the population over 65 years of age is expected to increase during the next decade, an increase that is expected to increase health care costs. The first section discusses the historical background of monitoring health levels to set prevention and promotion goals in the United States; the second section discusses the objectives and goals that decision makers have targeted for action over the coming decade. We emphasize those priority areas in *Healthy People 2000* that call for the health status objective to be measured in terms of years of healthy life. The third section discusses data sources and methods for monitoring progress for meeting the specified targets. Finally, we present estimates of costs and outcomes for prevention strategies and discuss the controversy about whether health promotion and disease prevention strategies can be used to control health care costs.

NATIONAL HEALTH LEVELS AND GOALS

The overall aim of health promotion and disease prevention activities is to improve health and reduce disease. To accomplish this, decision makers need to know both current population health and disease levels and effective promotion and prevention strategies. These strategies are often expressed in conjunction with a target level to be reached by a specific date. For example, the 1990 objective for death rates for motor vehicle accidents among children under 15 was set at 5.5 deaths per 100,000 children.

To identify national levels, analysts generally examine trends in health status measures such as mortality and disability days. These data may be organized by sociodemographic comparisons to identify groups at greater risk or by health condition or disease category to determine the burden placed on society. Traditionally, for example, mortality data have been used to plot the impact of selected diseases on national populations over time and to identify those diseases that seem to have increasing burdens. Since 1960, deaths attributed to cardiovascular disorders or diabetes mellitus have declined, whereas cancer deaths have risen over the same interval. Such information is important for making health policy decisions targeted to improving overall health using available resources.

Although mortality statistics in the United States can be traced back to colonial days, the compilation of national morbidity statistics is primarily a twentieth-century practice (Lawrence, 1976). Early in this century, public health officials experimented by using community-based health surveys to provide information on morbidity and disability (Goldberger et al., 1918). These surveys were designed to identify the causes of pellagra in rural villages in South Carolina. They formed the model for the first general population health survey, the Hagerstown Morbidity Survey, which was designed to collect information on all of the illnesses observed in a general population using continuous observation (Sydenstricker, 1925).

The first National Health Survey conducted in the United States in 1935–36 also used this methodology. Until they were superseded 20 years later, the data collected in this survey of about 750,000 families were used extensively by health decision makers. The need for current information on national health status led to enactment of the 1956 National Health Survey Act, which was intended to ensure that community-level information on morbidity and disability was available for policymaking. This act established a household interview survey, later named the National Health Interview Survey, for collecting information on the amount, distributions, and effects of illness and disability in the United States (Lawrence, 1976).

In 1960, the National Health Survey was combined with the National Office of Vital Statistics to create the National Center for Health Statistics (NCHS). Over the past three decades, NCHS has designed a number of different data systems and surveys to provide information on topics such as the extent and nature of illness and disability of the population in the United States, the impact of illness and disability on the economy and on other aspects of population well-being, determinants of health, and health care costs and financing (Pearce, 1981; Kovar, 1989).

The use of national data for monitoring trends and setting health goals had been informal until the passage of a 1974 law (Public Law 93–353) mandating that the secretary of the Department of Health and Human Services (DHHS) submit to the U.S. Congress an annual report on the health of the United States population—a report called *Health: United States.*

The initial volume, published in 1975, described health levels in terms of cross-sectional comparisons between population subgroups. More recent volumes have shifted toward trend analyses. For example, the health status tables in the current volume show trends in infant mortality, death rates for leading causes of death, incidence and prevalence of selected illnesses, limitation of activity caused by chronic conditions, disability days, and self-assessed health status (National Center for Health Statistics, 1991a).

The move toward systematic data compilation for monitoring population health levels in the United States was given another boost by a 1977 task force convened to review and analyze health promotion and disease prevention activities of the Department of Health and Human Services. The need for this task force review was stimulated by a number of important publications linking the role of health promotion and disease prevention to improved health status (Lalonde, 1974; Fogarty, 1976; Institute of Medicine, 1978).

U.S. Framework for Health Promotion

The task force report (Departmental Task Force on Prevention, 1978) proposed an analytic framework targeted at three areas that influence health: lifestyle, environment, and services. Lifestyle choices that an individual makes can increase risk of health problems in a series of behavioral areas. Settings and sources of hazard in an individual's environment may increase the risk of health problems. For example, lead-based paint in homes has been found to be associated with mental retardation in children. Availability of preventive services can influence the incidence or course of preventable disease and conditions for an individual.

Strategies for improving health status within this framework were developed around the following three areas: health promotion activities, health protection activities, and personal preventive health services. Health promotion activities are behaviors that have been shown to have significant impact in health-related quality of life, for example, smoking and alcohol use. Programs designed to assist individuals in trading harmful for healthy behaviors are thought to lead to substantial reductions in mortality.

Health protection programs directed at various population groups are basic public health activities, for example, regulation and enforcement and infectious disease control. The aim of these activities is to reduce exposure to a number of sources of hazard such as drugs, motor vehicles, and firearms. Clinical preventive services incorporate an extensive array of procedures and services available from medical providers and other health practitioners, for example, immunization and screening tests. These services are designed to prevent disease or slow its development.

Although all of the identified lifestyle, environment, and services activities were important, the 1977 Task Force recognized that action priorities would need to be set. High priority was given to activities meeting the following criteria: (1) they were important contributors to disability or death; (2) they were most likely to respond to intervention; (3) they were underfunded but required a relatively small addition of resources to produce a relatively large health benefit; and (4) they were deemed to be important to society.

Goals and Objectives

The analytic framework, action strategies, and criteria for prioritizing health promotion and disease prevention activities that were detailed by the Task Force set the background for the U.S. Surgeon General's report, *Healthy People* (Department of Health, Education and Welfare [DHEW], 1979). This report identified health goals for five population subgroups. These subgroups were based on age and ranged from infants to

Table 12.1 National health promotion and disease prevention goals and targets for 1990

Goal	Target
Continue to improve infant health	Reduce infant mortality by at least 35%, to fewer than 9 deaths per 1,000 live births
Improve child health, foster optimal childhood development	Reduce deaths among children ages 1–14 by at least 20%, to fewer than 34 per 100,000
Improve the health and health habits of adolescents and young adults	Reduce deaths among people ages 15–24 by at least 20% to fewer than 93 per 100,000
Improve the health of adults	Reduce deaths among people ages 25–64 by at least 25% to fewer tan 400 per 100,000
Improve the health and quality of life for older adults	Reduce the average annual number of days of restricted activity due to acute and chronic conditions by 20% to fewer than 30 days per year for people aged 65 and older

Source: Department of Health, Education and Welfare, 1979.

older adults. The resulting national goals, as well as the targets for 1990, are presented in Table 12.1 for each of the subgroups.

By setting goals according to major life stages, the report takes into consideration that health risks are age-related. Diseases that affect young children are not, for the most part, major problems for adolescents. From adolescence through early adulthood, accidents and violence take the greatest toll. A few decades later these causes of death and ill health are superseded by chronic illnesses such as heart disease, stroke, and cancer. Among older adults, the concern is not so much with extending life (or reducing the risk of dying) but rather with improving the health-related quality of life of the remaining life years.

This life-stage orientation has been criticized as being misleading because many chronic diseases commonly regarded as adult health problems may begin earlier. Eating and exercise habits, as well as exposure to toxic agents, can affect the likelihood of developing disease many years later. The presence of risk factors at early ages, sometimes even in early childhood, suggests that health promotion and disease prevention need to be considered lifelong concerns. Despite the criticism of the life-stage orientation, the goals suggest that at each stage of life, different steps can be taken to improve health (DHEW, 1979).

In addition to goals related to the five major life stages, specific and quantified objectives for 15 priority areas were identified. They include high blood pressure control, family planning, pregnancy and infant health, immunization, sexually trans-mitted diseases, toxic agent control, occupational safety and health, accident preven-tion and injury control, fluoridation and dental health, surveillance and control of infectious diseases, smoking and health, misuse of alcohol and drugs, physical fitness and exercise, and control of stress and violent behavior (Department of Health and Human Services [DHHS], 1980). Specific objectives in each of these priority areas are thought to be necessary for meeting the five broad goals in *Healthy People*.

Goal-Setting Process

The objectives were set by a consensus process that involved input from more than 500 health professionals over a 12-month period. To turn ideas submitted by such a large number of experts into an action-oriented policy, the report set specific goals as policy targets. Specific topics were identified for attention if they could be addressed from a prevention context and if they were amenable to prevention-type intervention (DHEW, 1979). For example, hypertension is one health condition that can be controlled by weight loss or by reducing sodium and alcohol intake. Thus, the experts considered high blood pressure control as a possible policy target. After a review of the possible targets, a list of quantified targets were spelled out and proposed as operational targets for 1990 (DHHS, 1980).

Monitoring Progress

These goals and objectives have been monitored throughout the 1980s, and the progress toward meeting them has been published in the Prevention Profile (National Center for Health Statistics [NCHS], 1983, 1986, 1990). As reported in the 1990 Prevention Profile (NCHS, 1990), the infant mortality rate has decreased steadily since 1977. The five leading causes of infant death in 1987 were (1) congenital anomalies, (2) sudden infant death syndrome, (3) disorders relating to short gestation and unspecified low birth weight, (4) respiratory distress syndrome, and (5) affects of maternal complications of pregnancy. In 1989, the infant mortality rate was 9.8 deaths per 1,000 live births. New technologies for treating infants, especially respiratory distress syndrome, are being credited as the major reason for the decline in the death rate toward the 1990 goal (Sullivan, 1991).

The goal for children 1–14 years of age (fewer than 34 deaths per 100,000) was met by 1984. The rate has continued to decline since that time, reaching 33.3 deaths per 100,000 population in 1987. The major cause of deaths for children in this age group is "accidents and adverse effects." Within this category, motor vehicle crashes, drowning, fire and flames, and suffocation are the major causes of death. A partial explanation for the decline in deaths among children under 15 years of age is the decline in motor vehicle crashes that occurred from 1978 to 1987. During this interval, the death rate declined from 9 to 6.8 deaths per 100,000 population.

Death rates for adolescents and young adults from 15 to 24 years of age showed declines in the first half of the 1980s. In 1985, the rate was 95.9 deaths per 100,000. Since then, however, the rates have increased. In 1989, the death rate of 99.9 was 7.4 percent above the goal. Provisional data for 1990 indicate that this goal has not been met. As with younger children, "accidents and adverse effects" were the leading cause of death among adolescents and young adults. Within this category, motor vehicle crashes, suicides, and homicides were the most common causes of death.

For adults from 25 to 64 years of age, the death rate has steadily declined since 1977. In 1989, the rate was approximately 409.8 per 100,000 population; provisional data indicate that the goal was essentially met by 1990. Since 1977, the number of deaths from heart disease, especially among persons 55–64 years, and stroke has steadily declined. This trend offers a partial explanation for the overall decline. On the other hand, deaths from cancer are rising. This increase may reduce the rate of decline in the overall death rate for adults in the coming years. For adults 65 years of age and older, the 1990 goal was 30 restricted-activity days per year. The average number of restricted-activity days per person was 30.3 in 1987. In 1990, persons 65 years of age and over reported 31.4 restricted-activity days per person (Adams and Benson, 1990).

The Department of Health and Human Services continues to endorse the notion of raising population health levels through the promotion of health and the prevention of disease. As a reflection of this commitment, the Office of Health Promotion and Disease Prevention of the Department of Health and Human Services started in 1988 to draft the goals, objectives, priority areas, and targets to be reached by 2000.

GOALS AND OBJECTIVES FOR THE YEAR 2000

The first section of *Healthy People 2000* sets forth three global goals for Americans in the coming decade: to increase the span of healthy life, to reduce health disparities, and to achieve access to preventive services for all. *Healthy People 2000* recognizes the challenge facing health planners, decision makers, and health care providers due to the heterogeneity of the United States population and its health care system. By setting these goals the Department of Health and Human Services aims to improve the health of Americans.

By adopting the years of healthy life as a measure of healthy life span, the drafters of *Healthy People 2000* recognized the importance of the tradeoffs between quality of life and quantity of life. Years of healthy life are particularly important in health promotion and disease prevention because they are sensitive to both short-term and long-term tradeoffs in well-being that are likely to occur as a result of prevention initiatives. Figure 12.1 shows these tradeoffs for a prototypical individual. The dashed line illustrates the impact of health promotion and disease prevention activities on years of healthy life for a prototypical individual. The sizes and locations of the areas shown are

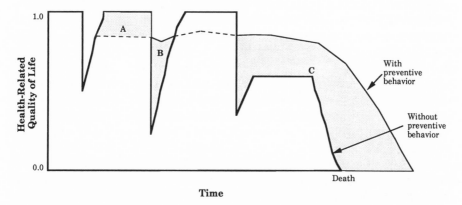

Figure 12.1 Years of healthy life with and without preventive/promotion behavior for a prototype individual. (A) Primary prevention may avoid the onset of illness but may result in lowered health-related quality of life because of the inconvenience of changing behavior or engaging in a preventive action. (B) Secondary prevention may reduce the incidence of secondary conditions. (C) Tertiary prevention may reduce disability and disadvantage.

hypothetical. Within a given population individuals will have alternative patterns. The areas as drawn, however, suggest the relationship between health promotion and disease prevention activities and years of healthy life.

Area A in the figure indicates reduced health-related quality of life that may be attributed to primary prevention. In this case, the individual is engaging in some behavior that will prevent illness but has a lowered health-related quality of life due to the inconvenience of the prevention activity. An attempt to stop smoking is an example of this type of behavior. Withdrawal symptoms as well as changing behavior patterns may cause lower health-related quality of life. Avoidance of lung cancer in the future, however, can lead to increased life expectancy.

Area B represents the impact of secondary prevention. In this situation, the health-related quality of life resulting from a health condition is maintained or improved because of a health promotion activity. For example, a person with diabetes mellitus may have reduced health-related quality of life because of the diabetes. Preventive care, however, may detect conditions secondary to the diabetes, such as hypertension or foot ulcers which may be treated, thereby maintaining the level of health-related quality of life and preventing unnecessary decline.

Area C represents the impact of tertiary prevention which reduces disability and extends healthy life. For example, behavior modification programs for chronic obstructive pulmonary disease may reduce some of the disability associated with this condition; they may also extend longevity. Thus both secondary and tertiary prevention would raise the level of health-related quality of life as measured by years of healthy life. With these programs, patients may also regain previously lost function and may also be able to slow the progression to more advanced stages of disability (Kaplan et al., 1984).

In addition to these global goals, *Healthy People 2000* is organized around the 22 priority areas listed in Table 12.2. In the report, the areas are grouped according to the strategy for action—health promotion, health protection, or preventive services. For example, priority areas 1–8 are related to individual lifestyle. Thus, health promotion programs are seen as a fundamental strategy for improving personal health by affecting personal choices such as use of alcohol and tobacco.

New priority areas for the year 2000 reflect these changes: the aging of the United States population, evolving health concerns, and expanding health promotion and disease prevention interventions. New topics in health promotion strategy include sexual behavior, vitality, and independence of older people. Environmental health is a new health protection strategy. Two former health protection strategies—toxic agent control and surveillance and the control of infectious diseases—are included in other strategies. Among the preventive services strategy for action, HIV infection, cancers, other chronic disorders, and mental and behavioral disorders have been added. In recognition of the role of and need for information in monitoring progress toward these goals, surveillance and data systems have been added as a priority in *Healthy People 2000* (DHHS, 1991b).

Within each priority area, there are specific objectives dealing with health status, risk reduction, and services and protection. Table 12.3 shows these objectives for priority area 8, Educational and Community-Based Programs. Some objectives may appear in more than one priority area. For example, the health status objective for

Table 12.2 Priority areas for promoting health and preventing disease in *Healthy People 2000*

Health promotion

1. Physical activity and fitness
2. Nutrition
3. Tobacco
4. Alcohol and other drugs
5. Family planning
6. Mental health and mental disorders
7. Violent and abusive behavior
8. Educational and community-based programs

Health protection

9. Unintentional injuries
10. Occupational safety and health
11. Environmental health
12. Food and drug safety
13. Oral health

Preventive services

14. Maternal and infant health
15. Heart disease and stroke
16. Cancer
17. Diabetes and chronic disabling conditions
18. HIV infection
19. Sexually transmitted diseases
20. Immunization and infectious diseases
21. Clinical preventive services

Surveillance and data systems

22. Surveillance and data systems

Source: Department of Health and Human Services, 1991b, p. 7.

priority area 8—to increase years of healthy life to at least 65—is also the objective for priority areas 17 (Diabetes and Chronic Disabling Conditions) and 21 (Clinical Preventive Services). In the following paragraphs we discuss each of these areas and indicate the rationale for selecting years of healthy life as the health status objective.

Educational and Community-Based Programs

In the United States, educational and community-based health promotion and disease prevention activities play an important role in reducing preventable illness, injury, disability, and premature death. Community-based interventions and programs attempt to reach and improve the health of many people who are outside of traditional health care settings. A community-based intervention is a single action intended to encourage or support change; a program is a planned, coordinated, ongoing effort that usually includes multiple interventions.

Although community-based programs may address a single risk factor or health problem, many are starting to take a more comprehensive and positive approach to

Table 12.3 Specific health status, risk reduction, and services and protection objectives for priority area 8, educational and community-based programs

Health status objective

8.1*ᵃ* Increase years of healthy life to at least 65 years. (Baseline: An estimated 62 years in 1980)

Years of healthy life	Special Population Targets	1980 baseline	2000 target
8.1a	Blacks	56	60
8.1b	Hispanics	62	65
8.1c	People aged 65 and older	12*ᵇ*	14*ᵇ*

Risk reduction objective

8.2 Increase the high school graduation rate to at least 90 percent, thereby reducing risks for multiple problem behaviors and poor mental and physical health. (Baseline: 79 percent of people aged 20–21 had graduated from high school with a regular diploma in 1989)

Services and protection objectives

8.3 Achieve for all disadvantaged children and children with disabilities access to high quality and developmentally appropriate preschool programs that help prepare children for school, thereby improving their prospects with regard to school performance, problem behaviors, and mental and physical health. (Baseline: 47 percent of eligible children aged 4 were afforded the opportunity to enroll in Head Start in 1990)

8.4 Increase to at least 75 percent the proportion of the nation's elementary and secondary schools that provide planned and sequential kindergarten through 12th-grade quality school health education. (Baseline data available in 1991)

8.5 Increase to at least 50 percent the proportion of postsecondary institutions with institutionwide health promotion programs for students, faculty, and staff. (Baseline: At least 20 percent of higher education institutions offered health promotion activities for students in 1989–90)

8.6 Increase to at least 85 percent the proportion of workplaces with 50 or more employees that offer health promotion activities for their employees, preferably as part of a comprehensive employee health promotion program. (Baseline: 65 percent of worksites with 50 or more employees offered at least one health promotion activity in 1985; 63 percent of medium and large companies had a wellness program in 1987)

8.7 Increase to at least 20 percent the proportion of hourly workers who participate regularly in employer-sponsored health promotion activities. (Baseline data available in 1991)

8.8 Increase to at least 90 percent the proportion of people aged 65 and older who had the opportunity to participate during the preceding year in at least one organized health promotion program through a senior center, lifecare facility, or other community-based setting that serves older adults. (Baseline data available in 1991)

8.9 Increase to at least 75 percent the proportion of people aged 10 and older who have discussed issues related to nutrition, physical activity, sexual behavior, tobacco, alcohol, other drugs, or safety with family members on at least one occasion during the preceding month. (Baseline data available in 1991)

8.10 Establish community health promotion programs that separately or together address at least three of the *Healthy People 2000* priorities and reach at least 40 percent of each state's population. (Baseline data available in 1992)

8.11 Increase to at least 50 percent the proportion of counties that have established culturally and linguistically appropriate community health promotion programs for racial and ethnic minority populations. (Baseline data available in 1992)

8.12 Increase to at least 90 percent the proportion of hospitals, health maintenance organizations, and large group practices that provide patient education programs, and to at least 90 percent the proportion of

(continued)

Table 12.3   (*Continued*)

community hospitals that offer community health promotion programs addressing the priority health needs of their communities. (Baseline: 66 percent of 6,821 registered hospitals provided patient education services in 1987; 60 percent of 5,677 community hospitals offered community health promotion programs in 1987)

8.13   Increase to at least 75 percent the proportion of local television network affiliates in the top 20 television markets that have become partners with one or more community organizations around one of the health problems addressed by the *Healthy People 2000* objectives. (Baseline data available in 1991)

8.14   Increase to at least 90 percent the proportion of people who are served by a local health department that is effectively carrying out the core functions of public health. (Baseline data available in 1992)

Source: Department of Health and Human Services, 1991b, pp. 250–62.
[a] This objective also appears as Objective 17.1 in *Diabetes and Chronic Disabling Conditions* and as Objective 21.1 in *Clinical Preventive Services.*
[b] Years of healthy life remaining at age 65

health and well-being. Community-based programs also increasingly recognize the importance of addressing the social and physical environment in which behavior occurs and which both shapes and is shaped by behavior. In keeping with the comprehensive nature of the community-based objectives, the drafters of *Healthy People 2000* have called for the use of years of healthy life to track the overall impact of the nation's efforts to implement more intensive and extensive educational and community-based interventions. Although other factors such as advances in treatment or increases in the use of clinical preventive services can influence this measure of the nation's health, achieving the risk reduction and services and protection objectives can contribute to a substantial increase in years of healthy life.

Diabetes and Chronic Disabling Conditions

The success of medical services and technology in reducing mortality allows the population to live to an age at which it is at risk of being afflicted with a variety of chronic diseases—diabetes, arthritis, or chronic disabling conditions. Although informative, mortality measures do not describe whether a population in which chronic diseases are prevalent is predominantly well or is heavily burdened with illness and disability. Furthermore, these measures understate the public health importance of conditions that result in more morbidity and disability than mortality.

To improve health status among persons with diabetes and chronic disabling conditions, *Healthy People 2000* proposes a strategy based on preventive services. Diabetes is a chronic metabolic disease that has been diagnosed in nearly 7 million persons in the United States. Another 5 million persons may have undiagnosed diabetes. Individuals with diabetes face not only a shortened life span but also the probability of incurring acute and chronic complications.

Chronic and disabling conditions have profound effects on the ability to function, whether the person is a child with mental retardation, a young adult with a spinal cord injury, or an older adult with osteoarthritis. For persons with diabetes or with chronic disabling conditions, quality of life, not merely quantity, has become the issue.

Clinical Preventive Services

Clinical preventive services, another type of health promotion and disease prevention activity, can also play an important role in extending years of healthy life by reducing preventable illness and premature death. These services include disease prevention and health promotion programs—immunizations, screening for early detection of disease or risk factors, and patient counseling—delivered in a health care setting. The effectiveness of preventive services in reducing morbidity and premature mortality is now well documented.

The dramatic declines in stroke mortality, cervical cancer mortality, and childhood infectious diseases are largely attributed to the widespread use of three preventive services: high blood pressure detection and control, Pap tests, and childhood immunizations. Other preventive services, such as screening mammography, have proved effective in controlled intervention trials. Like educational and community-based programs, clinical and preventive services are comprehensive. Thus, years of healthy life are being used as the global measure to track health improvements resulting from increased access to and use of clinical and preventive services.

The calculations described in Chapter 9 reflect the two ways to increase years of healthy life. One is to increase life expectancy; the other is to improve quality of life. The next section describes the data and calculations used to estimate possible increases in years of healthy life. It also suggests some impacts on years of healthy life that may result from increasing life expectancy, improving health-related quality of life, or increasing both quantity and quality of life.

DATA SOURCES AND TRACKING METHODS

Increasing years of healthy life is the number one goal set forth in *Healthy People 2000* for improving the health of the United States population. To derive baseline estimates of years of healthy life for *Healthy People 2000*, analysts used data primarily from the National Health Interview Survey (Erickson et al., 1989). Figure 12.2 shows average health-related quality of life scores for the civilian non-institutionalized United States population. Scores were calculated for males and females separately for selected age groups; they are measured according to the analogue of the Quality of Well-Being Scale developed from the retrospective analysis of NHIS data (Chapter 8). As shown here, there is a steady decline in average NHIS-QWB scores with age. The average scores range from 0.94 for persons aged 17 or less to approximately 0.80 for persons 65 years and older.

Because the NHIS represents the civilian noninstitutionalized population, these scores were supplemented with data from the National Nursing Home Survey and from the National Institute of Mental Health to estimate the quality of life of the total United States population using the methods presented in Chapter 9. Table 12.3 presents the health status, risk reduction, and services and protection objectives for priority area 8, Educational and Community-Based Programs. As shown, the overall health status goal is to raise years of healthy life from an estimate of 62 at the 1980 baseline to a target of 65 in 2000. Estimates for persons 65 years of age and older were calculated from the

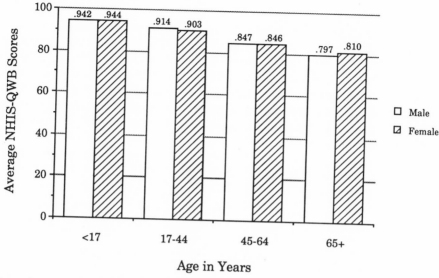

Figure 12.2 Average NHIS-QWB by gender and age, 1980 National Health Interview Survey. *Source:* National Center for Health Statistics. Unpublished data.

same data using comparable methods. These persons had an average of 12 years of healthy life remaining at the 1980 baseline.

Methods and data used to set baseline estimates and arrive at targets for years of healthy life for 2000 are now in developmental stages. Some of the problems in estimating quality of life using existing data were discussed in Chapter 8. Over the coming decade, limitations of both methods and data will be addressed. Even though the baseline and target estimates may change as a result of methodological refinements, years of healthy life was considered to be too important an indicator to be omitted from the process of setting and tracking goals and objectives.

Target levels of years of healthy life published in *Healthy People 2000* were determined by modeling the effects that changes in life expectancy and well-being would have on the number of years of healthy life. To estimate changes in life expectancy, analysts used data from 1987, the most recent available at the time the calculations were made. These estimated changes in years of healthy life over a seven-year interval were used to project the number of years of healthy life that might reasonably be expected by 2000.

Three scenarios could account for improvements in years of healthy life over the coming decade. Scenario 1 assumes that health-related quality of life improves while life expectancy remains constant. Scenario 2 shows that life expectancy improves while health-related quality of life remains constant. Scenario 3 assumes that both health-related quality of life and life expectancy improve. Because the goals and objectives set forth as national priorities for health promotion and disease prevention are aimed at improving health, these scenarios consider only positive changes in health status.

Table 12.4 illustrates the effect of these assumptions on the number of years of

Table 12.4 Three scenarios for assessing the impact of
improving quantity and quality of life

Baseline data, 1980	
Life expectancy (whites	74.4
Years of healthy life (YHL)	63.0
Life expectancy (whites), 1987	75.6
Scenario 1	
Quality of life improves 10%	
No change in life expectancy	$\Big\}$ = 72.9 YHL
Scenario 2	
No change in quality of life	
Life expectancy increases to 1987 level	$\Big\}$ = 67.3 YHL
Scenario 3	
Quality of life improves 10%	
Life expectancy increases to 1987 level	$\Big\}$ = 74 YHL

Source: National Center for Health Statistics, 1962–90 [1980, 1987]; National Health
Interview Survey, 1980.

healthy life for the white United States population. In this table, 1987 life expectancy data have been used to show the effect of reducing mortality (Scenarios 2 and 3). To illustrate the effect of improving health-related quality of life on years of healthy life, the quality-of-life estimates for 1980 have been assumed to increase 10 percent by 1987 for all age groups (Scenarios 1 and 3). Because there are as yet no trend data on the health-related quality of life of the general population, we used 10 percent to give an estimate of the percentage change that might be observed. As indicated by these three scenarios, the improvement in both quality and quantity of life leads to the highest number of years of healthy life.

The 10 percent increase in quality of life for all ages is one of the many assumptions that could be used to set future targets of years of healthy life. Scenarios could be developed in which the percentage of increase in quality of life varied by race or age group. For some age groups, the increase in life quality might be very small, less than 1 percent. For other age groups the increase in health-related quality of life might be large, say 10 percent. A new treatment for arthritis that resulted in alleviation of pain and joint tenderness and stiffness might result in a relatively large increase in quality of life for persons 65 years of age and older.

At the national level, decision makers set goals and specific targets for health promotion and disease prevention. These goals and targets do not specify which interventions to use. Rather, state and local health decision makers are responsible for selecting programs. To assist communities in translating the national objectives for action, the American Public Health Association is publishing *Healthy Communities 2000: Model Standards, Guidelines for Attainment of Year 2000 Objectives for the Nation* (DHHS, 1991a). This volume offers community implementation strategies for putting the national objectives into practice and encourages communities to establish achievable community health targets.

The National Center for Health Statistics is responsible for tracking the progress toward the goals and objectives in *Healthy People 2000*. Starting with the 1991 volume, annual progress reports will be published as a component of *Health: United States*. To prepare these reports, NCHS is developing a data base containing information relevant to the Year 2000 objectives. This data base will include the following: (1) an inventory with the proposed monitoring data sets and data set descriptors; (2) a list of the objectives with appropriate descriptors; (3) an assessment of each data set's appropriateness to monitor specific objectives; and (4) a list of persons and agencies responsible for the information contained in either the data sets or the objectives.

Current plans call for development of a classification system that can be used in the National Health Interview Survey to assess the health-related quality of life for the civilian noninstitutionalized population. The questionnaire is also being designed for use in a statewide telephone survey designed to monitor progress toward meeting the years of healthy life goal by 2000. One of the challenges in developing this classification system will be maintaining the ability to do trend analysis while adding measures to reflect the positive end of the health continuum.

These trend analyses illustrate the important policy-analytic uses of years of healthy life. Estimating the health status of cohorts of aging adults and projecting long-term care needs can suggest different interventions for different ages, new directions for health services research for aging and disabled population groups, and possibly new policy initiatives. The next section discusses how the Health Resources Allocation Strategy, incorporating both years of healthy life and costs for health promotion and disease prevention interventions, has already contributed and can continue to contribute to policy development.

COMPARING STRATEGIES FOR PREVENTION EFFECTIVENESS

The primary focus of *Healthy People 2000* is on setting health status and risk reduction objectives to improve population health levels. This focus reflects the Department of Health and Human Services' position that many chronic diseases and their health impacts can be prevented, leading to a higher level of health in the United States. A corollary to disease prevention and health promotion is that costly health care interventions may also be avoided. Table 12.5 shows selected preventable conditions, the magnitude of the problem, and the cost per patient for the avoidable intervention. For four examples given here—interventions for heart disease, cancer, injuries, and HIV infection—the cost savings from preventing these illnesses is considerable.

Although the national health promotion and disease prevention initiative does not express its goals and objectives in terms of cost–effectiveness analysis, a number of studies among target populations have evaluated the benefits and costs of disease prevention and health promotion programs. These interventions are evaluated in terms of the following criteria: (1) the effectiveness of the intervention; (2) cost effectiveness of the prevention or promotion intervention to treatment; and (3) the cost effectiveness of different preventive strategies for the same condition or population or for different conditions or populations. As costs and outcomes analysis becomes more common in assessing health promotion and disease prevention activities, these interventions will also need to be evaluated against alternatives more traditionally considered therapeutic.

A number of studies of elderly persons are being conducted to evaluate the effective-

Table 12.5 Costs of treatment for selected preventable conditions

Condition	Overall magnitude	Avoidable intervention[a]	Cost per patient[b]
Heart disease	7 million with coronary artery disease 500,000 deaths/year 284,000 bypass procedures/year	Coronary bypass surgery	$30,000
Cancer	1 million new cases/year 510,000 deaths/year	Lung cancer treatment Cervical cancer treatment	$29,000 $28,000
Stroke	600,000 strokes/year 150,000 deaths/year	Hemiplegia treatment and rehabilitation	$22,000
Injuries	2.3 million hospitalizations/year 142,500 deaths/year 177,000 persons with spinal cord injuries in the United States	Quadriplegia treatment and rehabilitation Hip fracture treatment and rehabilitation Severe head injury treatment and rehabilitation	$570,000 (lifetime) $40,000 $310,000
HIV infection	1–1.5 million infected 118,000 AIDS cases (as of January 1990)	AIDS treatment	$75,000 (lifetime)
Alcoholism	18.5 million abuse alcohol 105,000 alcohol-related deaths/year	Liver transplant	$250,000
Drug abuse	Regular users: 1–3 million, cocaine; 900,000, IV drugs; 500,000, heroin Drug-exposed babies: 375,000	Treatment of cocaine-exposed baby	$66,000 (5 years)
Low birth weight baby	260,000 LBWB born/year 23,000 deaths/year	Neonatal intensive care for LBWB	$10,000
Inadequate immunization	Lacking basic immunization series: 20–30%, aged 2 and younger; 3%, aged 6 and older	Congenital rubella syndrome treatment	$354,000 (lifetime)

Source: Department of Health and Human Services, 1991b, p. 5.

[a] Examples (other interventions may apply).

[b] Representative first-year costs, except as noted. Not indicated are nonmedical costs, such as lost productivity to society

ness of different promotion and prevention activities. These studies are motivated by the fact that the Medicare program, the primary source of health insurance for over 30 million elderly people in the United States, is prohibited by law from offering preventive services unless they are authorized by Congress through an amendment to the Medicare Act. To date, only four preventive services are covered by Medicare: vaccines for pneumococcal pneumonia and hepatitis B, screening mammography, and Pap smears (Office of Technology Assessment [OTA], 1990).

As a result of their exclusion from Medicare and private insurance packages, preventive services have been subject to more stringent standards for coverage than have most diagnostic and therapeutic procedures. Two major arguments are given for the tougher standards. The first is that because preventive services are offered to healthy people, their risks need to be evaluated more carefully. The second argument is that high-standards preventive services suggest that diagnostic and therapeutic services should be made more stringent (OTA, 1990).

One set of studies designed to assess the impact of preventive services on the Medicare population has been supported by the Health Care Financing Administration (HCFA). These demonstrations are being conducted at six sites in the United States (Table 12.6); sites in Washington, North Carolina, California, and Maryland are assessing prevention effectiveness in terms of years of healthy life. Therefore, it will be possible to use the Health Resource Allocation Strategy to assess the impact of the intervention on years of healthy life.

The study of Medicare beneficiaries enrolled in Group Health Cooperative (GHC) of Puget Sound, Seattle, Washington, provides an example of these studies. In the GHC study, the intervention consists of the following: (1) early identification of physical and mental conditions for which there are efficacious interventions available to modify risk factors for disease, disability, and dependency; (2) modifications of enrollee's social and physical environment to support health-promoting behaviors and maintain or increase independence; and (3) enhancement of enrollee autonomy to function independently and to make critical decisions about health behavior and health care.

The preventive services package consists of activities aimed at 15 major health concerns: exercise, nutrition, planning ahead, medication awareness, incontinence, hypertension, physical examination, laboratory testing, mental health, hearing, immunizations, injury prevention, alcohol use, smoking, and vision. The package has two parts. The health promotion component is directed toward those risk factors thought to predispose to loss of autonomy or decline in health-related quality of life. The disease prevention component is directed toward clinical screening, immunization, and further follow-up of chronic medical conditions as well as those conditions already detected through the health promotion component.

Patients are selected for participation in this prospective study from lists of Group Health Cooperative enrollees. At baseline, information is obtained on each individual's health-related quality of life, health risk, self-efficacy for behavioral change, preventive behaviors, social network and support, and plans for the future. The Quality of Well-Being Scale is used along with measures of health worry, depression, general health perceptions, and perceived quality of life to assess health status. Patients who agree to participate and who complete the baseline questionnaires are randomly assigned to either the experimental group receiving the preventive service or the control group receiving standard treatment (Patrick et al., 1991).

The hypothesis being tested is that use of preventive services leads to observable increases in quality and length of life. As shown in Figure 12.3, using hypothetical data, for the first two years of the program both groups have the same number of years of healthy life remaining. After this time, however, preventive services begin to have an observable impact on length and quality of life. The gap between the two groups widens as those who participate in preventive services experience both decreased mortality and increased quality of life compared to those who do not participate in the preventive services interventions.

The Office of Technology Assessment (OTA), the research arm of the U.S. Con-

Table 12.6 Characteristics of studies designed to assess the impact of preventive services on the Medicare population

Characteristic	Location					
	Seattle	Raleigh-Durham	San Diego	Los Angeles	Baltimore	Pittsburgh area
Directing organization	University of Washington	University of North Carolina	San Diego State University	University of California	Johns Hopkins University	University of Pittsburgh
Service provider	Group Health of Puget Sound (HMO)	Physicians' offices, clinics	Project team personnel in conjunction with Secure Horizon (HMO)	Health prevention clinic staff/allied health professions	Beneficiary's usual care provider	Rural hospitals, clinics, physicians' offices
Sample pool	Elderly HMO enrollees	Elderly patients of participating practices	Elderly HMO enrollees	Elderly patients of participating physicians	Elderly Medicare beneficiaries in local area	Elderly Medicare beneficiaries in local area
Sample size (total participants)	2,250	2,538	2,400	1,800	4,400	4,500
Control group	1,125	958	1,200	900	2,200	1,500
Experimental group(s)	Receive services (1,625)	Screening only (307) Health promotion only (317) Both screening and promotion (900)	Receive services (1,200)	Receive services (900)	Receive services at usual source of care (2,200)	Receive preventive services from clinic (2,000) Receive services from private physician (2,000)

Source: Office of Technology Assessment, 1990.

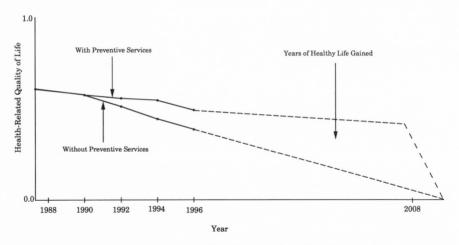

Figure 12.3 Hypothetical years of healthy life gained attributed to Medicare preventive services.

gress, is studying the costs and effects of health promotion and disease prevention strategies for older adults. OTA studies have evaluated the costs and effectiveness of breast cancer screening, pneumococcal vaccine, influenza vaccine, cholesterol screening, cervical cancer screening, and glaucoma screening. Of these six studies, the two that evaluated vaccines assessed costs and benefits in terms of the Health Resource Allocation Strategy. In 1983, the net discounted cost per year of healthy life gained ranged from a savings to a cost of $6,154, depending on the assumptions made concerning the prevalence and duration of pneumococcal pneumonia. In a retrospective analysis between 1972 and 1978, the cost per year of healthy life gained for all persons from influenza vaccination was $64. When costs for unrelated illnesses were included in the analysis, costs per year of healthy life gained was $1,782 (OTA, 1990).

Table 12.7 presents data on the OTA influenza vaccine study as well as selected other studies that evaluated health promotion and disease prevention activities using costs and outcomes analyses of the type included in the Health Resource Allocation Strategy. All of the studies selected for evaluation in this table use years of healthy life based on the preferences developed for the Quality of Well-Being Scale. Thus, net effects are measured in comparable gains in years of healthy life.

Two of the interventions shown in this table saved money, as indicated by negative costs. The first is an exercise intervention prescribed as a preventive activity for coronary heart disease for 35-year-old men who like to exercise. The other cost-saving preventive intervention is influenza vaccine for persons 65 years and older.

The rest of the interventions described in Table 12.7 have positive net costs, indicating that these cost more than the alternative intervention against which they were compared. Each of these studies seeks to determine the benefits of the specified intervention compared to "doing nothing" for the same condition. They calculate net costs and effects using the status quo as the comparison group, for example, exercise versus no exercise or vaccine versus no vaccine. The ratios of cost per year of healthy life range from $64 per year of healthy life for influenza vaccine among persons 25–44 years of age to $25,635 to screen for parasites among Indochinese refugees.

Table 12.7 Comparison of costs and outcomes for evaluating existing health promotion and disease prevention strategies

Intervention (1)	Study group (2)	Study design (3)	Health states preferences (4)	Net effect in terms of YHL (5)	Net costs (6)	Discount rate (7)	Cost/YHL (8)	Reference
Exercise prescribed to prevent coronary heart disease	35-year-old men who like exercise	Cohort analysis with 30-year follow-up (N = 1,000)	Based on QWB supplemented by expert judgment	354.4	$−2.66 million (1985)	3%	—[a]	Hatziandreu et al., 1988
Influenza vaccine	Persons 65+ years of age in general population	Cohort analysis using national survey data, 1970–78	Based on QWB	28 days	—[a]	5%	—[a]	OTA, 1981
Influenza vaccine	Persons 25–44 years of age in general population	Cohort analysis using national survey data, 1970–78	Based on QWB	30 days	$5	5%	$64	OTA, 1981
Influenza vaccine	Children under 3 years of age in general population	Cohort analysis using national survey data, 1970–78	Based on QWB	15 days	$10 (1978)	5%	$258	OTA, 1981
Exercise prescribed to prevent coronary heart disease	35-year-old men regardless of their like for exercise	Cohort anallysis with 30-year follow-up (N = 1,000)	Based on QWB supplemented by expert judgment	529.8	$6 million (1985)	3%	$11,313	Hatziandreu et al., 1988
Parasite screening	Indochinese refugees	Analysis of single specimen plus modeling for symptoms and dysfunction (N = 2,978 with 368 positive specimens)	Based on QWB	2.48	$63,576	0.233 pr 6% at 25 years	$25,635	Anderson and Moser, 1985

[a]Cost savings.

From the information provided in columns 2 and 3, we can assess the generalizability of results. For instance, the cost–effectiveness ratio for exercise intervention is based on 35-year-old men. Thus, these data give no indication of the effects and costs of such a program in men of other ages or in women of any age. Age can be an important variable in determining the ratio of cost per year of healthy life. As shown in this table, for influenza vaccine the ratio for children under 3 years of age is $258. This ratio is almost four times that of adults 25–44 years of age. Expansion of traditional costs and outcomes tables to include sociodemographic information about the study group can assist policymakers in more accurately estimating the total cost of a health intervention.

An overestimate of the cost of an influenza vaccine program might occur if the ratio supplied were based on data from children under 3 years of age and applied to the total population. If 1 million people of all ages were to be included in the vaccination program, the total cost would be $258 million. An underestimate of the program might occur if the ratio supplied was that for adults 65 years of age and older. In this case, the policymaker would be misled into thinking that cost savings would occur.

In analyses that compare the cost effectiveness of health promotion and disease prevention programs with medical- and technology-intensive interventions, such as neonatal care units and coronary artery bypass surgery, promotion and prevention programs rank at the top of the list, indicating that they are more cost effective. Total hip replacement surgery has been shown to be four times more costly per year of life gained than was advice to stop smoking. Coronary artery bypass graft surgery was five times more costly than smoking cessation programs.

The findings that prevention and promotion activities generally have low ratios of costs per year of healthy life are consistent with arguments in the late 1970s and early 1980s that these activities would lead to overall cost savings. It was argued that these savings would result from preventing disease rather than treating illness. For example, vaccinations were thought to cost less than treating influenzas and other infectious diseases. These arguments pertained to preventive activities not only among the young but also among the elderly population.

Somers (1984), for example, argued that the Medicare population was neither too old nor too debilitated to benefit from health promotion and disease prevention activities. She put forth four recommendations for introducing prevention programs into the Medicare program. The first was to improve consumer information about healthy behaviors, including self-care, and symptom recognition. The second was to increase federal excise taxes on cigarettes and alcohol as an incentive for healthy behaviors. The third was to establish a procedure for identifying cost-effective preventive services for Medicare coverage. The fourth was to encourage primary care practitioners to provide preventive services on a routine basis. These recommendations were considered to add only minimally to the costs of the Medicare program. Rather, it was envisioned that funds would be transferred from high-technology care to lower-cost primary care.

Other analysts have argued that the potential for cost savings through health promotion and disease prevention activities are not so straightforward. Russell (1986) suggests three complications that may make it difficult to realize cost savings from prevention and promotion programs. One of these is that prevention activities are not risk-free. For example, whooping cough vaccinations had been standard practice until the 1970s. At this time, several studies indicated that the vaccine was associated with neurologic illnesses and possibly brain damage in a small number of cases (Miller et al., 1982). Thus, patients and their families need to understand that some preventive activities result in risks that need to balanced against the alternatives.

Another factor affecting the potential cost savings of preventive activities is that the total cost of the activity may be much greater than the specific activity or intervention. For example, the blood pressure test is one of the least expensive of all the available medical tests. Yet current practice is to repeat the test every one to two years, a recommendation that does not improve health in and of itself but does result in costs. Additional tests will also be needed if the first test is high, again adding costs.

Of those persons identified as having hypertension, the costs of treating the condition exceed the savings. Weinstein and Stason (1977b, 1978) found that treating hypertension cost more money than it saved. The added cost of treating disease identified through a preventive activity is the third complication identified by Russell (1986).

Although it is becoming clear that disease prevention and health promotion may increase costs rather than save them, these activities are still considered important for reducing the rate of increase in health care costs in the United States (DHHS, 1991b). Decision makers tend to expect cost savings from prevention activities, although admitting that expensive medical technologies will continue to proliferate. This might be interpreted as something of a double standard.

The Health Resource Allocation Strategy provides policymakers with a framework for evaluating prevention and promotion activities against the same criteria as other types of health care interventions. Thus, the Strategy has the potential for allowing a more equitable allocation of resources across types of interventions by doing away with this double standard. In this way, the Strategy leads to a more equitable distribution of our increasingly scarce health care resources.

13

Improving Health-Related Quality of Life Through Technology

Medical care in the twentieth century has dramatically increased in accuracy of diagnosis and effectiveness of treatment. A major contributor to this capability is new technology, broadly defined as the application of an organized body of knowledge to practical purposes. Some of the uses for which health and medical care technologies have been developed include (1) preventing disease or other adverse consequences—poliomyelitis vaccine for disease prevention; (2) diagnosing diseases or health conditions—the CT scanner; (3) treating diseases and conditions—coronary artery bypass surgery; and (4) rehabilitating persons following accidental injury or major health event—prosthetic devices (Office of Technology Assessment [OTA], 1985).

The emergence of scientific medical care and its associated technologies in the United States has radically changed since the end of World War II. In 1945 the federal government began direct support of biomedical research. In addition to funding research, the government supported the construction of local hospitals and expanded physician supply by financing medical education. It also provided health insurance for older adults and poor persons which allowed hospitals to modernize and improve their treatment capabilities (Shannon, 1976).

As a result of almost 50 years of expanding biomedical research, the public expects enhancements in medical technology and application of these new techniques as desired. In addition, the increasing number of persons living to age 85 and beyond leads to greater use of medical services and technology. Further demand for medical care and medical technologies will come from an expanding pool of persons eligible to receive such treatment. One major source of increased demand will be policies to broaden Medicaid coverage to include these services (Ginzberg, 1990). Because of increased supply and demand for medical care, we can expect continued development and expanded application of health care technologies in the coming decades (Anbar, 1984).

In the first section of this chapter, we briefly review the emergence of effective diagnostic and therapeutic medical care, the kinds of new medical technologies, and the United States government's contribution to new technology development. Next is a review of some approaches to cost control using technology assessment techniques. The third section discusses procedures for collecting data and calculating years of healthy life associated with two different therapeutic technologies. We end by highlighting the contribution of the Health Resource Allocation Strategy to the costs and outcomes debates associated with health care technology.

TECHNOLOGY AND HEALTH CARE

Before this century, technology played a small role in the practice of medicine; most interventions that involved touching patients were administered by surgeons, who were considered to practice an inferior type of medicine. In that era, medicine, apart from surgery, was primarily practiced as an art of healing. Medical discoveries in the late 1800s, such as germ theory and antiseptic techniques, introduced the importance of using specific instruments and interventions in medical practice. Physicians were willing to adopt new technologies, hoping this would build respect within the scientific community (Reiser, 1984).

The twentieth century has seen rapid growth in health care technology. Initially, instruments were introduced to enhance patient care in the doctor's office. These tools included the microscope and the stethoscope. New therapeutic technologies were considered successful if they prolonged life. The major purpose for introducing a new surgical technique or medicine was to improve patient survival, as the Halstead radical surgery did for breast cancer and streptomycin did for tuberculosis.

The next wave of technologies involved larger instruments and processes of implementation. Thus, the new technologies were best used at specialized sites such as hospitals. Innovative technologies such as diagnostic imaging (computed tomography and nuclear medical procedures) and major surgeries like coronary artery bypass graft not only prolonged life but raised new issues relating to quality of life. This development was followed by the transfer of technologies previously used in hospitals and other health care facilities to use in the community. These innovations include portable oxygen masks and continuous ambulatory peritoneal dialysis.

The introduction and continued growth of technology have brought crucial problems to medicine. There is need for organizational structures capable of serving as geographic focal points for these emerging technologies as well as distributive mechanisms for allocating the benefits to patients (Reiser, 1984). The major solution to the structural problem has been to develop hospitals into technology centers. As a result, 39 percent of the total United States health care expenditures in 1988 were spent for hospital care (Office of National Cost Estimates, 1990). As costs continued to rise in the 1960s, the introduction of diagnostic and therapeutic technologies was coupled with an examination of costs. This trend is typified by the analysis that led to an expansion of Medicare to persons with end-stage renal disease (ESRD). In the debates that preceded enactment of the ESRD program two program objectives were stated: (1) to save lives by providing access to medical care to the large portion of the population covered by the Social Security Act who might fall ill with chronic kidney disease; and (2) to return these saved lives to economic productivity by providing dialysis. Estimates computed in 1972 indicated that these goals could be achieved at reasonable costs. The estimated cost of the program for its first year of operation was $75 million. It was estimated that after four years the ESRD program would cost $250 million (Plough and Berry, 1981).

After ten years of operation, the ability of the ESRD program to meet these aims at a reasonable cost began to be seriously questioned. In 1974, the first full year of the program, the expenditures were $229 million, almost triple the original estimate. Eight years later, expenditures were estimated at $1.8 billion (Eggers, 1984). This meant that

0.2 percent of the population covered under Medicare spent 5 percent of the total Medicare budget (OTA, 1984; Halper, 1985).

Additional direct costs attributed to the ESRD program are those associated with disability insurance. Qualification for the ESRD program is interpreted as qualification for benefits under the Social Security Administration's disability insurance program. Rettig and Marks (1983) estimate that income support "probably adds another $100 million to $250 million to the cost to the government of sustaining the lives of the ESRD Program beneficiaries."

Although the program has been more costly than originally estimated, it has been somewhat successful in saving lives. Data from the Medicare Statistical System and the ESRD Medical information System show that about 80 percent of persons treated with dialysis survive at least one year. First-year survival rates are higher for younger people than for older people. Survival rates after five years of dialysis vary from 22 percent for persons 75 and older to 64 percent for persons 15–24 years. The five-year survival rates also differ for various diagnoses: persons with polycystic kidney disease have the highest rate, 58 percent; persons with diabetic nephropathy have the lowest rate, 21 percent.

In meeting the ESRD's second objective of returning people to economic productivity, the data are less encouraging. According to a report issued by the United States Office of the Inspector General, the number of persons returning to work is lower than originally expected (Garrison et al., 1983). The relationship between chronic kidney disease and work status is complex. Empirical evidence has shown that the number of persons returning to work varies by type of treatment (see Table 13.1). Among the 859 patients included in the study by Evans and colleagues (1985), the percentage who were able to work while on dialysis or after undergoing transplant ranged from 27.80 to 62.30 percent. Those who had a kidney transplant were most able to work.

Other aspects of health-related quality of life—subjective assessment of well being, psychological affect, and life satisfaction—were assessed for these patients using the same measures as in Campbell and colleagues' general population survey (Campbell et

Table 13.1 Adjusted proportions and selected mean scores for objective and subjective indicators of quality of life, according to treatment for end-stage renal disease

Quality of life domain	Mean score adjusted for case mix				P value
	Home hemodialysis	In-center hemodialysis	CAPD[a]	Transplantation	
Ability to work (% of patients)	54.80	44.80	27.80	62.30	0.001
Subjective indicators of quality of life (mean score)	11.23	10.56	11.08	12.18	0.001
Psychological affect (mean score)	5.47	5.09	5.26	5.72	0.001
Life satisfaction (mean score)	5.25	4.99	5.30	5.90	0.001

Source: Evans et al., 1985.

[a]Continuous ambulatory peritoneal dialysis.

al., 1976). For all of these indicators, persons receiving kidney transplants had higher health-related quality of life scores than did persons receiving other types of treatment for end-stage renal disease; these differences were statistically significant ($P = 0.0001$). The quality of life data for kidney patients, both those on dialysis and those who received a transplant, were compared to similar data collected from the general population. Although scores for the kidney patients were lower than those from the general population, the scores were not statistically different. This lack of difference indicates that kidney patients perceived themselves to have health-related quality of life similar to that of the general population.

The introduction of erythropoietin has brought an overall improvement to the health-related quality of life for people undergoing dialysis (Delano, 1989; Evans et al., 1990; Lundin et al., 1990). The impact on return to work, however, is mixed. In two studies (Delano, 1989; Lundin et al., 1990), the majority of patients were able to return to work after receiving up to two years of erythropoietin treatment. However, a third study by Evans and colleagues (1990) found no change in return to work or employment status.

The recent analysis of the ESRD program that was conducted by the Institute of Medicine (IOM) studied the following aspects of the program: epidemiologic and demographic changes in the patient population; access to care for patients eligible and ineligible for Medicare; quality of care and the effects of reimbursement on this quality; and adequacy of data systems for monitoring these aspects (Rettig and Levinsky, 1991). The IOM Committee's concern that policies be developed that would increase the patients' levels of health-related quality of life within acceptable budgetary levels represented a continuation of the concern for both costs and outcomes that was associated with the debates that preceded the enactment of the initial Social Security Amendments which provided coverage for hemodialysis.

Cost–benefit assessment of the type performed for end-stage renal disease treatment is unusual. Most technologies have been introduced with no formal cost and benefit assessment. Table 13.2 shows the number of selected procedures per 1,000 population performed from 1980 through 1988. These procedures were selected from the list of

Table 13.2 Number of selected procedures performed per 1,000 persons in the United States, selected years

Procedure	ICD codes	1980	1982	1984	1986	1988
Coronary artery bypass	36.1	—[c]	170	202	284	353
Cardiac catheterization	37.21–37.23	348	471	570	775	930
Lens extraction	13.1–13.6	467	599	505	120	109
Caesarian section[a]	74.0–74.99	619	730	814	911	937
Disc/fusion	80.5, 81.0	204	227	277	337	340
Hip replacement	81.5, 81.6	—[c]	148	183	201	136
Knee replacement	81.41–81.47	—[c]	137	164	182	217
Prostatectomy[b]	60.2–60.6	335	358	361	366	449

Source: National Center for Health Statistics (1980–1988).

[a]Per 1,000 females.

[b]Per 1,000 males.

[c]Data not available for 1980.

technologies considered by the Priority-Setting Group (Lara and Goodman, 1990). The anecdotal approach was used to assess the success of coronary artery bypass surgery. When this surgery was first introduced, patients showed improvement and many reported relief of symptoms. From these anecdotal reports, the operation was considered successful and was used for increasing numbers of patients receiving cardiac catheterization and bypass surgery as reflected in Table 13.2 (Preston, 1989).

The increasing number of medical procedures performed has resulted in rising costs, which have led to several proposals for systematically assessing the application of new and existing technologies. These proposals have been necessary because health care operates outside of a market economy which would gradually identify and eliminate those technologies that were ineffective. Thus, different agencies within the federal government have been authorized to develop technology assessment programs. No agency, however, has oversight responsibility. This disjointed approach to monitoring the adoption of technological innovations is gradually giving way to more centralized oversight, discussed in the next section.

STRATEGIES FOR IDENTIFYING EFFECTIVE TECHNOLOGIES

Since the 1970s, federal agencies have used various tools to assess new technologies. The National Institutes of Health (NIH) has used the consensus development conference to assess the benefits of new technology. This procedure was formally started in the NIH in 1977 (Jacoby, 1985). Consensus building, which focuses on the safety, efficacy, and conditions for use of specific technologies, is used for technology assessment in Sweden (Calltorp, 1988; Johnsson, 1988) and the Netherlands (Caspirie and Everdingen, 1985) as well as in Norway, France, Canada, and the United Kingdom (Banta and Andreason, 1990). The goal of consensus development is to involve physicians and to have an impact on medical practice, rather than to serve as a mechanism for making policy recommendations.

Other approaches to technology assessment are more directly related to health policy. This is especially true of those programs implemented by the Office of Technology Assessment (OTA) and by the Agency for Health Care Policy and Research (AHCPR). Both of these organizations analyze health care outcomes and costs associated with various technologies. These analyses are used in general health decision making and specific resource allocation.

Office of Technology Assessment

For about 20 years, OTA has undertaken an extensive, systematic effort to assess benefits and costs of new technologies. In the 1970s, as health care costs continued to rise and methodologies for studying costs and health outcomes improved, OTA established its health program as a service provided to Congress. OTA is a nonpartisan analytical support agency of the U.S. Congress that provides congressional committees with analyses of emerging, difficult, and often highly technical issues. OTA's goals are to help Congress resolve uncertainties and conflicting claims, identify alternative policy options, and provide foresight or early alert to new developments that could have important implications for future federal policy. Rather than advocating particular policies or actions, OTA points out their strengths and weaknesses and sorts out the facts (OTA, 1986).

Since 1975, OTA has published more than 35 evaluations of the costs and benefits of various health technologies. These include assisting persons with speech impairments, dealing with alcohol abuse, and providing traditional health services through the use of nurse practitioners. OTA's health technology case study series includes studies on the following: computed tomography, upper gastrointestinal endoscopy, and magnetic resonance imaging; technologies for overcoming learning disabilities; devices to assist with speech and hearing impairments; and therapeutic technologies, including both pharmaceutical interventions (e.g., cimetidine) and surgical procedures (e.g., breast cancer surgeries and elective hysterectomy).

Although most of these studies used condition-specific measures to assess program benefit, the analysis of bone marrow transplantation and of orthopedic joint prostheses adjusted the health outcomes to account for changes in quality of life. In particular, the analysis of joint prostheses used years of healthy life as the outcome measure.

In addition to evaluating specific technologies, OTA reports may discuss the difficulties of conducting such analyses. For example, the study of automated multichannel chemistry analyzers points out the limitation of efficacy information needed for evaluation of this technology. The study discusses different ways of using the chemistry analyzers to achieve the greatest degree of efficiency. Formal data analyses and results are not presented in the OTA report. Rather, different ways of approaching the comparison of costs and outcomes are discussed along with the policy implications.

In addition to the studies in this technology series, OTA undertakes analyses targeted for special purposes. For example, OTA may undertake a study to justify amending the Medicare law to extend coverage to treatments or preventive services not currently covered. The preventive services evaluations and the pneumococcal vaccine studies discussed in Chapter 12 are examples of these types of OTA studies.

Agency for Health Care Policy and Research

The other major initiative for identifying effective technologies for policy purposes is the Medical Treatment Effectiveness Program (MEDTEP) implemented by the AHCPR in the U.S. Public Health Service. MEDTEP's major goal is to improve the effectiveness and appropriateness of medical practice by developing and disseminating scientific information regarding the effects of currently used health care services and procedures on patients' survival, health status, functional capacity, and quality of life. Research conducted under this program addresses fundamental questions about what difference medical care makes. Questions asked by MEDTEP research projects are "Do patients benefit?" "What treatments work best?" and "Are health care resources well spent?" MEDTEP research emphasizes the evaluation of outcomes rather than the processes of health services.

MEDTEP focuses on three areas of research: (1) medical effectiveness and patient outcomes research, (2) development of data bases for patient outcomes research and for clinical decision making, and (3) methods for disseminating research findings to lead to more informed clinical decision making and a more effective and efficient health care system.

This program is motivated by evidence that health care practitioners will voluntarily change their practice behavior when information about practice patterns and patient outcomes is available to them (Agency for Health Care Policy and Research, personal communication, 1990). This evidence on behavior change has led policymakers, providers, insurers, and consumers to emphasize the need for more and better information on costs and outcomes to guide policy-making. Thus, AHCPR is collaborating with other U.S. Public Health Service agencies, as well as the Health Care Financing Administration, to support combined research efforts of clinicians and health services researchers in collecting, analyzing, interpreting, and disseminating information on the outcomes of various health care services and procedures.

The principal form of this research effort is the Patient Outcomes Research Team (PORT) approach. PORT projects are large-scale, multifaceted, multidisciplinary projects that must meet special requirements. These include a large, diverse team consisting of members from both academic and community health care settings. The goals of a PORT project are to identify and analyze the outcomes and costs of current alternative practice patterns in order to determine the best treatment strategy and to develop and test methods for reducing inappropriate variations.

Criteria for selecting research topics appropriate for MEDTEP funding include the number of individuals affected, the extent of uncertainty or controversy surrounding the use of a procedure or its effectiveness, the level of related expenditure, and the availability of data. Studies that reflect the needs of the Medicare program and informational requirements for the development of practice guidelines are considered for support by AHCPR.

The following topics are among those being funded as part of the PORT initiative: back pain, treatment for acute myocardial infarction, biliary tract disease, and pneumonia. These selected projects illustrate the range of activities that are considered appropriate by the MEDTEP program. Since results from the first four PORT studies may be available shortly, they are discussed in greater detail next.

The back pain PORT assesses alternative types of lumbar spine surgery (fusion, laminectomy, and discectomy), a variety of nonsurgical interventions (e.g., traction and various therapeutic injections), and diagnostic tests (including myelography, computed tomography, magnetic resonance imaging, and thermography) commonly used for patients with back pain, especially pain due to spinal stenosis, the most common diagnosis leading to surgery among elderly patients. National and statewide hospital discharge data and Medicare claims data are being used to determine the frequency of poor outcomes. These outcomes included deaths, rehospitalizations, discharges to nursing homes, and in-hospital complications. A survey of patients with spinal stenosis and disc herniations is being conducted to obtain health outcome information not available from claims data. This survey will also be used to obtain information about individual preferences for certain outcomes. Data from the various sources will be combined and used in a formal decision analysis to aid patients and physicians in deciding when surgery is appropriate.

Findings from this assessment will be disseminated to physicians and hospitals in high-use areas. There will also be special materials for educating patients, whose decision-making role is especially important in these usually elective procedures. Since the goal is to improve practice patterns and, ultimately, the delivery of health care, approaches to dissemination will go beyond providing physicians with additional information. Alternative formats for conveying this information include interactive videodiscs, such as one developed for men contemplating surgery for benign prostatic hypertrophy (Deyo et al., 1990).

The PORT studying cataracts is assessing variations in short-term and long-term outcomes and costs for treatment of cataracts in the otherwise healthy eye, that is, where there is no indication of corneal, retinal, or optic nerve pathology. The analysis will include comparisons of the timing and type of surgical intervention (intracapsular cataract extraction, extracapsular extraction, and phacoemulsification), diagnostic procedures including ultrasound and speculomicroscopy, and differences in follow-up care. Data from Medicare enrollment and claims files as well as chart reviews and surveys of cataract patients and physicians at three sites will be analyzed. The data will then be used to estimate the probability that each of many potential outcomes will occur in specified patients. A panel of experts will define optimal management strategies for specified categories of cataract patients. Anticipated changes in demographic characteristics of the population over the next 25 years will be incorporated into a model. This model will project the clinical and economic impact of alternative strategies for cataract management (Steinberg et al., 1990).

The PORT studying prostate disease is assessing a variety of surgical and non-surgical interventions for benign prostatic hyperplasia (BPH) and localized adenocarcinoma of the prostate. BPH assessment will include variations in use and outcomes associated with transurethral resection, open prostatectomy, balloon dilation, bladder neck incision, transurethral incision of the prostate, prostatectomy, microwave diathermy, medical therapy, and watchful waiting. For prostate cancer, early diagnostic screening, radiation, radical prostatectomy, and watchful waiting will be compared. Outcome variables include survival, morbidity, symptoms, self-assessed functional status, and quality of life. Decision models based on probabilities of outcomes and associated patient utilities will be developed and used to analyze the effectiveness and cost effectiveness of treatment alternatives for patient subgroups (Fowler et al., 1988; Wennberg, 1990).

To aid in clinical decision making, this PORT study will incorporate practice guidelines, research, and health care policy findings into a "shared decision-making procedure" (SDP). The SDP combines video and computer technologies to allow patients to interactively review health scenarios relevant to their own condition. Symptoms and risks associated with a particular operative procedure are typically presented in this format (Wennberg, 1990).

The PORT studying myocardial infarction (MI) is establishing a national center to integrate information about medical technologies and processes of care for patients with acute MI. Four specific foci, selected through meta-analyses and recommendations of a national advisory panel, include controversies surrounding these topics:

1. Predischarge diagnostic tests for risk stratification (e.g., coronary angiography, exercise tolerance tests, echocardiography, Holter monitoring).
2. Acute interventions (especially thrombolytic therapy, streptokinase, and percutaneous transluminal coronary angioplasty [PTCA]).
3. Rehospitalization within three to six months post-MI.
4. Alternative procedures and medications used post-MI to reduce complications and recurrence (e.g., coronary arteriography, PTCA, aspirin, and cholesterol-reducing drugs).

Primary data will be obtained from an inception cohort of patients. Resource utilization, outcomes, and cost will be studied using Medicare data and comparable data from the Veterans Administration (VA). Recommendations will be developed and disseminated through direct physician education and distribution of printed materials in a series of interventions that target whole states, parts of states, and/or regions of the VA health care system (Pashos and McNeil, 1990).

The technology assessment programs operated by OTA and AHCPR are concerned with both the costs and outcomes of health care innovations. The inclusion of patient preferences as an important data element, as in the back pain and prostate PORT studies, reveals a growing trend toward measuring health outcomes in terms of years of healthy life. The next section describes the calculation of years of healthy life for two different technology assessments, the Disability/Distress Index and the Health Utility Index. These two examples illustrate how data for estimating years of life can be collected and how the calculations can be performed.

ESTIMATING YEARS OF HEALTHY LIFE FOR TECHNOLOGY ASSESSMENT

The two technologies introduced in this section are typical of therapeutic innovations that have become commonplace since the end of World War II. These treatments and others like them (listed in Table 13.2) will shape the health care policy debate over the coming decade, both in terms of effectiveness and affordability. Thus, neonatal intensive care units and coronary artery bypass graft surgery are good examples for discussing the use of the Health Resource Allocation Strategy for technology assessment.

Two different approaches to designing a study, collecting data, and conducting an analysis using years of healthy life for use in the Health Resource Allocation Strategy are described in this section; costs and outcomes comparisons based on these studies are discussed in the following section. The work of Boyle and colleagues (1983) is based on the Health Utilities Index system and uses primary data to study the impact of neonatal intensive care. The work of Williams (1985) uses the Disability/Distress Index and includes expert opinion to analyze the costs and outcomes of coronary artery bypass graft surgery.

Neonatal Intensive Care

The analysis by Boyle and colleagues (1983) was motivated by the need for costs and outcomes information on neonatal intensive care units (NICUs), which had not been previously subjected to economic evaluation. The very low birth weight infants were the focus of the study because NICUs are reported to be highly effective for this group (Sinclair et al., 1981). The effects of a NICU in a university medical center in Hamilton, Ontario, were studied separately for low (1,000–1,499 grams) and very low (500–999 grams) birth weight infants. Boyle et al. examined records of 213 low and 160 very low birth weight infants born in two other Hamilton hospitals before the NICU was installed and the records of 167 low and 98 very low birth weight infants born after the NICU was operational.

Medical records were reviewed for all infants included in this study. This review provided information on the infant's survival status on discharge, birth weight catego-

ry, Apgar score, and presence of respiratory distress syndrome. Maternal characteristics, including age at time of delivery and previous pregnancies and their outcomes, were also noted. Of the 301 infants who were discharged alive, approximately
85 percent were located for follow-up. Parents were mailed a questionnaire to assess
the morbidity of their child. The information collected in this questionnaire included
neurologic sequelae (cerebral palsy, hydrocephalus, epilepsy, and/or mental retardation), blindness, and deafness (Horwood et al., 1982).

In addition to the medical chart review and the postal questionnaire, data were
collected by household interview from a random sample of 148 adults in the community who had school-age children; of these, 112 completed the interview. This information was used to develop preferences for health states for the survivors. The health
states defined for this study are those in Appendix I.B. These states were based on
existing questionnaires developed for use in a general population (Eisen et al., 1979;
Patrick et al., 1973b; Kaplan et al., 1976). Special attention was paid to selecting
levels within each concept that pertained to the types of disabilities that might occur in
low birth weight infants.

To determine preferences for chronic states, the 112 respondents who completed
interviews were instructed to imagine that they were in a specific health state from birth
until death at age 70. Each respondent was asked about the same five health states. The
first four were the "corner" states required to calculate the multiattribute utilities, or
preferences. Each preference described the respondent being in the worst level in one
of the concepts and as healthy as possible in the other three. These levels are denoted as
P6, R5, S4, and H8 in Appendix I.B. For example, the respondent was asked to
consider needing help from another person in order to get around the house, yard,
neighborhood, or community and not being able to use or control the arms or legs but
otherwise being in normal, or average, health. The fifth state consisted of the worst
levels in all four concepts in the Health Utilities Index. The information collected in
response to this state was used to convert individual multiattribute utilities into social,
or group, preferences, as seen in Appendix I.B.

In 35 of the completed interviews, response to at least one item indicated confusion
about the measurement task; these interviews were excluded from further analysis.
Each of the 87 usable interviews provided information on preferences for health states
using both the category scaling and the time tradeoff methods (Chapter 6).

Using the information collected in the medical chart review, the postal questionnaire,
and the preference measurement sample, the investigators made separate computations
of life years and years of healthy life for low and very low birth weight babies who
were born before and after the introduction of the NICU (Table 13.3). The formulas
and examples at the bottom of the table indicate how the calculations were made. The
estimates of life years and years of healthy life were made using the cohort method that
was described in Chapter 9.

The NICU increased survival for three endpoints: to hospital discharge, to age 15,
and to time of death. For the very low birth weight babies, survival increased by almost
a factor of 2. However, when years of healthy life were considered, the gain attributed
to the NICU was less than when survival alone was the outcome measure. For example,
projections of survival to age 15 indicated a length of survival of 1.46 years before
intensive care and 3.37 years after. For the same two groups, the years of healthy life
were 1.22 and 1.80, respectively; the former represents a 130 percent increase in years

Table 13.3 Life years and years of healthy life for low and very low birth weight infants

	Birth weight 500–999 grams		Birth weight 1,000–1,499 grams	
	Pre-NICU	Post-NICU	Pre-NICU	Post-NICU
Total live births to age 15 (projected)	160	98	213	167
Life years (LY)/live births	1.46	3.37	9.0	11.1
Years of healthy life (YHL)/live birth	1.22	1.80	6.4	8.1
To death (projected)				
Life year (LY)/live birth	38.8	47.7	6.6	13.0
Years of healthy life (YHL)/live birth	27.4	36.0	5.5	9.1

Source: Boyle et al., 1983.

$$LY = \frac{\sum_{j}^{J} n_j t_j}{n}; YHL = \frac{\sum_{j}^{J} h_j n_j t_j}{n}$$

where n_j = the number of persons alive at time j; t_j = the duration of life at time j; h_j = the average quality of life score for individuals alive at time j; and n the total number of live births. The following examples, based on hypothetical data, illustrate the calculation of LY and YHL to obtain entries in this table.

$$LY = \frac{(15)\ 15\ +\ (8)\ 1\ +\ (0)\ 143}{160} = 1.46$$

$$YHL = \frac{15\ (h_1)\ (15)\ +\ 1\ (h_2)\ (8)\ +\ 1\ (h_3)\ (.6)\ +\ 143\ (0)\ (0)}{160} = 1.22$$

where $h_1 = 0.83$; $h_2 = 0.92$; and $h_3 = 0.65$.

of life; the latter is a 47 percent increase. For the low birth weight group, the comparable percentages are 23 and 26.5, respectively. Thus, for the very low birth weight babies, the NICU increased survival but did not result in a comparable increase in quality of life.

Boyle and colleagues' method of collecting preference estimates using community samples is rarely done. Instead, analysts usually adopt one of two approaches. The most frequently used approach is to adopt existing preference weights, that is, those identified in the literature. In the other method analysts estimate the values for two or three representative health states based on expert judgment. If expert opinion is used, the analyst must be careful to solicit these judgments from persons who are both knowledgeable and unbiased (Williams, 1988a).

Coronary Artery Bypass Graft Surgery

In evaluating the costs and benefits of coronary artery bypass graft (CABG) surgery against alternative therapies such as valve replacements and pacemakers, Williams (1985) used the published weights developed for the Disability/Distress Index (Rosser and Kind, 1978; Kind et al., 1982). Williams conducted this analysis to (1) ascertain whether the number of surgical graft procedures for coronary artery disease should be increased and (2) stimulate development of improved analytic techniques and data collection needed to implement the Health Resource Allocation Strategy.

To estimate quality of life of patients with angina, Williams asked three cardiologists to profile patients who either had already had a CABG surgery or who were being maintained by medical management. All were profiled in terms of disability and distress as characterized by the Disability/Distress Index (see Appendix I.A). Specifically, the cardiologists were asked to distinguish among mild, moderate, and severe cases of angina, and within each of these categories to distinguish between persons with left main disease or with one-, two-, or three-vessel disease. The cardiologists also estimated the prognoses for patients in each of these heart disease categories.

This classification allowed Williams to use the corresponding Disability/Distress Index weights to estimate the years of healthy life gained by surgery. In general, patients with severe angina and more serious disease benefited the most from surgery. These patients gained almost 6 years of healthy life, whereas those with one-vessel disease and moderate angina gained about 0.9 year of healthy life (Williams, 1985). The method of calculating years of healthy life is shown in Chapter 9 and is illustrated in Table 13.3. The quality of life score for each year is added to give the total years of health life. This summation is done separately for scores associated with medical management and with coronary artery bypass surgery. To estimate the years gained from surgery, the total years of healthy life for the two interventions are subtracted.

In both the neonatal intensive care and coronary artery bypass surgery studies years of healthy life were calculated as an intermediate step in evaluating the relative costs and outcomes of these two interventions against appropriate alternative courses of action.

The next section discusses the cost estimations used in each of these studies. Costs and health outcomes are combined to show the ranking by cost per year of healthy life. These ratios are then discussed in the context of the Health Resource Allocation Strategy.

COSTS AND OUTCOMES OF MEDICAL TECHNOLOGY

We selected the studies discussed here because both use years of healthy life as the measure of benefit attributed to the intervention. Also, both compare the gain in health to the cost of the intervention. Both conducted a cost–utility analysis, the core of the Health Resource Allocation Strategy. This section describes cost estimation, ranks cost per year of healthy life ratios, and discusses this analysis in the context of the stakeholders for each study.

Neonatal Intensive Care

To estimate the costs of care administered by the NICU, investigators first determined which service departments—neonatal, radiology, or operating room—were involved at each of the three hospitals. For each service, the most appropriate measure of service output was identified. These measures included patient days, radiology department work units, and operations. For each infant, the cost of care was found by recording the amount of each service used, multiplying this by the cost per service, and then adding all services used. This method of costing the NICUs resulted in cost estimates that include capital costs, supplies, and equipment as well as direct costs of care.

Other direct costs include the physician charges, community hospital charges, and cost of transport from the NICU to the community hospital if it was outside of Hamilton. Data on physician charges were obtained from health insurance records. Daily hospital rates were used to approximate the cost of care for infants treated outside the NICU (Boyle et al., 1983).

In addition to the costs incurred before hospital discharge, the investigators estimated follow-up costs. These costs included not only health care costs but also those associated with special services, institutionalization, appliances, and special education. Parents of the infants were interviewed to obtain information about these costs until the children reached age 15. Two developmental pediatricians projected lifetime costs by reviewing the health history of each child. For each child with disability who received parental care at home, the cost of food, shelter, clothing, and the opportunity cost for parental care was estimated at $8,462 in 1978 Canadian dollars. Using the same base, institutional care was estimated to cost $22,816 (Boyle et al., 1983).

The comparative costs and outcomes for the neonatal intensive care unit study are shown in Table 13.4. Columns 1 to 3 summarize essential features; columns 4 and 5 present information essential to the costs and outcomes comparison. The net effect of 8.6 (column 4) represents additional years of healthy life for the low birth weight group (1,000–1,499 grams) that can be attributed to use of the NICU. This number is reached by obtaining the difference between the years of healthy life for pre- and post-NICU groups projected over the lifetime of those infants who survived to discharge. The net effect of 3.6 years of healthy life represents the corresponding difference for the very low birth weight infants (500–999 grams). That both of these numbers are positive indicates that the NICU added years of life, or a positive health benefit.

For the low birth weight group, the total cost of care before the NICU was $92,500 (1978 Canadian dollars); after the introduction of the unit, the total costs were

Table 13.4 Ranking of costs and outcomes of a university medical center–based neonatal intensive care unit (NICU) using the Health Utilities Index with preferences from a community sample

Intervention (1)	Study group (2)	Design (3)	Net effects[a] (4)	Net costs (5)	C/YHL[b] (6)
NICU service for 1,000–1,499 gram infants	Infants born before and after NICU was introduced	Pre and post comparison Pre-NICU $n = 213$ Post-NICU $n = 167$	8.6	$7,600	$3,200
NICU service for 500–999 gram infants	Infants born before and after NICU was introduced	Pre and post comparison Pre-NICU $n = 160$ Post-NICU $n = 98$	3.6	$32,600	$22,400

Source: Boyle et al., 1983.

[a]Net effects are expressed in years of healthy life gained; these are based on the Health Utilities Index.

[b]Costs and effects are discounted at 5% per annum over the anticipated lifetime.

$100,100. The net increase in cost of care for these infants, $7,600, is recorded in column 5 of Table 13.4. The net increase in costs for treating the very low birth weight babies was $32,600. This figure is based on a total cost of care of $11,000 before the NICU was installed and $43,600 after intensive care was added.

The ratios for low and very low birth weight infants are ranked in ascending order according to cost per year of healthy life (C/YHL) (column 6). Ratios shown are based on a 5 percent discount rate and are calculated over the lifetime of the infants. NICU costs were $3,200 for the low birth weight infants, the NICU costs for each year of healthy life gained was $3,200 and $22,400 for the very low birth weights. In short, the NICU care for very low birth weight infants is seven times more expensive per year of healthy life gained than it is for low birth weight infants.

Table 13.4 summarizes Steps 2 through 7 of the Health Resource Allocation Strategy. An important aspect of the Strategy is the context. Analysts must consider the scope of the problem, alternative courses of action, stakeholders in the decision process, and budgetary constraints in which the health intervention is implemented. In the United States, approximately 5 percent of all newborns, or about 175,000 infants, are treated in NICUs each year. Of these, about one-half weigh 2,500 grams or less. In 1984, about 17,000 infants weighed less than 1,000 grams (OTA, 1987).

Data on the total population at risk, along with the cost per year of healthy life obtained by Boyle et al. (1983), can be used to set the context of any decision concerning the implementation of a NICU. In 1989 U.S. dollars, the cost per year of healthy life for very low birth weight infants was $27,767. For any given year, the total cost per year for these very low birth weight babies is almost $500 million. The total cost over their estimated lifetime of 13 years is about $6 billion.

Access to neonatal care varies by location in the United States; low birth weight infants born in rural areas are less likely to be treated in neonatal intensive care units than are such infants born in urban areas. Also, financial barriers may prevent some infants from receiving intensive care. Some hospitals may not serve cases covered by Medicaid, the health care plan that provides coverage to low-income persons. One explanation for the discrimination against these patients is that hospitals claim that Medicaid is a poor payer (OTA, 1987). Another explanation is that NICUs may be unavailable or of poor quality in hospitals whose principal clients are people living in poverty.

Thus, an element of the decision process may be to improve access to neonatal intensive care. One way of assuring access is to control geographic distribution of the units or to make them more widely available through emergency medical transportation. Another way of assuring access is to provide everyone with insurance coverage that is recognized and accepted by hospitals that provide the services. Clearly, one factor in a decision to make neonatal intensive care units more widely available is the total cost of such a program, especially when balanced against alternatives (OTA, 1987).

Neonatal intensive care is one of the most expensive types of care that a hospital can provide (OTA, 1987). Thus, it generally falls on the government to provide these services. In deciding whether or not to fund, the government needs to consider both stakeholders and programs that compete for resources. One group of stakeholders who will be proponents of a NICU program is likely to be potential parents known to have a high probability for use of this service. Two other groups who will pressure policymakers for the adoption of this intervention are persons with disabilities and activists who lobby for disability rights. They argue that it is possible to have a high quality of life despite obvious impairments (Hobbs et al., 1985) and that it is the government's responsibility to provide for people with disabilities. Government intervention is particularly important in the United States, where society may place low value on disability (Levin, 1990).

Stakeholders likely to oppose NICUs will be those who may be denied a needed service due to lack of resources. Resources spent on NICUs cannot be spent on another intervention, so people needing the other service will be opposed to allocating resources to intensive care units for high-risk infants. For example, mothers needing prenatal care will press for finite resources to be devoted to making this care available. In most policy decisions, stakeholders are rarely involved in determining which programs will be funded. Usually stakeholders become involved in the decision process when they need the service.

When a neonatal intensive care unit is available to a low birth weight infant, stakeholders focus on how to use the resources within the NICU. Parents, families, and health care providers frequently have to make survival decisions. If the quality of life of the infant might be lengthy survival with little enjoyment, the provider is likely to withhold or limit treatment. More aggressive treatment is applied to infants who have a chance for lengthy survival with a relatively high quality of life. The role of the parents and families may vary in different health care settings. Often their participation depends on the physician's acceptance of the parents' role in decision making (Levin, 1990).

This example based on the use of neonatal intensive care illustrates the role of the stakeholders when the health decision to offer a particular technology has already been made. In this case, the decision is how much of the intervention to use. In other situations, the technology may be unavailable because of a formal policy decision. For example, the State of Oregon decided that liver transplants would not be provided to people who received state-assisted health insurance. This policy decision was acceptable until people needing transplants pressured policymakers to rescind the decision (Welch and Larson, 1988); the Oregon legislature subsequently developed an alternative plan for allocating resources (Chapter 14).

Whether to support intensive care for low birth weight infants is one health decision facing the health policymaker. Key decision elements are the cost of care and the probability of extending infants' lives for relatively long periods at questionable quality. Other decisions may concern extending the lives of "productive" adults for possibly shorter periods but at probably higher quality and for less cost. An example of this type of decision is whether to fund surgical treatment for heart disease for middle-aged and older males. The Williams (1985) analysis of CABG surgery typifies this kind of decision.

Coronary Artery Bypass Graft Surgery

The Williams study used data from the British National Health Service to estimate direct inpatient costs of bypass surgery. On average, these costs were £3,580 in 1983–84. Neither outpatient direct nor indirect costs are included in the estimates used to compute cost per year of healthy life gained due to CABG. The direct inpatient costs were lower than those reported in the United States. This disparity was attributed to the difference in physician payment and in costs of acute inpatient care between the two countries.

In this analysis, CABG surgery was more cost effective among persons with severe angina than among persons with either left main vessel disease or triple-vessel disease; the ratios of costs per year of healthy life are £1,040 and £1,270, respectively. Among those with moderate angina, the most favorable ratio is for persons with left main disease, £1,330. Ratios of costs per year of healthy life for other combinations of degree of angina and vessel involvement are all over 2.0, indicating a cost of more than £2,000 for each year of healthy life gained. For one-vessel disease, regardless of degree of angina, the ratios are uniformly high, indicating a greater than sevenfold increase in cost for the same outcome as for the more severe cases (Williams, 1985).

In evaluating the relative cost per year of healthy life of CABG surgery compared to alternative treatments, Williams calculated the cost and years of healthy life for patients receiving other types of treatment for heart disease as well as for persons treated for selected non–heart conditions. The rankings of costs and outcomes for these conditions are shown in Table 13.5. In comparing other treatments for heart disease with coronary artery bypass graft, valve replacement and pacemaker implantations had lower cost–effectiveness ratios than did graft surgery. For example, £900 and £700 per year of healthy life, respectively compared to £1,040 for the most cost-effective use of CABG surgery. This suggests that these alternative procedures are of better monetary value for the treatment of heart disease than is coronary artery bypass surgery. In addition, percutaneous transluminal coronary angioplasty is more cost effective than CABG surgery for cases with one-vessel disease and severe angina with ratios of £2,400 and £11,400, respectively.

Williams also compared the cost effectiveness of heart disease treatment with treatments for hip fracture and end-stage renal disease. Hip replacement was one of the most cost-effective interventions considered, having a ratio of costs per year of healthy life of £750. With this small ratio, this treatment is almost at the top of the ranking. This ranking of interventions has led to comparisons with the standings of sporting teams or leagues. Some analysts even refer to such a table as a league table, or "QALY-league table."

Table 13.5 can be used in conjunction with the Health Resource Allocation Strategy to address one of the problems facing the medical community today: differentiating between effective and ineffective use of medical technologies. With respect to CABG surgery the ratio of cost per year of healthy life gained is more than five times greater for persons with one-vessel disease than for persons with left main disease or with double-vessel disease coupled with mild or severe angina. Furthermore, persons with less serious disease gain relatively short periods of years of healthy life above what would have been gained by medical management alone. For example, persons with one-vessel disease and mild angina gain three months of healthy life. The costs of surgery for patients with mild or with moderate to severe disease is roughly comparable.

From this analysis, policymakers might recommend that the preferred treatment for patients with double-vessel disease and mild angina is medical management rather than CABG surgery. This treatment would result in almost the same number of years of healthy life as would CABG surgery with a cost savings of £12,600 per year of healthy

Table 13.5 Ranking of costs and outcomes of existing health interventions using the Disability Distress Index with published preferences and expert judgments used to estimate years of healthy life

Intervention (1)	Study group (2)	Design (3)	Net effects[a] (4)	Net costs[a] (£000) in 1983–84 prices (5)	C/YHL[a] (£000) in 1983–84 prices (6)
Pacemaker implantation	Cases with atrioventricular heart block		5.0	3.5	0.7
Hip replacement			4.0	3.0	0.75
Valve replacement	Cases with aortic stenosis		5.0	4.5	0.9
Coronary artery bypass graft (CABG)	Cases with left main vessel disease and severe angina	Comparison of CABG with medical management	2.75	2.85	1.04
Coronary artery bypass graft (CABG)	Cases with left main vessel disease and moderate angina	Comparison of CABG with medical management	2.25	3.0	1.33
Coronary artery bypass graft (CABG)	Cases with double-vessel disease and severe angina	Comparison of CABG with medical management	1.25	2.85	2.28
Percutaneous transluminal coronary angioplasty (PTCA)	Cases with one-vessel disease and severe angina		1.0	2.4	2.40
Coronary artery bypass graft (CABG)	Cases with left main vessel disease and mild angina	Comparison of CABG with medical management	1.25	3.15	2.52
Kidney transplantation (cadaver)			5.0	15.0	3.0
Percutaneous transluminal coronary angioplasty (PTCA)	Cases with one-vessel disease and moderate angina		0.75	2.55	3.4
Coronary artery bypass graft (CABG)	Cases with double-vessel disease and moderate angina		0.75	3.0	4.0
Heart transplantation			4.5	23.0	5.0
Percutaneous transluminal	Cases with one-vessel disease and		0.25	2.68	10.72

(*continued*)

Table 13.5   *(Continued)*

Intervention (1)	Study group (2)	Design (3)	Net effects[a] (4)	Net costs[a] (£000) in 1983–84 prices (5)	C/YHL[a] (£000) in 1983–84 prices (6)
Coronary angioplasty (PTCA)	Mild angina				
Hemodialysis at home			6.0	66.0	11.0
Coronary artery bypass graft (CABG)	Cases with one-vessel disease and severe angina	Comparison of CABG with medical management	0.25	2.85	11.4
Coronary artery bypass graft (CABG)	Cases with one-vessel disease and moderate angina	Comparison of CABG with medical management	0.25	2.55	12.0
Coronary artery bypass graft (CABG)	Cases with double-vessel disease and mild angina	Comparison of CABG with medical management	0.25	3.15	12.60
Hemodialysis in hospital	Hemodialysis in hospital		5.0	70.0	14.0

Source: Williams, 1985.

[a] Net effects are expressed in years of healthy life gained; these are based on the Disability/Distress Index.

[b] Costs and effects are discounted at 5% per annum.

life per patient. The resources saved by this shift from surgical to medical treatment could then be reallocated to some other health intervention.

The ranking of costs and outcomes in Table 13.5 also illustrates the use of restricting access to expensive care, or rationing. Hospital hemodialysis, the most expensive intervention shown, costs an additional £14,000 per year of healthy life gained. Alternative treatments for end-stage renal disease—home dialysis and kidney transplant—are less expensive for the same or better benefit. Based on these data, the policymaker might decide that hospital dialysis would no longer be a service provided under a public health insurance program.

Under this recommendation and assuming patients receiving dialysis either in the hospital or at home were alike in all other ways, at least £3,000 per year of healthy life per patient would be freed for use in some other way. For each patient shifted from hospital to home hemodialysis, £3,000 per year of healthy life would be available to support some other health intervention(s).

Following this logic, even more resources would be available if the majority of those treated with hospital dialysis could receive a kidney transplant. For each person with end-stage renal disease who was shifted from hospital hemodialysis to a transplant, £11,000 per year of healthy life would be freed for use with other interventions.

Evaluating the Total Artificial Heart

The foregoing examples illustrate the use of the Health Resource Allocation Strategy for evaluating existing medical technologies. A recent study conducted by the Institute on Medicine analyzed the costs and outcomes associated with the development of a new technology, the total artificial heart (Hogness and VanAntwerp, 1991). This study addressed two issues: (1) the performance of the total artificial heart in routine use; and (2) the availability and cost of governmental support for the development of this device.

A complex simulation model which allowed for variations in assumptions about costs and outcomes was used to form a ranking of costs and outcomes for selected heart disease treatments, including the total artificial heart. Expert judgment was used to estimate of the probability of occurrence and mortality associated with clinical parameters such as device failure, infection, and thromboembolism.

As illustrated in Chapter 6, preferences for nine health states, ranging from successful implantation through various states of complications to device failure or death, were obtained using the time tradeoff method. The mean long-term health state for patients assumed to receive medical treatment only was 0.08; for those receiving a heart transplant, 0.75; and those receiving a total artificial heart, 0.66 (Hogness and VanAntwerp, 1991). In a ranking of costs and outcomes, the cost per year of healthy life gained for implantation of a total artificial heart was $105,000. The ratio for heart transplantation was $32,000. Ratios for other heart disease treatments considered in the analysis were also lower than for the total artificial heart.

As a result of this analysis, the National Heart, Lung, and Blood Institute, which sponsored the study, has a means of considering whether continued development of the total artificial hearts fits the overall goals for improving the cardiovascular health of the nation. This study is a good example of how the Health Resource Allocation Strategy can be used to analyze the impact of technological innovations.

From these examples, we see that the Health Resource Allocation Strategy can bring useful information into the debates surrounding technology assessment. The Strategy can be used to identify effective or ineffective treatments. In addition, as illustrated by the ranking of costs and outcomes attributed to coronary artery bypass surgery in relation to other types of treatments, the Strategy can assist decision making about public support for expensive medical treatments. By bringing stakeholder concerns into the process, the Health Resource Allocation Strategy goes beyond existing policy-analytic tools in assisting with the decision making.

14

Improving Access to Health Care

Despite many decades of public and private initiatives, a significant number of people in the United States do not have access to a satisfactory standard of health and medical care. *Access* is a shorthand term referring to the timely use of personal health services to achieve the best possible health outcomes (Millman, 1992). Some of these people may lack health insurance coverage or may not have financial entitlement. Others may live out of reach of current delivery systems, find available health services culturally inappropriate, or encounter other deterrents that interfere with their access to essential services. People with low income, children, some ethnic groups (in particular Hispanic and black persons), homeless people, and people with disabilities are among those who face such barriers.

Although there is increasing public awareness of the problem, no consensus has been achieved about the importance of improving access to health care versus addressing competing social priorities, such as education, defense, law enforcement, housing, and transportation. Since the enactment of Medicare and Medicaid in the 1960s, incremental strategies have been attempted, primarily at the state level, to expand public and private services to those who lack health care. A growing number of states—such as Oregon, Hawaii, Kansas, and New York—are attempting major reforms to their health care systems in hopes of improving access.

A significant impediment to large-scale reform is concern about the federal budget deficit. This concern is inextricably coupled with the public's reluctance to accept new taxes to fund the expansion of entitlement programs. The Medicaid program, which pays for the medical care of some very poor people, is expected to have the largest percentage increase of any major federal program in the next decade, in part because of the growing population of older and disabled poor persons residing in nursing homes. States are experiencing a similar strain on their revenues to fund Medicaid, with some states reducing benefits and changing eligibility criteria. Most states have even greater incentive to control increasing outlays for health care because they must have balanced budgets by law.

Another major concern is defining the *level* of health care that society judges "adequate" and is willing to fund. No consensus exists on the minimum basic package of benefits and services that should be available to all. Still another concern is conflict among different interest groups about who will win or lose under the different proposed policy alternatives. Many fear that medically fragile children or people with life-threatening diseases or long-term disabilities will not be covered under a universal insurance plan. Finally, legislators, employers, providers, and consumers all want some evidence that expanded access to health care will pay off in terms of improved health-related quality of life for *everyone* without escalating health care costs beyond their willingness or ability to pay.

The four interrelated challenges dominating the debate over America's health care system are improving access, reducing or slowing the rate of increase in costs, maintaining quality of care, and reducing health inequalities. The Health Resource Allocation Strategy provides one means for helping to address these challenges. Greater access to an agreed-upon level of services can be achieved through the social and political process of evaluating and ranking the cost and outcome ratios of different health interventions under consideration and making available those interventions that provide the largest benefit for the lowest cost. Funds would then be available to improve access to this basic level of service to all persons.

Funding only the most cost-effective health interventions implies that everyone will not be able to have access to every desired intervention. Thus, rationing, or the distribution of resources to individuals according to a specified rule, will occur. By rationing, the Health Resource Allocation Strategy recognizes fiscal limits to health care expenditures. By public discussion of health care interventions and their cost and benefits, the strategy permits every interested party to participate in the determination of the basic level of coverage to be provided to all.

In this chapter, we analyze the problem of providing universal access to health care. Rationing through a sociopolitical process is proposed as the necessary and fair approach to address both access and cost. We illustrate how the State of Oregon has used elements of the Health Resource Allocation Strategy as a means of developing a health care policy that could guarantee universal access to the health care system. In our view, the goal of improving access to health care should be linked to the objective of reducing health disparities. These disparities are examined with available data, including estimates of years of healthy life for persons belonging to different racial and ethnic groups. We examine the role of improved access to health care in reducing these disparities. Finally, we discuss the implications of rationing for the sociopolitical process.

RATIONING TO PROVIDE UNIVERSAL ACCESS TO HEALTH CARE

The United States faces a serious problem that promises to get worse: the inability of many residents to gain access to needed health care, primarily because of cost. Although geographic, cultural, and educational barriers limit access to care, financial barriers dominate. Poor people, near-poor people, and persons with chronic illness—especially those without public or private insurance—find it difficult to obtain health care services. Even persons with higher income may experience problems in access if their insurance does not cover certain conditions or needed services such as mental health services, drugs, durable medical equipment, or special devices.

The problem of health care access has increased in the United States over the last decade because the following four trends converged: (1) growth in the number of Americans without public or private health insurance; (2) rise in the price of medical care, prompting the attention of payers such as large corporations concerned that medical costs have grown more rapidly than inflation; (3) increasing price competition among hospitals and other health care providers; and (4) increasing recognition of and

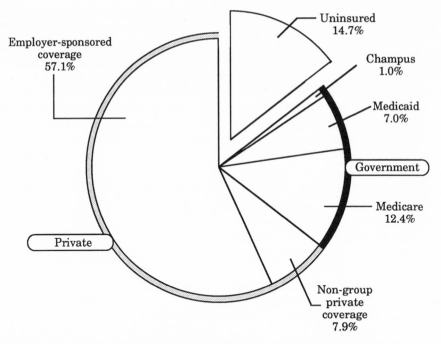

Figure 14.1 Primary source of health insurance, current population surveys, 1991. *Source:* Employee Benefit Research Institute, 1992

debate about the problem by politicians, the media, providers, and consumers. Figure 14.1 shows the primary sources of health insurance for persons in the United States in 1991. The majority of Americans continue to obtain health insurance coverage through their employers (57 percent) or government programs (20 percent) that serve older adults (Medicare), poor people (Medicaid), and the military (Veterans Administration).

The first trend is growth in the number of uninsured persons. An estimated 13.1 percent, or 33 million Americans, primarily lower-income workers or members of low-income families, do not have health insurance. Approximately 17 percent of the population under age 65 reported having no public or private health insurance at some time in 1987 (Moyer, 1989). Everyone age 65 and over is covered by Medicare; yet less than half of those under age 65 years living below the federal poverty line—that is, non-elderly poor people—are insured by Medicaid. Most workers are covered by health insurance, particularly those employed by companies with 500 or more employees. However, most companies with fewer than 10–20 employees do not offer health insurance. Currently, 87 percent of all companies in the United States have fewer than 20 employees.

Health insurance coverage is associated with age, employment, health, socioeconomic status, and racial and ethnic differences, and pre-existing health conditions. A higher than average percentage of persons under the age of 35 and a lower than average percent of persons over age 35 are uninsured. The age group 16–24 accounts for the greatest percentage of uninsured persons (General Accounting Office, 1991).

Private health insurance coverage among persons under 65 years of age is greatest for non-Hispanic white persons (Trevino et al., 1991). In contrast, less than 60 percent of non-Hispanic black Americans (58 percent), Mexican Americans (54 percent), and Puerto Rican Americans (51 percent) had private coverage. Medicaid was the major form of coverage for non-Hispanic black and Puerto Rican Americans. Thirty-five percent of Mexican Americans reported having no health insurance coverage during the period 1983–86.

Contrary to popular belief, the majority of uninsured persons in the United States live in households in which at least one member is employed full-time. Of all uninsured, 62 percent belong to families with at least one full-time employee, 23 percent are in families with only part-time employees, and 14.8 percent are unemployed (Foley, 1991). As health care costs have risen, employers have cut back benefits. This has forced employees to pay larger deductibles, higher copayments, and an ever-larger portion of their own premiums. Persons in lower income groups are more likely to be uninsured; for example, approximately 28 percent of adults earning $5.00 an hour or less are uninsured (Short et al., 1988).

The second trend, reviewed in Chapter 1, is rising health care expenditures that consume ever more of the nation's income. At the present rate of growth, these costs will amount to more than 13 percent of the 1993 gross national product. Figure 14.2 shows the primary sources of these health expenditures for 1989. Private expenditures (58 percent) still outstrip government expenditures (42 percent). Private health insurance accounts for 33 percent of health expenditures and out-of-pocket outlays for 20 percent. Federal sources pay for 29 percent of expenditures; state and local governments provide 13 percent. Most of these expenditures (39 percent) are for hospital

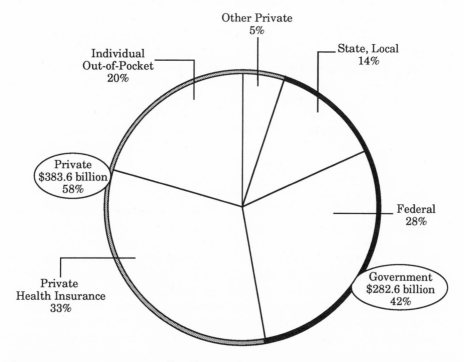

Figure 14.2 Primary sources of health expenditures, United States, 1990. *Source:* Levit et al., 1991

services, although approximately 20 percent goes for physician services. Many fear that escalating health expenditures threaten the chance of continuing prosperity for many individuals and employers.

The third trend, often labeled "uncompensated" care or, more properly, hospital revenue shifting, has existed since the advent of third-party insurance. Publicly owned hospitals (28 percent) provide the majority of charity care explicitly for poor people. Private, not-for-profit community hospitals (58 percent) and proprietary, for-profit hospitals (14 percent) also provide some nonreimbursable or discounted services, because many states require hospitals with emergency rooms to take emergency cases. Unreimbursed care prompts cost-shifting. Hospitals may raise charges to paying patients to subsidize unpaid care. The load falls unevenly on different hospitals. Purchasers of health care are challenging revenue shifting, asking for more favorable treatment. An oversupply of hospital beds and continuing price competition prompts hospitals to limit charity care. The result is reduced access to care for uninsured patients.

The fourth trend is increasing public concern over the state of health care in the United States. As Reinhardt points out, "Just like people in other industrialized nations, Americans proclaim, in survey after survey, that health care should be viewed as a social good accessible to every American, *at the same level of quality*, regardless of ability to pay" (1989, p. 339). Access to health care is beginning to appear in regular polls as one of "the most pressing problems facing Americans today."

The increase in public debate and public support for national health care reform does not mean that a public consensus is emerging on the specifics of such a proposal (Blendon and Donelan, 1991). In fact, a large majority of Americans are highly satisfied with their own health insurance and health care. An analysis of more than two decades of poll results identified six major trends in public opinion: Americans (1) are generally satisfied with the personal health care they receive, (2) favor more rather than less health spending, when the economy remains strong, (3) are influenced by economic downturns and reverse themselves to favor reduced spending, (4) are not in favor of cutting federal outlays to health to reduce deficit spending, (5) are in favor of limiting care to older persons, withholding "big-ticket" medical technology and reducing the future supply of physicians (if the nation faces a serious economic crisis), and (6) are losing their level of confidence in the leaders of the nations's major health institutions and professions (Blendon, 1988).

Sensing public unrest about health care, political campaigns at the state and national levels are beginning to focus on health care in America. Undoubtedly, public awareness that "something" needs to be done about the American health care system results from increased news media attention and increased public debate. Regardless of its origins, the future of health care is increasingly in the public's view.

In September 1990, the U.S. Bipartisan Commission on Comprehensive Health Care—the Pepper Commission—called for action to implement a system-wide health care reform that would guarantee all Americans health care coverage in an efficient, effective health care system (The Pepper Commission, 1990). The report stressed that universal health insurance coverage required major reform, and that expanding access must proceed hand in hand with controlling costs. The commission's mandate is for comprehensive national reform of the health care system. The responses and proposals, however, are primarily from state initiatives.

These forces—rising numbers of uninsured persons, rapid inflation of health care expenditures, increasing price competition that reduces unpaid care, and rising public awareness—have prompted state policymakers to attempt new approaches to financing and delivering care to poor people, uninsured persons, and underinsured groups. At least four major policy options have evolved to address the need for health care for these groups. These policy options include (1) a compulsory, employer-based private insurance program, with the government insuring nonworkers and the poor, primarily through expansion of Medicaid eligibility to persons without insurance; (2) a plan that requires employers to provide their employees with health insurance or pay a tax, with the government insuring nonworkers and the poor; (3) a program of income-related tax credits for individuals, independent of their employers, for the purchase of private insurance; and (4) an all-government insurance system (Blendon and Edwards, 1991).

In the first and second options, employers would be required either to offer insurance or to pay into a pool that would offer policies to uninsured workers. Tax incentives and new insurance regulations would be required to implement this solution. Small-business owners, the largest segment of employers not providing coverage, strongly oppose this approach. Medicaid expansion would cover the unemployed poor, but these programs would be financed through general revenues, and would require additional health resources.

In almost all options being pursued by states, significant increases in public spending would be required to aid smaller companies and to finance increases in Medicaid eligibility. Public insurance programs would be financed by income, payroll, or other taxes, and public payers would set uniform fees. The options to reforming our health system to improve access therefore raise the specter of increased costs. Although many have proposed a large number of ways to prevent increases in expenditures, primarily under the rubric of "cost containment," these have not succeeded to date in controlling costs or moderating public expectations for medical care. Increasing attention is being paid by states, the nation, and other countries, to medical effectiveness evaluations and rationing as major strategies for controlling costs and improving access to health care.

Limiting health care budgets and expenditures to cost-effective treatments is the major principle of resource allocation strategies, including the Health Resource Allocation Strategy. Medical effectiveness evaluations are based on the notion of not paying for inappropriate and unnecessary care, and thus involve rationing, though sometimes implicitly. Beneficial but not necessarily marginally cost-effective treatments are denied. Explicit rationing involves refusal by private or public insurers to pay for treatments "low in priority" in the eyes of the payers. Proponents of rationing propose that savings in health care outlays through medical effectiveness evaluations and rationing be used to improve access to health care for those currently outside the system.

Both implicit and explicit rationing impose limits on health care expenditures. Rationing to improve access requires acceptance that limits in expenditures are *necessary* and *desirable* to improve access to basic health care benefits for everyone. Rationing also requires denying payment for some costly procedures. When these procedures are clearly "useless," denying benefits is easy. More often, however, gains in health must be weighed against increases in costs. Refusing to pay for some kinds of care to hold down costs means not giving everything to everyone who wants it. These basic assumptions and elements of rationing are unpalatable, if not unacceptable, to many persons in the United States.

To accept rationing, one does indeed have to accept the necessity of fiscal limits to health care expenditures. It is highly seductive to believe that increasing the efficiency of the health care system or infusing the system with money, such as transfers from other sectors of the economy including defense, will solve the problem of improving access and answering the demand for health care. Increasing efficiency or increasing spending on health care, however, will *not* address two questions: "What is beneficial health care?" and "How should public monies be expended to provide this care to as many persons as possible?" Medical effectiveness evaluations and rationing are necessary for identifying cost-effective treatments, for more efficient allocation of public expenditures to the most beneficial treatments, and for improving access to persons who now do without a basic minimum level of health care.

Medical effectiveness evaluations and rationing should involve the community in debate over what is beneficial health care, what is the basic minimum level of health care that should be provided to all, what level of health is desired, and how public monies should be expended. The values to stakeholders for outcomes of care and their priorities for different services should be taken into account in the sociopolitical process. Steps 1 and 8 of the Health Resource Allocation Strategy are included to ensure that stakeholders and their values are prominently involved in health decisions.

The State of Oregon has embarked on a plan that incorporates such a sociopolitical process in allocating resources and rationing treatments in order to improve access to health care for uninsured persons. The Oregon Plan provides an important example of how the Health Resource Allocation Strategy could be used to free public monies for improving access to a basic level of health care and potentially to reduce health disparities.

THE OREGON PLAN

The State of Oregon has formulated a strategy for providing universal health services coverage for the poor and near-poor, an initiative that serves as a model for national policy. The state was motivated to enact legislation providing this coverage for two main reasons. First, nearly one-fifth (16 percent) of the state's population, between 400,000 to 450,00 Oregonians, have no health insurance, and approximately 230,000 are *underinsured*. Costs for caring for these patients are borne by third-party payers and paying patients; this is thought to increase the cost of insurance premiums by 30 percent. Second, the Oregon legislature faced a tax revolt in 1988 which limited state revenues. The state constitution calls for an annual balanced budget; thus, deficit financing of health care services is not permitted. Some strategy was needed to address budget constraints and the need to continue services. The Division of Adult and Family Services, the agency responsible for administering the state Medicaid program, realized that the program could either extend its funding for perinatal care to include about 1500 persons not covered previously, or continue to fund a program of organ transplantation for a projected 34 patients (Welch and Larson, 1988).

In 1989 the Oregon legislature, under the leadership of Senator John Kitzhaber (a physician), passed three bills (Senate Bills 27, 935, and 534) to establish a program to provide health care to all Oregon residents. Senate Bill 27, the centerpiece of the proposal, established the Oregon Plan, officially called the Basic Health Services Plan.

This legislation also created the 11-member Oregon Health Services Commission (5 physicians, 4 consumers, and 2 other health professionals) charged with reporting to the governor "a list of health services ranked by priority, from the most important to the least important, representing the comparative benefits of each service to the entire population to be served." Thus, the goal is a publicly defined, standard package of *effective* health care offered to all Oregonians (Oregon Health Services Commission, 1991)

Legislation passed in 1991 extended or modified the Basic Health Services Act of 1989. Medicaid-eligible elderly, disabled, and individuals in foster care or in state custody were originally exempt from the provisions of Senate Bill 27, but are now expected to be included in 1993. The Health Insurance Reform Act (SB 1076) passed in 1991 established limits and safeguards on employer-based insurance by constructing rate categories, limiting increases in small group plans, guaranteeing issue and renewability of policies, and regulating exclusion of pre-existing conditions. Finally, the Health Resources Commission Act (SB 1077) established a data and cost review commission designed to contain statewide health care costs in face of the expansion of insurance to new groups.

With the passage of Senate Bill 27 and the establishment of the Health Services Commission, the Oregon state legislature essentially mandated many elements of the Health Resource Allocation Strategy. Table 14.1 outlines the provisions of the Oregon Basic Health Services Act of 1989.

Universal Access to Care

Senate Bill 27 defines the population for which the state is responsible as all those with a family income below the federal poverty level. The amounts are recalculated each

Table 14.1 Provisions of the Oregon Basic Health Services Act of 1989

Universal access to care (less than 65 years old)
  Medicaid
  Employment-based coverage
  Insurance pool for "high-risk" Oregonians

Services assigned priorities by outcome
  Public process
    Clinical data
    Social values
  Funding based on effectiveness

Benefit level determined by society
  Benefits related to cost
  Applies across the board
    Forces explicit allocation decisions
    Mandated coverage in the workplace
  No cost-shifting for additional services

Reimbursement based on cost

Liability shield

Source: Oregon Health Services Commission, 1991.

year to reflect inflation and changes in the cost of living in the consumer price index. One or more persons are called a family, and income is gross income. Income does not include noncash benefits. For 1990, the federal poverty levels by family size ranged from $6,280 for one person to $21,260 for eight persons ($2,140 is added for each additional member above eight).

In Oregon, those with family income at or *below* the federal poverty level are to be guaranteed access to the state Medicaid program. Medicaid is a joint federal and state program which pays health expenses for low-income persons who are aged, blind, disabled, or members of families with dependent children. Medicaid operates under Title XIX of the Social Security Act within broad federal rules. Each state, however, has some flexibility in determining eligibility, optional services provided, and level of provider reimbursement.

Final implementation of Senate Bill 27 in Oregon requires waivers of federal Medicaid regulations. The first application for these waivers has been denied. The federal government pays 63 percent of the cost of Medicaid services in Oregon. Federal rules allow states to limit specific kinds of treatment, but not by disease categories. Organ transplants and vision, dental, and chiropractic services do not have to be offered. Except for certain groups of people, states are allowed to reduce income eligibility for the program. States are also prohibited, under current federal rules, from providing Medicaid insurance to adults without dependent children unless they are blind, aged, or disabled.

The private sector is covered under Senate Bill 935, which provides incentives for, and ultimately mandates, employer-based coverage to cover employers with 25 or fewer employees. If put into effect (this bill faces considerable legal opposition), those with a family income above the federal poverty level would be guaranteed access to an employment-based policy that must provide a benefit level equal to or greater than that offered by the state for those on Medicaid. The list of services established under Senate Bill 27 also determines the minimum package of benefits that employers must provide to qualify for state tax credits. In Oregon, all employers who do not offer health insurance benefits by 1995 are to pay 75 percent of the cost of insuring their workers and 50 percent of the cost of dependent coverage into a state insurance pool that will be used to insure those people. The amount that employers are to pay will be based on the cost of the Medicaid priority list established under Senate Bill 27. The law provides tax credits up to $25.00 a month for each employee.

The public and private sectors are thus linked by what the state determines is the benefit level for persons for whom the state is responsible. The state cannot mandate a benefit on the private sector, unless the benefit is important enough to offer to the public sector. The state thus defines the basic minimum level of service that will be available to all. These services are assigned priorities based on the following: (1) research and expert testimony on the effectiveness of treatments; (2) cost and outcomes comparisons based on a modified version of the Quality of Well-Being Scale; (3) public values obtained from community meetings; (4) priority categories of health services developed by the Commission and grouped as "essential," "very important," and "valuable to certain individuals" but significantly less likely to be cost effective or to produce substantial long-term gain; and (5) the independent judgment of commissioners.

Senate Bill 534 is intended to provide insurance for those people who want to buy insurance but who cannot because insurance companies will not sell it to them. Oregon residents with "high-risk" medical conditions often cannot purchase insurance from private insurers and will be eligible for a medical (high-risk) insurance pool established under Senate Bill 534. Persons who have been turned down for health insurance will be eligible to participate if they can afford the monthly premiums, which are to be set at 150 percent of a "normal" premium.

Services Prioritized by Outcome

The Oregon Health Services Commission was charged to seek testimony and information from advocates for selected target populations and to conduct community meetings to build consensus on the values used in reaching health resource allocation decisions. Values were elicited at community meetings and testimony was heard at public hearings; advocates for older adults, people with disabilities, consumers of mental health services, poor and near-poor citizens, and health care providers participated. The commission is also responsible for identifying which health services to assign priorities to, the basis for assigning priorities, and the specific means to involve the public. Therefore the commission had wide discretion and final authority in how to proceed in developing and implementing the process for assigning priorities to health services.

Oregon Health Decisions was established in 1983 as a private not-for-profit organization dedicated to educating citizens about ethical issues in health care (Crawshaw et al., 1990). Oregon Health Decisions conducted 19 public meetings, involving nearly 600 citizens, at key urban and rural locations. Using a structured priority-setting exercise, the Citizens' Health Care Parliament of 50 delegates prepared a list of 15 principles for allocating health care resources (Oregon Health Decisions, 1988). These principles have provided guidance for designing and implementing the Oregon Plan.

In implementing the provisions of Senate Bill 27, the Health Services Commission originally divided its task into three major areas: health outcomes and comparative benefits, social values, and mental health care and chemical dependency. As the commission's work proceeded, two additional subcommittees were appointed: ancillary services and alternative methodology.

The health outcomes/comparative benefits and social values subcommittees were assigned the original task of collecting and analyzing the data components of the Health Resource Allocation Strategy. The health outcomes subcommittee elicited judgments from licensed health providers in over 50 specialty areas on the consequences of designated treatments for specific conditions. The Oregon Health Services Commission defined health treatments largely in terms of categories of CPT codes, codes contained in the *Physicians' Current Procedural Terminology*. Diagnosed conditions were specified in relation to the *International Classification of Disease*, Ninth Revision (ICD-9-CM), for physical conditions and the *Diagnostic and Statistical Manual of Mental Disorders*, Third Edition–revised (DSMIII-R) for mental conditions. The treatments to which priorities are assigned are largely ICD-9/CPT code and DSMIII-R/CPT code categories.

In calculating cost–benefit ratios, each category was evaluated in terms of the cost of procedure, the probability of the success of the procedure, and the average health benefit and its duration resulting from a successful treatment. Health administration experts estimated costs, including the full costs of services, drugs, and durable medical equipment. The health outcomes panels projected the consequences of both treatment and nontreatment for each condition using the modified Quality of Well-Being Scale (QWB). This estimation procedure required health experts to indicate (1) what health services are appropriate for what diagnostic categories, and (2) what consequences are probable following treatment and nontreatment for each diagnosis. Experts estimated consequences using up to five scenarios defined in terms of the following: the health state classification system of the QWB (see Appendix I), the expected duration of the health state, and the probability of the scenario. Use of multiple scenarios made it possible to take into account the probability of return to usual health, the probability of death, and the probabilities of different levels of function including the side effects of treatment. The level of certainty for the outcomes was represented in the distribution of probabilities across the scenarios. Low probabilities reflected a relatively uncertain outcome, whereas high probabilities reflected a relatively certain outcome.

The difference between an estimate of a condition without treatment and with treatment was used to determine the level of benefit attributed to a condition/treatment pairing. These estimates from health care experts reflect the values and preferences of the specialty fields represented and the experts involved.

Benefit Level Determined by Society

The subcommittee on social values coordinated public involvement in the Oregon Plan. The public participated in (1) 12 public hearings held throughout the state at which 175 persons testified, (2) 47 community meetings held in every Oregon county and attended by 1,000 persons, and (3) a large-scale telephone survey administered to a random sample of 1,000 Oregon residents. A consortium of 73 citizens' groups coordinated by the Oregon Health Action Campaign was involved in obtaining public participation in the plan, and over 3,500 persons attended hearings and community meetings.

At the community meetings, participants completed a questionnaire designed to elicit health care process and outcome values. Table 14.2 summarizes the 13 values that resulted in the order of frequency with which they appeared (Garland and Hasmain, 1990; Oregon Health Services Commission, 1991). Prevention and quality of life were mentioned most frequently and personal responsibility and length of life were mentioned least frequently. The values expressed in these community meetings were incorporated in the final prioritization developed in Oregon. Commissioners grouped these health-related values into three attributes of health services: value to society (takes into account the costs to society if a health service is not provided), value to an individual at risk of needing the service (a service that is important to a person seeking it but that makes little difference on a societal level), and essential to basic health care (services every person should have).

Health benefit was also formally assessed by consumers in a telephone health survey using the QWB health state classification system. This classification system was selected because it has been widely used, has demonstrated measurement properties, is relatively easy to administer, and generates an overall score of health-related quality of life which places morbidity and mortality on the same continuum. To make this applicable in the Oregon context, the QWB was modified for use with persons with low levels of education. Four additional mental health and chemical dependency symp-

Table 14.2 Thirteen community values for health care elicited by Oregon health decisions

Value	Frequency of discussion (% of communities)	Summary description
Prevention	Very high (all)	Includes services which prevent (immunizations, prenatal care), detect symptoms at early stages (mammograms), or prevent deterioration (alcohol counseling).
Quality of life	Very high (all)	Services that enhance productivity and well-being, reduce pain, and promote independent function were considered higher priority than those that only extend life.
Cost effectiveness	High (>3/4)	Cost of a treatment through a cost-benefit ratio; not cost alone.
Ability to function	Moderately high (3/4)	Emotional well-being, productivity, independence, restored quality of life to pre-illness state.
Equity	Moderately high (3/4)	Based on premise that no person should be excluded from receiving health care when he/she needs it. Encompasses justice and humaneness.
Effectiveness of treatment	Medium high (>1/2)	The higher the likelihood of success (cure rate, improvement in quality of life, and duration of improvement), the higher the priority placed on the service.
Benefits many	Medium (1/2)	Services that benefit more members of the community should receive higher priority than those that benefit fewer.
Mental health and chemical dependency	Medium (1/2)	Education and awareness of alcohol and drugs, especially to pregnant women; must consider individual responsibility and environmental factors.
Community compassion	Medium low (<1/2)	Concern for life, preserving integrity of individual and family; compassion for vulnerable persons, including children and older adults; relief of pain and death with dignity.
Impact on society	Medium low (<1/2)	Services that potentially impact society, such as infectious diseases, alcoholism, drug abuse, and child abuse, should be given priority over those with more limited effects.
Length of life	Medium low (<1/2)	Extension of life beyond what would otherwise occur without intervention; simply extending life without consideration of quality of life was not considered valuable in the majority of the communities.
Personal responsibility	Medium low (<1/2)	Encouragement to take responsibility for health to promote individual autonomy and control over health and well-being; not to be construed as "victim blaming."

Source: Oregon Health Services Commission, 1991.

toms were added: (1) trouble falling asleep or staying asleep, (2) trouble with sexual interest or performance, (3) often worried, and (4) trouble with the use of drugs or alcohol.

For the modified QWB, value judgments were elicited using a variant of category scaling, the method used to weight the original version of the QWB. The QWB telephone survey asked respondents to assign preferences to health states using a scale from 0 to 100, with 0 representing death and 100, good health. Information was also obtained as to whether respondents had experienced the health state described in the scenario.

For feasibility, a select number of all possible health states was used in the scaling exercise. Rather than derive scale values for all of the possible health states, over 647 in total, the scaling study was designed to determine values for each of the symptoms and for each of the most extreme values of the mobility, physical activity, and social activity function subscales of the QWB. The procedure defined a number of states identical in content, except one state contained either the particular symptom or function level of interest and the other state did not. The value for the missing symptom or function level was found by subtracting the numerical value assigned to the scenario with the symptom or function level from the scenario without the missing attribute.

The health state preferences elicited by the telephone survey in Oregon were similar to those obtained for the QWB in other studies, including a household interview survey conducted in San Diego in 1975 (Kaplan and Anderson, 1988). Almost two-thirds of the preference weights obtained in Oregon do not differ by more than 20 percent with the San Diego weights. For some health states, estimates from the two scaling exercises differed by more than two standard deviations (Barry Anderson, personal communication). Two health states received a much higher dysfunction weighting in Oregon: (1) having to use a walker or wheelchair under own control ($-.373$ Oregon vs. $-.060$ San Diego), and (2) having to be in bed or in a wheelchair controlled by someone else ($-.560$ Oregon vs. $-.077$ San Diego). A third health state received much less severe weight in Oregon: losses of consciousness from seizures, blackouts, or coma ($-.114$ Oregon vs. $-.407$ California).

Possible explanations for these differences include differences in method of administration, scaling instructions, and response scale. Oregon used a telephone survey and a 100-point response scale on which respondents evaluated health states described as permanent. The San Diego study, completed in 1974–1975, used personal interview with an 11-point response scale on which respondents evaluated a single day spent in a particular health state. Another difference is that the preferences assigned to specific components in San Diego were derived by regression analyses with the convention that any variance shared by functions and symptoms was arbitrarily assigned to symptoms. Oregon did not use this assumption. Despite these different methodologies, the elicited health state values are strikingly similar.

Inconsistent responses in the Oregon survey were given by approximately 27 percent of respondents, not dissimilar to previous research with community respondents. The preference weights assigned by Oregon residents differed according to age, gender, and previous experience with the health state (Paige Sipes-Metzler, personal communication). Males viewed five states as significantly worse than did females, including trouble with sexual interest or performance. Females viewed four health states as significantly worse than males. Older respondents gave less favorable scores for ten of the health states. Most significantly, respondents who had experienced the health state viewed 12 health states more favorably than those who had not experienced them, which could significantly shift the ranking of condition/treatment pairs.

In initial analyses, a single formula brought the judgments of health experts and the QWB judgments of the public together and provided the basis for assigning priorities. The three principal factors taken into account were (1) how much a treatment costs, (2) what improvement in health-related quality of life the treatment is likely to produce, and (3) how many years that improvement will probably last. The original formula incorporated the full logic of cost–utility analysis and years of healthy life as described throughout this book:

$$\frac{\text{benefit}}{\text{cost}} = \frac{\sum P\text{YHL}^+ - \sum P\text{YHL}^0}{\text{costs}^+ - \text{costs}^0}$$

where $^+$ refers to years of healthy life or costs *with treatment*, and ^{0} means *without treatment*. Expected years of healthy life are computed by multiplying the probability P of each scenario by the years of healthy life for that scenario and summing over scenarios. The numerator is expected YHL with treatment minus expected YHL without treatment. The denominator is the cost of treatment minus the cost of nontreatment. This benefit–cost ratio is therefore the marginal expected benefits divided by marginal costs. The cost–benefit formula adopted by the commission did not include costs without treatment because these costs are not readily available. Thus cost was simply costs$^+$, or cost with treatment.

In the complete Health Resource Allocation Strategy, costs and benefits are discounted to take into account time preferences for costs and benefits; that is, people prefer to consume today rather than in the future. The principal departures of the Oregon formula from the cost and outcome formula of the Health Resource Allocation Strategy were forced by the unavailability of data on costs without treatment and on the distributions of costs over time. In most applications of the Strategy, cost without treatment data are estimated, and a discount rate is applied to take into account costs over time.

Preliminary Rankings Using Cost–Utility Ratios

Table 14.3 shows a selected subset of the preliminary cost–utility ratios for medical conditions and treatments ranked most and least worthwhile in May 1990 using the original formula and estimated cost–utility ratios obtained from the QWB. The formula was applied to 1,600 conditions/CPT codes. The cost–utility ratio of cost per year of healthy life gained ranged from $1.46 to over $300,000.

These preliminary rankings based on the original formula attracted national attention, including media coverage that spawned controversy not only about the rankings, but also about the wisdom of the overall Oregon Plan. The rankings themselves came under intense criticism by the commissioners immediately upon release (Morell, 1990). Treatments for acute headaches and thumbsucking were assigned more favorable rankings by the formula than treatments for cystic fibrosis and AIDS. Organ transplants were ranked close to the bottom, and a large number of uncommon and less

Table 14.3 Preliminary cost–utility ratios used to rank medical conditions and treatments most and least economically worthwhile, May 1990 (1,600 conditions evaluated)

Medical conditions	Treatment	Cost–utility ratio, $/year of healthy life gained
Highest benefit (lowest cost–utility ratio)		
Bacterial meningitis: Inflammation of the lining of the brain and central nervous system	Antibiotics	1.46
Phenylketonuria: Inherited metabolic problem that can causemental retardation; detectable by test at birth	Office visit	1.47
Non-Hodgkins: A type of cancer of the lymph system	Consultant, chemotherapy, drugs, treatment	1.50
Septicemia: Generalized bacterial or fungal blood infaction	Antibiotics, ventilation	1.54
Candidiasis: A fungal infection	Antibiotics	1.66
Salmonella: A bacterial infection spread by spoiled blood	Antibiotics IV	1.66
Wilms tumor: A type of cancer	Office visits, surgery, chemotherapy	1.68
Bacterial infection (general)	Outpatient visit, antibiotics	1.69
Listeriosis: A bacterial infection	Antibiotics	1.82
Lowest benefit (highest cost–utility ratio)[a]		
Alcoholic cirrhosis	Liver transplant	52,243.92
Other atherosclerotic embolism/thrombitis	Vascular surgery	60,797.28
Fulminant hepatic failure	Liver transplant	61,287.42
Aneurysm in artery of neck	Repair	65,214.43
ESOP varic in dis class	Repair/cannulization	65,657.74
Withdrawal	Hospitalization/outpatient therapy	68,091.84
Atherosclerosis in artery of extremity	Bypass graft	84,866.83
Phlebitis and thrombophlebitis	Legational division	88,803.44
Bursitis	Surgery	129,658.81
Phlebitis and thrombophlebitis, other site	Venous thrombectomy	301,879.59

Source: Oregon Health Services Commission, 1990.

[a] 191 conditions are listed as $999,998 representing net benefit of zero or $999,999 indicating missing data that did not permit calculation of a ratio (bottom 10 listed as dysmorphogenic goiter, internal hemorrhoids, impacted tooth, inflammatory condition of teeth, other unspecified, unspecified diseases of capillary, unspecified disorders of arteries, pelvic varices, umbilical with obstruction, and vulval varices.)

well-known conditions appeared on this preliminary list. The priority order of the draft list was deemed intuitively unacceptable.

Development of Health Services Priority Categories

The commission therefore found it necessary to revise the ranking based on the cost–benefit ratios because it "did not comprehensively reflect public values" (Oregon

Health Services Commission, 1991, p. 11). The preliminary ranking also made it clear that services which were not condition–treatment pairs, such as education and prevention, were difficult to compare to treatments for specific diagnoses. Therefore, an alternative methodology subcommittee was created to develop a plan that would take into account the full range of values expressed at community meetings and public hearings. This alternative methodology subcommittee focused on a "cost-free" or net-benefit method of assigning health care priorities. It adopted a categorization approach that consisted of 17 health services categories that were ranked in order of importance as shown in Table 14.4.

To assign condition–treatment pairs to the categories, commissioners first weighted on a scale from 0 to 100 the following attributes of health services: value to society, value to the individual needing the service, and how essential the service is to a basic health care package. Then commissioners assigned scores to each health service category on a scale from 1 to 10. Each category was rated three times by each commissioner, once for each attribute, and a modified Delphi technique was used to arrive at a consensus. Commissioners reviewed their own scoring to see if there were major discrepancies between their numbers and the numbers of other commissioners. The attribute weights were applied to the 1–10 category scoring, the weighted scores were summed (one score per commissioner), and they were averaged.

Condition–treatment pairs were classified as either acute or chronic by physicians on the commission and reviewed by health care providers. A computer algorithm sorted the chronic and acute conditions into the 17 defined health services categories by degrees of fatality and improvement in quality of life. Cost and duration were not included in this algorithm. Thus *net benefit,* defined as the difference between treatment (outcomes × probabilities) and no treatment (outcomes × probabilities) became the basis on which the final priorities were assigned. Net benefit was selected because earlier test runs had indicated that benefit alone generated the "most sensible priority order" (Hadorn, 1991). The commissioners reviewed the results of the computer algorithm and made final changes based on their judgment.

Final List of Prioritized Health Services

The final rank order reflects the clinical and public policy judgment of the commission. The list of prioritized health services resulted from the ranked categorization of health services with net benefit ranking within categories. Commissioners reranked "out-of-position" items on the draft list using a "reasonableness" criterion: it was not reasonable to rank preventable or readily treatable conditions in relatively unfavorable positions. Where severe or exacerbated conditions were ranked in a relatively favorable position compared to prevention of disease or disability using the computer algorithm, the commissioners reversed these rankings. Approximately 33 to 50 percent of the line items were rearranged; 24% of all CT pairs moved up or down at least 100 lines on the list (Hadorn, 1991; Office of Technology Assessment, 1992). Correlations between the cost–benefit ratios and the final ranking of treatment–condition pairs indicated that cost–benefit was significantly correlated at the 0.05 level but was not nearly as strong as the relationship between rank and net benefit alone (0.0001). The final revised ranking was submitted to the Oregon legislature and approved. Table 14.5 shows the revised rankings for the most and least worthwhile medical conditions and treatments published by the commission (Oregon Health Services Commission, 1991).

Table 14.4 Ranked list of 17 health services categories incorporating category weights and Oregon Health Services Commission judgment, May 1991

Health service category	Definition and examples
Most important or essential services	
1. Acute fatal	Treatment prevents death with full recovery: appendectomy for appendicitis; repair of deep, open wound in neck; medical therapy for myocarditis
2. Maternity care	Includes most disorders of the newborn: obstetrical care for pregnancy
3. Acute fatal	Treatment prevents death without full recovery: surgical treatment for head injury with prolonged loss of consciousness; medical therapy for acute bacterial meningitis; reduction of an open fracture of a joint
4. Preventive care for children	Immunizations; medical therapy for streptococcal sore throat and scarlet fever—reduce disability, prevents spread; screening for specific problems such as vision or hearing difficulties or anemia
5. Chronic fatal	Treatment improves life span and quality of life: medical therapy for Type I diabetes mellitus; medical and surgical treatment for treatable cancer of the uterus; medical therapy for asthma
6. Reproductive services	Excludes maternity and infertility services: contraceptive management; vasectomy; tubal ligation
7. Comfort care	Palliative therapy for conditions in which death is imminent
8. Preventive dental care	For adults and children: cleaning and fluoride applications
9. Proven effective preventive care for adults	Mammograms; blood pressure screening; medical therapy and chemoprophylaxis for primary tuberculosis
Very important services	
10. Acute nonfatal	Treatment causes return to previous health state: medical therapy for acute thyroiditis; medical therapy for vaginitis; restorative dental. Therapy for vaginitis; restorative dental service for dental care
11. Chronic nonfatal	One-time treatment improves quality of life; hip replacement; laser surgery for diabetic retinopathy; medical therapy for rheumatic fever
12. Acute nonfatal	Treatment without return to previous health state: relocation of dislocated elbow; arthroscopic repair of internal derangement of knee; repair of corneal laceration
13. Chronic nonfatal	Repetitive treatment improves quality of life: medical therapy for chronic sinusitis; medical therapy for migraine; medical therapy for psoriasis
Services valuable to certain individuals, least important or less likely to be cost effective	
14. Acute nonfatal	Treatment expedites recovery of self-limiting conditions: medical therapy for diaper rash; medical therapy for acute conjunctivitis; medical therapy for acute pharyngitis
15. Infertility services	Medical therapy for anovulation; microsurgery for tubal disease; in vitro fertilization

(continued)

Table 14.4 *(Continued)*

Health service category	Definition and examples
16. Less effective preventive care for adults	Dipstick urinalysis for hematuria in adults less than 60 years of age; signoidoscopy for persons less than 40 years of age; screening of nonpregnant adults for Type I diabetes mellitus
17. Fatal or nonfatal	Treatment causes minimal or no improvement in quality of life: repair fingertip avulsion that does not include fingernail; medical therapy for gallstone without cholecystitis; medical therapy for viral warts

Source: Oregon Health Services Commission, 1991.

In the revised ranking, the preliminary list of 1,600 conditions was reduced to 709 condition–treatment pairs. As shown in Table 14.5, terminal HIV disease with less than 10 percent chance of survival and several untreatable diseases are ranked in the bottom 10. AIDS detected in the early phases, where treatment is available, is ranked in the upper 25 percent of the list. Extremely low birth weight and anencephaly, conditions requiring extensive neonatal life-sustaining treatment, are at the bottom of the list. The commission recommended that only services that are "essential" (categories 1–9) and "very important" (categories 10–13) be included in the standard benefit package. Mental health and chemical dependency services not mandated by law are to be integrated into the list by 1993.

The final list was sent to an actuarial contractor who estimated the cost of providing services at various thresholds on the list. The Oregon plan provides services, within the constraints of limited revenue, to the Medicaid-eligible population starting at the top of the priority list and working down. When existing revenue has been exhausted, services on the margin will be debated.

The budgetary constraint and cutoff line below which no public funding would be provided was set by the Oregon legislature. The legislature decided to fund an initial benefits package consisting of all services included in the condition/treatment pairs listed from 1 through 587, leaving 122 pairs *below the line*. Some services that were previously uncovered were added above the line, such as hospice care and preventive services for adults. Other services, previously covered, were dropped below the line, such as treatments for temporomandibular joint disorder (line 620), bursitis (line 631), diaper rash (line 649), and the common cold (line 695).

Oregon now spends $700 million on public health care every two years; it gets 63 percent matching funds from the federal government. The new program is expected to increase health care expenditures by at least 20 percent, although some analysts estimate the proposed program will be at least 25 percent more costly than the current program (Eddy, 1991a).

Reimbursement Based on Cost

The state of Oregon is to enter into managed care contracts with providers to offer a package of health care benefits at a reimbursement rate determined by actuaries. These managed care contracts last for a one- or two-year period. The program is to reimburse

Table 14.5 List of health services assigned highest and lowest priorities by Oregon
Health Services Commission, May 1991[a]
(709 conditions evaluated)

Medical condition	Treatment
Highest benefit (10 most worthwhile)	
1. Several types of pneumonia: Including pneumococcal pneumonia, other bacterial pneumonia, bronchopneumonia, influenza with pneumonia	Medical therapy
2. Tuberculosis	Medical therapy
3. Peritonitis: An inflammation of the abdominal cavity	Medical and surgical treatment
4. Foreign body in the throat: Including the pharynx, larynx, trachea, bronchus, and esophagus	Removal of foreign body
5. Appendicitis	Appendectomy
6. Ruptured intestine	Repair
7. Hernia with obstruction and/or gangrene	Repair
8. Croup syndrome: An upper respiratory ailment	Medical therapy, intubation, tracheotomy
9. Acute orbital cellulitis: An inflammation of the tissue around the eye	Medical therapy
10. Ectopic pregnancy	Surgery
Lowest benefit (10 least worthwhile)	
700. Gynecomastia: Benign enlargement of the breast	Mastopexy
701. Cyst of kidney: A benign condition	Medical and surgical treatment
702. Terminal HIV disease: With less than 10% survival rate in 5 years	Medical therapy
703. Chronic pancreatitis: An untreatable ailment	Surgical treatment
704. Superficial wounds: Without infection and contusions	Medical therapy
705. Constitutional aplastic anemia (untreatable)	Medical therapy
706. Prolapsed urethral mucosa: A minor urinary condition	Surgical treatment
707. Blockage of the retinal artery	Paracentesis of aqueous humor
708. Extremely low birth weight: Less than 1.1 pounds and less than 23 weeks of gestation	Life support
709. Anencephaly: Including similar conditions, in which a child is born without a brain	Life support

Source: Oregon Health Services Commission, 1991.

[a]List did not contain mental health and chemical dependency conditions exempted by law from initial prioritization report.

providers for the cost of their services, but it does not subsidize cost shifting. It is
unlikely that Oregon will reimburse for "full costs" but will develop a formula that
limits reimbursements to some not yet defined level.

Liability Shield

The final provision of the Oregon Plan is a liability shield. This provision is intended to
safeguard practitioners if they do not provide a service which the Oregon Plan has

determined goes beyond its definition of basic and has chosen not to fund. Providers will not be liable for not providing care that is not on the priority list of services.

Implementation of the plan would undoubtedly change the Medicaid program in Oregon. Any changes to federal Medicaid rules could mean that more beneficiaries would be eligible under Senate Bill 27 than before passage of this law. Any such changes would require new funds to be added to the program, because savings secondary to the changes in health care delivery would not be sufficient to overcome the increased outlays for additional beneficiaries.

The final process of developing health services categories and relying on net benefit alone to produce a draft ranking of services departs significantly from the strategy. Debate on the preliminary cost–benefit ranking and revisions was not based initially on stakeholder challenge to the formula and sensitivity analyses in which the cost and outcomes components were varied to evaluate their effect on the ranking. An alternative process was created that relied much more heavily on their judgments of the benefit of health services and public testimony than on the social preferences contained in the formula. Costs and duration of benefit were also not included explicitly in this evaluation but were considered in the commissioners' subjective judgments. The final list of health services priorities therefore does not necessarily reflect tradeoffs between resource expenditure and health-related quality of life outcomes (Eddy, 1991b). As one observer has commented, "I'd trade all of the telephone surveys and public meetings for one seat on the Commission."

Before Oregon can implement the program, the state must receive 11 waivers to the Social Security Act as well as an agreement from the Health Care Financing Administration to provide the federal share of program costs. Most importantly, these waivers would permit the state to expand coverage to include low-income persons who currently do not meet categorical or financial requirements for Medicaid, and to redefine the basic package of services to be covered (Eddy, 1991c). In response to the application for waivers, the Office of Technology Assessment (OTA) was asked by the U.S. Congress to review and evaluate the Oregon plan.

The OTA evaluation, while praising the achievements of the Oregon plan, expressed serious reservations about assigning priorities to a comprehensive system of health services (Office Technology Assessment, 1992). Most notably, OTA's analysis suggests that classifying health care by general service categories and condition/treatment pairs is not an especially promising approach for assigning priorities to health services in order to ration. Outcomes and cost-effectiveness data are considered inadequate for constructing a ranking system of all services, even if better information on outcomes were available. Rather, the OTA suggests that such data are more useful in developing provider guidelines, quality-of-care screens, or for deciding whether specific individual services should be covered and under what circumstances. In essence, this evaluation recommends the Health Resource Allocation Strategy for medical effectiveness evaluations, but not for rationing.

The most critical aspect of the OTA evaluation concerned how the Oregon plan would work, if program expenditures are higher than predicted. No legislative mandate provides for a guaranteed core set of benefits below which coverage would not be allowed to fall. Under these circumstances, Medicaid recipients might lose benefits unless the federal government funded the difference. The expansion of coverage to all poor persons in Oregon is a clear benefit of the proposed plan. Any simplification of eligibility benefits that would deny coverage to some pregnant women and children is, however, a serious drawback. Advocacy organizations for people with disabilities also raised serious reservations about the Plan.

The waivers necessary to implement the Oregon plan were rejected by the Bush administration in 1992 because the plan was viewed as a violation of the Americans with Disabilities Act passed in 1990. The Oregon rankings were considered "illegal" because lower rankings were given to conditions affecting people with disabilities than to conditions affecting people without disabilities. Any rationing of health services on the basis of net benefits would almost certainly affect seriously ill persons, unless these persons were removed from consideration.

This initial rejection of the Oregon Plan reflects unwillingness, political or otherwise, to experiment with making the necessarily difficult choices to improve access to health services for those currently excluded from coverage. Without approval and implementation of programs such as that proposed by Oregon, it is impossible to evaluate the overall net impact of the proposed changes on current Medicaid participants. Oregon has used explicit outcomes and health state preference measurement methods to help set its health services priorities. A set of principles, methods, and results are open for critique, review, attempts at reversal, modification, and, most of all, improvement. Compared to the current system of rationing operating in the Medicaid program of most states, Oregon's bold attempt to apply method and data to a thorny political problem within the public view is to be commended.

THE ROLE OF ACCESS IN REDUCING HEALTH DISPARITIES

Improving access to health care is one means by which to reduce health disparities. This section examines the role of years of healthy life and the Health Resource Allocation Strategy in providing information that can assist in identifying disparities in health-related quality of life for different population groups and in improving access to reduce these disparities. Population groups are defined by racial and/or ethnic origins and poverty status. Poverty, sometimes defined broadly as lack of access to resources, is defined more narrowly here based on income level.

Although several programs have been implemented over the past 30 years to reduce the disparities in health-related quality of life between minority and majority populations in the United States, gaps still exist. Life expectancy and years of healthy life for whites, blacks, and Hispanics were estimated from 1980 data obtained in the National Health Interview Survey (Erickson et al., 1989). Average life expectancy at birth has risen into the upper seventies for white male babies, but the expected life span for their black counterparts has declined. Years of healthy life also reflect the gap between the ethnic and racial groups in the United States.

A particularly sensitive and compelling measure of disparity is infant mortality (Figure 14.3). Although these rates are improving and will continue to improve, a persistent gap remains. Black babies continue to die at twice the rate of white babies. The American Indian rate (13.9) and the black rate (18.7) were 1.5 and 2.1 times the rate for white mothers, respectively. Both the neonatal and postneonatal mortality rates for black and Puerto Rican Americans is high. By contrast, the infant mortality rate was lowest among the Japanese in the 1983–85 birth cohorts.

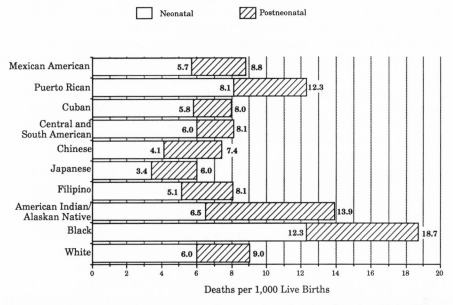

Figure 14.3   Infant mortality rates, according to color/ethnicity of mother, United States, 1983–85 birth cohorts. (Data on Hispanic origin of mother are from 23 states and the District of Columbia.) *Source:* National Center for Health Statistics, 1991a.

Low birth weight can contribute to the increased risk of infant mortality and morbidity. Infants born weighing less than 2,500 grams are known to be at increased risks; those weighing less than 1,500 grams are at greatest risk of death. In 1988, black mothers had the highest percentage of low birth weight births (13.3 percent), more than twice the rate for white mothers. Puerto Rican mothers ranked second highest, with 9.4 percent of infants weighing less than 2,500 grams. Low birth weight was less common among Chinese mothers.

In addition to higher mortality rates for selected conditions, minorities and low-income populations are more likely to rate themselves in either fair or poor health. Approximately 15 percent of the noninstitutionalized black population (compared to about 9 percent of the white population) report a general health rating of "fair" or "poor." The difference by income is even more striking. Over 20 percent of persons with family income less than $10,000 rated themselves in fair or poor health compared with 4 percent of persons in the highest income group.

Use of physician services can reflect both access to care and health-related quality of life. In general, persons who are less healthy have more contact with physicians than those who are more healthy. Respondent-assessed health status and physician utilization rates are compared among different ethnic groups. During 1985–88, physician use rates for persons 45–64 years of age were lower for Asians and higher for American Indian/Alaskan Natives. After adjusting for health status, physician use rates show a different ranking. Health status–adjusted use rates are estimates of the annual number of physician visits per person for each racial and ethnic group that would occur if the group had the same respondent-assessed health status as all persons. The adjusted physician use rate for non-Hispanic black persons was lower than for non-Hispanic white persons. Adjusting for health status, non-white persons do not use services at the same rate as white persons.

Early prenatal care is important, especially for women known to be at increased medical or social risk of adverse outcomes. Early prenatal care is therefore another index of access to services. In 1988 only 58 percent of American Indian and Mexican American mothers received early prenatal care. Black, Puerto Rican, and Central and South American mothers had the next lowest rates compared to other groups.

The trend for persons in poverty to have lower health-related quality of life can be expected to continue for a number of reasons. For one, the tendency in the last decade has been toward a widening income gap, with the poor losing income and the rich becoming relatively wealthier. For another, there continues to be a diversity of programs for access to health care through health insurance and entitlement programs. Thus, a large percentage of the population will continue to fall into the gaps of enrollment criteria between programs and will be without coverage for basic medical services. Third, the population will continue to age, with an increasing percentage of the population being over 85 years of age. Within this group, the trend is toward the feminization of poverty (Stone, 1989). The tendency for lower health status among these groups cannot be reversed without major changes in government policies.

The causal relationship between health status and poverty has been debated for decades. For some, however, the relationship is clear: "Poverty and powerlessness create circumstances in people's lives that predispose them to the highest indexes of social dysfunction, the highest indexes of morbidity and mortality, the lowest access to primary care, and little or no access to primary preventive programs" (Braithwaite and Lythcott, 1989). Others are less sure whether poverty causes poor health or poor health causes poverty, but they view the two as closely linked (Dutton, 1986).

Regardless of the causal relationships, it is clear that identifiable subsets of the population are in lower health status levels and are at higher risk for exposure to health hazards. This condition exists in spite of 30 years of government programs designed to improve access and opportunity. The data suggest the need to reexamine these programs.

The role of health care in reducing inequalities in health has also been debated in contrast to improvement in living standards, diet, sanitation, transportation patterns, and other social and economic changes (Levine et al., 1983). Policies to reduce health disparities should be based on causes, and interventions to support policies should be based on strategic points in the causal chain where the greatest impact can be made on reducing disparities (Illsley, 1990).

The determinants of health-related quality of life are multiple and interrelated. Illsley (1990) summarizes the causes of health inequalities as follows: (1) direct effects of the social and physical environment on health through nutrition, housing, hygiene, pollution, working conditions, and accidents; (2)indirect effects mediated by reproductive habits, lifestyles, consumption patterns, knowledge, values, and power; and (3) availability, accessibility, affordability, quality, use, and effectiveness of health services. Access to health services for everyone continues to be a major policy goal based on the assumption that improved access to health care will lead to improved health status.

Data on the relative contribution of direct effects, indirect effects, and health services do not exist. All factors contribute to health disparities, and all will likely need to be modified to eliminate disparities. Access to health services cannot be expected to compensate fully for the results of long-term socioeconomic inequities. Deprivation in early childhood can lead to years, and perhaps generations, of increased vulnerability and disadvantage. Decades may be necessary to reduce socioeconomic inequities and thereby reduce health disparities.

Access to health services for everyone continues to be a major policy goal in the United States. Health status has been used as a measure of need for health care because it will frequently trigger the use of services (Rosenstock and Kirscht, 1979). Studies incorporating health status as an indicator of need have used self-reported health status. For example, in a national telephone survey designed to examine access to health care for black and white Americans, Blendon and colleagues (1989) found that blacks had fewer ambulatory care and hospital visits than did whites even when health status was taken into consideration. This survey also found that the rate for blacks not receiving health care for economic reasons was almost twice that for whites.

As indicated by the national data presented in this chapter, equity in health status has been primarily examined in terms of limitations of activity, restricted activity days (including bed-disability days), and global, overall self-rating of health. The reliance on these data has been attributed to their availability, primarily in national sample surveys designed to be representative of the overall U.S. population (Patrick and Bergner, 1990). However, if health-related quality of life is to be used as an indicator of need, more comprehensive and sensitive measures of health-related quality of life are required for all populations in the United States, including minority groups who may have the greatest need for health services.

SOCIOPOLITICAL IMPLICATIONS OF RATIONING TO IMPROVE ACCESS

Two major questions reveal the sociopolitical implications of rationing to improve access: Whom will rationing affect? and Who gets to be involved in the decision process? The most vehement reaction against the Oregon Plan, and to most proposals to impose limits on spending, is that rationing will harm the groups to which it is applied. The Oregon Plan concerns a basic minimum level of health services for all Oregon residents. The Medicaid-eligible population, primarily poor, are subject to spending limits, because government outlays cover their health care. They are chiefly women and children who make up the poor and near-poor who use Medicaid benefits. Any reductions in a program that affects poor people, for whom health care resources are already low, appears unfair. Rationing to improve access, however, is based on the principle that limits are necessary to achieve a basic minimum level of health care for all persons, not just those currently eligible because of low income.

Millions of low-income people are not eligible for Medicaid and do not have access to private health insurance or an acceptable standard of health care. This results in a three-tier medical system in the United States: a top tier for those who can obtain access through private means, a middle tier for those who have access through public means, and a bottom tier for those who cannot obtain access at all. The lack of a national financing system to improve access maintains this three-tier system unless the public program is expanded to cover all those who cannot obtain insurance through private means. The only way to achieve a basic minimum under these circumstances is to define a mandated level of coverage, available either through the private system or through public expenditures.

Rationing public expenditures implies that those who can afford *more* benefits and services than the mandated basic minimum will pay for them if they choose. Rationing is therefore unlikely to affect the wealthy. Thus, the denial of benefits will be unequally experienced by poor and near-poor people, the majority of whom are employed. If one accepts the assumption that additional resources are not going to be pumped into the system, the tradeoff is clear: limit public expenditures on health care in order to improve access.

The second major sociopolitical implication in rationing to improve access is that public involvement is necessary to make the process work. Any health decision process that rests on value judgments as important as rationing health care demands high involvement on the part of the general public. This includes those who represent the public and experts who provide information for the rationing process.

In rationing to improve access, the entire community should be involved. In this sense, "community" is a cooperative endeavor aimed at achieving a better life for all through various social arrangements and joint labors. Health care should be viewed as a basic liberty, along with the rights to vote, speak, obtain an education, assemble, and hold property. Assuming that the availability of health services is associated with better health, society should attempt to achieve an equality in the distribution of health services or an equality in levels of health-related quality of life. Improving access affects the goal of providing the maximum possible level of well-being for the most disadvantaged members of the community.

The democratic process, as illustrated in the Oregon Plan, is one effective means to achieve a consensus on what is the social minimum of health care services that should be distributed to all. The entire community, as well as leaders and experts, should provide priorities. The preference-weighting judgments involved in the Health Resource Allocation Strategy permit the pooling of preferences for input into the collective decision-making process.

Experts make judgments of fact as well as judgments of priorities. The estimates of probability of benefit and of cost are derived from persons familiar with the treatments and conditions on which any rationing system must be based and the cost of the treatments. Because the actual work of these experts is likely to be affected by the results of the process, it is essential that a wide range of experts, health professionals, and administrators be involved in the rationing process.

Major changes in health policy are needed to address the continuing and unnecessary divergence in access to health services and in health status between the poor and the nonpoor. Solutions that are restricted to health resource distribution and the supply of medical care have failed. Both the costs and benefits of current treatments must be considered in choosing how to allocate and ration resources in order to achieve a better minimum of health care and health for all.

15

The Limits of Rationality in Allocating Health Resources

In the preceding chapters of this book we:

Advocate use of the Health Resource Allocation Strategy for distributing limited resources to competing health care programs based on anticipated benefits;

Describe eight steps in the Strategy that lead to a ranking of comparative health care costs and outcomes;

Identify how this ranking can be used in a sociopolitical process to assign priorities to health interventions based on community values; and

Apply the Strategy to three major health policy challenges: promoting health and preventing disease, using technology to improve health, and improving access to health care.

As advocates of the Strategy, we focus on its potential and on the positive aspects of using a rational approach to health decision making.

Application of the Strategy, however, is not without its shortcomings and detractors. Some criticisms stem from the unacceptance that health care resources are finite or the belief that elimination of ineffective medical treatments will release additional funds for reallocation to other more effective health care interventions. Others involve the underlying logic and technical procedures involved in using costs and years of healthy life to rank comparative costs and outcomes. Misunderstanding of the methods may account for some criticisms; others are important cautionary notes. We would be remiss if we did not address the concerns that decision makers, health services researchers, ethicists, health care providers, and consumers and their families have voiced about the approach proposed in the Health Resource Allocation Strategy.

In this chapter, we review the potential contributions of the Strategy to the health decision process with major attention to the roles of different stakeholders in these decisions, including legislators, government officials, administrators, clinicians, and consumers. Then we address the major political and ethical challenges to using the Strategy to allocate resources either through medical effectiveness evaluations or explicit rationing of health services based on heath care priorities. Even though we embed the analytic model of cost–utility in a sociopolitical process, a structured form of analysis can be overused or applied too literally. Limits exist to the application of rational choice theory to health decisions. These limits and the most common sources of potential abuses of the Strategy are considered. We then address some of the complex and unresolved issues that remain in developing and implementing the Strategy. Finally, we evaluate the role of the Strategy in reaching the overarching objective of the health care system, that of attaining equal opportunity for health.

CONTRIBUTIONS TO HEALTH DECISIONS

The current health care system in the United States has been characterized as being out of control because (1) health care needs of different population groups are met in a piecemeal fashion, (2) the "system" is virtually a nonsystem, and (3) expenditures are rapidly escalating. Adoption of the Health Resource Allocation Strategy as an input to health decision making responds to many of these criticisms. Under the assumptions of finite resources and economic efficiency, the Strategy provides a comprehensive and systematic approach to containing health care costs by evaluating health services according to their relative costs and benefits. With the goals of promoting equity of access and equal opportunity for health, the Strategy can be applied to maintain and improve the health of the community.

An important challenge to all communities in the 1990s, whether a nation, state, city, or township, is how to adjust to increasingly scarce resources in the face of continually rising demands. Citizens have steadily showed resistance over the past decade to paying higher taxes that would allow for the provision of more, and more costly, services, as witnessed by the current political debate, e.g., "read my lips." At the same time, citizens are reluctant to do without increasingly costly health care services. This trend of finite or scarce resources will continue. Not all publicly demanded goods and services, whether in health care, education, housing or some other market, will be provided. Thus, policy makers are increasingly called upon to make decisions affecting society's welfare by trading off desired services both within and between different sectors of the economy.

Health decisions involve difficult choices among preventing, caring, and curing objectives. These choices are made all the more difficult because of multiple stakeholders in the decisions, including insurers, providers, patients, and advocacy groups. Each player has a financial stake in the allocation of resources and stands to lose or gain with each "fix" to the system. These competing interests tend to perpetuate piecemeal delivery and decision making without paying explicit attention to the relationship between expenditures and outcomes.

Making these difficult choices requires the adoption of a common goal among all stakeholders in the community, namely that of increasing the healthy life span for the community as a whole. Attaining this goal requires honesty, compassion, and compromise between and among the stakeholders. Insurers, administrators, consumers, and physicians will need to forgo some freedom of behavior to assure universal access to health care at a price society is willing to pay. A dialogue between all stakeholders is needed to find a way for deciding how to limit choices where and when necessary. The Health Resource Allocation Strategy—with its inclusion of community values for health care, individual health state preferences, and stakeholder priorities, to the ranking of interventions to be funded—provides a forum for identifying socially acceptable limits to choice. In this way the Strategy makes an important contribution to decision making.

A Comprehensive Approach to Community Health Care

To date, policy makers in the United States have allocated health care resources by singling out either population groups or specific interventions in the health care sector in need of special consideration. Criteria for identifying either populations or interventions to "fix" have focused on socioeconomic characteristics of the population, such as age or income level, or features of the intervention, such as operational mortality rates for certain types of surgery.

One example of using age as a criterion is the Medicare program which provides health care to almost all Americans aged 65 years and older. The Medicaid program is an example of socioeconomic criteria. Use of socioeconomic characteristics to subdivide the population for special treatment ultimately leads to a lower overall level of health than if priorities were set based on the population as a whole. That is, the overall goal of increasing community health is lower than that which can be attained through a comprehensive allocation.

The same problem will occur if community priorities are set only by using criteria and guidelines for identifying medically ineffective interventions. As with priorities based on population characteristics, medical effectiveness criteria result in a piecemeal approach in that interventions are evaluated on an individual basis. Not all interventions for all conditions can be examined due to the enormity of the task. Thus, some ineffective procedures will continue to be used simply because they have not been evaluated.

The Health Resource Allocation Strategy goes beyond such piecemeal approaches by incorporating a comprehensive set of health care services associated with particular conditions for evaluation by all stakeholders in health decisions. The comprehensive approach used in the Strategy should extend health care to all members of the community, although not all will receive the most expensive and most intensive care. Rather, some persons who are terminally ill and for whom aggressive treatment will yield little or no additional benefit will receive palliative care and be allowed to face death with minimal discomfort and with dignity.

Hadorn (1991) suggests that the "Rule of Rescue" will impede any attempt *not* to save certain identifiable, highly visible lives; Americans place high value on lifesaving technologies. This moral imperative extends to almost all persons in obvious need of treatment. The benefits that accrue to these individuals, however, may detract from the benefits available to the entire community. The American ethos that supports heroic, high-technology treatments in the face of death will be difficult to change. However, a comprehensive system of health care priorities, even with its difficulties, makes the impact of the "Rule of Rescue" visible as a trade-off with other health care priorities supported by the community.

Socially Preferred Allocation

The Health Resource Allocation Strategy provides a formal structure in which to modify the more traditional routes to health decisions often characterized by implicit assumptions and hidden values. In the past, decision makers most often have assigned priorities and funded interventions without the formal input of community values and preferences or comparative cost and outcome data. Community input is sometimes elicited at the front-end of the allocation process. Rarely, however, have health care consumers and other stakeholders been consulted between the time that an analysis of interventions was completed and the final policy recommended and implemented. The Strategy makes explicit the tradeoffs between the costs and benefits attributed to health care interventions and mandates stakeholder review of the output of a cost-benefit formula. The Strategy includes the elicitation of community values for health services, the measurement of social preferences for health outcomes, and puts in public view the initial ranking of costs and outcomes, elicits stakeholder input to their revision, and permits a comparison of the analytic model with community values and goals in the assignment of health services priorities.

Resource allocation that omits community values or health state preferences may result in the wrong interventions being offered or funded. For example, decision makers may devote considerable resources to developing technology to prolong lives of persons who are terminally ill, even beyond that which many patients may desire or society may be willing to support. Without taking community values explicitly into account, resources may be allocated contrary to society's wishes. In the policy context, an expensive program that consumes most of the available budget may be funded; yet this intervention may not be responsive to the community's priorities for health services and preferences for health outcomes.

In the Oregon Plan, for example, the initial evaluation of cost per year of life gained for treatment–condition pairs resulted in higher ranking for conditions that were treated with antibiotics, such as bacterial meningitis, than for other conditions. Even though these treatments may yield the greatest expected gain according to the cost and outcome ranking, health decision makers may want to revise the ranking according to prevailing community values. Society may wish to allocate resources to chronic infectious diseases even though they may be relatively costly to treat in terms of years of healthy life gained, because they are treatable. For example, tuberculosis, originally ranked lower in Oregon's priority list, was moved up the list when commissioners considered community values and goals for treatment.

Hadorn (1991) cites two additional examples from the Oregon Plan based on the initial ranking of services in order of their ratios of costs per benefit. Dental caps for pulp exposure were assigned a higher priority than surgery for ectopic pregnancy, and splints for temporomandibular joints were ranked higher than appendectomies for appendicitis. These rankings are counterintuitive to most clinical observers, assigning a higher priority to some services that were clearly less important than other, lower ranked services. Strict reliance on a cost-effectiveness formula as contained in the ranking of comparative costs and outcomes may therefore conflict with prevailing community values for health services and for specific populations. In the end, some adjustments must be made "by hand," or as Oregon commissioners dubbed it, by "list jockeying," in order to achieve a socially preferred allocation.

Another reason for adjustment is that some health care interventions do not involve high-technology medicine and can be privately funded by a group or single individual. For example, with government assuming an advocacy role, consumers may take up jogging or aerobic walking on their own. Thus, there can be a gain in years of healthy life without the government devoting large amounts of its resources to providing equipment and facilities for exercise programs. Other interventions do not lend themselves to funding solely through private sources. For example, individuals needing a total hip replacement or a bone marrow transplant frequently cannot get treatment because of the cost of treatment and because of low availability of bone marrow donors. If the community wants to include these treatments as standard benefits, then government must provide the necessary funds and services.

No single element in the Health Resource Allocation Strategy can ensure close approximation of the final set of health care priorities to community values for health services and for health outcomes. By incorporating individually-assigned social preferences for health outcomes that define health benefits and by comparing the initial ranking of costs and outcomes with prevailing community values, resource allocation attains a higher degree of social consensus. By including consumers and providers explicitly in the ongoing decision process, power and responsibility can gradually shift from being more narrowly held by legislators and administrators to being more broadly held by all stakeholders in the decision. With a process of resource allocation open to community participation, individual stakeholders may also be more willing to accept tradeoffs among the difficult choices confronting health care decision makers and society in general.

Toward a More Equitable Allocation

A third contribution of the Strategy to the policy debate is in helping to provide a more equitable allocation of resources to the whole community. The Health Resource Allocation Strategy, by endorsing cost–utility analysis, goes beyond the strict welfare economic position based on economic efficiency and can incorporate a measure of equity into the decision process. Harris (1988) argues that years of healthy life lack distributive justice by being against the poor. This discrimination stems from the interpretation that cost per year of healthy life gained results in selecting the cheapest intervention. Kawachi (1989) points out that this is a misinterpretation of economic analysis. The goal of cost–utility analysis in particular is to identify the intervention that results in the lowest cost for a *gain* in years of healthy life.

Identifying a package of basic health services that are to be funded within the budget constraint and available to everyone in the community promotes equal access to health care services. The principle of equal access states that whenever a health service is available to any individual, it should be effectively available to any other person with a similar need (Gutmann, 1983). In essence, the Health Resource Allocation Strategy is a means of identifying a minimum level of care that can be claimed equally by everyone in the community with the assumption that all persons with a particular condition will benefit equally from a particular treatment.

In addition, resource allocation that is based on explicit preferences may overcome unfairness in the distribution of resources across different health interventions, which is associated with implicit preferences. Discrimination may be of particular concern when decisions are made by appointed, rather than elected, officials. With elected officials, such as members of Congress, voters have had the chance to choose their representatives in the decision-making process. Appointed officials and civil servants, however, are at least one step removed from direct voter choice and thus may be less likely to represent voters' preferences. For example, if the persons affected by policy decisions are poor and in the minority, and appointed officials are nonpoor and largely from the majority population, there may be large differences in values. Hence distribution of health care that is based on an implicit allocation process may not reflect the preferences of poor and minority constituents.

POLITICAL CHALLENGES

Broadly speaking, the role of government is to serve all the members it governs. Thus, through government direction, rich people help poor people, healthy people help sick people, and wise people help foolish people. Williams (1988c) calls this responsibility the government of "social solidarity." With the decision criteria elicited using community values and goals and made explicit through the costs and outcomes ranking, and the results reviewed by stakeholders, the Health Resource Allocation Strategy is a framework for assisting government in its role of providing social solidarity.

A major challenge to effective application of the Strategy is to merge its purposive, calculated steps with the diffuse process that characterizes decision making in the United States. Many decision makers are accustomed to a health decision process based on bargaining, administrative regulation, and political "moves and counter-moves." These approaches lead to decisions that sometimes do not follow a recognizable path, let alone being based on an assessment of the costs and benefits of different alternatives.

The successful merger of traditional approaches to decision making with the rational approach of the Strategy allows government to provide social solidarity in three areas that are necessary to assure that the Strategy serves all of members of society: (1) setting the balance between the individual and collective good; (2) representing disadvantaged and disenfranchised individuals; and (3) assuring that costs and outcomes rankings are based on current social values and goals.

Individual Versus Social Choice

When individual choice results in an imbalance of social welfare, as it does when individuals elect expensive treatments that deny basic minimum benefits to others, government may step in and readjust the balance to enhance the public good. Government restriction of individual choice involves a collective decision to override the sovereignty of individual choice to determine quality of life (Baldwin et al., 1990).

Analyses that incorporate years of healthy life for decision making are criticized as putting the quality and quantity tradeoff in the hands of "eager beavers" who purport to know what is best for individual members of society (O'Donnell, 1986). The eager beaver criticism misses the point that health decisions affecting the whole community are best made when they reflect a societal rather than an individual perspective. Policies are often made that are at odds with individual behavior. Laws requiring use of seat belts while in automobiles, use of safety helmets while riding a motorcycle, or not smoking on airplanes are examples of societal values that may contradict the wishes of some individuals in society. As long as people live in social groupings, there will be some individuals for whom the aggregate rules are unacceptable. This is minimized, albeit not eliminated, in the years-of-healthy-life approach to quantifying health benefits. Stakeholders are invited to participate in defining the values and goals on which resources are to be allocated, and they are encouraged to express their values in the preference weighting of health-related quality of life outcomes.

Community Representation

Public decision makers have a responsibility for evaluating the representativeness of community participation and of the social preferences included in social decisions. Given that one set of community values and social preferences for outcomes is needed, the logical choice is to collect them from a representative sample of the population. Using a representative sample within a societal perspective of socioeconomic evaluation, everyone has the chance to give input into the decision process. Unless decision makers use selective recruitment strategies and provide a sensitive and responsive listening environment, some members of society—cognitively impaired persons, children, or seriously mentally ill persons, for instance—will be unable to participate in community meetings, public hearings, or in preference elicitation schemes. Alternative recruitment strategies will be necessary if the values of all persons in the community are to be represented. In some circumstances advocacy groups will have to represent these often-disenfranchised persons. Regardless of the method of incorporation, the values and welfare of these persons must be considered in the allocation process.

Other members of society may be able but unwilling to participate for different reasons. People living in poverty, uninsured persons, and persons with disability may shun involvement in community affairs, because they do not trust the political process, feel unwelcome and stigmatized, or simply "have more important things to do." Even after the introduction of community meetings and other methods for determining community values, decision makers have a responsibility to serve as agents for those who are unable or unwilling to express their preferences.

Some barriers to broad participation in the elicitation of community values and preferences for health outcomes may be addressed with improved methods for mobilizing the community and for measuring their priorities. It is unlikely, however, that the problem of obtaining broad community representation will be overcome easily. Thus, government review and the continuing vigilance of advocacy groups will always be needed to adjudicate possible under- or overrepresentation or the total lack of involvement by different groups in the decision process.

Periodic Review and Revision

Another concern for practical implementation is periodic review. With diverse interventions and populations, annual readjustment of costs and outcomes may be unreasonable and costly. But interventions or populations not considered in the initial allocation process must be incorporated in subsequent revisions. A revision process every two or three years is practical. Congress or state legislatures could delegate stakeholder review and adjustment to an agency within the executive branch. Congress could conduct periodic oversight investigations, much as the Health Care Financing Administration now administers the Medicare program.

The Health Resource Allocation Strategy—particularly the incorporation of explicit values, use of a single index of outcomes, and ranking of costs and outcomes—will face considerable opposition from many analysts, decision makers, and consumers.

Possible sources of opposition, specifically resistance to change and underrepresentation of stakeholders in the community, have been addressed. We now turn to ethical issues that have been raised in allocating resources using costs and outcomes data.

ETHICAL CHALLENGES

As stated, the organization and structure of groups implies a tension between the rights of the individuals and the welfare of the majority of the members within the group. The major ethical issues concerning the Health Resource Allocation Strategy focus on the different ways in which critics see the Strategy violating the rights of individuals.

Group Versus Individual Measures

One ethical challenge concerns the basic assumption that the quality of life of individuals can be aggregated to obtain an overall measure of outcome for use in resource allocation. In this view, using years of healthy life to make decisions for individuals is incorrect. When averages are used for decision making, some individuals may get less treatment than they want or feel is necessary. For example, some people want extensive medical treatment regardless of their prognosis (La Puma and Lawlor, 1990). With any distribution of health resources, not everyone's needs or demands are met. To make these difficult social choices requires a community measure of health outcome and social preferences that may conflict with the particular choices of individuals. This conflict is inescapable.

In fact, this conflict exists with any application of averages to individuals. Any health-related quality of life data used for policy that affects the entire community are necessarily averages. Indicators such as infant mortality rates, life expectancy, mortality rates for selected causes of death, and prevalence of chronic conditions are aggregate data that summarize information into a single indicator. Thus, the use of averages in setting health policy is not unique to years of healthy life or the Health Resource Allocation Strategy.

Potential for Discrimination

Some critics oppose using years of healthy life on the grounds that this measure discriminates on the basis of age, functional capacity, and capacity to benefit. Some patients' lives—for example, the oldest-old (persons 85 years and older) and persons with some mental illness or cognitive dysfunction—may be judged to be of inadequate worth (Harris, 1988; Smith, 1987; La Puma and Lawlor, 1990). These authors argue that since years of healthy life are based on life expectancy, children with a longer expected life span will be more likely to receive treatment than elderly persons. This argument confuses life years with years of healthy life (Kawachi, 1989). Treatments for conditions that affect both older and younger populations, such as prostheses or medical devices for physically disabled persons as a result of injury, will have lower cost per year of healthy life gained ratios for younger persons than for older adults. Years of healthy life does not always, however, discriminate against older persons. In a study by the Office of Technology Assessment (1981), influenza vaccine is more cost effective for persons 65 years and older than it is for adults aged 25–44 years or for children under 3 years of age. Yet the expected number of life years remaining for both of these groups exceeds that for the older age group.

Another frequently voiced argument is that years of healthy life discriminate against persons who are in health states that are unlikely to benefit from additional care (La Puma and Lawlor, 1990). Persons in coma or in terminal stages of illness receive less care than persons with acute disease or with nonterminal chronic illnesses. Using cost per year of healthy life gained will give priority to treatments earlier in the course of disease, for example, early stages of HIV infection rather than later stages of AIDS. Palliative or comfort care is usually highly valued by some stakeholders in the community, such as hospice care for terminally ill cancer patients. These treatments are less intensive and less costly than high-technology heroic measures sometimes applied to terminally ill patients. The Strategy therefore does not deny *all* care to seriously ill persons but assigns higher priority to less intensive treatments.

If the community considers care for terminally ill persons more important than preventive or acute care, then this community value is likely to appear in the stakeholder challenges to the cost and outcome ranking. The health care delivery system, however, faces limits that must be set using some means and a set of community values (Callahan, 1990). It is likely that some outlays will be directed away from those with little or no ability to recover, for example, the permanently comatose and the terminally ill, based on community values and goals.

People with disabilities are another population group particularly concerned about the potential for discrimination using the Health Resource Allocation Strategy. Community advocacy groups for disabled persons have expressed the opinion that explicit rationing based on net benefit, such as proposed in the Oregon Health Plan, violates the Americans with Disabilities Act (ADA) (Marzen and Avila, 1991). The ADA prohibits state governments from excluding otherwise qualified individuals from government benefits or services on account of disability. These concerns are *real;* persons with disabilities, particularly those dependent upon government-funded health services, are threatened by the possible withholding of needed services. Rationing poses a special threat to disadvantaged persons struggling for the opportunities available to nondisadvantaged persons.

The calculation of benefits of health care in the Health Resource Allocation Strategy focuses on a definition of health-related quality of life that is value-based. The states defined in the health state classification system include many long-term disabilities, such as wheelchair mobility or permanent loss of extremities. These states are assigned less desirable weights in relation to perfect health. Thus, many persons with disabilities who enjoy a high quality of life live in health states that are given lower weights than persons without these disabilities. These weights do not necessarily mean that interventions for persons with disability will not be funded.

Interventions that have a high probability of raising the level of health-related quality of life of disabled persons, for example, physical therapy or corrective surgery, will result in a positive net health benefit, even in relation to costs. These interventions are likely to be funded within the budget constraint. Few services particular to persons with disability, for example, fall below the funding level in the Oregon Health Plan. Condition/treatment pairs that result in high cost and outcome ratios will not be included in the funding package. This will occur when the likelihood of benefit is low, the cost of treatment is high, and the number to be benefitted is low.

Similar to life-saving technologies and the "Rule of Rescue," these high-cost/low benefit services may be moved up the list when the community values of compassion and equity are considered. People with disabilities, like others in the community, will also have guaranteed access to a basic package of health care services. In this case, people with disabilities also have an equal stake in the common good of the entire community. The potential for discrimination exists for highly intensive treatments for disabled persons, but improvements in health care access to less intensive treatments for *all* persons with disabilities and the likelihood of special funding for "compassionate treatments" support the use of the Strategy in allocating health resources to the entire community, including persons with disabilities.

The concern of many persons in the United States is one of adding quality to life years, not just adding years to life. The Health Resource Allocation Strategy provides a systematic approach for making these difficult decisions. With the Strategy, the rationale and the basis on which the limits to health care get set are explicit and available for community review. This approach to setting limits is highly preferable and potentially less discriminating than one based on hidden information and unknown routes to decision making.

Utilitarianism

Finally, ethicists criticize the principle of utilitarianism in the Health Resource Allocation Strategy, that is, the distribution of society's resources to provide the greatest happiness to the greatest number of people. Those critics doubt that utilitarianism is the appropriate ethical theory for resolving resource allocation dilemmas (Smith, 1987; Harris 1988; La Puma and Lawlor, 1990).

The Health Resource Allocation Strategy does not necessarily assume or promote utilitarianism or any philosophical approach to the allocation of resources. Alternatively, the Strategy can be used according to principles of social justice such as those advocated by Rawls: that health care should be distributed equally unless an unequal distribution is to the advantage of the least favored (Rawls, 1971). Decision makers can choose to use comparative costs and outcomes information to maximize the expected welfare level of the worst off person, the "maximin" rule of justice. The challenge is in using information to make social arrangements that meet the fundamental rights of individuals while satisfying the principles of equality and social minimum.

Rawls has shown that a democracy can approximately satisfy his principles of justice, provided the government regulates a free economy in a certain way (Rawls, 1967, pp. 69–72). The principles of justice are balanced using an economic metric, most often average income per capita. The goals of economic policy—full employment, competition, price stability, appropriate rate of growth—are thus measured against income or dollars. A detailed weighting of output is thereby used in the political process for deciding policy.

Applying the same logic to social policy in the health sector, society is constantly making decisions about what is good and bad health, what is the social minimum, and how resources are distributed. Like economic indicators of worth, health-related quality of life, specifically years of healthy life, can be used to make collective decisions satisfying the principles of equality and social minimum. The difference is that health policy uses social preferences rather than dollars as the distribution metric.

A major question remains: Just how much priority must be given to the worst-off groups in society? In using comparative costs and outcomes in the sociopolitical process to maximize the welfare of the worst off in society, three positions are possible (Daniels, 1991). The strictest position is that improvements in the opportunity for health care and health status must never be made at the expense of the poorest groups. A modified position is that such decisions should not be made as long as there is a feasible alternative, such as investing more resources or increasing the efficiency of health services delivery. The weakest position would support denying access or making decisions at the expense of the worst off if they are not made much worse off and others who are not well off benefit significantly.

In applying the Health Resource Allocation Strategy, the last or weakest position must be adopted to improve the overall level of well-being of the community. No single allocation emerges that meets the demands of everyone. Access to services that are not high priority or part of the benefit available to everyone will be denied to persons who cannot afford to purchase the services. Although fairness cannot be guaranteed, the Strategy *can* and *should* be applied to guarantee a minimum benefit to all members of the community within the limits of available resources and according to community priorities. Although the resulting benefit may only approximate distributive justice, the process we advocate is surely better than the present alternative of investing more resources without evaluating their effect on the health-related quality of life of the whole community.

Many of the political and ethical challenges to the Health Resources Allocation Strategy can be met by decision makers' reasoned application of the Strategy. Uncaring or overzealous application, on the other hand, can lead to misguided resource allocation. Limiting potential abuses is important to all users and "beneficiaries" of the decisions made using the Strategy.

LIMITING POTENTIAL ABUSES

Many of the contributions of the Health Resource Allocation Strategy to the decision process stem from its incorporation of the theory of rational choice. As a normative theory, rational choice tells what we should do; it does not, however, tell us what our aims should be. Rational theory forms the basis of the costs and outcomes ranking. An allocation based solely on the ranking of costs and outcomes, however, may not meet overall societal aims or conform with the prevailing community values elicited Step 1 and reviewed in Step 8 of the Strategy. Thus, the limits of rationality may result in "abuses," or use of the Strategy in ways that were not originally intended. Three potential abuses are of particular concern: the use with special populations, the use as a technology, and use of selective inputs.

Selected Populations

Although the Health Resource Allocation Strategy adopts the societal perspective and is intended to be applied to all persons residing in the community, the potential exists to apply it selectively. For example, the Oregon Plan initially exempts older adults on

Medicaid from the ranking of services. Older, poor persons requiring long-term care, for instance, those living in nursing homes, place great demands on Medicaid resources. The remaining Medicaid recipients, children and their caretakers, constitute 75 percent of Medicaid recipients in Oregon and actually receive only 30 percent of the benefits in dollars (Daniels, 1991). This focus on special groups violates the ultimate goal of the Strategy: equality of opportunity for health to all persons in the community.

Although the Oregon Plan rations health care according to net benefit for poor mothers and children receiving Medicaid, Oregonians with private health insurance or elderly persons on Medicare are exempt from this rationing process. Thus, certain health care services that are available to other residents of Oregon may be denied to a select Medicaid population. This results in a two-tiered health care system both in terms of access to care and in health-related quality of life outcomes.

Selecting one group from the total population—whether that group be older persons, Medicaid recipients, or patients with end-stage renal disease—and allocating finite resources by means of rankings costs and outcomes will result in a lower level of health for the total population. Allocating resources to health services vertically—all services within one group—rather than horizontally—all services to all groups—gives higher priority to the allocation of less economically worthwhile services to the target group. Services with higher cost and outcomes ratios are more likely to be funded than if resources were allocated across all services and all groups in the population. Considering the whole population as the allocation target increases the probability that more economically worthwhile services with lower cost and outcomes ratios will be funded.

A Technological Bias

Another abuse is using the Strategy primarily as a technology rather than as a political tool. If Steps 1 and 8 are ignored or poorly implemented, then the Strategy is reduced to an analytic model that may well conflict with community values. No perfect computer algorithm exists for public decision making; the sociopolitical process and the values of stakeholders are always needed. Some persons see the use of cost–utility analyses and years of healthy life as an excessive move toward technologic policy, that is, toward standardized, quantified, and regulated protocols. Such methods lead away from the highly discretionary approaches to decision making, such as bargaining or implicit rules, that have characterized the politics of health throughout much of the twentieth century. In this critical view, the Health Resource Allocation Strategy makes health into just another commodity in the marketplace.

This criticism may apply to analytical models that use a measure of health that does not explicitly include the values that individuals place on health. Using years of healthy life as the measure of health outcome, however, incorporates the value that individuals gain from consuming health care. In this case, health care is the commodity and health is the valued outcome.

Sociopolitical input to the allocation of health care resources also limits rational choice in providing a mechanism for adjusting for imbalance of political power among different population groups. The review of the ranking by stakeholders as well as legislators and administrators helps overcome the potential abuse of rigorously attending to the methodology of economic analysis and can lead to more humanistic decision making.

Selected Inputs

Like the outcome of any decision-making process, the acceptability of the recommended priority list that results from applying the Strategy depends on the completeness and validity of the inputs. In particular, the values, definition of health, years of healthy life, costs, and the budget constraint may all be manipulated either intentionally or unintentionally to produce a priority list that is counter to the community's overall well-being.

The successful application of the Health Resource Allocation Strategy depends on the involvement of stakeholders and community representatives in the elicitation of community values and goals and in the assignment of preferences to health care outcomes. If participation is selective or incomplete, the Strategy will result in rankings of costs and outcomes that are biased. The direction of the bias will depend on who is included and who is excluded from the sociopolitical process and value elicitation scheme. This bias would most likely lead to a less-than-optimal allocation of resources.

Another selection bias is the definition of health-related quality of life that is used. Health states may be defined in ways that exclude the domains of health that are relevant to some persons in the community. For example, a questionnaire that focuses on collecting information on physical function and impairments will be insensitive for evaluating interventions that aimed at treating affective disorders such as depression. Methods for collecting this information can also lead to selectivity. For example, self-administered questionnaires may exclude blind persons and others who have limited manual dexterity. As a result, treatment benefit of these individuals will be omitted from the Strategy.

The two other major components of years of healthy life—preferences and prognosis—are also subject to abuse. Different methods of collecting preferences for health states may bias the results in one direction or another. For example, methods of preference elicitation that lead to a high nonresponse rate among a selected group of the population, say a particular ethnic group, effectively disenfranchise this group from participating in the ranking of costs and outcomes. The fundamental issue is one of whose preferences are used and how they are collected and included in the estimation of years of healthy life.

Similarly, selecting one set of transition probabilities over another can lead to bias in the years of healthy life gained for one intervention relative to another. Using life tables for the general population, for example, to estimate prognosis can underestimate the health benefit for interventions that prevent death among persons with diabetes. Even life tables based on diabetes as a cause of death will underestimate the impact of life-saving interventions since diabetes results in many deaths that are attributed to cardiovascular disease.

Inclusion of health care costs in the Strategy is another potential source of abuse. The selection of which direct and indirect costs to include is subject to the analyst's discretion. Because of the difficulty of collecting data on economic costs and the need to use charges and other forms of accounting data, the analyst may be unaware of biases introduced in estimating the incremental costs associated with a given intervention. Lack of data may also hinder the analyst from including some desired or necessary costs in the costs and outcomes ratios.

Problems with availability of data and selected inputs can be identified by the use of sensitivity analysis. By changing the assumptions made for handling incomplete data and recalculating the costs and outcomes ratios, the impact of each of the inputs on the final ranking can be assessed.

Decision makers may contribute to the abuse of the Strategy by their choice of the budget constraint. If too few resources are allocated and health care interventions that the community values are denied or not included as a benefit, then political challenges to the allocation should be, and will be, formidable. Also, if decision makers publish the final list of priorities in a form that radically differs from that of the ranking of costs and outcomes, then stakeholders will be unable to compare the changes that result from the decision makers' deliberations and negotiations. Modification of the format will obscure information thereby adversely affecting stakeholder confidence in the participatory decision-making process that is integral to the Strategy.

Some of the ethical considerations and possible abuses may be resolved by experience in implementing the Strategy as well as by further investigation. In particular, more conceptualization and empirical research are needed on components of the strategy.

ADDRESSING UNRESOLVED ISSUES

The Health Resource Allocation Strategy approach to policy analysis is relatively new, and many unresolved issues remain. Some of these are conceptual or methodological in nature. For example, the validity of the questionnaires used for collecting quality of life data needs to be demonstrated for the populations in which they are to be used. Also, in relation to the definition of health states, most of the existing measures focus on physical health, impairments, and symptoms, with less emphasis on affective well-being and concepts of positive health. How to include more positive domains such as satisfaction with health and well-being in composite health status measures requires a reexamination of social science theory and the development of new operational definitions. Other unresolved issues that are practical in nature include the reproducibility and stability of social preferences. These issues can be resolved by more empirical research.

Validity of Measurement

Questionnaires and methods for rapid and straightforward collection of both health status and the health state preferences used in the Health Resource Allocation Strategy have yet to be developed. Existing classification systems and measures have been, for the most part, developed using small populations and research settings or large populations of care-seekers, the exception being the Ontario Health Survey instrument described in Appendix I. Before the Strategy can be adopted for repeated use in allocating resources, particularly at a regional or national level, currently available methods need to be adapted for use in large-scale general population surveys.

The changes to be made vary with the classification system. They include modification of the wording of individual items in the questionnaire for comprehension by community respondents using interviews or self-administration; altering questionnaire answer categories for ease of response; and restructuring of the format to minimize the burdens of data collection.

The validity of the resulting methods for collecting information on both health-related quality of life and values needs to be rigorously tested. Special validity studies should be conducted using representatives from groups that might be expected to respond to the questionnaire differently from the majority of respondents: older persons, disabled persons, persons from different ethnic groups, and so on. Questionnaires need to be translated into the primary languages of the respondents. Such groups should be used to assure that the concepts and domains as well as individual questionnaire items are indeed measuring health-related quality of life (Carr-Hill, 1991).

Positive Health

A number of instruments that measure what is generally considered as positive health have been developed and empirically tested over the past 15 years (Stewart et al., 1988; Dupuy, 1984; Ware, 1984b). Items from these assessments have been shown to be significantly related to health outcome. For example, depressed persons tend to recover more slowly than do persons who are not depressed (Berwick, 1989; Wells, Stewart, et al., 1989). Longitudinal analysis of data from the NHANES Epidemiological Follow-Up Study (NHEFS) indicates that health perceptions are important predictors of mortality. Persons who were in fair or poor health in 1971–75 were more likely to have died by 1982–84 than were persons who perceived themselves to be in better health. Other researchers have posited that a significant factor in an individual's health-related quality of life is the discrepancy between one's actual and expected state, or one's satisfaction with health (Najman and Levine, 1981).

Concepts of positive health are gradually being incorporated into classification schemes for calculating years of healthy life. Torrance developed a socioemotional attribute that includes feeling happy or depressed and feeling relaxed and tense. These aspects of affective well-being are combined with a number of social concepts (Torrance, 1984). The EuroQol Group (1990) included mood as one of its domains. More work is needed on how to incorporate concepts such as depression, satisfaction, and health perceptions into states of health-related quality of life.

Preferences

One methodological, and still unresolved, issue has to do with the robustness of the preferences. That is, do the same preferences obtain across disease groups, or do the preferences change depending on the socio-demographic characteristics, socioeconomic level, and the health condition of respondents? Although this issue can be resolved with empirical testing, a few studies have been conducted to date with conflicting results. A great deal of research is necessary to address these potential differences.

Another area of robustness of preferences is whether they remain constant over time. Some researchers hypothesize that preferences may be stable in the short run but that they will change over the long run. Stability or change may depend on the health state descriptors. That is, preferences may not change for physical functioning, such as physical activity and mobility, in the long run and may change for health perceptions, including satisfaction and expectation for health. Stability properties of preferences can be assessed through empirical research.

A third area is the stability of health state preferences across cultures. Although preliminary evidence suggests that preferences are culturally robust, more studies are needed to determine if these results can be replicated and to determine if the results generalize to other disease-specific and cultural populations. The work of the EuroQol group (Brooks et al., 1991; Nord, 1991) in comparing preferences across different European countries begins to address this issue.

Some persons disagree with a fundamental premise of the Health Resource Allocation Strategy, namely, that preferences for health states can be measured at a level beyond ordinal measurement (i.e., interval or ratio). Even among those who agree that preferences can be measured, there are those who doubt that the resultant indexes can or should be used for policy purposes. To add across individuals, that is, to calculate an estimate of years of healthy life for the population, implies that preferences for health and quality of life can be compared between individuals. Most people, led by the economic formulation of the utility function as being multiattribute rather than additive, tend to agree that there are problems making interpersonal comparisons of utility.

On a practical level, methods are needed for collecting preference data on large samples of the population. To accomplish this, methods must be easy to administer so that preferences can be collected as part of ongoing national surveys. Thus, scaling techniques will need to be easily understood so that the response rate will be acceptably high and the data of high quality. The scaling will need to be understandable to a wide variety of individuals with diverse ethnic and educational backgrounds. Finally, the information, once collected, will need to be easy to score.

As with most concepts that are measured, empirical estimates of preferences are influenced by the measurement methods used. That is, preferences obtained by the use of category scaling may not be the same as those obtained by using the time tradeoff method, even though the health states were the same. The degree of difference, and whether or not the relationship is linear, needs to be thoroughly tested.

Child Health

Another unresolved issue is that of the sensitivity of existing conceptual frameworks to assess child health. Most of the health status outcome measures—measures of health-related quality of life—were developed for adults. Even in the cases where the developers claim the measures apply to children and adolescents, the questions included in the individual instruments are the same for youth as for adults; this assumes that the same aspects and levels of functioning are appropriate across the age spectrum. This assumption ignores the different stages of development of childhood.

Several efforts are under way to develop overall profiles or indexes of child health. These measures are being designed to evaluate a wide range of interventions targeted at children and young adults. Some of the conceptual problems yet to be resolved with these measures are testing content validity in samples of children and adolescents, assessing reliability and construct validity of the measures, and examining the ability of the measures to detect changes in children's health (Patrick and Bergner, 1990).

For policy purposes, however, measures of child health must include universal health states to allow for the comparison across population groups. Concentration on major activity—playing, going to school, working, or maintaining a household—remains the major means whereby costs and outcomes comparisons of interventions for children can be compared with those for adults and older persons.

Prognosis

The ethical criticism that years of healthy life are ageist speaks to the need to better estimate prognosis. In Chapter 9 we discussed the ideal—a matrix with as many states in future periods as in the present period. With the current lack of information about the movement between states, we use life expectancy as proxy data for future health. If probabilities of change over time could be estimated from population data, the trajectories of function could be incorporated. For example, a young person in a car accident may initially be critically injured but recover to full functioning after treatment in the intensive care unit.

Not only is more empirical research required to obtain estimates of transition probabilities; more conceptual research on how to forecast the movement between states is also needed. Several mathematical approaches have been used to date; each has some limitation in terms of representing the dynamic features of health. If these methods are to be used in the future, more needs to be known about their strengths and weaknesses. Also, research is needed to learn if there are more appropriate methods available for use in health care research.

Linking Interventions to Outcomes

The optimal way to use costs and outcomes to inform decision making is to have these data collected at the individual level for each of the interventions to be included in the allocation package. For example, if resources may be devoted to hospital hemodialysis, then costs and outcomes of a representative sample of persons receiving this treatment need to be obtained. Studies, using the same methods for determining costs and outcomes, should be conducted for other interventions and the data should be available for use in the Strategy. Such data directly link the treatment with its associated costs and outcomes.

The current reality is that such data are available on selected populations for only a few interventions. Although many data sources are available, for example, the health surveys and registration systems of the National Center for Health Statistics, the data frequently reflect either health outcomes or the use of services and interventions. That is, the vast majority of these sources have data either on costs or outcomes but not both. In the absence of other information, these data may be used. The lack of direct linkage among costs, outcomes, and interventions greatly weakens the measure of association of these three.

Time Preference for Health

With regard to people's time preference for health we have adopted the standard economic approach of discounting in the Health Resource Allocation Strategy for convenience. Yet research is needed to determine whether this assumption is appropriate. We have already raised questions about the assumption of positive time preference for health. Although the limited empirical research conducted to date suggests that the assumption of positive time preference holds, this research must be replicated. In addition, the validity of the reasons for discounting should be examined.

Community Involvement

The potential abuses of the Strategy in excessive use of rationality in allocating resources emphasize the importance of including the values of health care consumers and their agents in the setting and implementing of social goals. More study of the decision-making process is needed to identify the optimal time and method to involve the community in the Health Resource Allocation Strategy. For example, is the use of community members in testimonials before legislative committees effective in eliciting social values? Or do these forums bring forth "politically correct" responses that bear little relationship to society's true values? How do the values elicited in community meetings get disseminated and reviewed?

Cost of Implementation

We have shown that the use of the Strategy results in a more efficient allocation of existing resources. We have also argued that it is preferable to the present piecemeal methods of making tough decisions surrounding health care delivery. The administrative costs of implementing a strategy for allocating resources based on costs and outcomes for a wide range of interventions over a large population are largely unknown. It is possible that the costs for developing and implementing the strategy outweigh or are balanced by the savings.

One possibility for estimating the costs of implementing the Strategy is a congressional study. For example, the Office of Technology Assessment might investigate sources and levels of administrative costs associated with wider use of the Strategy, whether at state or national level. Simulation modeling can be used to examine upper and lower bounds on anticipated costs of implementation. Modeling provides the opportunity for testing the impact of different implementation formats. For example, the cost impact of large versus small review committees can be assessed. These models could also be used to identify sources of economies of scale.

Another possibility for implementation is that the responsibility for applying the Strategy can be subsumed by agencies already charged with administering health care insurance programs. For example, the Medicare and Medicaid programs might be merged with the Strategy and the combined program operated by the Health Care Financing Administration (HCFA). This merger and focusing of health care delivery in the United States might mean a change in function for HCFA staff at little or no additional cost for implementation.

Although unresolved conceptual, methodological, and practical issues remain, the basic elements of the Health Resource Allocation Strategy have been tested over the past 25 years. Both the conceptual and theoretical foundations and their empirical testing indicate that the Strategy can be applied with our existing technologies. Progress need not be deterred by the need for further research; knowledge and understanding will proceed incrementally with increased adoption and use of the Strategy.

TOWARD EQUALITY OF OPPORTUNITY FOR HEALTH

The health care system of the United States, as well as those in other developed countries, is being challenged to produce a high level of health-related quality of life within reasonable funding constraints. The technology and population dynamics that have produced this situation over the past 30 years are expected to continue. In proposing the Health Resource Allocation Strategy, we adopt the egalitarian view that access to health care is every citizen's right. This perspective fits with the notion that the output of the health care delivery system is equality of opportunity for health.

Provision of health care has received considerable attention in the last 20 years. Over this time, the success and failure of different health services delivery schemes in the United Kingdom and Canada, as well as in the United States, have been observed. This experience indicates that a private-based insurance system has strong incentives to control costs at the level of the individual patient, physician, and other health care providers. The private system has problems, however, of controlling supply at the aggregate level. On the other hand, public systems are more able to control costs in the aggregate but have problems at the individual level. Thus, most proposals for modifying existing health care systems are looking at a mixture of public and private systems (Williams, 1988c).

The potential for equal access and equal opportunity that follows from the application of the Health Resource Allocation Strategy requires a publicly supported, national health care plan. This plan, whatever mix of public and private financing mechanisms it comprises, must cover all persons, the young and the old, the ill and the well, and the rich and the poor. As argued in this book, a national focus to health care will assure the highest level of health within an expenditure level that society finds acceptable. We have shown that a piecemeal approach to allocation of resources can result in a lower level of health for a given level of funding. We advocate a central organizing structure to health care delivery as the way to generate the highest level of health and equality of opportunity.

A national plan is necessary to change the U.S. health care ethos from one that rations health care based on price to one that rations based on a sociopolitical mechanism. The current use of price, or ability to pay, to decide which members of society receive what types of health care is embedded in our strong belief in liberty and freedom of choice. These beliefs are fundamental to the U.S. character. Thus, there is strong resistance to ceding any freedom, the loss of which is implied by a societal approach to health care rationing.

Yet some individual freedom of choice in health care will need to be surrendered if we are to solve our current problems. These problems can be characterized by increasing health care costs that may threaten continued prosperity for some persons, employers, and businesses. Also, some individual freedom will need to yield if the United States is to address future health care problems associated with chronic illness, an aging population, and the growth of expensive medical technologies.

This shift from price as a rationing agent to some societal mechanism will take some adjustment of the collective American personality. This adjustment will be less painful if a systematic and visible approach is adopted by decision makers, rather than allowing decisions to be made in an ill-defined, "muddling through" fashion. We recommend that the Health Resource Allocation Strategy be used as the basic structure to replace the price mechanism for two main reasons. First, like price, the Strategy places an explicit statement of value on various health care interventions. Instead of using monetary units, however, the Strategy uses preferences. Second, the Strategy goes beyond economic efficiency to incorporate a sociopolitical process that can lead to equity in the allocation process.

In this book we addressed major issues facing health policymakers in the 1990s. We propose that the Health Resource Allocation Strategy be used in conjunction with a national plan for health care to improve the equality of opportunity for health. The health decisions that lie ahead are difficult. We recognize that difficulties abound in putting a price on additional years of life, on the joy of going to a daughter's wedding, or on the satisfaction that seriously ill patients and their families derive even when facing impending death. The route we propose is intended to help frame and make the hard choices necessary to maximize society's use of health care resources for increasing the opportunity for health of the community. In our view, making these hard choices explicit and addressing them in a public decision process based on cost and outcome data is the best strategy to achieve this goal.

APPENDIX I

Four Measures of Health-Related Quality of Life for Implementing the Health Resource Allocation Strategy

A. DISABILITY/DISTRESS INDEX

Contacts/Developers

Rachel M. Rosser, MA, MB, PhD
Department of Psychiatry
University College and
  Middlesex Medical School
University of London
London England W1N 8AA
Telephone: 011-44-71-636-8333
FAX: 011-44-71-323-1459

Alan Williams, PhD
Centre for Health
  Economics
University of York
Heslington, York Y01 5DD
England
Telephone: 011-44-904-433-651

Level	Definition of HRQOL concept		Preference weight
	Disability	**Distress**	
I-A	No disability	No distress	1.000
I-B	"	Mild distress	0.995
I-C	"	Moderate distress	0.990
I-D	"	Severe distress	0.967
II-A	Slight social disability	No distress	0.990
II-B	"	Mild distress	0.986
II-C	"	Moderate distress	0.973
II-D	"	Severe distress	0.932
III-A	Severe social disability and/or slight impairment of performance at work. Able to do all housework except very heavy tasks.	No distress	0.980
III-B	"	Mild distress	0.972
III-C	"	Moderate distress	0.956
III-D	"	Severe distress	0.912

(*continued*)

Level	Definition of HRQOL concept		Preference weight
	Disability	**Distress**	
IV-A	Choice of work or performance at work severely limited. Housewives and old people able to do light housework only, but able to go out shopping.	No distress	0.964
IV-B	"	Mild distress	0.956
IV-C	"	Moderate distress	0.942
IV-D	"	Severe distress	0.870
V-A	Unable to undertake any paid employment. Unable to continue any education. Old people confined to home except for escorted outings and short walks and unable to do shopping. Housewives able to perform only a few simple tasks.	No distress	0.946
V-B	"	Mild distress	0.935
V-C	"	Moderate distress	0.900
V-D	"	Severe distress	0.700
VI-A	Confined to chair or to wheelchair or able to move around in the home only with support from an assistant.	No distress	0.875
VI-B	"	Mild distress	0.845
VI-C	"	Moderate distress	0.680
VI-D	"	Severe distress	0.000
VII-A	Confined to bed	No distress	0.677
VII-B	"	Mild distress	0.564
VII-C	"	Moderate distress	0.000
VII-D	"	Severe distress	−1.486
VIII-A	Unconscious	No distress	−1.028
VIII-B	"	Mild distress	—[a]
VIII-C	"	Moderate distress	—[a]
VIII-D	"	Severel distress	—[a]

Source: Adapted from Williams, 1985.

[a]Not applicable.

Disability/Distress Index (Simplified) Self-Completed Questionnaire[1]
GM   General Mobility

Which one of these statements best describes your situation?

1. I can move around indoors and outdoors on my own easily with no aids or help. ☐

2. I can move around indoors and outdoors on my own with a little difficulty but with no aids or help. ☐

3. I can get about indoors and outdoors on my own *but* I have to use a walking aid, e.g., stick, frame, crutches, wheelchair. ☐

4. I can move around the house without anyone's help, but I need someone's help to get outdoors. ☐

Potential users of these measures are advised to contact the developers listed herein to enquire about copyright and the permission and instructions for using them.

5. I spend nearly all my time confined to a chair (other than a wheelchair).

6. I have to spend nearly all my time in bed.

UA   Usual Activity

During the past week, has your health affected any of the things you usually do (e.g., at work or study or at home)?

1. Not at all. ☐

2. Slightly affected. ☐

3. Severely affected. ☐

4. Unable to do usual activities at all. ☐

Self-Care

Do you need help with

1. Washing yourself?   Yes ☐   No ☐

2. Dressing?   Yes ☐   No ☐

3. Eating or drinking?   Yes ☐   No ☐

4. Using the toilet?   Yes ☐   No ☐

Social and Personal Relationships

Does your state of health seriously affect any of the following?

1. Your social life?   Yes ☐   No ☐

2. Seeing friends or relatives?   Yes ☐   No ☐

3. Your hobbies or leisure activities?   Yes ☐   No ☐

4. Your sex life?   Yes ☐   No ☐

Distress

How much does your state of health distress you overall? Mark a cross on the line.

NO DISTRESS   EXTREME
AT ALL   DISTRESS

├──┤

Conversion of (Simplified) Self-Completed Questionnaire Responses to Disability/Distress Categories
Disability

Coding.

"General Mobility" responses are already coded (GM) 1 to 6 in the questionnaire.
Patients who are not conscious will simply be so recorded.
"Self-care" responses are scored 1 for each "YES" response (possible range of scores is thus 0 to 4).

"Usual activities" responses are already coded (UA) 1 to 4 on the questionnaire.

"Social and personal relationships" responses are scored 1 for each "YES" response (possible range of scores is thus 0 to 4).

Assignment Rules

In the table below, first move to the appropriate *column*, using the General Mobility response (or "not conscious"). For GM4 to GM6 and for "not conscious," no further information is required, the Rosser disability categories being V, VI, VII, and VIII, respectively.

For GM1 to GM3, start with the "usual activity" response. If UA = 1 (i.e., not affected), one of the first three rows will be relevant. If UA = 2 (i.e., slightly affected), one of the next two rows will be relevant. If UA = 3 or UA = 4, the Rosser disability category will be IV and V, respectively.

For the first five rows, the scores on Self-Care and Social and Personal Relationships will be relevant, as indicated in the table.

Table for assigning respondents to disability categories

Other responses	General mobility:						
	1	2	3	4	5	6	Not conscious
UA = 1 SC = 0 *and* SP = 0	I	II	III				
UA = 1 SC = 1 or 2 *or* SP 1 or 2	II	II	III				
UA = 1 SC = 3 or 4 *or* SP 3 or 4	III	III	IV	V	VI	VII	VIII
UA = 2 *but* SC < 3 *and* SP < 3	III	III	III				
UA = 2 SC ≥ 3 *or* SP ≥ 3	III	III	IV				
UA = 3	IV	IV	IV				
UA = 4	V	V	V				

Coding. Measure position of cross on the 10-cm visual analogue scale in mm, with 0 at left end and 100 mm at right end. Treat this as the distress "score."

Assignment rules

Score	Rosser category
≤10	A
>10 but ≥50	B
>50 but ≤90	C
>90	D

Source: Gudex and Kind, 1988.

B. HEALTH UTILITIES INDEX

Contacts/Developers

George W. Torrance, PhD
Health Science Center
McMaster University, 3HIC
1200 Main Street, West
Hamilton, Ontario L8N 3Z5
Canada
Telephone: (416) 525-9140
    Ext. 2143
FAX: (416) 546-5211

Michael H. Boyle, PhD
Department of Psychiatry
McMaster University
1200 Main Street, West
Hamilton, Ontario L8N 3Z5
Canada
Telephone: (416) 521-2100 Ext. 7359

David Feeny, PhD
Departments of Economics and Clinical
    Epidemiology and Biostatistics
McMaster University
1200 Main Street, West
Hamilton, Ontario L8N 3Z5
Canada
Telephone: (416) 525-9140 Ext. 2131

I. Health Utilities Index (Mark I) (age ≥ 2 years)

Classification System

Level	Definition of HRQOL concept	Preference weight
Physical function: Mobility and physical activity (P)[a]		
P1	Being able to get around the house, yard, neighborhood, or community *without help* from another person; *and* having *no* limitation in physical ability to lift, walk, run, jump, or bend.	1.00
P2	Being able to get around the house, yard, neighborhood, or community *without help* from another person; *and* having *some* limitations in physical ability to lift, walk, run, jump, or bend.	0.91
P3	Being able to get around the house, yard, neighborhood, or community *without help* from another person; *and needing* mechanical aids to walk or get around.	0.81
P4	*Needing help* from another person in order to get around the house, yard, neighborhood, or community; *and* having *some* limitations in physical ability to lift, walk, run, jump, or bend.	0.80
P5	*Needing help* from another person in order to get around the house, yard, neighborhood, or community; *and needing* mechanical aids to walk or get around.	0.61
P6	*Needing help* from another person in order to get around the house, yard, neighborhood, or community; *and not* being able to use or control the arms and legs.	0.52
Role function: Self-care and role activity (R)[a]		
R1	Being able to eat, dress, bathe, and go to the toilet *without help; and* having *no* limitations when playing, going to school, working, or in other activities.	1.00

(*continued*)

Level	Definition of HRQOL concept	Preference weight
R2	Being able to eat, dress, bathe, and go to the toilet *without help; and* having *some* limitations when working, going to school, playing, or in other activities.	0.94
R3	Being able to eat, dress, bathe, and go to the toilet *without help; and not* being able to play, attend school, or work.	0.77
R4	*Needing help* to eat, dress, bathe, or go to the toilet; *and* having *some* limitations when working, going to school, playing, or in other activities.	0.75
R5	*Needing help* to eat, dress, bathe, or go to the toilet; *and not* being able to play, attend school or work.	0.50

Social-emotional function: Emotional well-being and social activity (S)

S1	Being happy and relaxed most or all of the time, *and* having an average number of friends and contacts with others.	1.00
S2	Being happy and relaxed most or all of the time, *and* having very few friends and little contact with others.	0.96
S3	Being anxious or depressed some or a good bit of the time, *and* having an average number of friends and contacts with others.	0.86
S4	Being anxious or depressed some or a good bit of the time, *and* having very few friends and little contact with others.	0.77

Health problem (H)[b]

H1	Having no health problem.	1.00
H2	Having a minor physical deformity or disfigurement such as scars on the face.	0.92
H3	Needing a hearing aid.	0.91
H4	Having a medical problem which causes pain or discomfort for a few days in a row every two months.	0.91
H5	Needing to go to a special school because of trouble learning or remembering things.	0.86
H6	Having trouble seeing even when wearing glasses.	0.84
H7	Having trouble being understood by others.	0.83
H8	Being blind *or* deaf *or* not able to speak.	0.74

[a]Multiple choices within each description are applied to individuals as appropriate for their age. For example, a 3-year-old child is not expected to be able to get around the community without help from another person.

[b]Individuals with more than one health problem are classified according to the problem they consider the most serious.

Calculating Formula

The formula gives utility values on the standard scale where healthy is 1.00 and dead is 0.00. However, since some of the health states were judged to be worse than death, some of the utility values are less than zero. The least utility value, for health state (P6, R5, S4, H8), is −0.21.

$$U = 1.42 \ (P_i \ R_i \ S_i \ H_i) - 0.42$$

where U = utility of health state; P_i = preference weight for the level on mobility and physical activity; R_i = preference weight for the level on role function, etc.

Example calculations[a]

$$U(P1,R1,S1,H1) = 1.42(1.00 \times 1.00 \times 1.00 \times 1.00) - 0.42 = 1.00$$
$$U(P1,R1,S1,H4) = 1.42(1.00 \times 1.00 \times 1.00 \times 1.91) - 0.42 = 0.87$$
$$U(P3,R2,S1,H1) = 1.42(0.81 \times 0.94 \times 1.00 \times 1.00) - 0.42 = 0.66$$
$$U(P1,R2,S4,H1) = 1.42(1.00 \times 0.94 \times 0.77 \times 1.00) - 0.42 = 0.61$$
$$U(P3,R2,S2,H5) = 1.42(0.81 \times 0.94 \times 0.96 \times 0.86) - 0.42 = 0.47$$
$$U(P5,R4,S3,H1) = 1.42(0.61 \times 0.75 \times 0.86 \times 1.00) - 0.42 = 0.14$$
$$U(P5,R5,S4,H7) = 1.42(0.61 \times 0.50 \times 0.77 \times 0.83) - 0.42 = -0.14$$
$$U(P6,R5,S4,H8) = 1.42(0.52 \times 0.50 \times 0.77 \times 0.74) - 0.42 = -0.21$$

Source: Adapted from Drummond et al., 1987.

[a] Although the formula produces a single utility value for each health state, the measurements on which the formula is based are not precise. Measurement uncertainty includes both sampling error and measurement imprecision. These are combined in the standard error $S_{\bar{x}} = 0.06$. A sensitivity analysis of $\pm 2S_{\bar{x}}$ would give an upper bound utility value of $U + 0.12$, not to exceed 1.00, and a lower bound of $U - 0.12$.

2. Health Utilities Index (Mark II)

Table 1.   Multiattribute health status system

Attribute	Level	Description
Sensory	1	Able to see, hear, and speak normally for age.
	2	Requires equipment to see or hear or speak.
	3	See, hears, or speaks with limitations, even with equipment.
	4	Blind, deaf, or mute.
Mobility	1	Able to walk, bend, lift, jump and run normally for age.
	2	Walks, bends, lifts, jumps, or runs with some limitations, but does not require help.
	3	Requires mechanical equipment (such as canes, crutches, braces, or wheelchair) to walk or get around independently.
	4	Requires the help of another person to walk or get around and requires mechanical equipment as well.
	5	Unable to control or use arms and legs.
Emotion	1	Generally happy and free from worry.
	2	Occasionally fretful, angry, irritable, anxious, depressed, or suffering "night terrors."
	3	Often fretful, angry, irritable, anxious, depressed, or suffering "night terrors."
	4	Almost always fretful, angry, irritable, anxious, depressed.
	5	Extremely fretful, angry, irritable, or depressed, usually requiring hospitalization or psychiatric institutional care.
Cognitive	1	Learns and remembers schoolwork normally for age.
	2	Learns and remembers schoolwork more slowly than classmates, as judged by parents and/or teachers.
	3	Learns and remembers very slowly and usually requires special educational assistance.
	4	Unable to learn and remember.
Self-care	1	Eats, bathes, dresses, and uses the toilet normally for age.

(continued)

Table 1. (*continued*)

Attribute	Level	Description
	2	Eats, bathes, dresses, or uses the toilet independently with difficulty.
	3	Requires mechanical equipment to eat, bathe, dress, or use the toilet independently.
	4	Requires the help of another person to eat, bathe, dress, or use the toilet.
Pain	1	Free of pain and discomfort.
	2	Occasional pain. Discomfort relieved by nonprescription drugs or self-control activity without disruption of normal activities.
	3	Frequent pain. Discomfort relieved by oral medicines with occasional disruption of normal activities.
	4	Frequent pain; frequent disruption of normal activities. Discomfort requires prescription narcotics for relief.
	5	Severe pain. Pain not relieved by drugs and constantly disrupts normal activities.
Fertility	1	Able to have children with a fertile spouse.
	2	Difficulty in having children with a fertile spouse.
	3	Unable to have children with a fertile spouse.

Table 2. Multiattribute functions for value and utility—simplified format

2.1 Multiattribute value function (MAVF)

Sensory		Mobility		Emotional		Cognitive		Self-Care		Pain		Fertility	
x_1	a_1	x_2	a_2	x_3	a_3	x_4	a_4	x_5	a_5	x_6	a_6	x_7	a_7
1	1.00	1	1.00	1	1.00	1	1.00	1	1.00	1	1.00	1	1.00
2	0.73	2	0.78	2	0.69	2	0.72	2	0.88	2	0.77	2	0.79
3	0.57	3	0.54	3	0.51	3	0.59	3	0.81	3	0.54	3	0.61
4	0.33	4	0.42	4	0.40	4	0.34	4	0.73	4	0.34		
		5	0.30	5	0.27					5	0.17		

$$v^* = 1.02 \, (a_1 * a_2 * a_3 * a_4 * a_5 * a_6 * a_7) - 0.02$$

where v^* is the value of the health state on a value scale where dead has a value of 0.00 and healthy has a value of 1.00. Because the worst possible health state was judged by respondents as worse than death, it has a negative value of -0.02.

2.2 Multiattribute utility function (MAUF)

Sensory		Mobility		Emotional		Cognitive		Self-Care		Pain		Fertility	
x_1	b_1	x_2	b_2	x_3	b_3	x_4	b_4	x_5	b_5	x_6	b_6	x_7	b_7
1	1.00	1	1.00	1	1.00	1	1.00	1	1.00	1	1.00	1	1.00
2	0.95	2	0.97	2	0.93	2	0.95	2	0.97	2	0.97	2	0.97
3	0.86	3	0.84	3	0.81	3	0.88	3	0.91	3	0.85	3	0.88
4	0.61	4	0.73	4	0.70	4	0.65	4	0.80	4	0.64		
		5	0.58	5	0.53					5	0.38		

$$u^* = 1.06 \, (b_1 * b_2 * b_3 * b_4 * b_5 * b_6 * b_7) - 0.06$$

where u^* is the utility of the health state on a utility scale where dead has a utility of 0.00 and healthy has a utility of 1.00. Because the worst possible health state was judged by respondents as worse than death, it has a negative utility of -0.02.

3. Health Utilities Index (Mark III)

The Health Utilities Index has been modified recently to include the following eight attributes. No classification for this version is available yet, but the attributes are:

1. Vision
2. Hearing
3. Speech
4. Getting around (mobility)
5. Hands and fingers (dexterity)
6. Feelings (emotional function)
7. Memory and thinking (cognitive function)
8. Pain and discomfort

A questionnaire from the Ontario Health Survey that can be used to collect data for this Index follows. Utility weights for this eight-attribute index are currently being collected. For further information about the utility weights and calculating formulas available in the future, please contact Dr. George Torrance.

Ontario Health Survey Interviewing Schedule
for Health Utilities Index (Mark III)

The following set of questions asks about each person's usual ability in certain areas, such as vision, hearing and speech. (Do not ask questions 2 to 32 for children less than 6 years old.)

1. INTERVIEWER CHECK ITEM:
   Person 6 years or older ⟶ ◯ Go to question 2

   Person less than 6 years old ⟶ ◯ Go to question 33

Vision

2. Are/Is _____usually able to see well enough to read ordinary newsprint *without* glasses or contact lenses?

   ◯ Yes ⟶ Go to 5
   ◯ No

3. Are/Is_____usually able to see well enough to read ordinary newsprint *with* glasses or contact lenses?

   ◯ Yes ⟶ Go to 5
   ◯ No

4. Are/Is_____able to see at all?

   ◯ Yes
   ◯ No ⟶ Go to 7

5. Are/Is _____ able to see well enough to recognize a friend on the other side of the street *without* glasses or contact lenses?

   ◯ Yes ⟶ Go to 7
   ◯ No

6. Are/Is _____ usually able to see well enough to recognize a friend on the other side of the street *with* glasses or contact lenses?

   ◯ Yes
   ◯ No

Hearing

7. Are/Is _____ usually able to hear
   what is said in a group conversation with
   at least three other people *without* a
   hearing aid?

   ○ Yes ➤ Go to 12
   ○ No

8. Are/Is _____ usually able to hear
   what is said in a group conversation with
   at least three other people *with* a hearing
   aid?

   ○ Yes ➤ Go to 10
   ○ No

9. Are/Is _____ able to hear at all?

   ○ Yes
   ○ No ➤ Go to 12

10. Are/Is _____ usually able to hear
    what is said in a conversation with one
    other person in a quiet room *without* a
    hearing aid?

    ○ Yes ➤ Go to 12
    ○ No

11. Are/Is _____ usually able to hear
    what is said in a conversation with one
    other person in a quiet room *with* a
    hearing aid?

    ○ Yes
    ○ No

Speech

12. Are/Is _____ usually able to be
    understood completely when speaking
    with strangers?

    ○ Yes ➤ Go to 17
    ○ No

13. Are/Is _____ able to be under-
    stood partially when speaking with
    strangers?

    ○ Yes
    ○ No

14. Are/Is _____ able to be under-
    stood completely when speaking with
    those who know _____ well?

    ○ Yes ➤ Go to 17
    ○ No

15. Are/Is _____ able to be under-
    stood partially when speaking with
    those who know _____ well?

    ○ Yes ➤ Go to 17
    ○ No

16. Are/Is _____ able to speak at all?

    ○ Yes
    ○ No

Getting Around

17. Are/Is _____ able to walk around
    the neighborhood without difficulty
    and without mechanical support such
    as braces, cane, or crutches?

    ○ Yes ➤ Go to 24
    ○ No

18. Are/Is _____ able to walk at all?

    ○ Yes
    ○ No ➤ Go to 21

19. Do/Does _____ require mechanical support such as braces, cane or crutches to be able to walk around the neighborhood?

○ Yes
○ No

20. Do/Does _____ require the help of another person to be able to walk?

○ Yes
○ No

21. Do/Does _____ require a wheelchair to get around?

○ Yes
○ No → Go to 24

22. How often do/does _____ use a wheelchair?

○ Always
○ Often
○ Sometimes
○ Never

23. Do/Does _____ need the help of another person to get around in the wheelchair?

○ Yes
○ No

Hands and Fingers

24. Do/Does _____ usually have the full use of two hands and ten fingers?

○ Yes → Go to 28
○ No

25. Do/Does _____ require the help of another person because of limitations in the use of hands or fingers?

○ Yes
○ No → Go to 27

26. Do/Does _____ require the help of another person with some tasks, most tasks, almost all tasks, or all tasks?

○ Some tasks
○ Most tasks
○ Almost all tasks
○ All tasks

27. Do/Does _____ require special equipment, for example, devices to assist in dressing because of limitation in the use of hands or fingers?

○ Yes
○ No

Feelings

28. Would you describe _____ as being usually:

(Mark one only)

(a) happy and interested in life?   a) ○

(b) somewhat happy?   b) ○

(c) somewhat unhappy?   c) ○

(d) unhappy with little interest in life?   d) ○

(e) so unhappy that life is not worthwhile?   e) ○

Memory

29. How would you describe _____   (Mark one only)
    usual ability to remember things?
    Are/Is _____:

    (a) able to remember most things?   a) ◯

    (b) somewhat forgetful?   b) ◯

    (c) very forgetful?   c) ◯

    (d) unable to remember anything at all?   d) ◯

Thinking

30. Would you describe _____ usual   (Mark one only)
    ability to think as:

    (a) able to think clearly and solve   a) ◯
        problems?

    (b) having a little difficulty when trying   b) ◯
        to think or solve problems?

    (c) having some difficulty when trying to   c) ◯
        think or solve problems?

    (d) having a great deal of difficulty when   d) ◯
        trying to think or solve problems?

    (e) unable to think or solve any problems?   e) ◯

Pain and Discomfort

31. Are/Is _____ usually free of   ◯ Yes → Finished
    pain and discomfort?
         ◯ No

32. Which one of the following sentences   (Mark one only)
    best describes the effect of the pain
    and discomfort _____ usually
    experiences?

    a) pain and discomfort that does not   a) ◯
       prevent any activities?

    b) pain and discomfort that prevents   b) ◯
       a few activities?

    c) pain and discomfort that prevents   c) ◯
       some activities?

    d) pain and discomfort that prevents   d) ◯
       most activities?

For information on the Ontario Health Survey (1990) contact:

Dave Bogart, Director
User Support Branch
Information & Systems Division
Ministry of Health Ontario
15 Overlea Boulevard
Toronto, Ontario M4H 1A9
Canada
Telephone: (416) 327-7610
FAX: (416) 327-7611

Larry Chambers, PhD
Department of Clinical Epidemiology
 and Biostatistics
McMaster University
1200 Main Street, West
Hamilton, Ontario L8N 3Z5
Canada
Telephone: (416) 525-9140, Ext. 2136

C. QUALITY OF WELL-BEING SCALE AND GENERAL HEALTH POLICY MODEL

Contacts/Developers

Robert M. Kaplan, PhD, or John P. Anderson, PhD
Division of Health Care Sciences
Department of Community Medicine
School of Medicine, M-022
University of California, San Diego
La Jolla, California 92093
Telephone: (619) 534-6058
FAX: (619) 534-4642

Level	Definition of HRQOL concept	Preference weight
Mobility Scale (MOB)		
5	No limitations for health reasons	−0.000
4	Did not drive a car, health related; did not ride in a car as usual for age (younger than 15 years), health related	−0.062
3	Did not use public transportation, health related	−0.062
2	Had or would have used more help than usual for age to use public transportation, health related	−0.062
1	In hospital, health related	−0.090
Physical Activity Scale (PAC)		
4	No limitations for health reasons	−0.000
3	In wheelchair, moved or controlled movement of wheelchair without help from someone else	−0.060
2	Had trouble or did not try to lift, stoop, bend over, or use stairs or inclines, health related; limped, used a cane, crutches, or walker, health related; had any other physical limitation in walking, or did not try to talk as far or as fast as others the same age are able, health related	−0.060
1	In wheelchair, did not move or control the movement of wheelchair without help from someone else, or in bed, chair, or couch for most or all of the day, health related	−0.077

(*continued*)

Level	Definition of HRQOL concept	Preference weight
Social Activity Scale (SAC)		
5	No limitations for health reasons	−0.000
4	Limited in other (e.g., recreational) role activity, health related	−0.061
3	Limited in major (primary) role activity, health related	−0.061
2	Performed no major role activity, health related, but did perform self-care activities	−0.061
1	Performed no major role activity, health related, and did not perform or had more help than usual in performance of one or more self-care activities, health related	−0.106
23	Standard symptom/problem	−0.257
22	No symptoms or problem (not on respondent's card)	−0.000
21	Breathing smog or unpleasant air	−0.101
20	Wore eyeglasses or contact lenses	−0.101
19	Taking medication or staying on a prescribed diet for health reasons	−0.144
18	Pain in ear, tooth, jaw, throat, lips, tongue; several missing or crooked permanent teeth—includes wearing bridges or false teeth; stuffy, runny nose; or any trouble hearing—includes wearing a hearing aid	−0.170
17	Overweight for age and height or skin defect of face, body, arms, or legs, such as scars, pimples, warts, bruises, or changes in color	−0.188
16	Pain or discomfort in one or both eyes (such as burning or itching) or any trouble seeing after correction	−0.230
15	Trouble talking, such as lisp, stuttering, hoarseness, or being unable to speak	−0.237
14	Burning or itching rash on large areas of face, body, arms, or legs	−0.240
13	Headache, or dizziness, or ringing in ears, or spells of feeling hot, or nervous, or shaky	−0.244
12	Spells of feeling upset, being depressed, or of crying	−0.257
11	Cough, wheezing, or shortness of breath, with or without fever, chills, or aching all over	−0.257
10	General tiredness, weakness, or weight loss	−0.259
9	Sick or upset stomach, vomiting or loose bowel movement, with or without fever, chills, or aching all over	−0.290
8	Pain, burning, bleeding, itching, or other difficulty with rectum, bowel movements, or urination (passing water)	−0.292
7	Pain, stiffness, weakness, numbness, or other discomfort in chest, stomach (including hernia or rupture), side, neck, back, hips, or any joints or hands, feet, arms, or legs	−0.299
6	Any combination of one or more hands, feet, arms, or legs either missing, deformed (crooked), paralyzed (unable to move), or broken—includes wearing artificial limbs or braces	−0.333
5	Trouble learning, remembering, or thinking clearly	−0.340
4	Pain, bleeding, itching, or discharge (drainage) from sexual organs—does not include normal menstrual (monthly) bleeding	−0.349
3	Burn over large areas of face, body, arms, or legs	−0.387
2	Loss of consciousness such as seizure (fits), fainting, or coma (out cold or knocked out)	−0.407
1	Death (not on respondent's card)	−0.727

Source: Adapted from Kaplan and Anderson, 1988.

Calculating formulas: Formula 1: Point-in-time well-being score for an individual (*W*):

$$W = 1 + (\text{CPX}wt) + (\text{MOB}wt) + (\text{PAC}wt) + (\text{SAC}wt)$$

(*continued*)

Level	Definition of HRQOL concept	Preference weight

where wt is the preference-weighted measure for each factor and CPX is symptom–problem complex.

Formula 2: Well-years (*WY*) as an output measure:

$$WY = \text{number of persons} \times (1 + CPXwt + MOBwt + PACwt + SACwt) \times \text{time}$$

Example: The *W* score for a person with the following description profile may be calculated for one day as:

Level	Definition of HRQOL concept	Preference weight
CPX-11	Cough, wheezing, or shortness of breath, with or without fever, chills, or aching all over	−0.257
MOB-5	No limitations	−0.000
PAC-1	In bed, chair or couch for most or all of the day, health related	−0.077
SAC-2	Performed no major role activity, health related, but did perform self-care	−0.061

$$W = 1 + (-0.257) + (-0.077) + (-0.061) = 0.605$$

Interview Schedule for Quality-of-Well-Being Scale

Contact:

Pennifer Erickson
Clearinghouse on Health Indexes
Centers for Disease Control
Room 1070, National Center for Health Statistics
6525 Belcrest Road
Hyattsville, Maryland 20782
Telephone: (301) 436-7035
FAX: (301) 436-8459

ID Number: _____   Date of Interview: _____

Interviewer Number: _____   Time Began: _____ am pm

                                    Time Ended: _____ am pm

HELLO, I'm _____ , calling for _____ .

We're doing a study of the health-related quality of life of residents.

Your telephone number has been chosen randomly by _____ to be included in the study, and we'd like to ask some questions related to health and disability, which may affect quality of life.

Is this (___) _____? NO: Thank you very much, but I seem to have dialed the wrong number. It's possible that your number may be called at a later time. STOP.

Is this a private residence? NO: Thank you very much, but we are only interviewing private residences. STOP.

Any information which you give us in response to our questions will be kept strictly confidential and will be used only for routine statistical research purposes. [Your participation in this survey is voluntary.]

Call Disposition Codes: Final disposition: _____

01 Completed interview.
02 Refused interview.
03 Nonworking number.
04 No answer (multiple times).
05 Business phone.
06 No eligible respondent at this number.
07 No eligible respondent could be reached during time period.
08 Language barrier prevented completion of interview.
09 Interview terminated within questionnaire.
10 Line busy (multiple tries).
11 Selected respondent unable to respond because of physical or mental impairment.

Part 1

1. Do you now have — [Check "Yes" or "No" as you read each item.]

A.	To wear eyeglasses or contact lenses?	1 [ ] Yes	2 [ ] No
B.	Any trouble seeing with or without glasses or contact lenses? [If No, go to d.]	1 [ ] Yes	2 [ ] No
C.	Blindness in one or both eyes?	1 [ ] Yes	2 [ ] No
D.	Trouble hearing with or without a hearing aid?	1 [ ] Yes	2 [ ] No
E.	Speech problems such as lisping, stuttering, or being unable to speak clearly?	1 [ ] Yes	2 [ ] No
F.	Trouble learning, remembering, or thinking clearly?	1 [ ] Yes	2 [ ] No
G.	General tiredness or weakness?	1 [ ] Yes	2 [ ] No
H.	A problem with losing weight when you don't want to lose weight?	1 [ ] Yes	2 [ ] No
I.	A PROBLEM with being overweight or underweight?	1 [ ] Yes	2 [ ] No
J.	A PROBLEM with missing teeth or very crooked teeth?	1 [ ] Yes	2 [ ] No
K.	A hernia or rupture?	1 [ ] Yes	2 [ ] No
L.	Any very noticeable skin imperfections, such as bad acne, many warts, or large scars?	1 [ ] Yes	2 [ ] No
M.	Any back deformities?	1 [ ] Yes	2 [ ] No
N.	Any missing hands, feet, arms or legs?	1 [ ] Yes	2 [ ] No
O.	Any deformity or paralysis of the fingers, hand or arm, toes, foot, or leg?	1 [ ] Yes	2 [ ] No
P.	Any burns over large areas of the face, body, arms, or legs?	1 [ ] Yes	2 [ ] No

(continued)

393

Now I am going to read a list of symptoms, health complaints, and pains. These questions refer to only the past 4 days, (*day*), (*day*), (*day*), and (*day*).

2a. During the past 4 days, did you have (*item*)? [Check box as you read each item.] [Enter reference days on lines provided.]

2b. Which days? Any other days?
[Circle appropriate day code(s) for items and repeat 3a with the next item.]

	No days	Day 1	Day 2	Day 3	Day 4	All four days
A. Burning, itching, or pain in one or both eyes?	0	1	2	3	4	5
B. A headache?	0	1	2	3	4	5
C. Dizziness or ringing in the ears?	0	1	2	3	4	5
D. An earache?	0	1	2	3	4	5
E. A stuffy or runny nose?	0	1	2	3	4	5
F. A sore throat?	0	1	2	3	4	5
G. Cough or wheezing?	0	1	2	3	4	5
H. Hoarseness?	0	1	2	3	4	5
I. Shortness of breath?	0	1	2	3	4	5
J. A toothache or pain in the jaw?	0	1	2	3	4	5
K. Sore lips, tongue, or gums?	0	1	2	3	4	5
L. An upset stomach, vomiting, or diarrhea?	0	1	2	3	4	5
M. Pain in the stomach?	0	1	2	3	4	5
N. A burning or itching rash on large areas of the face or body?	0	1	2	3	4	5
O. Trouble sleeping?	0	1	2	3	4	5
P. Spells of feeling hot, nervous, or shaky?	0	1	2	3	4	5
Q. Spells of feeling upset, depressed, or crying?	0	1	2	3	4	5
R. Excessive worry or anxiety?	0	1	2	3	4	5
S. A broken hand, arm, foot, or leg?	0	1	2	3	4	5

		0	1	2	3	4	5
T.	Pain or other discomfort in the chest?	0	1	2	3	4	5
U.	Pain, stiffness, weakness, or numbness in the neck or back?	0	1	2	3	4	5
V.	. . . in the hips or side?	0	1	2	3	4	5
W.	. . . in any joints of the hands, feet, arms, or legs?	0	1	2	3	4	5
X.	Difficulty with bowel movements or any pain or discomfort in the rectal area?	0	1	2	3	4	5
Y.	Pain, burning or other difficulty with urination (passing water)?	0	1	2	3	4	5
Z.	Genital pain, itching, burning, or abnormal discharge?	0	1	2	3	4	5
AA.	Loss of consciousness, fainting, or seizures?	0	1	2	3	4	5
BB.	Enough alcohol to drink that you became intoxicated?	0	1	2	3	4	5
CC.	Any problems with sexual interest or performance?	0	1	2	3	4	

In the past 4 days, did you . . .

		0	1	2	3	4	5
DD.	Take prescribed medication?	0	1	2	3	4	5
EE.	Stay on a medically prescribed diet for health reasons?	0	1	2	3	4	5
FF.	Breathe smog or unpleasant air?	0	1	2	3	4	5

3a. During the past 4 days, did you have any symptoms, health complaints, or pains that have not been mentioned?

1 [ ] Yes   2 [ ] No (4)

[Enter reference days on lines provided.]

3b. What were they?

	Day 1	Day 2	Day 3	Day 4	All four days
A: _____	1	2	3	4	5
B: _____	1	2	3	4	5
C: _____	1	2	3	4	5

(continued)

3c. Which days? [Circle appropriate day code(s) in 3b.]

3d. Anything else? [Enter on lines provided in 3b and reask 3c and 3d.]

4. On which of the past 4 days, if any, did you spend any part of a day or night as a bedpatient in a hospital? [Circle appropriate day codes, 0 if none.]

    0   1   2   3   4   5

5. During the past 4 days, because of any impairment or health problem, did you use help from another person with your personal care needs, such as eating, bathing, dressing, or getting around your home?

    1 [ ] Yes   2 [ ] No (6a)

5b. Which day(s): [Circle appropriate day codes.]

6a. During the past 4 days, because of any impairment or health problem, did you use help from another person in handling your routine needs, such as everyday household chores, doing necessary business, shopping, or getting around for other purposes?

    1 [ ] Yes   2 [ ] No (Part II)

6b. Which day(s)? [Circle appropriate day codes.]

    1   2   3   4   5

Part 2. Mobility

1. Do you now have a driver's license?

    1 [ ] Yes (3)
    2 [ ] No

2. Are the reasons that you do not now have a driver's license related in any way to your health?

    1 [ ] Yes, health-related ⎱
    2 [ ] No, not health-related ⎰ (4)

[Enter reference days on lines provided.]

	None	Day 1	Day 2	Day 3	Day 4	All four days
	0	1	2	3	4	5 (4)

3a. On which of the past 4 days, if any, did you drive a car?
[Circle appropriate day codes, 0 if none.]

[Ask for each day NOT circled in 3a.]

3b. On (*day*), was the reason you did not drive related in any way to your health?

	Day 1	Day 2	Day 3	Day 4
	1 [ ] Yes	1 [ ] Yes	1 [ ] Yes	1 [ ] Yes
	2 [ ] No	2 [ ] No	2 [ ] No	2 [ ] No

4. On which of the past 4 days, if any, did you use public transportation such as a bus, subway, taxi, train, or airplane?

None	Day 1	Day 2	Day 3	Day 4	All four days
0 (6)	1	2	3	4	5

[Ask for each day circled in 4.]

5. On (*day*), because of health reasons, did you use help from another person in order to use public transportation?

	Day 1	Day 2	Day 3	Day 4
	1 [ ] Yes	1 [ ] Yes	1 [ ] Yes	1 [ ] Yes
	2 [ ] No	2 [ ] No	2 [ ] No	2 [ ] No

[Ask for each day *not* circled in 4.]

6a. On (*day*), were the reasons you did not use public transportation related in any way to your health?

	None	Day 1	Day 2	Day 3	Day 4
	1 [ ] Yes (nd)	1 [ ] Yes (nd)	1 [ ] Yes (nd)	1 [ ] Yes (nd)	1 [ ] Yes (Part III)
	2 [ ] No	2 [ ] No	2 [ ] No	2 [ ] No	2 [ ] No

6b. If you HAD used public transportation on (*day*), would you have used help from another person because of health reasons?

	None	Day 1	Day 2	Day 3	Day 4
	1 [ ] Yes	1 [ ] Yes	1 [ ] Yes	1 [ ] Yes	1 [ ] Yes

[Repeat 6a and 6b for all days NOT circled in 4.]

(*continued*)

Part 3. Physical Activity

[Enter reference days on lines provided below.]

	None	Day 1	Day 2	Day 3	Day 4	All four days
1a. On which of the past 4 days, if any, did you spend more than half the day in a wheelchair? [Circle appropriate day codes, 0 if none.]	0 (2)	___ 1	___ 2	___ 3	___ 4	5
1b. On (*day*), did you move or control the movement of the wheelchair without help most of the time?	1 [ ] Yes 2 [ ] No	1 [ ] Yes 2 [ ] No	1 [ ] Yes 2 [ ] No	1 [ ] Yes 2 [ ] No		
	[If ALL FOUR DAYS circled in 1a, go to number 9.]					
2. On which of the past 4 days, if any, did you spend more than half the day in bed because of health reasons?	0 (3)	1	2	3	4	5
3. On which of the past 4 days, if any, did you spend more than half the day in a chair or couch because of health reasons?	0 (4)	1	2	3	4	5
4. On which of the past 4 days, if any, did you have trouble lifting, or not try to lift because of health reasons?	0 (5)	1	2	3	4	5
5. On which of the past 4 days, if any, did you have trouble bending over, or not try to bend over because of health reasons?	0 (6)	1	2	3	4	5

6.	On which of the past 4 days, if any, did you have trouble using stairs or inclines because of health reasons?	0 (7)	1	2	3	4	5
7.	On which of the past 4 days, if any, did you limp or use a cane, crutches or walker?	0 (8)	1	2	3	4	5
8.	On which of the past 4 days, if any, did you have trouble walking, or NOT TRY to walk because of health reasons?	0 (9)	1	2	3	4	5
9.	On which of the past 4 days, if any, did you have any (other) physical limitations in movement?	0 (Part IV)	1	2	3	4	5

Part 4. Usual Activity

1. At the present time, are you primarily . . . [Read responses.]

   1 [ ] Working at a job or business, (3)
   2 [ ] Retired, (2)
   3 [ ] Keeping house, (2)
   4 [ ] Going to school, or (2)
   5 [ ] Doing something else? (2)

   [Priority if two or more activities reported: 1—Spent the most time doing; 2—Considers the most important.]

2. At the present time, are you working 20 or more hours a week for pay?

   1 [ ] Yes (3)   2 [ ] No (UA1)

UA1   Usual activity

   1 [ ] Going to school [Go to number 6.]
   2 [ ] Other [Go to number 10.]

(continued)

[Questions 3–5 are asked of employed persons.]

[Enter reference days on lines provided below.]

	None	Day 1	Day 2	Day 3	Day 4	All four days
	0 (5)	1	2	3	4	5

3. On which of the past 4 days, if any, did you work any time at your job or business?
[Circle appropriate day codes, 0 if none.]

[Ask for each day circled in 3.]

4. On (*day*), were you limited in any way in the amount or kind of work done, such as not doing certain tasks, taking special rest periods, or working only part of the day?

	Day 1	Day 2	Day 3	Day 4
	1 [ ] Yes	1 [ ] Yes	1 [ ] Yes	1 [ ] Yes
	2 [ ] No	2 [ ] No	2 [ ] No	2 [ ] No

[If all days checked in 4, go to number 14.]

[Ask for each day NOT circled in 3.]

5a. On (*day*), was the reason you did not work at your job or business related in any way to your health?

	Day 1	Day 2	Day 3	Day 4
	1 [ ] Yes (nd)	1 [ ] Yes (nd)	1 [ ] Yes (nd)	1 [ ] Yes (14)
	2 [ ] No	2 [ ] No	2 [ ] No	2 [ ] No

5b. If you HAD worked at your job on (*day*), would you have been limited in any way in the amount or kind of work done, such as taking special rest periods, working only part of the day, or not doing certain tasks?

	Day 1	Day 2	Day 3	Day 4
	1 [ ] Yes	1 [ ] Yes	1 [ ] Yes	1 [ ] Yes (14)
	2 [ ] No	2 [ ] No	2 [ ] No	2 [ ] No (14)

[Questions 6–9 are asked of students.]

6. Is the reason you are not now working (more hours) for pay related in any way to your health?   1 [ ] Yes   2 [ ] No

[Enter reference days on lines provided below.]

	None	Day 1	Day 2	Day 3	Day 4	All four days
	0 (9)	----- 1	----- 2	----- 3	----- 4	5

7. On which of the past 4 days, if any, did you attend classes or do any school activities at all? [Circle appropriate day codes, 0 if none.]

[Ask for each day circled in 7.]

8. On (*day*), were you limited in any way in the amount or kind of school activities you did because of health reasons? For example, were you excused for certain courses, have special tutoring or courses at home, attend a special school or classes, or not carry a full schedule?

	None	Day 1	Day 2	Day 3	Day 4	All four days
	[Check for each day circled in 7.]					
	1 [ ] Yes	1 [ ] Yes	1 [ ] Yes	1 [ ] Yes	1 [ ] Yes	1 [ ] Yes
	2 [ ] No	2 [ ] No	2 [ ] No	2 [ ] No	2 [ ] No	2 [ ] No

[If all days checked in 8, go to number 14.]

[Ask for each day NOT circled in 7.]

9a. On (*day*), was the reason you did not attend classes or do school activities related in any way to your health?

9b. If you HAD (attended classes/done school activities on (*day*), would you have been limited in any way in the amount or kind of activities done because of health reasons?

	None	Day 1	Day 2	Day 3	Day 4	All four days
	[Check for each day NOT circled in 7.]					
9a.	1 [ ] Yes (nd)	1 [ ] Yes (nd)	1 [ ] Yes (nd)	1 [ ] Yes (nd)	1 [ ] Yes (14)	
	2 [ ] No	2 [ ] No	2 [ ] No	2 [ ] No	2 [ ] No	
9b.	1 [ ] Yes	1 [ ] Yes	1 [ ] Yes	1 [ ] Yes	1 [ ] Yes (14)	
	2 [ ] No	2 [ ] No	2 [ ] No	2 [ ] No	2 [ ] No (14)	

(continued)

401

[Questions 10–13 are asked of homemakers, retired persons, and others.]

10. Is the reason you are not now working (more hours) for pay related in any way to your health?

1 [ ] Yes   2 [ ] No

11. On which of the past 4 days, if any, did you do any household activities such as working in or around the house or yard, caring for children, cooking, or cleaning? [Circle appropriate day codes, 0 if none.]

[Enter reference days on lines provided below.]

None	Day 1	Day 2	Day 3	Day 4	All four days
0 (13)	1	2	3	4	5

[Ask for each day circled in 11.]

12. On (day), were you limited in any way in the amount or kind of household activities you did, such as not doing periods, or working only part of the day?

[Check for each day circled in 11.]

	Day 1	Day 2	Day 3	Day 4	All four days
	1 [ ] Yes	1 [ ] Yes	1 [ ] Yes	1 [ ] Yes	1 [ ] Yes
	2 [ ] No	2 [ ] No	2 [ ] No	2 [ ] No	2 [ ] No

[If all days checked in 12, go to number 14.]

[Ask for each day NOT circled in 11.] [Check for each day NOT circled in 11.]

13a. If you HAD done household activities on (*day*), would you have been limited in any way in the amount or kind of work done, such as not doing certain tasks or strenuous work, or taking special rest periods?	1 [ ] Yes (nd) 2 [ ] No	1 [ ] Yes (nd) 2 [ ] No	1 [ ] Yes (nd) 2 [ ] No	1 [ ] Yes (nd) 2 [ ] No	1 [ ] Yes (14) 2 [ ] No
13b. If you HAD done household activities on (*day*), would you have been limited in any way in the amount or kind of work done, such as not doing certain tasks or strenuous work, or taking special rest periods?	1 [ ] Yes 2 [ ] No	1 [ ] Yes 2 [ ] No	1 [ ] Yes 2 [ ] No	1 [ ] Yes 2 [ ] No	1 [ ] Yes 2 [ ] No
14. On which of the past 4 days, if any, were you limited because of health reasons in any activities OTHER THAN work/school/household activities, such as hobbies, shopping, recreational, social, or religious activities?	0 (15)	1	2	3	4	5
15. On which of the past 4 days, if any, did you have to CHANGE any of your plans or activities because of your health?	0	1	2	3	4	5

403

D. EUROQOL INSTRUMENT

Contacts/Developers

Martin Buxton, Brunel University
Rosalind Rabin, Middlesex Hospital
Paul Kind, Center for Health Economics
University of York
York YO1 5DD
Heslington, England
Telephone: 011-44-904-433653
FAX: 011 44 904 433 644

Markku Pekurinen
National Public Health Institute
Elimaenkatu 25 A
SF-00510 Helsinki
Finland

Stefan Bjork
Swedish Institute for Health Economics
P.O. Box 1207
S-22105 Lund
Sweden

Gouke Bonsel
Institute for Medical Technology Assessment
Department of Public Health and Social Medicine
Erasmus University
Rotterdam
The Netherlands

Erik Nord
National Institute of Public Health
Geitmyrsveien 75
0462 Oslo 4
Norway

Original Classification		Revised Classification	
Level	Definition of HRQOL concept	Level	Definition of HRQOL concept
	Mobility		**Mobility**
1	No problems walking about	1	No problems in walking about
2	Unable to walk about without a stick, crutch, or walking frame	2	Some problems in walking about
3	Confined to bed	3	Confined to bed
	Self-care		**Self-care**
1	No problems with self-care	1	No problems with self-care
2	Unable to dress self	2	Some problems washing or dressing self
3	Unable to feed self	3	Unable to wash or dress self
	Main activity		**Usual activities**
1	Able to perform main activity (e.g., work, study, housework)	1	No problems with performing usual activities (e.g., work, study, housework, family or leisure activities)
2	Unable to perform main activity	2	Some problems with performing usual activities
		3	Unable to perform usual activities
	Pain		**Pain/discomfort**
1	No pain or discomfort	1	No pain or discomfort

(*continued*)

Original Classification		Revised Classification	
Level	Definition of HRQOL concept	Level	Definition of HRQOL concept
2	Moderate pain or discomfort	2	Moderate pain or discomfort
3	Extreme pain or discomfort	3	Extreme pain or discomfort
	Mood		**Anxiety/depression**
1	Not anxious or depressed	1	Not anxious or depressed
2	Anxious or depressed	2	Moderately anxious or depressed
		3	Extremely anxious or depressed
	Social relationships		
1	Able to pursue family and leisure activities		
2	Unable to pursue family and leisure activities		

Source: Adapted from EuroQol Group, 1990.

Questionnaire for EuroQol Instrument Revised Classification

We are trying to find out what people think about health. We are going to describe a few health states that people can be in. We want you to indicate how good or bad each of these states would be for a person like you. There are no right or wrong answers. Here we are interested only in your personal view.

But first of all, we would like you to indicate (on the next page) the state of your own health today.

By placing a tick (thus $\boxed{\checkmark}$) in one box in each group below, please indicate which statements best describe your own health state today.

Mobility

- I have no problems in walking about
- I have some problems in walking about
- I am confined to bed

Self-Care

- I have no problems with self-care
- I have some problems washing or dressing myself
- I am unable to wash or dress myself

Usual Activities

- I have no problems with performing my usual activities (e.g., work, study, housework, family or leisure activities)
- I have some problems with performing my usual activities
- I am unable to perform my usual activities

Pain/Discomfort

- I have no pain or discomfort
- I have moderate pain or discomfort
- I have extreme pain or discomfort

Anxiety/Depression

- I am not anxious or depressed
- I am moderately anxious or depressed
- I am extremely anxious or depressed

Compared with my general level of health over the past 12 months, my health state today is: (Please tick one box)

- Better
- Much the same
- Worse

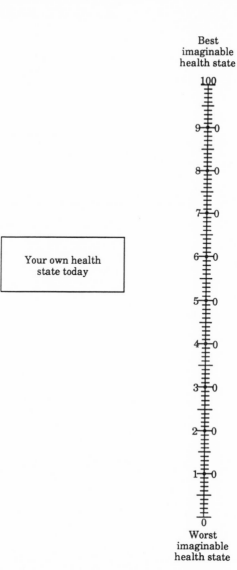

Best
imaginable
health state

Your own health
state today

Worst
imaginable
health state

To help people say how good or bad a health state is, we have drawn a scale (rather like a thermometer) on which the best state you can imagine is marked by 100 and the worst state you can imagine is marked by 0. We would like you to indicate on this scale how good or bad is your own health today, in your opinion. Please do this by drawing a line from the box above to whichever point on the scale indicates how good or bad your current health state is.

Health state valuations on original classifications

| Health state | | | | | | Median valuations | | | Medial valuations (standard deviations) | | |
Mobility	Self-care	Main activity	Social relationships	Pain	Mood	Sweden	United Kingdom	Netherlands	Sweden	United Kingdom	Netherlands
1	1	1	1	1	1	100	99	95	93 (13)	95 (10)	93 (13)
1	1	1	1	2	1	86	84	86	83 (16)	81 (14)	81 (19)
1	1	1	1	1	2	75	70	75	69 (21)	67 (18)	71 (22)
1	1	1	1	2	2	70	68	70	64 (20)	65 (17)	69 (21)
1	1	2	1	2	1	65	70	65	61 (22)	67 (18)	63 (23)
1	1	2	1	3	1	50	59	60	51 (21)	56 (19)	56 (22)
1	1	2	2	2	2 (a)	35	40	43	36 (20)	41 (17)	43 (21)
1	1	2	2	2	2 (b)	39	40	40	38 (19)	40 (16)	41 (21)
1	1	2	2	3	2	35	35	33	36 (20)	36 (17)	37 (23)
2	1	2	2	3	2	22	25	20	26 (20)	26 (16)	26 (20)
2	2	2	2	3	2	10	10	7	14 (19)	12 (12)	12 (15)
2	3	2	2	3	2	7	5	6	12 (19)	8 (9)	10 (16)
3	2	2	2	3	2	4	2	5	9 (18)	5 (7)	10 (18)
3	3	2	2	3	2	1	1	4	8 (19)	4 (6)	7 (12)
being dead (a)						0	0	3	10 (24)	10 (20)	19 (25)
being dead (b)						0	1	2	10 (23)	10 (21)	18 (25)

Source: Adapted from EuroQol Group, 1990.

408

APPENDIX II

Sources of Information About Measures of Health-Related Quality of Life

A. BOOKS

Baldwin S, Godfrey C, Propper C, eds. *Quality of Life: Perspectives and Policies*. London: Routledge, 1990.

> Discusses a number of different issues ranging from the philosophical question concerning the definition of the good life, to studies of quality of life in specific patient groups, to implications of using quality of life assessments to determine resource allocation

Drummond MF, Stoddard GL, Torrance GW. *Methods for the Economic Evaluation of Health Care Programmes*. Oxford, England: Oxford University Press, 1987.

> Considers quality of life assessment in the economic context of resource allocation, including chapters on cost–effectiveness, cost–utility, and cost–benefit analyses. The text focuses on methodological issues that policymakers need to consider in conducting an economic evaluation.

Fallowfield L. *The Quality of Life: The Missing Measurement in Health Care*. London: Souvenir Press, 1990.

> Contains discussions of philosophical and methodological issues in assessing quality of life, including brief reviews of several generic and disease-specific assessments. Individual chapters are devoted to cancer, AIDS, cardiovascular disease, arthritis, the elderly, and the terminally ill.

Frank-Stromborg MF. *Instruments for Clinical Nursing Research*. Norwalk, Conn.: Appleton & Lange, 1988.

> Contains descriptions of selected questionnaires for assessing health and function and clinical problems, including concepts such as spirituality, body image, bowel function, skin integrity, and vaginitis.

Kane RA, Kane RL. *Assessing the Elderly: A Practical Guide to Measurement*. Lexington, Mass.: Lexington Books, 1981.

> Contains descriptions and analytic reviews of a large number of questionnaires and rating scales for use in long-term care settings organized under the following headings: Measures of Physical Functioning; Measures of Mental Functioning; Measures of Social Functioning; and Multidimensional Measures.

McDowell I, Newell C. *Measuring Health: A Guide to Rating Scales and Questionnaires*. New York: Oxford University Press, 1987.

> Contains descriptions and actual questionnaires for measures organized into the following headings: Functional Disability and Handicaps; Psychological Well-Being; Social Health; Quality of Life and Life Satisfaction; Pain; and General Health.

Smith GT, ed. *Measuring Health: A Practical Approach*. New York: John Wiley & Sons, 1988.

> Contains chapters on various approaches to measuring health-related quality of life and chapters on specific diseases and health problems such as rheumatoid arthritis, cancer, Parkinson's disease, and irritable bowel syndrome.

Spilker B, ed. *Quality of Life Assessments in Clinical Trials*. New York: Raven Press, 1990.

> Contains chapters on various approaches to quality of life measurement, information on psychosocial, economic, and other measures, applications to special populations such as pediatric, geriatric, and surgery, and applications to specific problems or diseases such as diabetes, cancer, and lung disease.

Stewart AL, Ware JE. *Measuring Functioning and Well-Being: The Medical Outcomes Study Approach*. North Carolina: Duke University Press, 1992.

> This edited volume contains chapters on various steps in the development and application of measures of health-related quality of life used in the Medical Outcomes Study. Particular attention is paid to the use of the 20-item Short Form health assessment.

Walker SR, Rosser RN, eds. *Quality of Life Assessment: Key Issues in the 1990s*. London: Kluwer Academic Publishing, 1992.

> Contains discussion of principles underlying assessment of quality of life and application of such assessments to specific clinical conditions.

Wenger NK, Mattson ME, Furberg CD, Elinson J, eds. *Assessment of Quality of Life in Clinical Trials of Cardiovascular Therapies*. New York: LeJacq, 1984.

> Contains descriptions and selected questionnaires for the following composite measures: Sickness Impact Profile; Quality of Well-Being Scale; McMaster Index Questionnaire; Nottingham Health Profile; Psychological General Well-Being Schedule; and General Health Rating Index. Applications to cardiovascular disease are described.

B. RECENT JOURNAL ISSUES

Feeny D, Guyatt G, Patrick D, eds. "Proceedings of the International Conference on the Measurement of Quality of Life as an Outcome in Clinical Trials." *Controlled Clin Trials* 12(4), 79S–280S, 1991.

Katz S, guest editor. The Portugal Conference: Measuring Quality of Life and Functional Status in Clinical and Epidemiological Research. *J Chronic Dis* 40(6):459–650, 1987.

Lohr KN, guest editor. Advances in Health Status Assessment: Conference Proceedings. *Med Care* 27(3 suppl), March 1989.

Lohr KN, guest editor. Advances in Health Status Assessment: Conference Proceedings. *Med Care* 30(5 suppl), 1–293,1992.

Lohr KN, Ware JE, guest editors. Proceedings of the Advances in Health Assessment Conference, Palm Springs, California, 19–21 February 1986. *J Chronic Dis* 40(suppl 1), 1987.

Spilker B, Tilson H, guest editors. *Med Care* 28(12 suppl), December 1990.

C. SELECTED JOURNALS PUBLISHING HEALTH-RELATED QUALITY OF LIFE ARTICLES

American Journal of Public Health
Gerontologist
Health Policy

Health Psychology
Health Services Research
International Journal of Epidemiology
International Journal of Technology Assessment in Health Care
Journal of the American Geriatrics Society
Journal of Clinical Epidemiology (formerly *Journal of Chronic Diseases*)
Journal of Epidemiology and Community Health
Journal of General Internal Medicine
Medical Care
Medical Decision Making
Milbank Quarterly
Social Science and Medicine

D. REFERENCE SERVICES

Clearinghouse on Health Indexes

Searching: No computer data base currently available

Content: Health and medical care research on the development and application of measures of health-related quality of life (mostly English-language material from 1950s forward)

Output: Annotated bibliography, *Bibliography on Health Indexes*, published quarterly.

Address: Clearing House on Health Indexes
              National Center for Health Statistics
              Room 1070, 6525 Belcrest Road
              Hyattsville, MD 20782
              Telephone: (301) 436-7035

Health and Psychosocial Instruments (HAPI)

Searching: Text and key work searching to identify assessments

Content: Health and psychosocial assessments (assessments published in the English language since 1985, many older measures are also included)

Output: Brief abstract of each assessment, followed by several articles describing the development or use of the assessment

Address: BRS Information Technologies
              8000 Westpark Drive
              McLean, VA 22102
              Telephone: (703) 442-0900
                           1 (800) 289-4277
              FAX: (703) 893-4632

National Library of Medicine (NLM)

Searching: Text and key word searching to identify articles that discuss quality of life assessment

Content: Health and medical care research, ethical concerns and medical history (6.5 million articles from 3,600 journals published around the world)

Output: Citations, including author, title and source, key words, and, for most English-language articles, author-supplied abstracts

Address: National Library of Medicine
            8600 Rockville Pike
            Bethesda, MD 20894
            Telephone: 1-800-272-4787

The On-Line Guide to Quality-of-Life Assessment (OLGA)

Searching: Decision-theoretic programs to aid in the selection of quality of life
    assessments and their applications, as well as key work searching to identify
    assessments and their applications
Content: Quality of life assessments and empirical literature describing their applications
    (over 150 quality of life assessments and over 1,000 references to their development
    and application)
Output: Summaries of assessments in standardized format, plus a bibliography
    documenting the development of each assessment and citations, quality of life
    measures, and, in selected cases, quality of life–specific abstracts of references to
    applications
Address: On-Line Guide to Quality of Life Assessment
            11404 Lund Place
            Kensington, MD 20895
            Telephone: (301) 933-2312

E. MEDLINE KEYWORDS FOR LITERATURE SEARCHES

Cost–benefit analysis
Disability evaluation
Health status indicators
Quality of life

F. A FRAMEWORK FOR LITERATURE REVIEW[1]

The framework serves as a guideline for searching for information about instruments for
assessing health-related quality of life that may be available in the professional literature. The
categories identify the most important conceptual, measurement, and practical considerations
that are to be considered in selecting or developing a strategy for assessing health-realted quality
of life. The Sickness Impact Profile (SIP) is used to illustrate the type of information that might
be identified in each of the categories.

Purpose: Health outcome, or diagnosing or screening for a particular disease or condition
    SIP: Assesses health outcome from a wide range of interventions on a common scale
Age Range: Concepts of health-related quality of life are measured differently, depending
    on age of the target population
    SIP: 20–99 years
Concepts: Major concepts included in health-related quality of life assessments are death;
    impairments; mental, physical, and social function; perceptions; and potential
    SIP: Alertness behavior, ambulation, body care and movement, communication,
    eating, emotional behavior, home management, mobility, recreation and pastimes,
    sleep and rest, social interaction, and work

[1] Source: The On-Line Guide to Quality-of-Life Assessment (OLGA). (C) Copyright 1991 Jeffrey Scott

Weighting: Investigator-assigned weighting, frequency weighting (e.g., Likert, Visual Analog), and preference weighting (e.g., category rating, magnitude estimation, time tradeoff, standard gamble)

SIP: Preference weighting based on magnitude estimation

Scoring: Method of scoring, availability of overall score, range of scores, typical values, direction

SIP: Overall scores range from 0 to 100, with lower scores indicating less dysfunction

Reliability/validity: Types of reliability and validity used and which populations

SIP: Test–retest reliability for the interviewer-administered format is 0.97. Construct validity using self-assessed dysfunction is 0.69.

Administration: Self administered or assisted self-administered questionnaires, face-to-face interview, telephone interview, observation/rating by health professional

SIP: Can be administered in face-to-face interview or assisted-self-administered format

Time to administer: Average length time the typical respondent needs to complete the assessment

SIP: 20–30 minutes for face-to-face interviewer-administered version

Languages: Language in which developed and those into which translations have been made

SIP: Developed in English, also available in Danish, Dutch, Chicano, and Swedish

Copyright: Assessments may be copyrighted by the developer, the journal that publishes them, or in the public domain, if developed with government funds

SIP: Marilyn Bergner, Ph.D., Johns Hopkins University

Glossary

Access to Health Care.   Implies at least four levels of health care coverage: availability of personnel and services; ability to use services through insurance or entitlement; affordability, or ability to purchase insurance or services; and acceptability, or the perceived value of and barriers to care.

Active Life Expectancy.   A term that refers to the adjustment of life expectancy according to the presence of dependent functioning on one or more activities of daily living. Different types of dependencies, such as unable to get to the toilet, eat, or dress, are given equal weight in making the adjustment to life expectancy. The term *disability-free life expectancy* is sometimes used when morbidity is more broadly defined to include activity limitations and disability days as adjustments to life expectancy.

Activities of Daily Living.   Measures of independence in the performance of five personal care activities: bathing, dressing, using the toilet, getting in or out of bed or chair, and eating.

Activity Limitations.   Any long-term reduction in a person's capacity to perform the average activities associated with his or her age group.

Activity Restrictions.   Behavior usually associated with a reduction in activity because of chronic or acute conditions. These are reductions in a person's activities below his or her usual capacity and/or performance, e.g., mobility, self-care, sleep, rest, and communication.

Attribute, Health.   Term used to describe the states, behaviors, or perceptions included in an operational definition of health-related quality of life. All domains may be considered as possible attributes for the purposes of developing and weighing health states to create the measure.

Bed Days.   A day during which a person stayed in bed more than half a day because of illness or injury. All hospital days for inpatients are considered bed days even if the patient was not in bed more than half a day.

Budget Constraint.   The level of funding available to the health care sector of an economy that is defined by geographical or political boundaries.

Selected terms are adapted from Guyatt G, Patrick D, and Feeny D (1991). Glossary. Pp. 274S–280S in: Feeny D, Guyatt G, Patrick D, eds., Proceedings of the International Conference on the Measurement of Quality of Life as an Outcome in Clinical Trials, *Controlled Clinical Trials,* Volume 12 (4 Supplement).

Cohort Method. With this approach to calculating years of healthy life, the number of years survived by each member of the target population is adjusted by each individual's health-related quality of life. The adjusted life years are summed to give an estimate of the years of healthy life for this population.

Construct. An idea developed or constructed through informed scientific theory. Health status and quality of life are terms understood or inferred from a network of interrelationships such as the correlation between a measure of physical functioning and increasing age, number of chronic conditions, or a physiological measure.

Construct Validation. Involves specifying the factors or constructs that account for variance in a proposed measure as well as the hypothesized relations among constructs. Empirical evidence is sought according to the logic of scientific inquiry to give meaning to the measure. If different measures of the same construct of health-related quality of life are logically related and highly correlated, then convergent validity has been achieved (e.g., depression and anxiety for psychological distress); if a logically different measure is not as highly correlated as a more logically related measure, then discriminant validity is evident (depression versus happiness as compared to anxiety).

Cost Per Year of Healthy Life Gained Ratio. A number that expresses the relationship between the additional costs attributed to an intervention, that is, the net costs, and the net health effect gained from the same intervention. Lower cost per year of healthy life ratios indicate more cost-effective interventions.

Costs and Outcomes Table. A table that shows an array of different health interventions according to their cost per unit of outcome gained and usually expressed as a ratio. When costs and outcomes associated with different interventions are quantified using the same metrics, then different interventions can be compared to assess their relative effectiveness. See also cost per year of healthy life gained.

Cronbach's Alpha. A statistic to quantify internal consistency. Cronbach's alpha ranges from -1 to +1; when internal consistency is an important instrument property, as in discriminating between different groups, high values are better. Cronbach's alpha varies directly with the mean interitem correlation and the number of items. Thus, one can increase alpha by deleting items that do not correlate highly with other items in a questionnaire, or by adding more items that correlate as well with existing items as those items correlate with one another.

Cumulative Scaling. A means of determining if the interrelationships among three or more items in a health status measure constitute a unidimensional scale (component items move toward or away from a single underlying attribute) and are cumulative (component items can be ordered by degree of difficulty). Also referred to as *Guttman scaling*.

Cut-Down Days. A day on which a person cuts down for more than half a day on the things he or she usually does.

Determinants of Health-Related Quality of Life. Includes all the factors and processes that influence health and quality of life outcomes of an individual or community. Outside the health system, these determinants include the environment (social, personal, and physical), as well as the culture, economy, and politics of the community. Determinants within the health care system include the resources, structure, services, quality of care, efficacy, effectiveness, and ethics of health care delivery as well as population characteristics, access to services, and health, illness, and sick role behavior.

Direct Costs.   Organizing and operating costs that are associated with developing and operating a health care program. Direct health care costs include the costs of health care providers' (e.g., physicians, nurses, and pharmacists) services and the costs of supplies and equipment used in providing services. Direct costs plus indirect costs are used to determine the cost estimates used in the costs and outcomes table. *See also* Health care costs.

Disability-Free Life Expectancy.   A term that refers to the adjustment of life expectancy according to limitations in activity. Different types of activity limitations, such as unable to work, problems moving about the community, and hospitalizations, are given equal weight in making the adjustment to life expectancy. The term *active life expectancy* is sometimes used when limitations are measured as activities of daily living.

Discounting.   A process used to convert future dollars to their present value. For policymaking, future dollars are discounted to present terms for two reasons: (1) money available today has a higher value than the same amount of money that is available in the future; and (2) individuals have a positive time preference, that is, they would rather consume today than delay consumption until some time in the future. Although developed to account for intertemporal decision making regarding money, the method of discounting is also applied to health to express future outcomes in terms of their present value.

Disease-Specific Measure.   Designed to assess patient populations or specific diagnostic groups, most often with the goal of detecting minimally important differences or changes in health-related quality of life. These are changes that clinicians, patients, or significant others think are discernible and important, have been detected with an intervention of known efficacy, or are related to well-established physiological measures (e.g., grip strength for arthritis patients or spirometry for those with chronic obstructive lung disease).

Domain.   A state, attitude, perception, behavior, or other sphere of action or thought related to health or quality of life. All the entities in a single domain have some property in common. Domain theory is one of the major ways of viewing reliability and test construction in social and behavioral science. Domains can be viewed as infinitely large, so when one measures the domain, one draws only a sample. Health-related quality of life is therefore composed of an infinitely large domain from which one can draw different samples of behaviors and traits for measurement.

Dysfunction.   See functional status.

Economic Efficiency.   According to economic theory an allocation of resources is considered efficient when no one can be made better off without making someone worse off. This situation is also referred to as *Pareto optimality* or a *Pareto efficient allocation*. An efficient allocation is not necessarily an equitable one.

Effect Size.   Effect size is an estimate of change in health-related quality of life. Effect sizes are used to translate the before-and-after changes into a standard unit of measurement to provide a clearer understanding of results. Standardized effect sizes are defined as the mean change found in a variable divided by the standard deviation of that variable at baseline. Effect sizes must be interpreted, and this can be accomplished using global ratings of change or importance of improvement, relating effects to treatments of known effectiveness, relating changes to clinical measures or large changes in clinical condition, or interpreting observed changes in terms of elements of those measures more meaningful to stakeholders. Effect sizes for generic measures are usually established over a long period of using the measure resulting in a consensus on what constitutes a significant change score or effect size.

Equality of Opportunity.   The ultimate goal of the health care system. This goal includes both equity in access to health care for all members of the community and equity in health-related quality of life. Equal access does not guarantee equal health outcomes, because many determinants of health-related quality of life fall outside the health care system. Nevertheless, opportunity for health care and health are the most important outputs of the health care system.

Expected Utility Theory.   An approach used by economists to model choice when made under conditions of uncertainty, that is, when the outcome of a choice cannot be known in advance. Von Neumann and Morgenstern generalized the axioms of individual choice under conditions of certainty to conditions of uncertainty.

Functionalism.   Involves the analysis of social and cultural phenomena in terms of the functions they perform in a sociocultural system. Functionalism is the theoretical foundation for most definitions of health based on the performance of major social roles and valued activities and tasks.

Functional Status.   An individual's effective performance of or ability to perform those roles, tasks, or activities that are valued, e.g., going to work, playing sports, maintaining the house. Most often functional status is divided into physical, emotional, mental, and social domains, although much finer distinctions are possible. Deviations from usual performance or ability indicate dysfunction.

Game Theory.   A theory proposed by von Neumann and Morgenstern that centers on the assumption that the utility of two objects or outcomes is reflected by the relative expectations for the occurrence or acquisition of the two outcomes. Thus, the issue of assigning utilities to outcomes expands to the problem of assigning values to gambles, i.e., choices about outcomes that are not a sure thing.

Generic Measure.   Measures of health-related quality of life designed to be broadly applicable across types and severities of disease, across different medical treatments or health interventions, and across demographic and cultural subgroups. These measures summarize a spectrum of the concepts and domains of health-related quality of life that apply to many different impairments, illnesses, patients, and populations.

Global Ratings of Change.   Respondents' evaluation of changes in one or more domains of health-related quality of life indicating whether they are better, about the same, or worse. This three-point rating is sometimes expanded to a five- or seven-point scale. Global ratings are useful in defining the minimally important differences in the score obtained from a health-related quality of life questionnaire. Global ratings are used to present mean differences in health-related quality of life scores corresponding to small, moderate, or large degrees of change. *See also* Effect size.

Health Care.   A special collection of personnel, facilities, services, and goods devoted to the prevention and curing of disease as well as the care of illness.

Health Care Costs.   In the Health Resource Allocation Strategy, costs are defined in the economic sense, namely, as the value of a resource in its alternative use, i.e., opportunity cost. *See also* Direct costs; Indirect costs.

Health Decision.   Consists of all the alternative courses of action to improve the health-related quality of life of an individual or population. To specify health decisions, one should list alternatives, identify possible outcome of alternatives and their determinants, stakeholders in the decision, and the values and preferences of these stakeholders. If socioeconomic evaluation is involved, then the logic and assumptions of this evaluation should be specified, including the budgetary constraint.

Health Disparities.   Inequality, inequities, or differences in the health-related quality of life of different population groups, including age groups (children or older adults), members of certain racial and ethnic groups (African Americans, Hispanics, Asians, and Pacific Islanders), people with low income (below the poverty level), and people with disabilities (developmental disabilities, injuries, and chronic conditions). A major goal of the health care system is to reduce health disparities by promoting equal opportunity for health.

Health Policy.   The way nations, states, cities, and communities distribute resources to competing interventions and competing populations based primarily on anticipated benefits. Health policy reflects the values of the society or community in terms of how and to whom health resources are distributed.

Health Profile.   A health status measure that produces multiple scores using the same metric or scoring system. Health profiles generally consist of scores for different health domains such as physical well-being, role functioning, and mental health. Some profiles also yield an overall or index score (*see* Health status index). Well-known examples include the Sickness Impact Profile, Nottingham Health Profile, and Medical Outcomes Study Short-Form Health Survey.

Health-Related Quality of Life.   The value assigned to duration of life as modified by the impairments, functional states, perceptions, and social opportunities that are influenced by disease, injury, treatment, or policy.

Health Resource Allocation.   A process by which decision makers determine the assignment of available resources to a diverse set of competing programs to maximize health-related quality of life of a target population. Two strategies for allocating health resources are medical effectiveness evaluations and rationing. *See also* Economic efficiency.

Health Resource Allocation Strategy.   A conceptual and sociopolitical process for comparing health outcomes with health care costs across all programs in the health sector of an economy. In eight steps, the strategy aids policymakers in making health decisions based on the sociopolitical analysis of cost per year of healthy life gained ratios for different health interventions. This analysis, informed by community goals and values, yields a ranking of health interventions to be included in a funding package according to the budgetary constraint.

Health Services Priority or Ranking. A listing of health services or interventions in order of their priority for funding according to the budgetary constraint. Initially this ranking is based solely on the cost per year of healthy life gained ratios in the costs and outcomes table. It is revised according to the decision makers' interpretation of community objectives and values for health services. The final priority list should also indicate the line at which services are considered to have lowest priority and thus may fall outside the budget constraint.

Health State. The combination of one or more concepts, domains, or indicators that describes the health-related quality of life of an individual. Every individual can be classified at any point in time on each attribute into one and only one level of health-related quality of life. Health states can be holistic/multiattribute (combinations of different domains) or decomposed/single attribute (contain a single domain or construct). They can be written in narrative form (as a descriptive paragraph with sentences) or taxonomic form (as short descriptive phrases).

Health State Classification System. A mutually exclusive and exhaustive set of health states used to describe and measure health-related quality of life. The classification system consists of one or more concepts, domains, or indicators and is used to generate health states. Health states are used for assigned preference weights that reflect the relative desirability of that state to the person(s) providing the weights.

Health Status. Most often defined by the World Health Organization's definition: "A state of complete physical, mental, and social well-being, and not merely the absence of disease or infirmity" (1948). Not included in this definition are physiological phenomena, the probability of health in the future, or the means for determining which states of well-being are more healthy or desirable than others. Nonetheless, WHO's popular definition encompasses most of the usual meanings given to health status, including functional status, morbidity, and well-being. A complete representation of health includes a definition of health states, weights for these states, and prognosis, or the probability of movement to future states based on all the evidence.

Health Status Batteries. Collections of different health status and quality of life measures that are scored independently and reported as individual scores.

Health Status Index. An aggregation of two or more domains of health-related quality of life into a single number that purports to represent the health of either an individual or group of individuals. The concept for developing a health status index stems from the desire to have an overall measure of health much as the gross national product gives a summary of the economic status of a nation.

Health Status Instrument. The constellation of questionnaires, interview schedules, administration procedures, and scoring instructions for a measure of health-related quality of life.

Healthy-Year Equivalents. A measure of health-related quality of life that incorporates two sets of preferences. One set reflects individuals' preferences for life years, or duration of life. The other set reflects individuals' preferences for states of health.

Human Capital. The knowledge and health status that an individual has to invest in producing goods and services. Human capital is generally valued by using employment earnings. *See also* Willingness to pay.

Impairment. Includes the classic category of morbidity indicative of disease as defects in the structure or biological functioning of the body. Measures of impairment include symptoms, signs, tissue alterations, reports of disease, and diagnoses.

Indicator, Health Status. A measure indicating the presence, absence, or degree of health-related quality of life. Indicators are sometimes single concepts or domains, such as all-cause mortality. In other instances, health status indicators may be composed of indexes, profiles, or batteries.

Indirect Costs. The value of resources lost. Indirect costs of morbidity include reduced levels of work output, time spent to obtain health care, loss of productivity occurring due to employment change caused by illness, and lost leisure time. Indirect costs plus direct costs are used to determine the cost estimates used in the costs and outcomes table. *See also* Health care costs.

Instrumental Activities of Daily Living. Generally consists of an evaluation of independence in performing six home management activities: preparing meals, shopping for personal items, managing money, using the telephone, doing light housework, and doing heavy housework.

Internal Consistency. A measurement property of an instrument assessing the extent to which each item, or each section of a questionnaire, is measuring the same thing. The intercorrelation among a number of different questions or items that are supposed to reflect the same concept is used to assess internal consistency (sometimes referred to as *reliability*). *See also* Cronbach's alpha.

Interobserver or interrater reliability. Refers to the correlation between responses to the same items obtained by different observers, raters, or interviewers.

Intervention. A health care program or treatment that is applied to either an individual or group of individuals for the purpose of improving health-related quality of life.

Intraclass Correlation Coefficient. An intraclass correlation coefficient is a ratio of variances. The most commonly used intraclass correlation coefficient is the reliability coefficient, which is the ratio of the variance between subjects to the total variance. The reliability coefficient is used so often that it is sometimes referred to as "the" intraclass correlation coefficient. When a single instrument is administered repeatedly, the reliability coefficient not only will decrease with random variation between replicate measures (as will the product–moment correlation coefficient) but also will decrease as a result of systematic differences between the first and second administration.

Life Expectancy. The number of years remaining for persons who have attained a given age. This is the most frequently used life table statistic.

Life Table. A statistical method for summarizing the mortality experience of a population to obtain measures of comparative longevity. The current life table considers a hypothetical cohort that is subject to the age-specific death rates that have been observed for an actual population for a given time period. Complete life tables provide information for single years of age; abridged life tables provide information by five-year age groups.

Life Years.   The number of years lived. The number can be either real, as in observed; or expected or hypothetical, as when derived from life table analysis.

Major Activity.   Refers to a person's participation in daily activities in the workplace, in the household, in the community, or at school. Classified according to age groups that correspond to the national status transitions from infancy to old age. In the National Health Interview Survey, major activities by age groups are (1) ordinary play for children under 5 years of age, (2) attending school for those 5–17 years of age, (3) working or keeping house for persons 18–69 years of age, and (4) capacity for independent living (e.g., the ability to bathe, shop, dress, eat, etc., without needing the help of another person) for those 70 years of age and over. For some retired persons, volunteer or community service might also be considered their major activity. Each person is classified into one of four categories: unable to perform the major activity; able to perform the major activity but limited in the kind or amount of this activity; not limited in the major activity but limited in the kind or amount of other activities; and not limited in any way.

Measurement.   The assignment of numbers to aspects of objects or events according to a rule of some kind. The rules scientists commonly employ for assigning numbers are defined by types of scales: nominal (nonoverlapping classification), ordinal (numbers assigned corresponding to order of magnitude), interval or cardinal (operationally defined distance between ranks), and ratio (absolute zero as well as equal intervals in quantity being measured). Health-related quality of life can be measured at any of these levels. For the Health Resource Allocation Strategy, health-related quality of life must be an interval or ratio measure.

Measurement Objectives.   In the context of health-related quality of life measures, four objectives can be identified: description (to describe the behaviors, opinions, attitudes, perceptions defining health status and quality of life of a person or group); discrimination (to distinguish between persons or populations with or without the trait, behavior, or disease); prediction (as a screening test to predict a more costly or intrusive outcome or "gold standard"); and evaluation (to measure change over time). These objectives determine the desired measurement properties of health-related quality of life assessments, e.g., responsiveness is important for evaluation but not for other objectives and internal consistency is not relevant to the assessment of change.

Medical Effectiveness Evaluations.   The evaluation of one or more health programs, clinical interventions, or regulatory practices to establish the magnitude of benefits, disseminate the results, and eliminate ineffective interventions.

Meta-Analysis.   A formal set of statistical techniques for combining results of previous research to test for treatment effects. This form of analysis has been proposed as a systematic and rigorous method of reviewing and summarizing the results of a body of scientific literature. Although techniques for pooling data from multiple studies have been around from the early part of this century, they have been used primarily in studies of agricultural and physical data since these sciences tend to use the same units of measurement between studies.

Minimally Important Difference.   That difference in score on a health-related quality of life instrument which corresponds to the smallest change in status that stakeholders (persons, patients, significant others, or clinicians) consider important. The minimally important difference is the smallest difference that would lead to the initiation or change in a course of action, such as prescription of medication, change in behavioral regimen, or modification of reimbursement formula. The assessments of minimally important difference need not, and do not always, agree among different stakeholders in the health decision.

Multiattribute Utility Theory (MAUT). In measuring preferences or utilities for health states, multiple attributes are often involved: mobility, ambulation, emotional dysfunction, physical activity, etc. In MAUT the evaluation task is broken down into attributes, and single attributes are evaluated using different numerical estimation methods such as category scaling, standard gamble, or time tradeoff. Then tradeoffs among attributes are quantified as importance weights or other scaling factors. Finally, formal models are applied to reaggregate the single-attribute evaluations. *See* Utility measurement.

National Health Level. The stock of health-related quality of life within a given country. Years of healthy life measures the level of health in a single number, trading off mortality and morbidity experienced by the population.

Net Health Effect. The difference between benefits attributed to the alternative interventions being compared. In clinical studies, this difference may result from a comparison of outcomes obtained among persons receiving placebo compared to those receiving an experimental treatment. Or the net effect may result from a comparison of persons receiving two different treatments. This difference is referred to as the *net benefit* or *net effect.* Years of healthy life gained is a net health effect.

Opportunity. The chance or potential for optimal performance of the valued roles and tasks of living influenced by disease, injuries, treatment, or policy. Often assessed as the disadvantage associated with ill health, such as inability to obtain an education or employment. Alternatively assessed as capacity or potential for health. *See* Positive health.

Outcomes. A term used synonymously with health-related quality of life. *See also* Costs and outcomes table.

Out-of-Pocket Expenditures. Health care costs that are paid for by consumers directly, as opposed to being covered by health insurance. Most out-of-pocket expenditures are for drugs and other medical nondurables and physician services. Out-of-pocket spending does not include health insurance premiums.

Perceptions, Health. Psychological conceptions of health and well-being, including past, present, and future health, worries and concerns about health, satisfaction with health, or some other quality of life associated with health.

Pilot Study. Large pretests usually involving 75 or more respondents and making a complete study including data collection, scoring, and analysis; these are often small investigations in their own right and are published separately.

Positive Health. The upper end of the health–illness continuum that might be considered desirable deviations from expected or usual functions, activities, or perceptions, such as physiologic reserve, feelings of well-being, or ability to withstand stress, and resilience. Positive health may be viewed as optimum capacity for health or wellness.

Preferences.   Judgments of the desirability of a particular set of outcomes or situations that describe what is labeled "good" or "bad." Connotes the exact meaning of value, desirability, or utility of health states. *See also* Utility; Utility measurement.

Pretest.   Generally small investigations involving 5–75 administrations of a measure or battery of measures. This helps investigators estimate the length of time the assessment takes to complete, respondent reactions to different measures, completeness of instructions and other instrumentation, format and flow of the questionnaire, and other considerations in health survey research.

Prognosis.   In measuring health-related quality of life, prognosis is the foretelling of the course of health status after an original health state has been determined. *See also* Transition probability.

Proxy Respondent.   Person who responds to a health survey by providing information about another person who is in the survey sample and who cannot respond for himself or herself. Sometimes called a surrogate respondent.

Psychophysical Methods.   Methods of quantifying judgments derived from the field of psychophysics. These methods include newer ones such as discriminating and matching judgments (to an existing standard) and interval or partition judgments (equal subjective spacing by bisection or equisection) and older methods such as category rating (using numbered categories) and numerical magnitude estimation (unlimited range of numerical judgments). Category scaling and magnitude estimation are the most commonly applied psychophysical methods to the measurement of health state preferences.

Psychophysics.   The study of the relationship between physical stimuli and psychological sensation or perception. Psychophysics is most commonly concerned with the correlation between psychological scales and the physical measurements of stimuli. With nonphysical stimuli such as health states, psychophysics is concerned with the most reproducible and valid representation of psychological perceptions of different dimensions or attributes of stimuli.

Quality of Life.   Encompasses the entire range of human experience, states, perceptions, and spheres of thought concerning the life of an individual or a community. Both objective and subjective, quality of life can include cultural, physical, psychological, interpersonal, spiritual, financial, political, temporal, and philosophical dimensions. Quality of life implies a judgment of value placed on the experience of communities, groups such as families, or individuals.

Rationing.   The distribution of health care resources to services or individuals according to rules based on one or more of the following: personal characteristics, disease status, cost of intervention, and outcomes.

Ratio of Cost Per Year of Healthy Life Gained.   A single number obtained by dividing the net costs by the net health effect expressed in years of healthy life gained.

Reliability.   A generic way to refer to the extent to which, when one repeatedly administers a health-related quality of life measure or test to persons who are stable, one gets the same results (referred to as test-retest reliability in the psychometric literature). Reliability is also used in a much more specific fashion to refer to the extent to which a single observation can consistently distinguish between members of a population. This latter property can be quantified as the ratio of the variance attributable to between-person differences to the total variance. This ratio, an intraclass correlation coefficient, is often referred to as the *reliability coefficient*. The word "reliability" is used to refer to internal consistency. *See also* Cronbach's alpha; Internal consistency; Reproducibility.

Reproducibility or Test–Retest Reliability.   Refers to the correlation between responses to the same items administered to the same respondents at different times. A health-related quality of life measure administered two or more times to the same group of individuals that results in high intercorrelations among scores would have high reproducibility.

Responsiveness.   Responsiveness refers to the extent to which a valuative instrument (one designed to measure within-person change over time) can detect differences in score which are important, even if those differences are small. *Sensitivity to change* is a term that has been used synonymously with responsiveness. Responsiveness can be conceptualized as the ratio of a signal (the real change over time that has occurred) to the noise (the variability in score seen over time which is not associated with true change in status).

Restricted-Activity Days.   Refers to the number of days a person experienced any one of the four types of activity restriction (bed days, work-loss days, school-loss days, and cut-down days). The number of restricted-activity days is the number of days a person experienced at least one of the four types of activity restriction. It is the most inclusive measure of disability days and the least descriptive. Restricted-activity days may be associated with either persons or conditions. It is a frequently used measure to assess the health and activity of older adults.

Risk Aversion.   Persons are said to be risk averse if they prefer a certain rather than an uncertain outcome. Persons may also be risk lovers; i.e., they may prefer uncertain outcomes rather than certain outcomes. Persons who are risk neutral are indifferent to certain and uncertain outcomes.

Rule of Rescue.   The moral imperative that prompts the use of technologies and services that rescue endangered life. People view it as their perceived duty to save an identified person's life when it is visibly threatened, if effective rescue measures are available. The Rule of Rescue operates most often when life is endangered, but it also applies to identified persons in need of treatments that are not necessarily life-saving but are readily available, such as emergency care or injuries.

School-Loss Days.   Reports from students from 5 to 17 years of age who have missed more than half of a day from the school in which they are currently enrolled

Self Report.   Respondent-supplied information on health status gathered through written questionnaires or oral interviews. In self-administration, the respondent independently completes the questionnaire according to written or oral instructions.

Sensitivity Analysis.   A procedure for determining the robustness of an analytic result by systematically varying the values assigned to important variables in the analysis.

The goal of sensitivity analysis is to identify variables whose values are most likely to change the results and to find a solution that is relatively stable for the most commonly occurring values of these variables. In the Health Resource Allocation Strategy, the health state preference weights, the discount rate, and prognostic estimates might be varied to determine their impact on the analytic result. Challenges to the costs and outcomes table might also be treated as sensitivity analyses to determine changes in the cost-per-year-of-healthy-life ratios and relative ranking of alternative interventions in the table.

Socioeconomic Evaluation.   Analysis of health care costs and outcomes in a standard format for the purpose of comparing alternative health care interventions. Evaluation is usually conducted under the assumption of finite resources.

Sociopolitical Process.   Relating to or concerned with the interaction between health decision makers and stakeholders in decisions about the allocation of resources to health care through rationing or medical effectiveness evaluations. The process involves groups and communities (social) and often concerns the state, its government, or public affairs in general (political).

Stability.   Refers to reproducibility of health status measures over relatively long periods of time, i.e., more than six months. If a measure is intended to represent the relatively enduring status of a trait in people, such as intelligence, it needs to remain stable over the period in which scores are employed for the purpose of measurement.

Stakeholders.   All the individuals and groups interested in or having a stake in health decisions. Stakeholders include the person or patient, family members or significant others, clinicians, administrators, government officials, public interest groups, lobbyists, and the entire community when affected by health decisions.

Standard Gamble.   *See* Utility measurement.

Standardized Measure.   Measurement scales with known reliability and validity that have been applied repeatedly to different populations such that comparative scores are available.

Summative Ratings.   Measures based on these rating scales assume that individual items in a measure are monotonically related to underlying attributes and that a summation of item scores is approximately linearly related to the attribute. Also referred to as *Likert scales*.

Survival.   The duration of life as measured by life years, life expectancy, or remaining years of life. Survival is modified by the different domains of health and quality of life to indicate a tradeoff between quantity and quality of life as health-related quality of life.

Technology Assessment.   A form of policy research that evaluates technology for providing decision makers with information on different policy options. These options may include the allocation of resources to research and development, development of regulations or legislation, and setting standards or guidelines for health planning and health practice.

Theory of Rational Choice.   The assumptions that economists make about the way that individuals make choices. The theory consist of three basic assumptions, or axioms, about individuals' behavior: (1) individuals can rank alternative bundles of goods according to their preferences for the goods; (2) individuals are consistent in their choices; and (3) individuals prefer more rather than less.

Time Preference for Health. *See* Discounting.

Transition Probability. Likelihood that an individual's or a population's current level of health will increase, stay the same, or decrease. Transition is a function of the current level of health and all determinants. Probabilities are obtained empirically by monitoring health states over time. Health status transitions have been estimated using stochastic models.

Unintended Outcomes. The adverse effects or experiences associated with an intervention or treatment. These undesirable outcomes may be known in advance of the intervention or unanticipated. All interventions ranging from focused pharmacologic treatment to broad social interventions may have unintended outcomes.

Utilitarianism. A theory of social justice that holds that policies that produce the greatest good for the greatest number improve social welfare. This theory incorporates everyone's well-being into the social process by balancing the utility of persons who gain from a given policy with the utility of those who lose as a result of the same policy.

Utility. A concept in economics, psychology, and decision analysis referring to the preference for, or desirability of, a particular outcome. In the context of health-related quality of life measurement, utility refers to the preference of the rater (usually a patient or a member of the general public) for a particular health outcome or health state. The health state being evaluated may be a state that has been recently experienced by the patient, is being experienced by the patient at the time the instrument is administered, or may be described as a hypothetical health state. It is important to distinguish between utility scores obtained from interviews of patients (especially for states they have experienced or are experiencing) and scores obtained from interviews of members of the general public for whom the health states are, in general, hypothetical. Scores obtained from members of the general public for hypothetical states are sometimes called social preference (or utility) scores. If the respondent evaluates the desirability of the health state on behalf of herself, as if she was experiencing the health state, then the resulting score is not strictly a social utility. If, on the other hand, she evaluates the desirability of the health state on behalf of members of society in general, then the score may accurately be labeled as a social utility or social preference.

Utility Measurement. By convention utility is usually measured on a 0.0- to 1.0-scale in which 0.0 is the least desirable state, associated with death, and 1.0 is the most desirable state, associated with perfect health. In some instances, states of health may be considered worse than death, yielding negative utilities. The most commonly used methods for measuring health state utilities are the standard gamble or time tradeoff, although there are a number of variations on and combinations of these approaches. In the standard gamble approach judges are asked to compare life in a particular health state to a gamble with a probability p that perfect health is the outcome and $1 - p$ that death is the outcome. The probability p is varied until preference for the sure thing, the certainty of the particular health state, is equal to the preference for the gamble. The probability p for which the expected utility of the two choices is equal is then a measure of the preference for the health state. (In the standard gamble the lottery is comprised of a more preferred and a less preferred state versus an intermediately ranked state as the sure thing. The choices in the gamble need not be perfect health and death.) In the time tradeoff approach, patients are asked to trade off life years in a state of less than perfect health for a shorter life span in a state of perfect health. The ratio of the number of years of perfect health that is equivalent to longer life span in less than perfect health provides a measure of the preference for that health state.

Validity. A descriptive term used to mean that a measure accurately reflects the concept that it is intended to measure. *Face validity* is that quality of health status measure such that it seems to be a reasonable measure of some domain of health-related quality of life. *Content validity* refers to the degree to which a measure covers the range of meanings included within the concept. For health-related quality of life measures, this means the range of domains covered in the measure such as survival, impairment, physical/psychological/social function, perceptions, and opportunity.

Values. Standards of the desirable which influence selective behavior. In this view, "a value is a conception, explicit or implicit, distinctive of an individual or characteristic of a group, of the desirable which influences the selection from available modes, means and ends of action" (Kluckhohn, 1951).

Willingness to Pay. A method of valuing health that is based on the amount of money that individuals would be willing to pay either to reduce the probability of death due to a given disease or to increase the probability of cure for a given disease. The willingness-to-pay approach is an alternative to the human capital method for expressing health benefits in monetary units.

Work-Loss Days. A day on which a currently employed person 18 years of age or over missed more than half a day from a job or business.

Years of Healthy Life (YHL). The duration of life discounted by some fraction between 0 and 1 that estimates the quality of life during a given period. If duration of life is 1 year and the health-adjustment factor for a given health state is 0.5, then the years of healthy life is 0.5 year. This is interpreted as equivalent to being alive for half a year in perfect health. Note that the terms "well years," "well life expectancy," "health life years," and "quality-adjusted life years" are synonyms for years of healthy life.

References

Aaron HJ (1991). *Serious and unstable condition: financing America's health care*. Washington DC: Brookings Institution.

Aaron HJ, Schwartz WB (1984). *The painful prescription: rationing hospital care*. Washington DC: Brookings Institution.

Aaron HJ, Schwartz WB (1990). "Rationing health care: the choice before us." *Science*: 247 (4941), 418–22.

Aaronson NK, Ahmedzi S, Bullinger M (1991). The EORTC core quality of life questionnaire: interim results of an international field study. In *The effect of cancer on quality of life*. Osoba, D, ed. New York: CRC Press.

Achenbach TM, Edelbrock C (1983). *Manual for the child behavior checklist and revised behavioral profile*. Burlington: University of Vermont, Department of Psychology.

Acton JP (1973). *Evaluating public health programs to save lives: the case of heart attacks*. Rand Report R-950-RC. Santa Monica, CA: Rand Corporation.

Ad Hoc Committee of the U.S. National Committee on Vital and Health Statistics (1958). *Report on the possibility of measuring positive health*. Washington DC: U.S. Department of Health, Education and Welfare.

Adams PF, Benson V (1990). "Current estimates from the National Health Interview Survey: United States, 1989. National Center for Health Statistics." *Vital Health Stat*: 10 (176), 1–221.

Adams PF, Benson V (1991). "Current estimates from the National Health Interview Survey: United States, 1990. National Center for Health Statistics." *Vital Health Stat*: 10 (181), 1–212.

Aday LA (1989). *Designing and conducting health surveys*. San Francisco: Jossey-Bass.

Aday LA, Andersen R (1975). *Development of indices of access to medical care*. Ann Arbor, MI: Health Administration Press.

Aday LA, Chiu GY, Andersen R (1980). "Methodologic issues in health care surveys of the Spanish heritage population." *Am J Public Health*: 70, 367–74.

Affleck JW, Aitken RC, Hunter JA, McGuire RJ (1988). "Rehabilitation status: a measure of medicosocial dysfunction." *Lancet*: 230–33.

Alexander FG (1950). *Psychosomatic medicine: its principle and applications*. New York: Norton.

Allison GT (1971). *Essence of decision: explaining the Cuban missile crisis*. Boston: Little, Brown.

Alonso J, Anto JM, Moreno C (1990). "Spanish version of the Nottingham Health Profile: translation and preliminary validity." *Am J Public Health*: 80 (6), 704–8.

Amberg JM, Schneiderman LJ, Berry CC, Zettner A (1982). "The abnormal outpatient chemistry panel serum alkaline phosphatase: analysis of physician response, outcome, cost and health effectiveness." *J Chron Dis:* 35(2), 81–88.

American Psychological Association (1974). *Standards for educational and psychological tests*. Washington DC: American Psychological Association.

Anbar M (1984). Penetrating the black box: physical principles behind health care technology. In *The machine at the bedside: strategies for using technology in patient care*. Reiser SJ, Anbar M, eds. New York: Cambridge University Press, 23–34.

Anderson JP, Moser RJ (1985). "Parasite screening and treatment among Indochinese refugees: cost-benefit/utility and the General Health Policy Model." *JAMA:* 253 (15), 2229–35.

Anderson JP, Bush JW, Berry CC (1977). *Performance versus capacity: a conflict in classifying function for health status measurement. Meeting of the American Public Health Association*. San Diego: University of California.

Anderson NH (1976). "How functional measurement can yield validated interval scales of mental qualities." *J Appl Psych*: 61 (6), 667–92.

Andrews F, Withey SB (1974). "Developing measures of perceived life quality: results from several national surveys." *Soc Indic Res*: 1, 1–26.

Andrews FM, Withey SB (1976). *Social indicators of well-being: Americans' perceptions of life quality*. New York: Plenum.

Aristotle (circa 335–323 B.C./1976). *Ethics*. Thomson JAK, trans. Harmondsworth, England: Penguin Books.

Arrow KJ (1951). *Social choice and individual values*. New York: Wiley.

Augustinsson LE, Sullivan L, Sullivan M (1986). "Physical, psychologic, and social function in chronic pain patients after epidural spinal electrical stimulation." *Spine*: 11 (2), 111–19.

Bachrach P, Baratz MS (1963). "Decisions and nondecisions: an analytical framework." *Am Pol Sci Rev*: 57, 632–42.

Balaban DJ, Sagi PC, Goldfarb NI, Nettler S (1986). "Weights for scoring the quality of well-being instrument among rheumatoid arthritics: a comparison to general population weights." *Med Care*: 24 (11), 973–80.

Baldwin S, Godfrey C, Propper C (1990). *Quality of life: perspectives and policies*. London: Routledge.

Bandura A (1982). "Self-efficacy mechanism in human agency." *Am Psychol*: 37, 122–47.

Banta HD, Andreasen PB (1990). "The political dimension in health care technology assessment programs." *Int J Technol Assess Health Care*: 6, 115–23.

Barker DC, Kabcenell A, Weisfeld V (1991). *Challenges in health care: a chartbook perspective 1991*. Princeton, NJ: The Robert Wood Johnson Foundation.

Basset SS, Magaziner J, Hebel JR (1990). "Reliability of proxy response on mental health indices for aged, community-dwelling women." *Psychol Aging*: 2 (1), 127–32.

Bebbington AC (1977). "Scaling indices of disablement." *Br J Prev Soc Med*: 31 (2), 122–26.

Beck AT (1967). *Depression: causes and treatment*. Philadelphia: University of Pennsylvania Press.

Beck AT, Ward CH, Mendelson M, Mock J, Erbaugh J (1961). "An inventory for measuring depression." *Arch Gen Psychiat*: 4, 561–71.

Bentham J (1789/1948). *An introduction to the principles of morals and legislation*. New York: Hafner.

Bergner L, Hallstrom AP, Eisenberg M (1984). "Health status of survivors of out-of-hospital cardiac arrest six months later." *Am J Public Health*: 74 (5), 508–10.

Bergner LH, Hallstrom AP, Bergner M, Eisenberg M, Cobb LA (1985). "Health status of survivors of cardiac arrest and of myocardial infarction controls." *Am J Public Health* 75:1321–3.

Bergner M (1984). The Sickness Impact Profile. In *Assessment of quality of life in clinical trials of cardiovascular therapies*. Wenger NK, Mattson ME, Furberg CD, Elinson J, eds. New York: LeJacq, 152–59.

Bergner M (1985). "Measurement of health status." *Med Care*: 23 (5), 696–704.

Bergner M, Bobbitt RA, Carter WB, Gilson BS (1981). "The Sickness Impact Profile: development and final revision of a health status measure." *Med Care*: 19 (8), 787–805.

Bergner M, Bobbitt RA, Kressel S, Pollard WE, Gilson BS, Morris JR (1976). "The Sickness Impact Profile: conceptual formulation and methodological development of a health status index." *Int J Health Serv*: 6, 393–415.

Bergner M, Hudson LD, Conrad DA, Patmont CA, McDonald GT, Perrin EB, Gilson BS (1988). "The cost and efficacy of home care for patients with chronic lung disease." *Med Care*: 26 (6), 566–79.

Berry CC, Bush JW (1978). Estimating prognosis for a dynamic health index, the weighted life expectancy, using the multiple logistic with survey and mortality data. In *Proceedings of the American Statistical Association, Social Science Section,* 716–21. Washington, DC: American Statistical Association.

Berwick D (1989). "Depression: down-hearted and blue." Presented at the annual meeting of the Medical Decision Society, Minneapolis, Minnesota.

Berwick DM, Cretin S, Keeler EB (1980). *Cholesterol, children, and heart disease: An analysis of alternatives.* New York: Oxford University Press.

Bess FH, Lichtenstein MJ, Logan SA, Burger MC (1989). "Comparing criteria of hearing impairment in the elderly: a functional approach." *J Speech Hear Res*: 32 (4), 795–802.

Bindman AB, Keane D, Lurie N (1990). "Measuring health changes among severely ill patients: the floor phenomenon." *Med Care*: 28, 1142–52.

Blaug M (1983). *Economic theory in retrospect.* Cambridge, England: Cambridge University Press.

Blazer D (1991). "Spirituality and aging well." *Generations*: 61–65.

Blendon RJ (1988). "The public's view of the future of health care." *JAMA:* 259 (24), 3587–93.

Blendon RJ, Donelan K (1991). "Interpreting public opinion surveys." *Health Aff*: 10 (2), 166–69.

Blendon RJ, Edwards JN (1991). "Caring for the uninsured: choices for reform." *JAMA*: 265 (19), 2563–65.

Blendon RJ, Aiken LH, Freeman HE, Corey CR (1989). "Access to medical care for black and white Americans: a matter of continuing concern." *JAMA*: 261 (2), 279–81.

Blessed G, Tomlinson BE, Roth M (114). "The association between quantitative measures of dementia and of senile change in the cerebral gray matter of elderly subjects." Br J Psychiatr 797–811.

Blischke WR, Bush JW, Kaplan RM (1975). "Successive intervals analysis of preference measures in a health status index." *Health Serv Res*: 10 (2), 181–98.

Bock RD, Jones LV (1968). *The measurement and prediction of judgment and choice.* San Francisco: Holden-Day.

Bombardier C, Ware J, Russell IJ, Larson M, Chalmers A, Read JL (1986). "Auranofin therapy and quality of life in patients with rheumatoid arthritis: results of a multicenter trial." *Am J Med*: 81 (4), 565–78.

Bonham GS (1983). *Procedures and questionnaires of the National Medical Care Utilization and Expenditure Survey.* Hyattsville, MD: National Center for Health Statistics.

Bonica JJ (1990). *The management of pain.* Phildelphia: Lea and Febiger.

Boyle MH, Torrance GW (1984). "Developing multiattribute health indexes." *Med Care*: 22 (22), 1045–57.

Boyle MH, Torrance GW, Sinclair JC, Horwood SP (1983). "Economic evaluation of neonatal intensive care of very-low-birth-weight infants." *N Engl J Med*: 308 (22), 1330–37.

Bracht N (1990). *Health promotion at the community level.* Newbury Park, CA: Sage Publications.

Bradburn NM (1969). *The structure of psychological well-being.* Chicago: Aldine.

Braithwaite RL, Lythcott N (1989). "Community empowerment as a strategy for health promotion for black and other minority populations." *JAMA*: 261 (2), 282–83.

Branch LG, Jette AM (1981). "The Framingham Disability Study: social disability among the aging." *Am J Public Health*: 1202

Brandt J, Spencer M, Folstein M (1988). "The telephone interview for cognitive status." *Neuropsychiat, Neuropsychol, Behav Neurol*: 1 (2), 111–17.

Brickman P, Campbell DT (1971). Hedonic relativism and planning the good society. In *Adaptation-level theory: a symposium*. Appley MH, ed. New York: Academic Press, pp. 287–304.

Brislin R, Lonner W, Thorndike R (1973). *Cross cultural research methods*. New York: Wiley, 32–81.

Britten N, Davies JM, Dolley JR (1987). "Early respiratory experience and subsequent cough and peak expiratory flow rate in 36 year old men and women." *Br Med J*: 294, 1317–20.

Broadhead WE, Kaplan BH, James SA, Wagner EH, Schoenbach VJ, Grimson R, Heyden S, Tibblin G, Gehlbach SH (1983). "The epidemiologic evidence for a relationship between social support and health." *Am J Epidemiol*: 117, 521–37.

Brook RH, Ware JE, Davies-Avery A, Stewart AL, Donald CA, Rogers WH, Williams KN, Johnston SA (1979). "Overview of adult health status measures fielded in Rand's health insurance study." *Med Care*: 17 (7 suppl), iii–x, 1–131.

Brook RH, Ware JE, Rogers WH, Keeler EB, Davies ER, Donald CA, Goldberg GA, Lohr KN, Masthay PC, Newhouse JP (1983). "Does free care improve adults' health? Results from a randomized controlled trial." *N Engl J Med*: 309 (23), 1426–34.

Brooks C, Richards J, Bailey W, Martin B, Winsor R, Soong S (1989). "Subjective symptomatology of asthma in an outpatient population." *Psychosom Med*: 51, 102–8.

Brooks RG, Jedteg S, Lindgren B, Persson U, Bjork S (1991). "EuroQol: health-related quality of life measurement. Results of the Swedish questionnaire exercise." *Health Policy* 18: 37–48.

Brown GW, Bifulco A, Harris TO (1987). "Life events, vulnerability and onset of depression: some refinements." *Br J Psychiat*: 150, 30–42.

Brown GW, Harris TO (1978). *Social origins of depression: a study of psychiatric disorder in women*. London: Tavistock.

Brownell A, Shumaker SA (1984). "Social support: an introduction to a complex phenomenon." *J Soc Issues*: 40 (4), 1–11.

Bruhn JG, Philips BU (1984). "Measuring social support: a synthesis of current approaches." *J Behav Med*: 7 (2), 151–69.

Bulpitt CJ, Fletcher AE (1987). "Measurement of the quality of life in angina." *J Hypertension Suppl*: 5 (1), S41–S45.

Burckhardt CS, Woods SI, Schults AA, Ziebarth DM (1989). "Quality of life of adults with chronic illness: a psychometric study." *Res Nurs Health*: 12 (6), 347–54.

Burton RM, Damon WW, Dellinger DC (1975). "Patient states and the technology matrix." *Interfaces*: 5 (4), 43–53.

Bush JW (1984a). General Health Policy Model/Quality of Well-Being (QWB) scale. In *Assessment of quality of life in clinical trials of cardiovascular therapies*. Wenger NK, Mattson ME, Furberg CD, Elinson J, eds. New York: LeJacq, 189–99.

Bush JW (1984b). Invited discussion: relative preference versus relative frequencies in health-related quality of life evaluation. In *Assessment of quality of life in clinical trials of cardiovascular therapies*. Wenger NK, Mattson ME, Furberg CD, Elinson J, eds. New York: LeJacq, 118–39.

Bush JW, Chen MM, Patrick DL (1973). Health Status Index in cost-effectiveness: analysis of PKU program. In *Health status indexes*. Berg R, eds. Chicago: Hospital Research and Educational Trust, 172–208.

Bush JW, Fanshel S, Chen MM (1972) "Analysis of a tuberculin testing program using a health status index." *Socio-Econ Plan Sci* 6, 49.

Callahan D (1987). *Setting limits: medical goals in an aging society*. New York: Simon and Schuster.

Callahan D (1990). *What kind of life: the limits of medical progress*. New York: Simon and Schuster.

Calltorp J (1988). "Consensus development conferences in Sweden: effects on health policy and administration." *Int J Technol Assess Health Care*: 4, 75–88.

Calman KC (1984). "Quality of life in cancer patients—an hypothesis." *J Med Ethics*: 10, 124–27.

Calman KC (1987). Definitions and dimensions of quality of life. In *The quality of life of cancer patients*. Aaronson NK, Beckman J, eds. New York: Raven Press, 1–9.

Campbell A (1981). *The sense of well-being in America: recent patterns and trends*. New York: McGraw-Hill.

Campbell A, Converse PE, Rodgers WL (1976). *Quality of American life: perceptions, evaluations and satisfaction*. New York: Russell Sage Foundation.

Campbell DT, Fiske DW (1959). "Convergent and discriminant validation by the multitrait–multimethod matrix." *Psychol Bull*: 56, 85–105.

Canadian Erythropoietin Study Group (1990). "Association between recombinant human erythropoietin and quality of life and exercise capacity of patients receiving haemodialysis. Canadian Erythropoietin Study Group." *Br Med J:* 300 (6724), 573–78.

Cantor JC, Morisky DE, Green LW, Levine DM, Horwood SP (1985). "Cost-effectiveness of education interventions to improve patient outcomes in blood pressure control." *Prev Med*: 14 (6), 782–800.

Caradoc-Davies TH, Wilson BD, Anson JG (1990). "The rehabilitation of injured workers in New Zealand: a pilot study." *N Z Med J*: 103 (888), 179–82.

Carey RG, Posavac EJ (1977). Program evaluation of a physical medicine and rehabilitation unit: a new approach. *Arch Physical Med Rehab* 330–337.

Carlson RJ (1975). *The end of medicine*. New York: Wiley.

Carlsson P, Pedersen KV, Varenhorst E (1990). "Costs and benefits of early detection of prostatic cancer." *Health Policy* 16, 241–53.

Carr-Hill RA, Morris J (1991). "Current practice in obtaining the 'Q' in QALYs: a cautionary note." *Br Med J:* 303, 699–701.

Carter WB, Bobbitt RA, Bergner M, Gilson BS (1976). "Validation of an interval scaling: the Sickness Impact Profile." *Health Serv Res*: 11 (4), 516–28.

Caspirie AF, Everdingen JJE (1985). "Consensus development conferences in the Netherlands." *Int J Technol Assess Health Care*: 1, 905–12.

Cassel J (1975). Social science in epidemiology: psycho-social processes and 'stress': theoretical formulation. In *Handbook of evaluation research*. Struening EL, Guttentag M, eds. Beverly Hills, CA: Sage Publications.

Chambers LW (1982). *The McMaster Health Index Questionnaire (MHIQ): methodologic documentation and report of second generation of investigations*. Hamilton, Ontario: Department of Clinical Epidemiology and Biostatistics.

Charlton JR, Patrick DL, Peach H (1983). "Use of multivariate measures of disability in health surveys." *J Epidemiol Community Health*: 37 (4), 296–304.

Charlton JRH (1989). Approaches to assessing disability. In *Disablement in the community*. Patrick DL, Peach H, eds. Oxford, England: Oxford University Press, 39–61.

Chen MK (1973). The G-Index for program priority. In *Health status indexes: proceedings of the Conference on a Health Status Index*. Berg RL, ed. Chicago: Hospital Research and Educational Trust, 28–39.

Chen MK (1976). "The K-Index: a proxy measure of health care quality." *Health Serv Res*: 11 (4), 452–63.

Chen MM, Bush JW (1976). "Maximizing health system Output with Political and Administrative Constraints Using Mathematical Programming." *Inquiry:* 13 (3), 215–227.

Chen MM, Bush JW (1979). Health status measures, policy, and biomedical research. In *Health:*

what is it worth: measures of health benefits. Mushkin SJ, Dunlop DW, eds. New York: Pergamon Press, 15–42.

Chen MM, Bush JW, Patrick DL (1975). "Social indicators for health planning and policy analysis." *Policy Sci*: 6, 71–89.

Chiang CL (1965). An index of health: mathematical models. In *Public Health Services Publication No. 1000, Series 2, No. 5*. Washington, DC: National Center for Health Statistics.

Churchill DL, Torrance GW, Taylor DW, Barnes CC, Ludwin D, Shimizu A, Smith EKM (1987). "Measurement of quality of life in end-stage renal disease: the time trade-off approach." *Clin Invest Med*: 10 (1), 14–20.

Churchill DN, Morgan J, Torrance GW (1984). "Quality of life in end-stage renal disease." *Peritoneal Dialysis Bull*: Jan–Mar, 20–23.

Churchill L (1987). *Rationing health care in America*. Notre Dame, IN: University of Notre Dame Press.

Clearinghouse on Health Indexes (1973–1991, qtrly.). *Bibliography on health indexes*. Washington, D.C.: U.S. Government Printing Office, Public Health Service. DHHS Publication no. (PHS) 86–1225.

Clipp EC, Elder GH (1987). "Elderly confidants in geriatric assessment." *Compr Gerontol (B)*: 35–40.

Coates A, Gebski V, Bishop JF, Jeal PN, Woods RL, Snyder R, Tattersall MH, Byrne M, Harvey V, Gill G (1987). "Improving the quality of life during chemotherapy for advanced breast cancer." *N Engl J Med*: 317 (24), 1490–95.

Cohen BB, Erickson P, Powell A (1984). Does length of recall affect the number of reported doctor visits? In *Proceedings of the American Statistical Association, Social Statistics Section*. Washington, DC: American Statistical Association.

Cohen BB, Barbano HE, Cox CS, Feldman JJ (1987). "Plan and operation of the NHANES I epidemiologic followup study: 1982–1984." *Vital Health Stat*: 1 (22), 1–142.

Cohen J (1977). *Statistical power analysis for the behavioral sciences*. New York: Academic Press.

Collins, JG (1986). "Prevalence of selected chronic conditions: United States 1979–1981." *Vital Health Stat* 10(155), 1–66.

Colvez A, Blanchet M (1981). "Disability trends in the United States population 1966–1976: analysis of reported causes." *Am J Public Health*: 71 (5), 464–71.

Colvez A, Robine JM (1986). "Problems encountered in using the concepts of impairment, disability, and handicap in a health assessment survey of the elderly in Upper Normandy." *Int Rehabil Med*: 8 (1), 18–22.

Commission on Professional and Hospital Activities (1978). *International Classification of Diseases 9th Revision—Clinical modification*. Ann Arbor, MI: Commission on Professional and Hospital Activities.

Conte HR (1986). "Multivariate assessment of sexual dysfunction." *J Consult Clin Psychol*: 54 (2), 149–57.

Cornoni-Huntley JC, Huntley RR, Feldman JJ, (eds.) (1990). *Health status and well-being in the elderly*. New York: Oxford University Press.

Costa PT, McCrae RR, Locke BZ (1990). Personality factors. In *Health status and well-being in the elderly*. Cornoni-Huntley JC, Huntley RR, Feldman JJ, eds. New York: Oxford University Press, 210–20.

Crawshaw R, Garland M, Hines B, Anderson BG (1990). "Developing principles for prudent health care allocation: the continuing Oregon experiment." *West J Med*: 152, 441–46.

The Criteria Committee of the New York Heart Association, Inc. (1964). *Disease of the heart and blood vessels: nomenclature and criteria for diagnosis*, 6th ed. Boston: Little, Brown.

Cronbach LJ (1951). "Coefficient alpha and the internal structure of tests." *Psychometrika*: 16, 297.

Croog SH, Levine S, Testa MA, Brown B, Bulpitt CJ, Jenkins CD, Klerman GL, Williams GH (1986). "The effects of antihypertensive therapy on the quality of life." *N Engl J Med*: 314 (26), 1657–64.

Curtin LR, Armstrong R (1988). *Cause eliminated life tables for the United States*. Hyattsville, MD: National Center for Health Statistics.

Danchik KM, Drury TF (1985). Evaluating the effects of survey design and administration on the measurement of subjective phenomena: the case of self-assessed health status. *Proceedings of the American Statistical Association, Social Statistics Section*. Washington, DC: American Statistical Association.

Daniels N (1985). *Just health care*. Cambridge, England: Cambridge University Press.

Daniels N (1991). "Is the Oregon rationing plan fair?" *JAMA:* 265, 2232–35.

Danis M, Patrick DL, Southerland LI, Green ML (1988). "Patients' and families' preferences for medical intensive care." *JAMA*: 260 (6), 797–802.

Davies AR, Ware JE (1981). *Measuring health perceptions in the health insurance experiment*. Santa Monica, CA: Rand Corporation.

DCCT Research Group (1987). "Diabetes Control and Complications Trial (DCCT): results of feasibility study." *Diabetes Care*: 10 (1), 1–19.

de Haes JC, van Knippenberg FC, Neijt JP (1990). "Measuring psychological and physical distress in cancer patients: structure and application of the Rotterdam Symptom Checklist." *Br J Cancer:* 62(6), 1034–38.

DeJong R, Osterlund OW, Roy GW (1989). "Measurement of qualty-of-life changes in patients with Alzheimer's disease." *Clin Ther*: 11 (4), 545–54.

Del Greco L, Walop W, Eastridge L (1987). "Questionnaire development. 3. Translation." *Can Med Assoc J:* 136, 817–18.

Delano BG (1989). "Improvements in quality of life following treatment with r-HuEPO in anemic hemodialysis patients." *Am J Kidney Dis*: 14 (2 suppl 1), 14–18.

Department of Health and Human Services (1980). *Promoting health/preventing disease: objectives for the nation*. Washington DC: U.S. Government Printing Office.

Department of Health and Human Services (1981). *User's manual: The National Death Index*. Washington DC: U.S. Government Printing Office.

Department of Health and Human Services (1985). *Report of the Secretary's Task Force on Black and Minority Health*, Vol. 1. Washington DC: U.S. Government Printing Office.

Department of Health and Human Services (1990). *Healthy people 2000: national health promotion and disease prevention objectives*. Washington DC: U.S. Government Printing Office.

Department of Health and Human Services (1991a). *Healthy communities 2000: model standards, quidelines for attainment of year 2000 objectives for the nation*. Washington DC: U.S. Government Printing Office.

Department of Health and Human Services (1991b). *Healthy people 2000*. Washington DC: U.S. Government Printing Office.

Department of Health, Education and Welfare (1973). *The Framingham study: an epidemiological investigation of cardiovasuclar disease. Some characteristics related to the incidence of cardiovascular disease and death, 18-year follow-up. Section 30*. Bethesda, MD: U.S. Public Health Service.

Department of Health, Education and Welfare (1979). *Healthy people: the surgeon general's report on health promotion and disease prevention*. Washington DC: U.S. Department of Health, Education and Welfare, U.S. Public Health Service. Publication no. DHEW (PHS) 79–55071.

Departmental Task Force on Prevention (1978). *Disease prevention and health promotion: federal programs and prospects*. Washington DC: U.S. Department of Health, Education and Welfare, Public Health Service. Publication no. DHEW (PHS) 79–55071B.

Derogatis LR (1980). "Psychological assessment of psychosexual functioning." *Psychiat Clin North Am*: 3 (1), 113–31.

Derogatis LR (1986). "The psychosocial adjustment to illness scale (PAIS)." *J Psychosom Res*: 30, 77–91.

Derogatis LR, Lipman RS, Covi L (1973). "SCL-9: an outpatient psychiatric rating scale: preliminary report." *Psychopharmacol Bull*: 9 (1), 13–28.

Derogatis LR, Lipman RS, Uhlenhuth EH (1974). "The Hopkins Symptom Checklist (HSCL): a self-report symptom inventory." *Behav Sci:* 19, 1–15.

Detsky AS, Naglie IG (1990). "A clinician's guide to cost-effectiveness analysis." *Ann Intern Med:* 113 (2), 147–54.

Deyo R, Patrick D (1989). "Barriers to the use of health status measures in clinical investigation, patient care, and policy research." *Med Care*: 27 (3 suppl), S254–68.

Deyo RA (1984). "Measuring functional outcomes in therapeutic trials for chronic disease." *Controlled Clin Trials*: 5 (3), 223–40.

Deyo RA (1986). "Comparative validity of the Sickness Impact Profile and shorter scales for functional assessment in low-back pain." *Spine*: 11 (9), 951–54.

Deyo RA (1988). Measuring the quality of life of patients with rheumatoid arthritis. In *Quality of life: assessment and application*. Walker SR, Rosser RM, eds. Lancaster, England: MTP Press, 205.

Deyo RA, Centor RM (1986). "Assessing the responsiveness of functional scales to clinical change: an analogy to diagnostic test performance." *J Chronic Dis*: 39 (11), 897–906.

Deyo RA, Diehl AK (1983). "Measuring physical and psychosocial function in patients with low-back pain." *Spine*: 8, 635.

Deyo RA, Cherkin D, Conrad D (1990). "The back pain outcome assessment team." *Health Serv Res*: 25 (5), 733–37.

Deyo RA, Diehr P, Patrick D (1991). "Reproducibility and responsiveness of health status measures: statistics and strategies for evaluation." *Controlled Clin Trials*: 12(4), 142S–158S.

Deyo RA, Inui TS, Leininger J, Overman S (1982). "Physical and psychosocial function in rheumatoid arthritis: clinical use of a self administered health status instument." *Arch Intern Med*: 142 (5), 879–82.

Diener E (1984). "Subjective well-being." *Psychol Bull*: 95, 542–75.

Dohrenwend BP, Dohrenwend BS, Gould MS (1980). *Mental illness in the United States*. New York: Praeger, 163.

Donabedian A (1966). "Evaluating the quality of medical care." *Milbank Mem Fund Q*: 44, 166–206.

Donald CA, Ware JE (1982). *The quantification of social contacts and resources*. Santa Monica, CA: Rand Corporation.

Dratcu L, DaCosta Ribeiro L, Calil HM (1987). "Depression assessment in Brazil. The first application of the Montgomery-Ashberg Depression Rating Scale." *Br J Psychiat*: 150, 797–800.

Drossman DA, Patrick DL, Mitchell CM, Zagami EA, Appelbaum MI (1989). "Health-related quality of life in inflammatory bowel disease. Functional status and patient worries and concerns." *Dig Dis Sci*: 34 (9), 1379–86.

Drummond MF (1980). *Principles of economic appraisal in health care*. New York: Oxford Medical Publications.

Drummond MF, Stoddart GL, Torrance GW (1987). *Methods for the economic evaluation of health care programmes*. New York: Oxford University Press.

Dublin LI, Lotka AJ (1930). *The money value of a man*. New York: Ronald Press.

Dubos R (1976). "The state of health and the quality of life." *West J Med*: 125 (1), 8–9.

Dupuy HJ (1973). The psychological section of the current Health and Nutrition Examination Survey. In *Proceedings of the Public Health Conference on Records and Statistics*. Rockville, MD: National Center for Health Statistics, 508–15.

Dupuy HJ (1974). Utility of the National Center for Health Statistics General Well-Being Schedule in the assessment of self-representations of subjective well-being and distress. In *The National Conference on Evaluation in Alcohol, Drug Abuse and Mental Health Programs*. Washington DC: Alcohol, Drug Abuse and Mental Health Administration.

Dupuy HJ (1984). The Psychological General Well-Being (PGWB) Index. In *Assessment of quality of life in clinical trials of cardiovascular therapies*. Wenger NK, Mattson ME, Furberg CD, Elinson J, eds. New York: Le Jacq, 170–83.

Durkheim E (1897/1951). *Suicide*. Spaulding JA, Simpson G, trans. New York: The Free Press.

Dutton DB (1986). Social class, health, and illness. In *Applications of social science to clinical medicine and health policy*. Aiken LH, Mechanic DM, eds. New Brunswick, NJ: Rutgers University Press.

Dworkin R (1981). "What is equality? Part 1. Equality of welfare." *Philos Public Aff*: 10, 185–246.

Ebrahim S, Barer D, Nouri F (1986). "Use of the Nottingham Health Profile with patients after a stroke." *J Epidemiol Community Health*: 40 (2), 166–0.

Eddy DM (1991a). "What's going on in Oregon?" *JAMA:* 266 (3), 417–20.

Eddy DM (1991b). "Oregon's methods: did cost-effectiveness fail?" *JAMA:* 266 (15), 2135–41.

Eddy DM (1991c). "Oregon's plan: should it be approved?" *JAMA:* 266 (17), 2439–45.

Edwards WS, Berlin M (1989). *Questionnaires and data collection methods for the household survey and the survey of American Indians and Alaska natives: methods 2*. Rockville, MD: National Center for Health Services Research and Health Care Technology Assessment. DHHS Publication No. (PHS) 89–3450.

Edwards WS, Edwards B (1989). *National Medical Expenditure Survey: questionnaires and data collection methods for the institutional population component: methods 1*. Rockville, MD: National Center for Health Services Research and Health Care Technology Assessment.

Eggers PW (1984). "Trends in Medicare reimbursement for end-stage renal disease: 1974–1979." *Health Care Financ Rev*: 6 (1), 31–38.

Eisen M, Donald C, Ware JE (1980). *Conceptualization and measurement of health for children in the Health Insurance Study, R-2313-HEW*. Santa Monica, CA: Rand Corporation.

Eisen M, Ware JE, Donald CE, Brook RH (1979). "Measuring components of children's health status." *Med Care*: 17 (9), 902–21.

Eisenberg JM, Kitz DS (1986). "Savings from outpatient antibiotic therapy for osteomyelitis: economic analysis of a therapeutic strategy." *JAMA*: 255 (12), 1584–88.

Eisenberg JM, Glick H, Hillman AL, Baron J, Finkler SA, Hershey JC, Lavazzo-Mourey R, Buzby GP (1988). "Measuring the economic impact of perioperative total parenteral nutrition: principles and design." *Am J Clin Nutr*: 47, 382–91.

Ellison GW (1983). "Spiritual well-being: conceptualization and measurement." *J Psychol Theol*: 11 (4), 330–40.

Ellwood P (1990). *Outcomes management system*. Excelsior, MN: Interstudy.

Elster J (1991). "Local justice and interpersonal comparisons." In *Interpersonal comparisons of well-being*. Elster J Roemer JE, eds. New York: Cambridge University Press.

Employee Benefit Research Institute (1992). EBRI Issue Brief 123.

Epstein AM, Hall JA, Tognetti J, Son LH, Conant L (1989). "Using proxies to evaluate quality of life: can they provide information about patients' health status and satisfaction with medical care?" *Med Care*: 27 (3), S91–98.

Epstein KA, Schneiderman LJ, Bush JW, Zettner A (1981). "The 'adnormal' screening serum thyroxine (T4): analysis of physician response, outcome, cost and health effectiveness." *J Chronic Dis*: 34 (5), 175–90.

Erickson P, Golden PM (1991). "Defining the disparities: old and new measures." Working Paper, National Center for Health Statistics.

Erickson P, Anderson JP, Kendall EA, Kaplan RM, Ganiats T (1988). "Using retrospective data for measuring quality of life: National Health Interview Survey and the Quality of Well-Being Scale." *Qual Life Cardiovasc Care*: 4 (4), 179–84.

Erickson PE, Kendall EA, Anderson JP, Kaplan RM (1989). "Using composite health status measures to assess the nation's health." *Med Care*: 27 (3 suppl), S66–S76.

EuroQol Group (1990). "EuroQol—a new facility for the measurement of health-related quality of life." *Health Policy:* 16, 199–208.

Evans RG, Stoddart GL (1990). "Producing health, consuming health care." *Soc Sci Med*: 31(12), 1347–63.

Evans RW, Manninen DL, Garrison LP, Hart LG, Blagg CR, Gutman RA, Hull AR, Lowrie EG (1985). "The quality of life of patients with end-stage renal disease." *N Engl J Med* 312 (9), 553–59.

Evans RW, Rader B, Manninen DL, The Cooperative Multicenter EPO Clinical Trial Group (1990). "The quality of life of hemodialysis recipients treated with recombinant human erythropoietin." *JAMA*: 263 (6), 825–30.

Fabrega H (1974). *Disease and social behavior: an interdisciplinary perspective*. Cambridge: Massachusetts Institute of Technology Press.

Fairbank J, Couper J, Davies JB, O'Brien JP (1980). "The Oswestry low back pain disability questionnaire." *Physiotherapy*: 66 (8), 271–73.

Fallowfield L (1990). *The quality of life: the missing measurement in health care*. London: Souvenir Press.

Fanshel S, Bush JW (1970). "A health-status index and its application to health-services outcomes." *Oper Res*: 18 (6), 1021–66.

Fazio AF (1977). "A concurrent validational study of the NCHS General Well Being Schedule." *Vital Health Stat:* ser. 2 (73).

Feeny D, Guyatt G, Patrick D eds. (1991). "Proceedings of the international conference on the measurement of quality of life as an outcome in clinical trials." *Controlled Clinical Trials: Design, Methods, and Analysis* 12 (4), 1S–280S.

Feinstein AR, Josephy BR, Wells CK (1986). "Scientific and clinical problems in indexes of functional disability." *Ann Intern Med*: 105 (3), 413–20.

Feldstein PJ (1988). *Health care economics,* 3rd ed. New York: Wiley.

Fienberg SE, Loftus EF, Tanur JM (1985). "Cognitive aspects of health survey methodology: an overview." *Milbank Mem Fund Q*: 63 (3), 547–64.

Fink AL (1985). "Social Dependency and Self Care Agency: a descriptive-correlational study of ALS patients." Master of Nursing Thesis, University of Washington.

Fink R (1989). "Issues and problems in measuring children's health status in community health research." *Soc Sci Med*: 29 (6), 715–19.

Finkler SA (1982). "The distinction between costs and charges." *Ann Intern Med*: 96, 102–9.

Fischer GW (1979). "Utility models for multiple objective decisions: do they accurately represent human preferences?" *Decis Sci*: 10, 451–79.

Fletcher RH, Fletcher SW, Wagner EH (1982). *Clinical epidemiology: the essentials*. Baltimore: Williams and Wilkins.

Fogerty International Center for Advanced Study in the Health Sciences (1976). *Preventive Medicine, USA*. New York: Prodist.

Foley JD (1991). Uninsured in the United States: the non-elderly population without health insurance. In *Current population survey*. Washington DC: Employee Benefit Research Institute.

Folkman S, Lazarus RS, Dunkel-Schetter C, DeLongis A, Given RJ (1986). "The dynamics of a stressful encounter: cognitive appraisal, coping, and encounter outcomes." *J Pers Soc Psychol*: 50, 992–1003.

Follick MJ, Smith TW, Ahern DK (1985). "The Sickness Impact Profile: a global measure of disability in chronic low back pain." *Pain*: 21, 67–76.

Folstein MF, Folstein SE, McHugh PR (1975). "Mini-mental state. A practical method for grading the cognitive state of patients for the clinician." *J Psychiatr Res*: 12 (3), 189–98.

Fowler FJ, Mangione TW (1990). *Standardized survey interviewing*. Newbury Park, CA: Sage Publications.

Fowler FJ, Wennberg JE, Timothy RP, Barry MJ, Mulley AG, Hanley D (1988). "Symptom status and quality of life following prostatectomy." *JAMA*: 259 (20), 3018–22.

Frank-Stromborg MF (1988). *Instruments for clinical nursing research*. Norwalk, CT: Appleton & Lange.

Frankenburg WK, Camp BW, eds. (1975). *Pediatric screening tests*. Springfield, IL: Charles C Thomas.

Frankenburg WK, Dodds JB (1967). "The Denver Developmental Screening Test." *J Pediatr*: 171, 181–91.

Frankl V (1990). "Facing the transitoriness of human existence." *Generations*: Fall, 7–10.

Freud S (1920). *A general introduction to psychoanalysis*. New York: Liveright.

Freyd M (1923). "The graphic rating scale." *J Educ Psychol:* 14, 83–102.

Fries JF, Spitz PW, Young DY (1982). "The dimensions of health outcomes: the Health Assessment Questionnaire, disability and pain scales." *J Rheumatol*: 9 (5), 789–93.

Fries JF, Spitz P, Kraines RG, Holman HR (1980). "Measurement of patient outcome in arthritis." *Arthritis Rheum*: 23 (2), 137–45.

Froberg DG, Kane RL (1989a). "Methodology for measuring health-state preferences. I. Measurement strategies." *J Clin Epidemiol*: 42 (4), 345–54.

Froberg DG, Kane RL (1989b). "Methodology for measuring health-state preferences. II. Scaling methods." *J Clin Epidemiol*: 42 (5), 459–71.

Froberg DG, Kane RL (1989c). "Methodology for measuring health-state preferences. III. Population and context effects." *J Clin Epidemiol*: 42 (6), 585–92.

Froberg DG, Kane RL (1989d). "Methodology for measuring health-state preferences. IV. Progress and a research agenda." *J Clin Epidemiol*: 42 (7), 675–85.

Fromm E (1979). The nature of hypnosis and other altered states of consciousness: an ego-psychological theory. In *Hypnosis: developments in research and new perspectives*. Fromm E, Shor RE, eds. New York: Aldine.

Fuchs VR (1974). *Who shall live? Health, economics, and social choice*. New York: Basic Books.

Furlong W, Feeny D, Torrance GW, Barr R, Horsman J (1990). *Guide to design and development of health-state utility instrumentation*. Hamilton, Ontario: McMaster University. CHEPA working paper series 90–9.

Ganiats TG, Humphrey JDC, Tares HL, Kaplan RM (1991). "Routine neonatal circumcision: a cost-utility analysis." *Med Decision Making:* 11, 282–93.

Ganz PA, Schag CA, Cheng HL (1990). "Assessing the quality of life: a study in newly-diagnosed breast cancer patients." *J Clin Epidemiol*: 43 (1), 75–86.

Garber AM, Littenberg B, Sox HC, Gluck ME, Wagner JL, Duffy BM (1989). *Costs and effectiveness of cholesterol screening in the elderly*. Washington DC: U.S. Congress, Office of Technology Assessment.

Garland M, Hasmain R (1990). "Health care in common: setting priorities in Oregon." *Hastings Center Rep*: 20 (5), 16–18.

Garrison LP, Evans RW, Mannien DL (1983). *Labor force participation among end-stage renal disease patients: results from the National Kidney Dialysis and Kidney Transplantation Study*. Seattle: Battelle Human Affairs Research Centers.

Gell C, Elinson J (1969). "The Washington Heights Master Sample Survey." *Milbank Mem Fund Q*: 47, 13–301.

General Accounting Office (1991). *Health insurance: a profile of the uninsured in selected states*. Washington DC: U.S. General Accounting Office.

George LK (1981). Subjective well-being: conceptual and methodological issues. In *Annual review of gerontology geriatrics*. Eisdorfer C, ed. New York: Springer, J45–J82.

George LK, Bearon LB (1980). *Quality of life in older persons*. New York: Human Sciences Press.

George LK, Fillenbaum GG (1985). "OARS methodology: A decade of experience in geriatric assessment." *J Am Geriatr Soc:* 33, 607–15.

George LK, Gwyther L (1986). "Caregiver well-being: a multidimensional examination of family caregivers of demented adults." *Gerontologist*: 26, 253–59.

George LK, Landerman R (1984). "Health and subjective well-being: a replicated secondary data analysis." *Int J Aging Hum Dev:* 19, 133–56.

Geronimus AT, Neidert JL, Bound J (1990). "A note on the measurement of hypertension in NHANES." *Am J Public Health*: 80 (12), 1437–42.

Ghoneim MM, Hinrichs JV, O'Hara MW, Mehta MP, Pathak D, Kumar V, Clark CR (1988). "Comparison of psychologic and cognitive functions after general or regional anesthesia." *Anesthesiology*: 69 (4), 507–15.

Gilson BS, Bergner M, Bobbitt R, et al. (1979). *The Sickness Impact Profile: final development and testing 1975–1978*. Seattle: Department of Health Services, School of Public Health, University of Washington. 2 vols.

Gilson BS, Erickson D, Chavez CT, Bobbitt RA, Bergner M, Carter WB (1980). "A Chicano version of the Sickness Impact Profile (SIP): a health care evaluation instrument crosses the language barrier." *Cult Med Psych*: 4, 137–50.

Gilson BS, Gilson J, Bergner M, Bobbitt RA, Kressel S, Pollard WE, Vesselago M (1975). "The Sickness Impact Profile: development of an outcome measure of health care." *Am J Public Health*: 65 (12), 1304–10.

Ginzberg E (1990). "High-tech medicine and rising health care costs." *JAMA:* 263 (13), 1820–22.

Glass GV (1976). "Primary, secondary, and meta-analysis of research." *Educ Res:* 5, 3–8.

Goffman E (1963). *Stigma: notes on the management of spoiled identity*. Englewood Cliffs, NJ: Prentice-Hall.

Goldberg D (1972). *The detection of psychiatric illness by questionnaire*. London: Oxford University Press.

Goldberg DP, Cooper B, Eastwood MR (1970). A standardized psychiatric interview for use in community surveys. *Brit J Prev Soc Med:* 18–23.

Goldberg KC, Hartz AJ, Jacobsen SJ, Krakauer H, Rimm AA (1992). "Racial and community factors influencing coronary artery bypass graft surgery rates for all 1986 Medicare patients." *JAMA:* 267, 1473–77.

Goldberger J, Wheeler GA, Sydenstricker E (1918). "A study of the diet of nonpellagrous and of pellagrous households in textile mill communities in 1916." *JAMA*: 71, 944–99.

Goldman J, Stein CL, Guerry S (1983). *Psychological methods of child assessment*. New York: Brunner/Mazel.

Goldman L, Cook WEF, Mitchell N, Flatley M, Sherman H, Cohn P (1982). "Pitfalls in the serial assessment of cardiac functional status: how a reduction in 'ordinary' activity may reduce the apparent degree of cardiac compromise and give a misleading impression of improvement." *J Chron Dis:* 35, 763–71.

Goldman L, Hashimoto B, Cook EF, Loscalzo A (1981). "Comparative reproducibility and validity of systems for assessing cardiovascular functional class: advantages of a new specific activity scale." *Circulation*: 64 (6), 1227–34.

Good BJ, Good MD (1980). The meaning of symptoms: a cultural hermeneutic model for clinical practice. In *The relevance of social science for medicine*. Eisenberg L, Kleinman A, eds. Dordrecht, Holland: D. Reidel, 165–96.

Goodenough WH (1944). "A technique for scale analysis." *Educ Psychol Meas:* 179–90.

Gramlich EM (1981). *Benefit-cost analysis of government programs*. Englewood Cliffs, NJ: Prentice-Hall.

Green LW, Krueter MW (1991). *Health promotion planning: an educational and environmental approach* (2nd ed.). Mountain View, CA: Mayfield Publishing.

Grogono AW, Woodgate DS (1971). "Index for measuring health." *Lancet:* 2, 1024–26.

Gudex C (1986). *QALYs and their use by the Health Service*. York: Centre for Health Economics, University of York. Discussion paper no. 20.

Gudex C, Kind P (1988). *The QALY toolkit*. York: Centre for Health Economics, University of York. Discussion paper no. 38.

Gundarov IA (1991). "The rose of quality of life." Paper presented at the Conference on Advances in Health Status Assessment held in Washington, D.C., September 12–14, 1991.

Gurin G, Veroff J, Feld S (1960). *Americans view their mental health: a nationwide interview survey: a report to the staff director, Jack E. Ewalt, 1960*. New York: Basic Books.

Gurland BJ, Kuriansky J, Sharpe L, Simon R, Stiller P, Birkett P (1977). "The comprehensive assessment and referral evaluation (CARE): rationale, development and reliability. *Int J Aging Hum Dev:* 8, 9–42.

Gutmann, A (1983). "For and against equal access to health care." *Securing Access to Health Care*, Vol. 2. President's Commission for the Study of Ethical Problems in Medicine and Biomedical and Behavioral Research. Washington, D.C.: Government Printing Office, pp. 51–66.

Guttman LA (1944). "A basis for scaling qualitative data." *Am Sociol Rev:* 91, 139–50.

Guyatt G, Feeny D, Patrick D (1991). "Issues in quality-of-life measurement in clinical trials." *Controlled Clin Trials:* 12 (4 Suppl), 81S–90S.

Guyatt G, Mitchell A, Irvine EJ, Singer J, Williams N, Goodacre R, Tompkins C (1989). "A new measure of health status for clinical trials in inflammatory bowel disease." Gastroenterology: 96 (3), 804–10.

Guyatt GH, Nogradi S, Halcrow S, Singer J, Sullivan MJ, Fallen EL (1989). "Development and testing of a new measure of health status for clinical trials in heart failure." *J Gen Int Med:* 4 (2), 101–07.

Guyatt G, Townsend M, Berman L, Keller J (1987). "A comparison of Likert and Visual Analog scales for measuring change in function." *J Chronic Dis:* 40 (12), 1129–33.

Guyatt G, Walter S, Norman G (1987). "Measuring change over time: assessing the usefulness of evaluative instruments." *J Chronic Dis:* 40 (2), 171–78.

Guyatt GH, Berman LB, Townsend M, Rugsley SO, Chambers LW (1987a). "A measure of quality of life for clinical trials in chronic lung disease." *Thorax:* 42 (10), 773–78.

Guyatt GH, Deyo RA, Charlson M, Levine MN, Mitchell A (1989). "Responsiveness and validity in health status measurement: a clarification." *J Clin Epidemiol:* 42 (5), 403–8.

Guyatt GH, Townsend M, Berman LB (1987b). "Quality of life in patients with chronic airflow limitation." *Br J Dis Chest* 45–54.

Guyatt GH, Veldhuyzen Van Zanten S, Feeny DH, Patrick DL (1989). "Measuring quality of life in clinical trials: a taxonomy and review." *Can Med Assoc J:* 140 (12), 1441–48.

Haber LD (1970). *The epidemiology of disability. 2. The measurement of functional capacity limitations*. Washington DC: Social Security Administration. Research report no. 10.

Hadorn D (1991). "Setting health care priorities in Oregon: cost-effectiveness meets the rule of rescue." *JAMA:* 265, 2218–25.

Haig THB, Scott DA, Wickett LI (1986). "The rational zero point for an illness index with ratio properties." *Med Care:* 24 (2), 113–24.

Halper T (1985). "Life and death in a welfare state: end-stage renal disease in the United Kingdom." *Milbank Mem Fund Q:* 63 (1), 52–93.

Hamilton M (1959). "The assessment of anxiety states by rating." *Br M Med Psychol:* 32, 50–5.

Hamilton M (1960). "A rating scale for depression." *J Neurol Neurosurg Psychiat:* 23, 56–62.

Hamilton M (1967). "Development of a rating scale for primary depressive illness." *Br J Soc Clin Psychol:* 278–296.

Harlan WR, Murt HA, Thomas JW, Lepkowski JM, Gure KE, Parsons PE, Berki SE, Landis JR (1986). *Incidence, utilization, and costs associated with acute respiratory conditions, 1980.* Hyattsville, MD: National Center for Health Statistics. Publication no. (DHHS) 86-20404.

Harlan WR, Murt HA, Thomas JW, Lepkowski JM, Guire KE, Berki SE, Landis JR (1989). *Health care utilizations and costs of adult cardiovascular conditions, United States, 1980.* Hyattsville, MD: National Center for Health Statistics. Publication no. (DHHS) 89-20407.

Harris J (1988). "Life, quality, value and justice." *Health Policy:* 10, 259–66.

Harris RE, Mion LC, Patterson MB, Frengley JD (1987). "Severe illness in older patients: the association between depressive disorders and functional dependency during the recovery phase." *J Am Geriatr Soc:* 36 (10), 890–96.

Hart LG, Evans RW (1987). "The functional status of ESRD patients as measured by the Sickness Impact Profile." *J Chronic Dis:* 40 (suppl 1), 117S–36S.

Hatziandreu EI, Koplan JP, Weinstein MC, Caspersen CJ, Warner KE (1988). "A cost-effectiveness analysis of exercise as a health promotion activity." *Am J Public Health:* 78 (11), 1417–21.

Hedges LV, Olkin I (1985). *Statistical methods for meta-analysis.* Orlando, FL: Academic Press.

Heithoff KA, Lohr KN (1990). *Hip fracture: setting priorities for effectiveness research.* In Report of a study by a committee of the Institute of Medicine. Washington DC: National Academy Press.

Helewa A, Goldsmith CH, Smythe HA, et al. (1982). "Independent measurement of functional capacity in rheumatoid arthritis." *J Rheumatol:* 9 (5), 794–97.

Helmes EM (1988). "Multidimensional observation scale for elderly subjects." *Psycholopharmacol Bull:* 24 (4), 733–45.

Hendricson WD, Russell IJ, Prihoda TJ, Jacobson JM, Rogan A, Bishop GD (1989). "An approach to developing a valid Spanish language translation of a health-status questionnaire." *Med Care:* 27 (10), 959–66.

Hillier FS, Lieberman GJ (1986). *Introduction to operations research,* 4th ed. San Francisco: Holden-Day.

Himmelfarb S, Murrel SA (1983). "Reliability and validity of five mental health scales in older persons." *J Gerontol:* 38 (3), 333–39.

Hobbs N, Perrin JM, Ireys HT (1985). In: *Chronically ill children and their families.* San Francisco: Jossey-Bass, 62–101.

Hochstim JR (1964). *The California Human Population Laboratory for Epidemiologic Studies. Series A, No. 6.* San Francisco: State of California Department of Public Health.

Hodgson TA (1988). "Annual costs of illness versus lifetime costs of illness and implications of structural change." *Drug Inf J:* 22, 323–41.

Hodgson TA (1992). "Cigarette smoking and lifetime medical expenditures." *Milbank Q:* 70 (1): 81–125.

Hodgson TA, Meiners MR (1982). "Cost-of-illness methodology: a guide to current practices and procedures." *Milbank Mem Fund Q:* 60 (3), 429–62.

Hogness J, Van Antwerp M. (1991). *The artificial heart: its development and use*. Washington DC: National Academy Press.

Hollandsworth JG Jr (1988). "Evaluating the impact of medical treatment on the quality of life: a 5-year update." *Soc Sci Med*: 26 (4), 425–34.

Hornquist JO (1982). "The concept of quality of life." *Scand J Soc Med*: 10 (2), 57–61.

Horwood SP, Boyle MH, Torrance GW, Sinclair JC (1982). "Mortality and morbidity of 500- to 1,499-gram birth weight infants live-born to residents of a defined geographic region before and after neonatal intensive care." *Pediatrics*: 69 (5), 613–20.

Hughes CP, Berg L, Danziger WL, Coben LA, Martin RL (1982). "A new clinical scale for the staging of dementia." *Br J Psychiat*: 140, 566–72.

Hunt SM (1986). "Cross-cultural issues in the use of socio-medical indicators." *Health Policy*: 6, 149–58.

Hunt SM, Wiklund I (1987). "Cross-cultural variation in the weighting of health statements: a comparison of English and Swedish valuations." *Health Policy*: 8, 227.

Hunt SM, McEwen J, McKenna SP (1986). *Measuring health status*. London: Croom Helm.

Hunt SM, McKenna SP, McEwen JA (1980). "A quantitative approach to perceived health status: a validation study." *J Epidemiol Community Health*: 34, 281–85.

Hurst JW, Mooney GH (1983). Implicit values in administrative decisions. In *Health indicators: an international study for the European Science Foundation*. Culyer AJ, ed. New York: St. Martin's Press, 174–85.

Hyde E (1989). "Acupressure therapy for morning sickness. A controlled clinical trial." *J Nurse Midwifery*: 34 (4), 171–78.

Hyland ME (1991). "Living with asthma questionnaire." *Respir Med:* 85 (Suppl B), 13-6; 33-7.

IASP Subcommittee on Taxonomy (1979). "Pain terms: a list with definitions and notes on usage." *Pain* 6 (3), 249–52.

Idler EL, Kasl S (1991). "Health perceptions and survival: do global evaluations of health status really predict mortality?" *J Gerontol*: 46 (2), 555–65.

Illich I (1976). *Medical nemesis: the expropriation of health*. New York: Pantheon Books.

Illsley R (1990). "Comparative review of sources, methdology and knowledge." *Soc Sci Med*: 31(3), 229–36.

Institute of Medicine (1978). *Perspectives on health promotion and disease prevention in the United States*. Washington DC: National Academy of Sciences.

Jacoby I (1985). "The consensus development program of the National Institutes of Health." *Int J Technol Assess Health Care*: 1, 420–32.

Jaeschke R, Guyatt GH, Keller J, Singer J (1991). "Interpreting changes in quality-of-life score in *N* or 1 randomized trials." *Controlled Clin Trials:* 12, 226S–33S.

Jaeschke R, Singer J, Guyatt GH (1989). "Measurement of health status. Ascertaining the minimal clinically important difference." *Controlled Clin Trials*: 10 (4), 407–15.

Jahoda M (1958). From ideas to systematic research. In *Current concepts in positive mental health: a report to the staff director, Jack R. Ewalt, 1958*. New York: Basic Books.

Jecker NS, Pearlman RA (1992). "An ethical framework for rationing health care." *J Med Philosophy:* 17, 72–96.

Jenkinson C (1990). "Health status and mood state in a migraine sample." *Int J Soc Psychiat*: 36 (1), 42–48.

Jenkinson C, Fitzpatrick R, Argyle M (1988). "The Nottingham Health Profile: an analysis of its sensitivity in differentiating illness groups." *Soc Sci Med*: 27 (12), 1411–14.

Jennett B, Bond M (1975). "Assessment of outcome after severe brain damage." Lancet 480–484.

Jette AM (1980). "Functional Status Index: reliability of a chronic disease evaluation instrument." *Arch Phys Med Rehab*: 61, 395.

Jette AM, Davies AR, Cleary PD, Calkins DR, Rubenstein LV, Fink A, Kosecoff J, Young RT, Brook RH, Delbanco Tl (1986). "The Functional Status Questionnaire: reliability and validity when used in primary care." *J Gen Intern Med.* 1, 143–49.

Jette AM, Deniston OL (1978). "Inter-observer reliability of a functional status assessment instrument." *J Chronic Dis*: 31, 573–80.

Johnsson M (1988). "Evaluation of the consensus development program in Sweden: its impact on physicians." *Int J Technol Assess Health Care*: 4, 89–94.

Jones FN (1974). History of psychophysics and judgment. In *Handbook of perception, Vol. II: Psychophysical judgment and measurement.* Carterete EC, Friedman MP, eds. New York: Academic Press, 2–22.

Jonsen A (1986). "Bentham in a box: technology assessment and health care allocation." *Law Med Health Care:* 14, 172–4.

Kaasa S, Mastekaasa A, Stokke I, Naess S (1988). "Validation of a quality of life questionnaire for use in clinical trials for treatment of patients with inoperable lung cancer." *Eur J Cancer Clin Oncol*: 24 (4), 691–701.

Kahn RL, Goldfarb AI, Pollack M, Peck A (1960). "Brief objective measures for the determination of mental status in the aged." *Am J Psych*: 117, 326–28.

Kahn S (1982). *A guide for grassroots leaders: organizing.* New York: McGraw-Hill.

Kalton G, Kasprzyk D (1982). Imputing for missing survey responses. In *Proceedings of the ASA survey research section.* Washington DC: American Statistical Association.

Kamlet MS (1992). *A framework for cost-utility analysis of government health care programs.* Washington DC: Department of Health and Human Services, Office of Disease Prevention and Health Promotion.

Kandel ER (1979). "Psychotherapy and the single synapse: the impact of psychiatric thought on neurologic research." *New Engl J Med*: 301 (9), 1028–37.

Kane RL, Kane RA (1981). *Assessing the elderly: a practical guide to measurement.* Lexington, MA: Lexington Books.

Kaplan A (1964). *The conduct of inquiry: methodology for behavioral science.* San Francisco: Chandler.

Kaplan RM (1989). "Health outcome models for policy analysis." *Health Psychol* 8(6), 723–35.

Kaplan RM, Anderson JP (1988). "A general health policy model: update and applications." *Health Serv Res*: 23 (2), 203–35.

Kaplan RM, Bush JW (1982). "Health-related quality of life measurement for evaluation research and policy analysis." *Health Psych*: 1, 61–80.

Kaplan RM, Ernst JA (1983). "Do category rating scales produce biased preference weights for a health index?" *Med Care*: 21 (2), 193–207.

Kaplan RM, Atkins CJ, Timms RM (1984). "Validity of a Quality of Well-Being Scale as an outcome measure in chronic obstructive pulmonary disease." *J Chronic Dis*: 37 (2), 85–95.

Kaplan RM, Atkins CJ, Wilson DK (1988). "The cost-utility of diet and exercise interventions in non-insulin dependent diabetes mellitus." *Health Promotion:* 2 (4), 331–40.

Kaplan RM, Bush JW, Berry CC (1976). "Health status: types of validity and the Index of Well-being." *Health Serv Res*: 11 (4), 478–507.

Kaplan RM, Bush JW, Berry CC (1978). "The reliability, stability, and generalizability of a health status index." In *Proceedings of the American Statistical Association.* Washington, DC: Social Statistics Section, pp. 704–09.

Kaplan RM, Bush JW, Berry CC (1979). "Health Status Index: category rating versus magnitude estimation for measuring levels of well-being." *Med Care*: 17 (5), 501–25.

Kaplan RM, Anderson JP, Wu A, Mathews WC, Kozin F, Orenstein D (1989). "The Quality of Well-Being Scale: applications in AIDS, cystic fibrosis, and arthritis." *Med Care*: 27 (3 suppl), S27–S43.

Karnofsky DA, Burchenal JH (1949). The clinical evaluation of chemotherapeutic agents. In *Evaluation of chemotherapeutic agents*. MacLeod CM, ed. New York: Columbia University Press, 191–94.

Karnofsky DA, Abelmann WH, Burehenal JH, Craver LF (1948). "The use of nitrogen mustards in the palliative treatment of cancer." *Cancer*: 1, 634–56.

Kasl S (1983). Social and psychological factors affecting the course of disease: an epidemiological perspective. In *Handbook of health, health care, and the health professions*. Mechanic D, ed. New York: Free Press, 683–708.

Katz S (1987). "The Portugal conference: measuring quality of life and functional status in clinical and epidemiological research." *J Chronic Dis:* 40 (6), 459–650.

Katz S, Akpom CA (1976). "A measure of primary sociobiological functions." *Int J Health Serv:* 6, 493–507.

Katz S, Ford AB, Moskowitz RW (1963). "The Index of ADL: a standardized measure of biological and psychosocial function." *JAMA*: 185 (12), 914–19.

Katz S, Branch LG, Branson MH, Papsidero JA, Beck JC, Greer DS (1983). "Active life expectancy." *New Engl J Med*: 309 (20), 1218–24.

Katzman R, Brown T, Thal L, Fuld P, Aronson M, Butters N, Klauber M, Wiederholt W, Pay M, Renbing X, Ooi W, Hofstetter R, Terry R (1988). "Comparison of rate of annual change of mental status score in four independent studies of patients with Alzheimer's disease. *Ann Neurol:* 24 (3), 384–89.

Kawachi I (1989). "QALYs and justice." *Health Policy:* 13 (2), 115–20.

Kazis LE, Anderson JJ, Meenan RF (1989). "Effect sizes for interpreting changes in health status." *Med Care*: 27 (3 suppl), S178–S189.

Keeney R, Raiffa H (1976). *Decisions with multiple objectives: preferences and value tradeoffs*. New York: Wiley.

Kellner R, Sheffield B. (1973). "A self-rating scale of distress." *Psychol Med*: 3, 88–100.

Kind P, Rosser R, Williams A (1982). "Valuation of quality of life: some psychometric evidence." In *The value of life and safety*. Jones-Lee MW, ed. Amsterdam: North Holland, 159–70.

Kirschner B, Guyatt G (1985). "A methodological framework for assessing health indices." *J Chronic Dis*: 38 (1), 27–36.

Kitzhaber J (1989). *The Oregon Basic Health Services Act (SB-27)*. Salem, Oregon.

Kleinman A, Eisenberg L, Good B (1978). "Culture, illness and care: clinical lessons from anthropologic and cross-cultural research." *Ann Int Med*: 88, 251–58.

Kleinman JC (1977). "Age-adjusted mortality indexes for small areas: applications to health planning." *Am J Public Health*: 67 (9), 834–40.

Kluckhohn CK (1951). Values and value orientations in the theory of action. In *Toward a general theory of action*. Parsons T, Shils EA, eds. Cambridge, MA: Harvard University Press.

Knobloch H, Stevens F, Malone AF (1980). *Manual of developmental diagnosis: the administration and interpretation of the revised Gesell and Amatruda developmental and neurologic examination*. Hagerstown, MD: Harper and Row.

Kobasa S (1979). "Stressful life events, personality, and health: an inquiry into hardiness." *J Pers Soc Psychol*: 37, 1–11.

Kovar MG (1989). "Data systems of the National Center for Health Statistics." *Vital Health Stat:* 1 (23), 1–21.

Kozma A, Stones MJ (1989). "The measurement of happiness: development of the Memorial University of Newfoundland Scale of Happiness (MUNSH)." *J Gerontology:* 35, 906–12.

Kroenke K, Wood DR, Mangelsdorff AD, Meier NJ, Powell JB (1988). "Chronic fatigue in primary care: prevalence, patient characteristics, and outcome." *JAMA*: 260 (7), 929–34.

Kuriansky JB, Gurland B (1976). "Performance test of activities of daily living." *Int J Aging Hum Dev:* 7 343–52.

Kurtzke JF (1983). "Rating neurologic impairment in multiple sclerosis: an expanded disability status scale (EDSS). *Neurology:* 33, 1444–53.

LaPlante MP (1988). *Data on disability from the National Health Interview Survey, 1983–1985.* Washington, DC: National Institute on Disability and Rehabilitation Research.

La Puma J, Lawlor EF (1990). "Quality-Adjusted Life Years: ethical implications for physicians and policymakers." *JAMA:* 263 (21), 2917–21.

LaCroix AZ (1987). "Determinants of health: exercise and activities of daily living." In *Health statistics on older persons, United States, 1986. Vital and Health Stat:* 3 (25), 41–55.

Laird N, Mosteller F (1990). "Some statistical methods for combining experimental results." *Int J Technol Assess Health Care:* 6, 5–30.

Lalonde M (1974). *A new perspective on the health of Canadians.* Ottawa: Government of Canada.

Land KC, Spilerman S (1975). *Social indicator models: an overview.* New York: Russell Sage Foundation.

Lara ME, Goodman C, eds. (1990). *National priorities for the assessment of clinical conditions and medical technologies: report of a pilot study.* Washington DC: National Academy Press.

Lawrence PS (1976). "The health record of the American people." In *Health in America: 1776–1976.* Washington DC: U.S. Government Printing Office, 16–36.

Lawton MP (1972). Assessing the competence of older people. In *Research Planning and Action for the Elderly.* Kent DP, Kastenbaum R, Sherwood S, eds. New York: Behavioral Publications, 122–43.

Lawton MP, Brody EM (1969). "Assessment of older people: self-maintaining and instrumental activities of daily living." *Gerontologist:* 9, 179–86.

Levin BW (1990). "International perspectives of treatment choice in neonatal intensive care unit." *Soc Sci Med:* 30 (8), 901–12.

Levine MN, Guyatt GH, Gent M, De Pauw S, Goodyear MD, Hryniuk WM, Arnold A, Findlay B, Skillings JR, Bramwell VH (1988). "Quality of life in stage II breast cancer: an instrument for clinical trials." *J Clin Oncol:* 6 (12), 1798–810.

Levine S, Croog SH (1984). "The primary care physician and the patient's quality of life." *Qual Life Cardiovasc Care:* 1, 29–36.

Levine S, Croog SH, Sudilovsky A, Testa MA (1988). "Antihypertensive therapy and life satisfaction." *Qual Life Cardiovasc Care:* 5–19.

Levine S, Elinson J, Feldman J (1983). Does medical care do any good? In *Handbook of health, health care and the health professions.* Mechanic DM, ed. New York: Free Press, 394–406.

Levit KR, Lazenby HC, Letsch SW, Cowan CA (1991a). "National health care spending, 1989." *Health Affairs:* 10 (1), 117–30.

Levit KR, Lazenby HC, Cowan CA, Letsch SW (1991b). "National health expenditures." *Health Care Financ Rev:* 13(1), 29–54.

Lewis CC, Pantell RH, Kieckhefer GM (1989). "Assessment of children's health status: field test of new approaches." *Med Care:* 27 (3 suppl), S54–S65.

Liang MH, Larson MG, Cullen KE, Schwartz JA (1985). "Comparative measurement efficiency and sensitivity of five health status instruments for arthritis research." *Arthritis Rheum:* 28, 542–47.

Liang MH, Cullen KE, Larson MG, Thompson MS, Schwartz JA, Fossell AH, Roberts WN, Sledge CB (1986). "Cost-effectiveness of total joint arthroplasty in osteoarthritis." *Arthritis Rheum.:* 29 (8), 937–43.

Light RJ, Pillemer DB (1984). *Summing up: the science of reviewing research*. Cambridge, MA: Harvard University Press.

Likert R (1932). "A technique for the measurement of attitudes." *Arch Psychol*: 140.

Linder FE (1966). "The health of the American people." *Sci Am*: 214 (6), 21–29.

Lipscomb J (1982). Value preferences for health: meaning, measurement, and uses in program evaluation. In *Values and long term care*. Kane RL, Kane RA, eds. Lexington, MA: Lexington Books, 27–84.

Lipscomb J (1989). "Time preference for health in cost-effectiveness analysis." *Med Care*: 27 (3 suppl), S233–S254.

Liu K, Manton KG (1989). "The effect of nursing home use on Medicaid eligibility." *Gerontologist:* 29(1), 59–66.

Llewellyn-Thomas H, Sutherland HJ, Tibshirani R, Ciampi A, Till JE, Boyd NF (1982). "The measurement of patients' values in medicine." *Med Decis Making*: 2 (4), 449–62.

Llewellyn-Thomas H, Sutherland HJ, Tibshirani AC, Ciampi A, Till JE, Boyd NF (1984). "Describing health states: methodologic issues in obtaining values for health states." *Med Care*: 22 (6), 543–53.

Lohr K (ed.) (1992). "Advances in health status assessment: conference proceedings." *Med Care* 30 (5 suppl), 1–293.

Lohr KN (1989). "Advances in health status assessment: overview of the conference." *Med Care*: 27 (3 suppl), 51–11.

Lohr KN, Ware JE (1987). "Proceedings of the advances in health assessment conference, Palm Springs, California, 19–21 February 1986." *J Chronic Dis:* 40 (suppl 1).

Lonner WJ, Berry JW (1986). *Field methods in cross-cultural research*. Beverly Hills, CA: Sage Publications.

Luce BR, Elixhauser A (1990a). "Estimating costs in the economic evaluation of medical technologies." *Int J Technol Assess Health Care*: 6, 57–75.

Luce BR, Elixhauser A (1990b). *Standards for socioeconomic evaluation of health care products and services*. Berlin: Springer-Verlag.

Lundin AP, Delano BG, Quinn-Cefaro R (1990). "Perspectives on the improvement of quality of life with epoetin alpha therapy." *Pharmacotherapy*: 10 (2 Part 2), 22S–26S.

MacKenzie CR, Charlson ME, DiGioia D, Kelley K (1986). "A patient-specific measure of change in maximal function." *Arch Intern Med*: 146 (7), 1325–29.

Madans JH, Kleinman JC, Cox CS, Barbano HE, Feldman JJ, Cohen B, Finucane FF, Cornoni-Huntley J (1986). "Ten years after NHANES I: report of initial followup, 1982–84." *Public Health Rep*: 101 (5), 465–73.

Magaziner J, Simonsick EM, Kashner TM, Hebel JR (1988). "Patient-proxy response comparability on measures of patient health and functional status." *J Clin Epidemiol:* 41 (11), 1065–74.

Mahler DA, Weinberg DH, Wells CK, Feinstein AR (1984). "The measurement of dyspnea: contents, interobserver agreement, and physiologic correlates of two new clinical indexes." *Chest*: 85 (6), 751–58.

Mahoney FI, Barthel DW (1965). "Functional evaluation: the Barthel Index." *Md State Med J*: 14, 61–65.

Manton KG (1987). "Forecasting health status changes in an aging U.S. population: assessment of the current status and some proposals." *Clim Change*: 11 (1/2), 179–210.

Manton KG (1988). *Chronic disease modelling*. New York: Oxford University Press.

Manton KG (1989). "Epidemiological, demographic, and social correlates of disability among the elderly." *Milbank Q:* 67 (suppl 2, pt 1), 13–58.

Manton KG, Soldo BJ (1985). "Dynamics of health changes in the oldest old: new perspectives and evidence." *Milbank Mem Fund Q Health Soc:* 63(2), 206–85.

Marzen TJ, Avila D (1991). Correspondence between the National Legal Center for the Medically Dependent and Disabled, Inc., and the Honorable Christopher H. Smith, United States Representative in Congress, December 5, 1991.

Maslow AH (1943). "A theory of human motivation." *Psychol Rev*: 50, 370–96.

Matarazzo JD, Weiss SM, Herd JA, Miller NA, Weiss SM, eds. (1984). *Behavioral health: a handbook of health enhancement and disease prevention.* New York: Wiley.

McCorkle R, Young K (1978). "Development of a symptom distress scale." *Cancer Nurs:* 1, 373–78.

McDowell AJ, Engel A, Massey JT, Maurer K (1981). Plan and operation of the second National Health and Nutrition Examination Survey. *Vital Health Statistics.* Series 1, No. 15.

McDowell I, Newell C (1987). *Measuring health: a guide to rating scales and questionnaires.* New York: Oxford University Press.

McKeown T (1976). *The role of medicine: dream, mirage, or nemesis?* Princeton, NJ: Princeton University Press.

McLean A, Dikmen S, Temkin N, Wyler AR, Gale JL (1984). "Psychosocial functioning at 1 month after head injury." *Neurosurgery*: 14 (4), 393–99.

McNair DM, Lorr M, Droppleman LF (1981). *EITS Manual for the Profile of Mood States.* San Diego, CA: Educational and Industrial Testing Service.

Meenan RF (1982). "The AIMS approach to health status measurement: conceptual background and measurement properties." *J Rheumatol*: 9 (5), 785–88.

Meenan RF, Gertman PM, Mason JM (1980). "Measuring health status in arthritis: the Arthritis Impact Measurement Scales." *Arthritis Rheum:* 23 (2), 146–52.

Meenan RF, Gertman PM, Mason JH, Dunaif R (1982). "The arthritis impact measurement scales: further investigators of a health status measure." *Arthritis Rheum*: 25 (9), 1048–53.

Meenan RF, Mason JH, Anderson JJ, Guccione AA, Kazis LE (1992). "AIMS2. The content and properties of a revised and expanded Arthritis Impact Measurement Scales Health Status Questionnaire." *Arthritis Rheum:* 1–10.

Mehrez A, Gafni A (1989). "Quality-adjusted life years, utility theory, and healthy-years equivalent." *Med Decis Making*: 9 (2), 142–49.

Merton R (1968). *Social theory and social structure,* enlarged ed. New York: Free Press.

Miller DL, Alderslade R, Ross EM (1982) "Whooping cough vaccine: the risks and benefits debate." *Epidemiol Rev:* 4, 1–23.

Miller GA (1956). "The magical number seven plus or minus two: some limits on our capacity to process information." *Psychol Rev*: 63, 81–97.

Miller J (1970). "An indicator to aid management in assigning program priorities." *Public Health Rep*: 85 (8), 725–31.

Millman M (ed.) (1992). *Access to Personal Health Services: Report of the IOM Committee on the Monitoring of Access to Personal Health Care Services.* Washington, D.C.: National Academy Press.

Million R, Hall W, Nilsen K, Baker R, Jayson M (1982). "Assessment of the progress of the back-pain patient." *Spine*: 7 (3), 204–12.

Mills CW (1959). *The sociological imagination.* New York: Grove Press.

Mitchell BD, Stern MP, Haffner SM, Hazuda HP, Patterson JK (1990). "Functional impairment in Mexican Americans and non-Hispanic whites with diabetes." *J Clin Epidemiol*: 43 (4), 319–27.

Monks J (1988). "Interpretation of subjective measures in a clinical trial of hyperbaric oxygen therapy for multiple sclerosis." *J Psychosom Res*: 32 (4–5), 365–72.

Moore JT (1978). "Functional disability of geriatric patients in a family medicine program: implications for patient care, education and research." *J Fam Pract*: 7 (6), 1159–66.

Moos R (1977). *Coping with physical illness*. New York: Plenum.

Morell V (1990). "Oregon puts bold health plan on ice." *Science*: 249, 268–71.

Morgan M (1989). "Social ties, support, and well-being." In: *Disablement in the Community*, Patrick DL and Hedley P, eds. Oxford: Oxford Medical Publications, 152–175.

Moriyama IM (1968). Problems in the measurement of health status. In *Indicators of social change*. Sheldon EB, Moore WE, eds. New York: Russell Sage Foundation, 573–600.

Morrow GR (1984). "The assessment of nausea and vomiting: past problems, current issues, and suggestions for future research." *Cancer*: (suppl), 2267.

Mossey J, Shapiro E (1982). "Self-rated health: a predictor of mortality among the elderly." *Am J Public Health*: 72(6), 800–809.

Moyer EM (1989). "A revised look at the number of uninsured Americans." *Health Aff*: 8 (2), 102–10.

Mullen B (1989). *Advanced BASIC meta-analysis*. Hillsdale, NJ: Lawrence Erlbaum Associates.

Mulley AG (1990). "Supporting the patient's role in decision making." *J Occup Med*: 32, 1227–28.

Mulley AG Jr (1989). "Assessing patients' utilities: can the ends justify the means?" *Med Care*: 27 (3 suppl), S269–S281.

Najman JM, Levine S (1981). "Evaluating the impact of medical care and technologies on quality of life: a review and critique." *Soc Sci Med*: 15F, 107–15.

National Center for Health Statistics (1962–90). *Vital statistics of the United States. Vol. II—Mortality, Part B*. Washington DC: U.S. Government Printing Office.

National Center for Health Statistics (1970). *Current estimates from the Health Interview Survey: United States 1968*. Washington DC.: National Center for Health Statistics. Public Health Service Pub. no. 1000, ser. 10, no. 63.

National Center for Health Statistics (1973–91). "Current estimates from the National Health Interview Survey: United States." *Vital and Health Statistics*. Washington DC: U.S. Government Printing Office.

National Center for Health Statistics (1980–88). "Detailed diagnosis and procedures, National Hospital Discharge Survey." *Vital and Health Statistics*. Washington DC: U.S. Government Printing Office.

National Center for Health Statistics (1979). A reason for visit classification for ambulatory care. *Vital Health Stat*: 78.

National Center for Health Statistics (1983). *Health: United States and prevention profile, 1983*. Hyattsville, MD: Department of Health and Human Services. DHHS Pub. no. (PHS) 84-1232.

National Center for Health Statistics (1985). *United States life tables. U.S. decennial life tables for 1979–1981*. Washington DC: U.S. Government Printing Office. DHHS Pub. no. (PHS) 85-1150-1.

National Center for Health Statistics (1986). *Health: United States and prevention profile, 1986*. Washington DC: United States Department of Health and Human Services. DHHS Pub. no. (PHS) 87-1232.

National Center for Health Statistics (1988a). *Health, United States, 1987*. Hyattsville, MD: Department of Health, Education and Welfare. DHHS Pub. no. (PHS) 88-1232.

National Center for Health Statistics (1988b). *Vital statistics of the United States. Vol. II—Mortality*. Washington DC: U.S. Government Printing Office.

National Center for Health Statistics (1989). *Health, United States: 1988*. Washington DC: U.S. Government Printing Office. Publication no. (PHS) 89-1232.

National Center for Health Statistics (1990). *Health, United States, 1989*. Hyattsville, MD: Department of Health, Education and Welfare. DHHS Pub. no. (PHS) 90-1232).

National Center for Health Statistics (1991a). *Health, United States, 1990*. Hyattsville, MD: Department of Health and Human Services. DHHS Pub. no. (PHS) 91-1232.

National Center for Health Statistics (1991b). *Vital statistics of the United States, 1988. Vol.II. Sec. 6, life tables.* Washington DC: Public Health Service.

National Center for Health Statistics (1992). "Advance report of final mortality statistics, 1989." *Monthly Vital Statistics Report:* 40 (8), Supplement 2.

National Health Interview Survey (1990). Unpublished data, personal communication.

National Opinion Research Center (1991). *General social surveys, 1972–1991: cumulative codebook.* Chicago: National Opinion Research Center, University of Chicago.

Nelson EC, Landgraf JM, Hays RD, Wasson JH, Kirk JW (1990). "The functional status of patients: how can it be measured in physicians' offices?" *Med Care:* 28 (12), 1111–26.

Neugarten BL, Havighurst RJ, Tobin SS (1961). "The measurement of life satisfaction." *J Gerontol:* 16, 134–43.

Newhouse JP (1974). "A design for a health insurance experiment." *Inquiry:* 11, 5–27.

Newman SC (1988). "A Markov process of interpretation of Sullivan's index of morbidity and mortality." *Stat Med:* 7 (7), 787–94.

Nissinen A, Tuomilehto J, Kottke TE, Puska P (1986). "Cost-effectiveness of the North Karelia Hypertension Program. 1972–1977." *Med Care:* 24 (8), 767–80.

Nocturnal Oxygen Therapy Trial Group (1980). "Continuous or nocturnal oxygen therapy in bypoxemic chronic obstructive lung disease." *Ann Intern Med:* 93 (3), 391–98.

Nord E (1991). "EuroQol: health-related quality of life measurement. Valuations of health states by the general public in Norway." *Health Policy:* 18, 25–36.

Nozick R (1974). *Anarchy, state and utopia.* New York: Basic Books.

Nunnally JC (1978). *Psychometric theory,* 2nd ed. New York: McGraw-Hill.

O'Brien BJ, Banner NR, Gibson S, Yacoub MH (1988). "The Nottingham Health Profile as a measure of quality of life following combined heart and lung transplantation." *J Epidemiol Community Health:* 42 (3), 232–34.

O'Brien BJ, Buxton MJ, Ferguson BA (1987). "Measuring the effectiveness of heart transplant programmes: quality of life data and their relationship to survival analysis." *J Chron Dis:* 40 (Supp.), 137S–153S.

O'Donnell M (1986). "One man's burden." *Br Med J:* 293, 59.

O'Dowd TC, Pill R, Smail JE, Davis RH (1986). "Irritable urethral syndrome: follow up study in general practice." *Br Med J Clin Res:* 292 (6512), 30–32.

Office of National Cost Estimates (1990). "National health expenditures, 1988." *Health Care Financ Rev:* 11 (4), 1–54.

Office of Technology Assessment (OTA) (1981). *Cost effectiveness of influenza vaccination.* Washington DC: U.S. Government Printing Office.

Office of Technology Assessment (OTA) (1985). *Abstracts of case studies in the health technology case study series.* Washington DC: U.S. Government Printing Office.

Office of Technology Assessment (OTA) (1986). *Assessment activities.* Washington DC: U.S. Government Printing Office.

Office of Technology Assessment (OTA) (1987). *Neonatal intensive care for low birthweight infants: costs and effectiveness.* Washington DC: U.S. Government Printing Office.

Office of Technology Assessment (1990). *Preventive health services for medicare beneficiaries: policy and research issues.* Washington DC: U.S. Government Printing Office.

Office of Technology Assessment (1992). *Evaluation of the Oregon Medicaid proposal.* Washington DC: U.S. Government Printing Office, Publication no. OTA-H-532.

Olafsson K, Korner A, Bille A, Jensen HV, Thiesen S, Andersoon J (1989). "The GBS scale in multi-infarct dementia and senile dementia of Alzheimer type." *Acta Psychiatr Scand:* 79, 94–97.

Oldridge N, Guyatt G, Jones N, Crowe J, Singer J, Feeny D, McKelvie R, Runions J, Streiner D, Torrance G (1991). "Effects on quality of life with comprehensive rehabilitation after acute myocardial infraction." *Am J Cardiology:* 67 (13): 1084–1089.

Olson M (1965). *The logic of collective action*. Cambridge, MA: Harvard University Press.

Olson M, Bailey MJ (1981). "Positive time preference." *J Polit Econ:* 89 (1), 1–25.

Ontario Ministry of Health (1990). "An overview of the survey content of the Ontario Health Survey." *Ontario Health Survey Bulletin,* February 1990.

Oregon Health Decisions (1988). *Quality of life in allocating health care resources: Principles adopted by the Citizens' Health Care Parliament*. Portland: Oregon Health Decisions.

Oregon Health Services Commission (1990a). "Preliminary list of cost-utility ratios: test computer run." Salem, OR: Health Services Commission.

Oregon Health Services Commisssion (1990b). *Preliminary rank ordering of health services*. Salem: Health Services Commission.

Oregon Health Services Commission (1991). *Prioritization of health services: a report to the governor and legislature*. Salem: Oregon Health Services Commission.

Organic HN, Goldstein S (1970). The Brown University, Rhode Island, Population Laboratory: its purposes and initial progress. In *The community as an epidemiologic laboratory: a casebook of community studies*. Kessler II, Levin ML, eds. Baltimore, MD: Johns Hopkins Press.

Oster G, Huse DM, Delea TE, Colditz GA (1986). "Cost-effectiveness of nicotine gum as an adjunct to physician's advice against cigarette smoking." *JAMA:* 256 (10), 1315–18.

Ott CR, Sivarajan ES, Newton KM, Almes M, Bruce RA, Bergner M, Gilson G (1983). "A controlled randomized study of early cardiac rehabilitation: the Sickness Impact Profile as an assessment tool." *Heart Lung:* 12 (2), 162–70.

Ouweneel P, Veenhoven R (1989). "Cross national differences in happiness: cultural bias or societal quality?" Paper presented at the Regional Congress for Cross Cultural Psychology, Amsterdam, June 1989. Unpublished manuscript, Rotterdam, Erasmus Universiteit.

Overall JE, Gorham DR (1962). "The Brief Psychiatric Rating Scale." *Psychol Rep:* 10, 799–802.

Paffenbarger RS, Hyde RT, Wing AL, Hsieh CC (1986). "Physical activity, all-cause mortality, and longevity of college alumni." *New Engl J Med:* 314, 605–13.

Parducci A (1974). Contextual effects: a range of frequency analysis. In *Handbook of perception, Vol. II: Psychophysical judgment and measurement*. Carterette E, Friedman M, eds. New York: Academic Press, 127–41.

Pareto V (1917). *Traite de sociologie generale*. Boven P, ed. Lausanne: Payot et Cie. Cited in Parsons, T. (1937). *The structure of social action, Vol. 1*. New York: Free Press, 241–49.

Paringer L, Berk A (1977). *Costs of illness and disease fiscal year 1975. Report 2*. Washington DC: Georgetown University.

Parkerson GE, Gehlbach SW, Wagner EH, James SA, Clapp NE, Muhlbuier LH (1981). "The Duke–UNC Health Profile: an adult health status instrument for primary care." *Med Care:* 19, 806–28.

Parr G, Darekar B, Fletcher A, Bulpitt CJ (1989). "Joint pain and quality of life: results of a randomized trial." *Br J Clin Pharmacol:* 27 (2), 235–42.

Parsons T (1951). *The social system*. Glencoe, IL: Free Press.

Parsons T (1958). Definition of health and illness in the light of American values and social structure. In *Patients, physicians, and illness: a sourcebook in behavioral science and health*. Gartly JE, ed. New York: Free Press, 165–87.

Pashos CL, McNeil BJ (1990). "Consequences of variation in treatment for acute myocardial infarction." *Health Serv Res:* 25 (5), 718–22.

Paterson M (1984). Measuring the socio-economic benefits of auranofin. In *Measuring the social benefits of medicine*. Teeling-Smith G, ed. London: Office of Health Economics, 97–111.

Patrick D (1984). Quality of life measures for assessing disablement. In *Assessment of quality of life in clinical trials of cardiovascular therapies*. Wenger NK, Mattson ME, Furbert CD, Elinson J, eds. New York: LeJacq, 232–41.

Patrick D (1985). Sociological investigations. In *Oxford textbook of public health*, Vol. 3. Holland W, Knox G, Detels R, eds. New York: Oxford University Press, 189–206.

Patrick D, Green S, Locker D, Darby S, Wiggins D, Horton G (1981). "Screening for disability in the inner city." *J Epidemiol Community Health*: 35 (1), 65–70.

Patrick D, Sittampalam Y, Somerville S, Carter WB, Bergner M (1985). "A crosscultural comparison of health status values." *Am J Public Health*: 75 (12), 1402–7.

Patrick DL (1972). *Measuring social preference for function levels of health status*. PhD dissertation, Columbia University.

Patrick DL (1976). "Constructing social metrics for health status indexes." *Int J Health Serv*: 6 (3), 443–53.

Patrick DL (1979). *Health and care of the handicapped in Lambeth: description of objectives and proposed research*. London: St. Thomas's Hospital Medical School, Department of Community Medicine. (Unpublished)

Patrick DL (1987). "Commentary: patient reports of health status as predictors of physiologic health in chronic disease." *J Chronic Dis*: 40 (Suppl 1), 37S–40S.

Patrick DL, Bergner M (1990). "Measurement of health status in the 1990s." *Annu Rev Public Health*: 11, 165–83.

Patrick DL, Elinson J (1979). Methods of sociomedical research. In *Handbook of medical sociology*, 3rd ed. Freeman HE, Levine S, Reeder L, eds. Englewood Cliffs, NJ: Prentice-Hall, 437–59.

Patrick DL, Elinson J (1984). "Sociomedical approaches to disease and treatment outcomes in cardiovascular care." *Qual Life Cardiovasc Care*: 1 (2), 53–62.

Patrick DL, Erickson P (1992). "Assessing health-related quality of life for clinical decision making. In *Quality of Life Assessment: Key Issues in the 1990s*, Walker SR, Rosser RN, eds. London: Kluwer Academic Publishing, pp. 11–62.

Patrick DL, Guttmacher S (1983). Socio-political issues in the uses of health indicators. In *Health indicators*. Oxford, England: Martin Robertson and Company, 165–73.

Patrick DL, Peach H, eds. (1989). *Disablement in the community*. Oxford, England: Oxford University Press.

Patrick DL, Bush JW, Chen MM (1973a). "Towards an operational definition of health." *J Health Soc Behav*: 14 (11), 6–23.

Patrick DL, Bush JW, Chen MM (1973b). "Methods for measuring levels of well-being for a health status index." *Health Serv Res*: 8, 228–45.

Patrick DL, Danis ML, Southerland LI, Hong G (1988). "Quality of life following intensive care." *J Gen Intern Med*: 3 (3), 218–23.

Patrick DL, Grembowski DE, Beery W, Durham M, Odle K (1991). *A healthy future: can preventive care improve your health and quality of life?* Seattle: University of Washington, School of Public Health and Community Medicine.

Patrick DL, Stein J, Porta M, Porter CQ, Ricketts TC (1988). "Poverty, health services, and health status: lessons from rural America." *Milbank Q*: 66 (1), 105–36.

Pauker SG, Pauker SP, McNeil BJ (1981). "The effect of private attitudes on public policy. Prenatal screening for neural tube defects as a prototype." *Med Decis Making*: 1 (2), 103–14.

Pauly M, Kissick W, eds. (1988). *Lessons from the first twenty years of Medicare*. Philadelphia: University of Pennsylvania Press.

Pearce D (1983). *Cost-benefit analysis*, 2nd ed. New York: St. Martin's Press.

Pearce N (1991). Health information resources: United States—Health and social factors. In

Oxford textbook of public health, Vol. 2, 2nd ed. Holland WW, Detels R, Knox G eds. New York: Oxford University Press.

The Pepper Commission (1990). *A call for action: final report of the Pepper Commission.* Washington DC: U.S. Government Printing Office.

Pfeiffer E, ed. (1975). *Multidimensional functional assessment: the OARS methodology. A manual.* Durham, NC: Duke University, Center for the Study of Aging and Human Development.

Plough AL, Berry RE (1981). Regulating medical uncertainty policy issues in end-stage renal disease. In *Federal health programs.* Altman SH, Spapolsky HM, eds. Lexington, MA: Lexington Books.

Pope AM, Tarlov AR, eds. (1991). *Disability in America: toward a national agenda for prevention.* Washington DC: National Academy Press.

Poulton EC (1989). *Bias in quantifying judgments.* Hillsdale, NJ: Lawrance Erlbaum Associates.

Preston TA (1989). "Assessment of coronary bypass surgery and percutaneous transluminal coronary angioplasty." *Int J Technol Assess Health Care:* 5 (3), 431–42.

Public Law 93-353 (July 23, 1974). *Medical Libraries Act of 1974. United States Statutes at Large,* Vol. 88, 362.

Radloff LS (1977). "The CES-D Scale: a self-report depression scale for research in the general population." *Appl Psychol Meas:* 1 (3), 385–401.

Rappaport J (1977). *Community psychology.* New York: Holt, Rinehart and Winston.

Rawls J (1967). *Distributive justice. In philosophy, politics, and society,* 3rd ser. Laslett P, Runciman WG, eds. Oxford: Basil Blackwell, 58–82.

Rawls J (1971). *A theory of justice.* Cambridge, MA: Belknap Press of Harvard University Press.

Read JL, Quinn RJ, Berwick DM, Fineberg HV, Weinstein MC (1984). "Preferences for health outcomes: comparisons of assessment methods." *Med Decis Making:* 4 (3), 315–29.

Rector TS, Kubo SH, Cohn JN (1987). "Patients' self-assessment of their congestive heart failure." *Heart Failure:*Oct/Nov (part 1).

Rector TS, Kubo SH, Cohn JN (1987). "Patients' self-assessment of their congestive heart failure." *Heart Failure:*Oct/Nov (part 2).

Rees GJG (1985). "Cost-effectiveness in oncology." *Lancet:* 2 (8469–70), 1405–8.

Reichenbach H (1963). *The rise of scientific philosophy.* Berkeley: University of California Press.

Reinhardt UE (1989). Economists in health care: saviors, or elephants in a porcelain shop? In *AEA Papers and Proceedings,* Nashville: American Economics Association, May 1989.

Reisberg B, Ferris SJ, deLeon MJ, Crook T (1982). "The Global deterioration Scale for assessment of primary degenerative dementia." *Am J Psychiatry:* 9, 1136–39.

Reisberg B, Schneck MK, Ferris SH, Schwartz GE, deLeon MJ (1983). "The Brief Cognitive Rating Scale (BCRS): findings in primary degenerative dementia (PDD). *Psychopharmacol Bull:* 47–50.

Reiser SJ (1984). The machine at the bedside: technological transformations of practices and values. In *The machine at the bedside: strategies for using technology in patient care.* Reiser SJ, Anbar M, eds. New York: Cambridge University Press, 1–22.

Rettig RA, Levinsky NG, eds. (1991). *Kidney failure and the federal government.* Washington DC: National Academy Press.

Rettig RA, Marks E (1983). *The federal government and social planning for end-stage renal disease: past, present, and future.* Santa Monica, CA: Rand Corporation.

Reynolds CF, Frank E, Thase ME, Houck PR, Jennings JR, Howell JR, Lilienfeld SO, Kupfer DJ (1988). "Assessment of sexual function in depressed, impotent, and healthy men: factor analysis of a Brief Sexual Function Questionnaire for men." *Psychiatry Res:* 24 (3), 132–50.

Rice DP, Hodgson TA (1981). *Social and economic implications of cancer in the United States.* Hyattsville, MD: National Center for Health Statistics.

Richards J, Bailey W, Windsor R, Martin B, Soong S (1988). "Some simple scales for use in asthma research." *J Asthma*: 25 (6), 363–71.

Ringsberg KC, Wiklund I, Wilhelmsen L (1990). "Education of adult patients at an "asthma school": effects on quality of life, knowledge and need for nursing." *Eur Respir J*: 3, 33–37.

Robert Wood Johnson Foundation (1987). *Special Report on Access to Medical Care.* Robert Wood Johnson Foundation, Princeton, NJ.

Rockey PH, Griep RJ (1980). "Behavioral dysfunction in hyperthyroidism: improvement with treatment." *Arch Intern Med*: 140 (9), 1194–97.

Rogers A, Rogers RG, Branch LG (1989). "A multistate analysis of active life expectancy." *Public Health Rep*: 104 (3), 222–26.

Rogers WH, Williams KN, Brook RH (1979). *Conceptualization and measurement of health for adults in the health insurance study, Vol. VII. Power analysis of health status measures.* Santa Monica, CA: Rand Corporation.

Roizen MF, Coalson D, Hayward RSA, Schmittner J, Thisted RA, Apfelbaum JL, Stocking CB, Cassel CK, Pompei P, Ford DE, Steinberg EP (1992). "Can patients use an automative questionnaire to define their current health status?" *Med Care:* 30 (5), suppl.

Roland MO, Morris RW (1983). "A study of the natural history of back pain: development of a reliable and sensitive measure of disability in low-back pain." *Spine*: 8, 141–44.

Rose GA (1965). "Ischemic heart disease. Chest pain questionnaire." *Milbank Memorial Fund Q*: 43, 32–39.

Rosenberg M (1965). *Society and the adolescent self-image.* Princeton, NJ: Princeton University Press.

Rosenberg M (1979). *Conceiving the self.* New York: Basic Books.

Rosenstock IM, Kirscht JP (1979). Why people seek health care. In *Health psychology: a handbook: theories, applications, and challenges of a psychological approach to the health care system.* Stone GC, Cohen F, Adler NE, eds. San Francisco: Jossey-Bass, 161–68.

Rosow I, Breslau N (1966). "A Guttman health scale for the aged." *J Gerontol*: 21 (4), 556–59.

Rosser RM (1983a). A history of the development of health indicators. In *Measuring the social benefits of medicine.* Smith GT, ed. London: Office of Health Economics, 50–62.

Rosser RM (1983b). Issues of measurement in the design of health indicators: a review. In *Health indicators: an international study for the European Science Foundation.* Culyer AJ, ed. New York: St. Martin's Press, 34–81.

Rosser RM (1988). A health index and output measure. In *Quality of life: assessment and application.* Walter SR, Rosser RM, eds. Lancaster, England: MTP Press.

Rosser RM (1990). From health indicators to quality-adjusted life years: technical and ethical issues. In *Measuring the outcomes of medical care.* Hopkins A, Costain B, eds. London: Royal College of Physicians, 1–17.

Rosser RM, Kind P (1978). "A scale of valuations of state of illness: is there a social consensus?" *Int J Epidemiol*: 7 (4), 347–58.

Rosser RM, Watts VC (1972). "The measurement of hospital output." *Int J Epidemiol*: 1 (4), 361–68.

Rothman ML, Hedrick SC, Bulcrot KA, Hickam DH, Rubenstein LZ (1991). "The validity of proxy-generated scores as measures of patient health status." *Med Care*: 29 (2), 115–24.

Russell LB (1986). *Is prevention better than cure?* Washington DC: Brookings Institution.

Russell LB (1987). *Evaluating preventive care: report on a workshop.* Washington DC: Brookings Institution.

Saaty TL (1980). *The analytic hierarchy process: planning, priority setting, resource allocation.* New York: McGraw-Hil.

Sackett DL, Torrance GW (1978). "The utility of different health states as perceived by the general public." *J Chronic Dis*: 31 (11), 697–704.

Saffir MA (1937). "A comparative study of scales constructed by three psychological methods." *Psychometrika*: 2, 179–98.

Sanazaro PJ (1965). "Research in patient care." *Science*: 148, 1489–90.

Sande IG (1982). "Imputation in surveys: coping with reality." *Am Stat:* 36 (3, part 1), 145–52.

Sanders B (1964). "Measuring community health levels." *Am J Public Health*: 54 (7), 1063–70.

Sayetta RB (1980). "Basic data on depressive symptomatology, United States, 1974–1975." *Vital Health Statistics:* 11 (216), 1.

Schipper H, Clinch J, McMurray A, Levitt M (1984). "Measuring the quality of life of cancer patients: the Functional Living Index—Cancer: development and validation." *J Clin Oncol*: 2 (5), 472–83.

Schwartz WB, Mendelson DN (1991). "Hospital cost containment in the 1980s: hard lessons learned and prospects for the 1990s." *New Engl J Med*: 324 (15), 1037–42.

Scitovsky AA (1985). "Changes in the costs of treatment of selected illnesses, 1971–1981." *Med Care* 23 (12), 1345–57.

Scott J, Huskisson EC (1977). "Measurement of functional capacity with visual analogue scales." *Rheum Rehabil:* 16, 257–59.

Seabright P (1989). "Social choice and social theories." *Philos Public Aff:* 18(4), 365–87.

Sen AK (1982). *Choice, welfare, and measurement.* Oxford, England: Basil Blackwell.

Shader RI, Harmatz JS, Salzman C (1974). A new scale for assessment in geriatric populations: Sandoz Clinical Assessment—geriatrics (SCAG). *J Am Geriatr Society:* 107–113.

Shannon JA (1976). The American experience with biomedical science. In *Health in America: 1776–1976.* Washington DC: U.S. Government Printing Office, 89–107.

Shapiro S (1967). "End-result measurements of quality of medical care." *Milbank Mem Fund Q*: 45, 7–30.

Shoemaker PJH (1982). "The expected utility model: its variants, purposes, evidence and limitations." *J Econ Lit*: 20, 529–63.

Short PF, Monheit A, Beauregard K (1988). *Uninsured Americans: a 1987 profile.* Rockville, MD: National Center for Health Services Research, National Medical Expenditures Survey.

Shryock HS, Siegel JS, Larmon EA (1975). *The methods and materials of demography,* Vol. 2, 3rd ed. Washington DC: U.S. Bureau of the Census.

Sinclair JC, Torrance GW, Boyle MH, Horwood SP, Saigal S, Sackett DL (1981). "Evaluation of neonatal-intensive-care program." *N Engl J Med*: 305 (9), 489–94.

Skelton JA, Pennebaker JW (1982). The psychology of physical symptoms and sensation. In *Social psychology of health and illness.* Hillsdale, NJ: Lawrence Erlbaum Associates.

Skinner DE, Yett DE (1973). Debility index for long-term care patients in Health Status Indexes. Berg RL, ed. Chicago: Hospital Research and Educational Trust, 69–89.

Slater RJ, LaRocca NG, Scheinberg LC (1984). "Development and testing of a minimal record of disability in multiple sclerosis." *Ann New York Acad Sci*: 436, 453–68.

Smith A (1987). "Qualms about QALYs." *Lancet*: 1 (8542), 1134–36.

Smith GT (1988). *Measuring health: a practical approach.* New York: Wiley.

Snedecor GW, Cochran WG (1989). *Statistical methods,* 8th ed. Ames: Iowa State University Press.

Somers AR (1984). "Why not try preventive illness as a way of controlling Medicare costs?" *N Eng J Med*: 311 (13), 853–56.

Sonnenfeld ST, Waldo DR, Lemieux JA, McKusick DR (1991). "Projections of national health expenditures through the year 2000." *Health Care Financ Rev:* 13(1), 1–27.

Speilberger C (1977). *STAI—self-evaluation questionnaire*. Palo Alto, CA: Consulting Psychologists Press.

Spilker B (ed.) (1990). *Quality of life assessments in clinical trials*. New York: Raven Press.

Spilker B, Schoenfelder J (1990). *Presentation of clinical data*. New York: Raven Press.

Spilker H, Tilson B, guest eds. (1990). *Med Care*: 28 (12 suppl).

Spitzer RL, Endicott J, Fleiss JL, Cohen J (1970). "The psychiatric status schedule: a technique for evaluating psychopathology and impairment in role functioning." *Arch Gen Psychiatry*: 35, 773–82.

Spitzer WO, Dobson AJ, Hall J, Chesterman E, Levi J, Shepherd R, Buttista RN, Catchlove BR (1981). "Measuring the quality of life of cancer patients: a concise QL-Index for use by physicians." *J Chronic Dis*: 34 (12), 585–97.

Starfield B (1974). "Measurement of outcome: a proposed scheme." *Milbank Mem Fund Q*: 52, 132–36.

Stein REK, Jessop DJ (1990). "Functional Status II(R): A measure of child health status." *Med Care*: 28 (11), 1041–55.

Steinberg EP, Topol EJ, Sakin JW, Kahane SN, Appel LJ, Powe NR, Anderson GF, Erickson JE, Guerci AD (1988). "Cost and procedure implications of thrombolytic therapy for acute myocardial infarction. *J Am Coll Cardiol*: 12 (5), 58A–68A.

Steinberg EP, Bergner M, Sommer A, Anderson GF, Bass EB, Canner J, Gittelsohn AM, Javitt J, Kolb MM, Powe NR, Steinwachs DM, Tielsch JM, Weiner JP (1990). "Variations in cataract management: Patient and economic outcomes." *Health Serv Res:* 25 (5), 727–31.

Steinbrocker O, Traeger CH, Batterman RC (1949). "Therapeutic criteria in rheumatoid arthritis." *JAMA*: 140, 659–62.

Stephens T, Craig CL (1989). Fitness and activity measurement in the 1981 Canada Fitness Survey. In *Assessing physical fitness and physical activity in population-based surveys*. Drury TF, ed. Washington DC: U.S. Government Printing Office, 401–21. DHHS Publ. no. (PHS) 89-1253.

Stephens T, Craig CL, Ferris BF (1986). "Adult physical activity in Canada: findings from the Canada Fitness Survey I." *Can J Public Health*: 77, 285–90.

Sternbach RA (1978). Clinical aspects of pain. In *The psychology of pain*. Sternbach RA, ed. New York: Raven Press.

Sternbach RA, Murphy RW, Timmermans G, Greenhoot JH, Akeson WH (1974). Measuring the severity of pain. In *Advances in neurology,* Vol. 4. Bonica JJ, ed. New York: Raven Press.

Stevens SS (1957). "On the psychophysical law." *Psychol Rev*: 64, 153–80.

Stevens SS (1960). "On the new psychophysics." *Scan J Psychol*: 1, 27–35.

Stevens SS (1961). "To honor Fechner and repeal his law." *Science*: 133, 80–86.

Stevens SS (1968). Ratio scales of opinion. In *Handbook of measurement assessment in behavioural sciences*. Whitla DH, ed. Reading, MA: Addison-Wesley, 171–99.

Stevens SS (1971). "Issues in psychophysical measurement." *Psychol Rev*: 77, 426–50.

Stevens SS, Galanter E (1957). "Ratio scales for a dozen perceptual continua." *J Exp Psychol*: 54, 377–411.

Stewart AL, Hays RD, Ware JE Jr (1988). "The MOS short-form general health survey: reliability and validity in a patient population." *Med Care*: 26 (7), 724–35.

Stewart AL, Greenfield S, Hays RD, Wells K, Rogers WH, Berry SD, McGlynn EA, Ware JE Jr (1989). "Functional status and well-being of patients with chronic conditions: results from the Medical Outcomes Study." *JAMA*: 262 (7), 907–13.

Stewart AL, Ware JE, eds. (1992). *Measuring functioning and well-being: the Medical Outcomes Study Approach*. Durham, NC: Duke University Press.

Stewart AL, Ware JE, Brook RH (1982). *Construction and scoring of aggregate functional status indexes*. Santa Monica, CA: Rand Corporation.

Stone D (1984). *The disabled state*. Philadelphia: Temple University Press.

Stone RI (1989). "The feminization of poverty among the elderly." *Women's Stud Q*: 17 (1/2), 20–34.

Stones MJ, Kozma A (1980). "Issues relating to the usage and conceptualization of mental health constructs employed by gerontologists." *Int J Aging Hum Dev*: 11, 269–81.

Strickland B (1984). Levels of health enhancement: individual attributes. In *Behavioral health: a handbook of health enhancement and disease prevention*. Matarazzo J, Weiss SM, Herd JA, Miller NA, Weiss SM, eds. New York: Wiley, 101–13.

Sugarbaker PH, Barofsky I, Rosenberg SA, Gianola FJ (1982). "Quality of life assessment of patients in extremity sarcoma clinical trials." *Surgery*: 91 (1), 17–23.

Sullivan DF (1966). *Conceptual problems in developing an index of health*. Washington DC: U.S. Department of Health, Education and Welfare. Publication no. (HRA) 74-1017, Series 2, No. 17.

Sullivan DF (1971). "A single index of mortality and morbidity." *HMSHA Health Rep*: 86 (4), 347–55.

Sullivan L (1991). Press conference for the release of *Health: United States, 1991*, April 8.

Sullivan M (1985). "Sickness Impact Profile: Introduktion av en Svensk version for matning av sjukdomskonsekvenser (Introduction of a Swedish Version of health status indicators)." *Lakartidningen*: 82 (20), 1861–62.

Sullivan ME, Sullivan L, Kral JG (1987). "Quality of life assessment in obesity: physical, psychological, and social function." *Gastroenterol Clin North Am*: 16 (3), 433–42.

Sunderland T, Alterman I, Yount D, Hill J, Tariot P, Newhouse P, Mueller E, Mellow A, Cohen R (1988). "A new scale for the assessment of depressed mood in demented patients." *Am J Psychiatry*: 145 (8), 955–59.

Sydenstricker E (1925). "The incidence of illness in a general population group." *Public Health Rep*: 40, 279–91.

Szalai A (1980). The meaning of comparative research on the quality of life. In *The quality of life: comparative studies*. Beverly Hills, CA: Sage Publications, 7–21.

Tandon PK, Stander H, Schwarz RP (1989). "Analysis of quality of life data from a randomized, placebo-controlled heart-failure trial." *J Clin Epidemiol*: 42 (10), 955–62.

Tarlov AR, Ware JE Jr, Greenfield S, Nelson EC, Perrin E, Zubkoff M (1989). "The Medical Outcomes Study: an application of methods for monitoring the results of medical care." *JAMA*: 262 (7), 925–30.

Taylor H, Curran NM (1985). *The Nuprin Pain Report*. New York: Louis Harris and Associates, Inc.

Taylor WC, Pass TM, Shepard DS, Komaroff AL (1987). "Cholesterol reduction and life expectancy: a model incorporating multiple risk factors." *Ann Int Med*: 106, 605–14.

Temkin N, McLean A Jr, Dikmen S, Gale J, Bergner M, Almes MJ (1988). "Development and evaluation of modifications to the Sickness Impact Profile for head injury." *J Clin Epidemiol*: 41 (1), 47–57.

Temkin NR, Dikmen S, Machamen S, McLean A (1989). "General vs. disease specific measures: further work on the Sickness Impact Profile for head injury." *Med Care*: 27 (3 suppl), S44–S53.

Tenney JB, White KL, Williamson JW (1974). *National Ambulatory Medical Care Survey: background and methodology. United States, 1967–72*. NCHS Series Report, Series 2, No. 61.

Testa MA, Sudilovsky A, Rippey RM, Williams GH (1989). "A short form for clinical assessment of quality of life among hypertensive patients." *Am J Prev Med*: 5 (2), 82–89.

Thaler R, Rosen S (1975). The value of saving a life: evidence from the labor market. In *Household production and consumption*. Terleckyj N, ed. New York: National Bureau of Economic Research.

Thoits P (1982). "Conceptual, metholodological, and theoretical problems in studying social support as a buffer against life stress." *J Health Soc Behav:* 22, 324–36.

Thomas WI, Znaniecki F (1958). *The Polish peasant in Europe and America,* 2nd ed. New York: Dover.

Thompson E, Doll W (1982). "The burden of families coping with the mentally ill: an invisible crisis." *Fam Relat:* 31, 379–88.

Thompson MS, Read JL, Hutchings HC, Paterson M, Harris ED Jr (1988). "The cost effectiveness of auranofin: results of a randomized clinical trial." *J Rheumatol:* 15 (1), 35–42.

Thompson MS, Read JL, Liang M (1984). "Feasibility of willingness-to-pay measurement in chronic arthritis." *Med Decis Making:* 4 (2), 195–216.

Thould AK (1985). "Costs of health care: experience of one department of rheumatology." *Br Med J:* 291, 957–59.

Thurstone L (1959). *The measurement of value.* Chicago: University of Chicago Press.

Thurstone LL (1927). "A law of comparative judgement." *Psychol Rev:* 34, 273–86.

Tibblin G, Tibblin B, Peciva S, Kullman S, Svardsudd K (1990). " 'The Göteborg Quality of Life Instrument'—An assessment of well-being and symptoms among men born 1913 and 1923: methods and validity." *Scand J Prim Health Care:* suppl 1, 33–38.

Toevs CD, Kaplan RM, Atkins CJ (1984). "The costs and effects of behavioral programs in chronic obstructive pulmonary disease." *Medical Care:* 22 (12), 1088–1100.

Torgerson WS (1958). *Theory and methods of scaling.* New York: Wiley.

Torrance GW (1976a). "Toward a utility theory foundation for health status index models." *Health Serv Res:* 11 (4), 349–69.

Torrance GW (1976b). "Health status index models: a unified mathematical view." *Manage Sci:* 22 (9), 990–1001.

Torrance GW (1976c). "Social preferences for health states: an empirical evaluation of three measurement techniques." *Socio-Econ Plan Sci:* 10, 129–36.

Torrance GW (1982). Multiattribute utility theory as a method of measuring social preferences for health states in long-term care. In *Values and long-term care.* Kane RL, Kane RA, eds. Lexington, MA: D.C. Heath and Company.

Torrance GW (1986). "The measurement of health state utilities for economic appraisal." *J Health Econ:* 5 (1), 1–30.

Torrance GW (1987). "Utility approach to measuring health-related quality of life." *J Chronic Dis:* 40 (6), 593–600.

Torrance GW, Feeny D (1989). "Utilities and quality-adjusted life years." *Int J Technol Assess Health Care:* 5, 559–78.

Torrance GW, Boyle MH, Horwood SP (1982). "Application of multi-attribute utility theory to measure social preferences for health states." *Operations Research:* 30 (6), 1043–69.

Torrance GW, Sackett DL, Thomas WH (1973). Utility maximization model for program evaluation: a demonstration application. In *Health status indexes.* Berg RL, ed. Chicago: Hospital Research and Educational Trust, 156–72.

Torrance GW, Thomas WH, Sackett DL (1972). "A utility maximization model for evaluation of health care programs." *Health Serv Res:* 7 (2), 118–33.

Torrance GW, Zipursky A (1977). "Cost-effectiveness analysis of treatment with anti-D." Rh Prevention Conference, McMaster University, Hamilton, Ontario.

Torrance GW, Zipursky A (1984). "Cost-effectiveness of antepartum prevention of Rh immunization." *Clin-Perinatol:* 11 (2), 267–81.

Townsend M, Feeny D, Guyatt G, Furlong W, Seip A, Dolovich J (1991). "Evaluation of the burden of illness for pediatric asthmatic patients and their parents." *Ann Allergy:* 10, 403–08.

Traver GA (1988). "Measures of symptoms and life quality to predict emergent use of institutional health care resources in chronic obstructive airways disease." *Heart Lung*: 17 (9), 689–97.

Trevino FM, Moyer ME, Valdez RB, Stroup-Benham CA (1991). "Health insurance coverage and utilization of health services by Mexican Americans, mainland Puerto Ricans, and Cuban Americans." *JAMA*: 265, 233–37.

Tugwell PX, Bombardier C, Buchanan W, Goldsmith CH, Grace E, Hanna B (1987). "The MACTAR patient preference disability questionnaire: an individualized functional priority approach for assessing improvement in physical disability in clinical trials in rheumatoid arthritis." *J Rheumatol*: 14 (3), 446–51.

Tugwell PX, Bombardier C, Buchanan W, Grace E, Southwell D, Bianchi F, Hanna B (1983). "The ability of the MACTAR disability questionnaire to detect sensitivity to change in rheumatoid arthritis." *Clin Res*: 31, 239A.

Tversky A, Kahneman D (1974). "Judgment under uncertainty: heuristics and biases." *Science*: 185, 1124–31.

Tversky A, Kahneman D (1981). "The framing of decisions and the psychology of choice." *Science*: 211, 453–58.

US Department of Commerce, Bureau of the Census (1988). *National health interview survey supplement booklet*. Washington DC: U.S. Department of Commerce, 86–111. Form HIS-1A.

Vandenburg MJ (1988). "Measuring the quality of life of patients with angina. Quality of life: assessment and application." Walker SR, Rosser RM, eds. Lancaster, England: MTP Press, 267.

Veit CT, Ware JE (1982). Measuring health and health care outcomes: issues and recommendations. In *Values and long-term care*. Kane RL, Kane RA, eds. Lexington, MA: Lexington Books, 233–60.

Verbrugge LM (1984). "Longer life but worsening health? Trends in health and mortality of middle-aged and older persons." *Milbank Mem Fund Q*: 62 (3), 475–519.

Verbrugge LM (1989). "Recent, present, and future health of American adults." *Ann Rev Public Health*: 10, 333–61.

Verbrugge LM, Balaban DJ (1989). "Patterns of change in disability and well-being." *Med Care:* 27 (3, suppl), S128–47.

Vertinsky I, Wong E (1975). "Eliciting preferences and the construction of indifference maps: A comparative empirical evaluation of two measurement methodologies." *Socio-Econ Plann Sci:* 9 (1), 15–24.

von Neumann J, Morgenstern O (1944). *Theory of games and economic behavior*. Princeton, NJ: Princeton University Press.

von Winterfeldt D, Edward W (1986). *Decision analysis and behavioral research*. New York : Cambridge University Press.

Waddell G, Main CJ (1984). "Assessment of severity in low-back disorders." *Spine*: 9, 204–8.

Walker SR, Rosser RM (1987). *Quality of life: assessment and application*. Lancaster, England: MTP Press.

Ware JE (1984a). "Conceptualizing disease impact and treatment outcomes." *Cancer*: 53 (suppl), 2316–23.

Ware JE (1984b). *The General Health Rating Index*. Wenger NK, Mattson ME, Furberg CD, Elinson J, eds. New York: LeJacq.

Ware JE (1984c). Methodological considerations in selection of health status assessment procedures. In *Assessment of quality of life in clinical trials of cardiovascular therapies*. Wenger NK, Mattson ME, Furberg CD, Elinson J, eds. New York: LeJacq, 87–111.

Ware JE (1987). "Standards for validating health measures: definition and content." *J Chronic Dis*: 40 (6), 473–80.

Ware JE (1990). "The MOS Short-Form 36: Conceptual Background and Method of Administration. In MAPI Quality-of-life Symposium, September 19–20, 1990, Paris, France.

Ware JE Jr (1991). *The use of health status and quality of life measures in outcomes and effectiveness research.* Unpublished paper, Rockville, MD: Agency for Health Care Policy and Research.

Ware JE, Brook RH, Davies-Avery A (1979). *Analysis of relationships among health status measures.* Santa Monica, CA: Rand Corporation.

Ware JE, Johnston SA, Davies-Avery A, Brook RH (1979). *Conceptualization and measurement of health for adults in the health insurance study," Vol. 3, mental health.* Santa Monica, CA: Rand Corporation.

Warner KE, Luce BR (1982). *Cost-benefit and cost-effectiveness analysis in health care: principles, practice, and potential.* Ann Arbor, MI: Health Administration Press.

Warner SC, Williams JI (1987). "The meaning in life scale: determining the reliability and validity of a measure." *J Chronic Dis*: 40(6), 503–12.

Weinberg E (1983). "Data collection; planning and management." In Rossi PH, Wirte DJ, Anderson AB, eds. *Handbook of Survey Research.* Orlando, FL: Academic Press.

Weinstein MC (1981). "Economic assessments of medical practices and technologies." *Med Decis Making*: 1 (4), 309–30.

Weinstein MC (1990). "Principles of cost-effectiveness resource allocation in health care organizations." *Int J Technol Assess Health Care*: 6, 93–103.

Weinstein MC, Coxson PG, Williams LW, Pass TM, Stason WB, Goldman L (1987). "Forecasting coronary heart disease incidence, mortaility, and cost: the Coronary Heart Disease Policy Model." *Am J Public Health*: 77 (11), 1417–26.

Weinstein MC, Stason WB (1977a). "Foundations of cost-effectiveness analysis for health and medical practices." *New Engl J Med*: 296 (13), 716–21.

Weinstein MC, Stason WB (1977b). *Hypertension: a policy perspective.* Cambridge, MA: Harvard University Press.

Weinstein MC, Stason WB (1978). "Economic considerations in the management of mild hypertension." *Ann New York Acad Sci:* 304 (March 30): 424–40.

Weinstein MC, Stason WB (1982). "Cost-effectiveness of coronary artery bypass surgery." *Circulation*: 66 (suppl 3), 56–66.

Weinstein MC, Stason WB (1985). "Cost-effectiveness of interventions to prevent or treat coronary heart disease." *Annu Rev Public Health*: 6, 41–63.

Weiss CH (1986). Research and policy-making: a limited partnership. In *The use and abuse of social science.* Heller F, ed. Beverly Hills, CA: Sage Publications, 214–35.

Welch HG, Larson EB (1988). "Dealing with limited resources: the Oregon decision to curtail funding for organ transplantation." *N Engl J Med*: 319 (3), 171–73.

Wells KB, Manning WG, Valdez RB (1989). *The effects of insurance generosity on the psychological distress and well-being of a general population: results from a randomized trial of insurance.* Santa Monica, CA: Rand Corporation.

Wells KB, Stewart A, Hays RD, Burnam MA, Rogers W, Daniels M, Berry S, Greenfield S, Ware J (1989). "The functioning and well-being of depressed patients: results from the Medical Outcomes Study." *JAMA*: 262 (7), 914–19.

Wenger NK, Mattson ME, Furberg CD, Elinson J (1984). *Assessment of quality of life in clinical trials of cardiovascular therapies.* New York: LeJacq.

Wennberg JE (1990). "On the status of the prostate disease assessment team." *Health Serv Res:* 25 (5), 727–31.

White K, Murnaghan J (1969). *International comparisons of medical care utilization: a feasibility study.* Washington DC: National Center for Health Statistics. Public Health Service publication no. 1000, ser. 2, no. 33.

Wiklund I, Herlitz J, Hjalmarson A (1989). "Quality of life in postmyocardial infarction patients in relation to drug therapy." *Scand J Prim Health Care*: 7 (1), 13–18.

Wiklund I, Romanus B, Hunt SM (1988). "Self-assessed disability in patients with arthrosis of the hip joint. Reliability of the Swedish version of the Nottingham Health Profile." *Int Disabilities Stud*: 10 (4), 159–63.

Wilkins R, Adams OB (1983). "Health expectancy in Canada, late 1970's: demographic, regional and social dimensions." *Am J Public Health*: 73 (9), 1073–80.

Williams B, Sen AK (eds.) (1982). *Utilitarianism and beyond.* Cambridge, England: Cambridge University Press.

Williams A (1985). "Economics of coronary artery bypass grafting." *Br Med J*: 291 (6491), 326–29.

Williams A (1988). "Priority setting in public and private health care: a guide through the ideologic jungle." *J Health Econ*: 7 (2), 173–83.

Williams A (1988a). Applications in management. In *Measuring health: a practical approach.* Teeling-Smith G, ed. New York: Wiley, 225–43.

Williams A (1988b). The importance of quality of life in policy decisions. In *Quality of life: assessment and application.* Walker SR, Rosser RM, eds. Lancaster, England: MTP Press, 279–90.

Williams ME, Hadler NM, Earp JA (1982). "Manual ability as a marker of dependency in geriatric women." *J Chronic Dis*: 35, 115.

Williams R (1983). Disability as a health indicator. In *Health Indicators.* Culyer AJ, ed. Oxford, England: Martin Robertson and Company, 150–64.

Williams RG, Johnston M, Willis LA, Bennett AE (1976). "Disability: a model and measurement technique." *Br J Prev Soc Med*: 30, 71–78.

Wilson A, Wiklund I, Lahti T, Wahl M (1991). A summary index for the assessment of quality of life in angina pectoris." *J Clin Epidemiol*: 981–88.

Wilson RW, Drury TF (1984). "Interpreting trends in illness and disability: health statistics and health status." *Annu Rev Public Health*: 5, 83–106.

Wilson RW, White EL (1977). "Changes in morbidity, disability, and utilization differentials between the poor and the nonpoor: data from the Health Interview Survey—1964 and 1973." *Med Care*: 15, 636–46.

Wolfson AD, Sinclair AJ, Bambardier C, McGeer A (1982). Preference measurements for functional status in stroke patients: interrater and intertechnique comparisons. In *Values and long-term care.* Kane RL, Kane RA, eds. Lexington, MA: Lexington Books, 191–214.

World Health Organization (1948). *Constitution of the World Health Organization. Basic documents.* Geneva, Switzerland: World Health Organization.

World Health Organization (1980). *International classification of impairments, disabilities and handicaps.* Geneva, Switzerland: World Health Organization.

Yesavage JA, Brink TL, Rose TL (1983). "Development and validation of a geriatric depression screening scale: preliminary report." *J Psych Research:* 37–49.

Zautra A, Goodhart D (1979). "Quality of life indicators: a review of the literature." *Community Ment Health Rev*: 4 (1), 1–10.

Zborowski M (1969). *People in pain.* San Francisco: Jossey-Bass.

Zeldow PB, Pavlou M (1988). "Physical and psychosocial functioning in multiple sclerosis: descriptions, correlations, and a tentative typology." *Br J Med Psychol*: 61 (Pt 2), 185–95.

Zigmond AS, Snaith RP (1983). "The hospital anxiety and depression scale." *Acta Psychiatr Scand*: 67, 361–70.

Zill N, Schoenborn CA (1990). Developmental, learning, and emotional problems: health of our nation's children, United States, 1988. *Advance data 190.* Hyattsville, MD: National Center for Health Statistics.

Zung W (1971). "A rating instrument for anxiety disorders." *Psychosomatics:* 12:371–379.

Zung W, Durham NC (1965). "A self-rating depression scale." *Arch Gen Psychiatry*: 12, 63–70.

Author Index

Subject Index